NEUROCRITICAL CARE

Very few hospitals have dedicated neurointensive care units for management of critically ill neurologic and neurosurgical patients. Frequently, these patients are managed in the medical or surgical ICU by non-neurologists, who have a difficult time appreciating the delicate needs of these patients. This book is a straightforward, practical reference for physicians who need to deal with a wide range of complex conditions and associated medical problems. Although comprehensive in scope, this book is designed for neurologists and physicians in the ICU who need a concise and thorough guide to management and treatment. It emphasizes practical state-of-the-art suggestions for management and treatment and provides accessible, easy-to-follow, highly structured, and focused protocols for the assessment, day-to-day management, and treatment of critically ill patients in various ICU divisions.

Michel T. Torbey, MD, MPH, FAHA, FCCM, is Associate Professor of Neurology and Neurosurgery, Director of the Stroke Critical Care Program, and Director of the Neurointensive Care Unit at the Medical College of Wisconsin, Milwaukee, Wisconsin. He is also coeditor of *The Stroke Book* with Dr. Magdy H. Selim, published in 2007.

NEUROCRITICAL CARE

Edited by

Michel T. Torbey

Medical College of Wisconsin
Milwaukee, Wisconsin

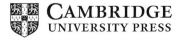
CAMBRIDGE
UNIVERSITY PRESS

CAMBRIDGE UNIVERSITY PRESS
Cambridge, New York, Melbourne, Madrid, Cape Town, Singapore,
São Paulo, Delhi, Dubai, Tokyo

Cambridge University Press
32 Avenue of the Americas, New York, NY 10013-2473, USA

www.cambridge.org
Information on this title: www.cambridge.org/9780521676892

First published 2010

Printed in the United States of America

A catalog record for this publication is available from the British Library.

Library of Congress Cataloging in Publication data
Neurocritical care / edited by Michel T. Torbey.
    p. ; cm.
Includes bibliographical references and index.
ISBN 978-0-521-67689-2 (hardback)
1. Neurological intensive care. I. Torbey, Michel T.
[DNLM: 1. Nervous System Diseases – therapy.   2. Critical Care – methods.
3. Intensive Care Units. WL 140 N49103 2009]
RC350.N49N443 2009
616.8′0428–dc22   2009008939

ISBN 978-0-521-67689-2 Hardback

Every effort has been made in preparing this book to provide accurate and up-to-date information that
is in accord with accepted standards and practice at the time of publication. Although case histories
are drawn from actual cases, every effort has been made to disguise the identities of the individuals
involved. Nevertheless, the authors, editors, and publishers can make no warranties that the information
contained herein is totally free from error, not least because clinical standards are constantly changing
through research and regulation. The authors, editors, and publishers therefore disclaim all liability for
direct or consequential damages resulting from the use of material contained in this book. Readers are
strongly advised to pay careful attention to information provided by the manufacturer of any drugs or
equipment that they plan to use.

Contents

Contributors

Riad Azar, MD
Division of Gastroenterology
Department of Internal Medicine
Washington University School of Medicine
St. Louis, Missouri

Andrew Beaumont, MD, PhD
Department of Neurosurgery
Medical College of Wisconsin
Milwaukee, Wisconsin

Jennifer L. Berkeley, MD, PhD
Neurosciences Critical Care Division
Johns Hopkins Medical Institutions
Baltimore, Maryland

Anish Bhardwaj, MD, FAHA, FCCM
Departments of Neurology, Neurological Surgery,
    Anesthesiology, and Peri-Operative Medicine
Oregon Health and Science University
Portland, Oregon

Lee Biblo, MD
Division of Cardiology
Department of Medicine
Medical College of Wisconsin
Milwaukee, Wisconsin

Ricardo Carhuapoma, MD
Division of Neurocritical Care
Departments of Neurology and Anesthesia/Critical
    Care Medicine
Johns Hopkins University School of Medicine
Johns Hopkins Hospital
Baltimore, Maryland

Veronica L. Chiang, MD
Department of Neurosurgery
Yale University School of Medicine
New Haven, Connecticut

Christian Compagnone, MD
Neurosurgical and Trauma
    Intensive Care Unit
Maurizio Bufalini Hospital
Cesena, Italy

Aaron Dall, MD
Division of Nephrology
Department of Medicine
Medical College of Wisconsin
Milwaukee, Wisconsin

Michael Frank, MD
Department of Medicine
Infectious Disease Clinic
Medical College of Wisconsin
Milwaukee, Wisconsin

Thomas A. Gennarelli, MD
Department of Neurosurgery
Neuroscience Center
Medical College of Wisconsin
Milwaukee, Wisconsin

Romergryko G. Geocadin, MD
Neurosciences Critical Care Division
Johns Hopkins Medical Institutions
Baltimore, Maryland

Todd Gienapp, MD
Division of Pulmonology
The Vancouver Clinic
Vancouver, Washington

Carmelo Graffagnino, MD, FRCPC
Departments of Medicine and Neurology
Duke Neuroscience Critical Care Unit
Duke University Medical Center
Durham, North Carolina

Mary Beth Graham, MD
Division of Infectious Disease
Department of Medicine
Medical College of Wisconsin
Milwaukee, Wisconsin

Angelos Katramados, MD
Department of Neurology
Henry Ford Hospital
Detroit, Michigan

Thomas Kerr, MD, PhD
Division of Gastroenterology
Department of Internal Medicine
Washington University School of Medicine
St. Louis, Missouri

Ahmed J. Khan, MD
Division of Pulmonary Medicine
Department of Medicine
Medical College of Wisconsin
Milwaukee, Wisconsin

May A. Kim, MD
Department of Neurology
Keck School of Medicine
University of Southern California
Los Angeles, California

James Kleczka, MD
Division of Cardiology
Department of Medicine
Medical College of Wisconsin
Milwaukee, Wisconsin

James A. Kruse, MD, FCCM
Critical Care Services
Bassett Healthcare
Cooperstown, New York

Dan Larriviere, MD, JD
Department of Neurology
University of Virginia School of Medicine
Program in Health Law
University of Virginia School of Law
Charlottesville, Virginia

Reed Levine, MD
Department of Neurology
Keck School of Medicine
University of Southern California
Los Angeles, California

John J. Lewin III, PharmD, BCPS
Department of Pharmacy
Neurosciences Critical Care Unit
Johns Hopkins Hospital
Baltimore, Maryland

Geoffrey S. F. Ling, MD, PhD
Medical Corps, U.S. Army
Departments of Neurology and Critical Care
    Medicine for Anesthesiology and Surgery
Uniformed Services University of the Health
    Sciences
Bethesda, Maryland

Marta Lopez-Vicente, MD
Department of Family and Community Medicine
Medical College of Wisconsin
Milwaukee, Wisconsin

Melissa Y. Macias, MD, PhD
Department of Neurosurgery
Medical College of Wisconsin
Milwaukee, Wisconsin

Dennis J. Maiman, MD, PhD
Spinal Cord Injury Center
Medical College of Wisconsin
Milwaukee, Wisconsin

Marc Malkoff, MD
Department of Neurology
Barrow Neurological Institute
Phoenix, Arizona

Edward M. Manno, MD
Department of Neurology
Mayo Clinic
Rochester, Minnesota

Scott Marshall, PharmD
US Army Medical Corps
Clinical Fellow, Neurosciences Critical Care
Johns Hopkins Hospital
Baltimore, Maryland
and Department of Neurology
Uniformed Services University of the Health
  Sciences
Bethesda, Maryland

Matthew Miller, MD
Department of Neurosurgery
Medical College of Wisconsin
Milwaukee, Wisconsin

Marek A. Mirski, MD, PhD
Departments of Neurology, Anesthesiology and
  Critical Care Medicine, and Neurosurgery
Johns Hopkins University School of Medicine
Baltimore, Maryland

Rahul Nanchal, MD
Division of Pulmonary Critical Care
Department of Medicine
Medical College of Wisconsin
Milwaukee, Wisconsin

Yume Nguyen, MD
Division of Gastroenterology
Department of Internal Medicine
Washington University School of Medicine
St. Louis, Missouri

Santiago Ortega-Gutierrez, MD
Department of Neurology
Medical College of Wisconsin
Milwaukee, Wisconsin

Kenneth Presberg, MD
Pulmonary and Critical Care Division
Department of Medicine
Medical College of Wisconsin
Milwaukee, Wisconsin

H. Adrian Püttgen, MD
Division of Neurocritical Care
Johns Hopkins Hospital
Baltimore, Maryland

Ahmed Raslan, MD
Division of Neurological Surgery
Oregon Health and Science University
Portland, Oregon

Andy J. Redmond, MD
Department of Neurosurgery
Yale University School of Medicine
New Haven, Connecticut

Jonathan Rosand, MD, MSc
Division of Vascular and Critical Care Neurology
Center for Human Genetic Research
Massachusetts General Hospital
Boston, Massachusetts

Natalia Rost, MD
Division of Vascular and Critical Care Neurology
Center for Human Genetic Research
Massachusetts General Hospital
Boston, Massachusetts

Rehan Sajjad, MD
Department of Neurology
Medical College of Wisconsin
Milwaukee, Wisconsin

Kristin Santa, PharmD
Pharmacy Department
Froedtert Memorial Lutheran Hospital
Milwaukee, Wisconsin

Rebecca Schuman, PharmD
Pharmacy Department
Froedtert Memorial Lutheran Hospital
Milwaukee, Wisconsin

Clif Segil, MD
Department of Neurology
University of Southern California
Los Angeles, California

Magdy Selim, MD, PhD
Division of Cerebrovascular Diseases
Department of Neurology
Beth Israel Deaconess Medical Center
Harvard Medical School
Boston, Massachusetts

Grant Sinson, MD
Department of Neurosurgery
Medical College of Wisconsin
Milwaukee, Wisconsin

Gene Y. Sung, MD, MPH
Neurocritical Care and Stroke Program
LAC+USC Neurology
University of Southern California
Los Angeles, California

Fernanda Tagliaferri, MD
Department of Anesthesiology and
    Intensive Care
Maurizio Bufalini Hospital of Cesena
Cesena, Italy

Michel T. Torbey, MD, MPH, FAHA, FCCM
Department of Neurology and Neurosurgery
Medical College of Wisconsin
Milwaukee, Wisconsin

Panayiotis N. Varelas, MD, PhD
Department of Neurology and Neurosurgery
Henry Ford Hospital
Detroit, Michigan

Justin Wagner, MD
Keck School of Medicine
University of Southern California
Los Angeles, California

Jeffrey Wesson, MD
Department of Veterans Affairs Medical Center
Medical College of Wisconsin
Milwaukee, Wisconsin

Michael A. Williams, MD, FAAN
Sandra and Malcolm Berman Brain and Spine
    Institute
and Adult Hydrocephalus Center
Sinai Hospital
Baltimore, Maryland

Timothy Woods, MD
Division of Cardiology
Department of Medicine
Medical College of Wisconsin
Milwaukee, Wisconsin

Wendy C. Ziai, MD, MPH
Division of Neurosciences Critical Care
Departments of Neurology, Neurosurgery,
    Anesthesia, and Critical Care Medicine
Johns Hopkins University School of Medicine
Baltimore, Maryland

Wendy Zouras, MD
Division of Pulmonary/Critical Care Medicine
Department of Medicine
Medical College of Wisconsin
Milwaukee, Wisconsin

Foreword

Twenty-two years ago, I wandered into an eight-bed ICU dedicated to caring for critically ill neurologic and neurosurgical patients to begin my fellowship training in Neurosciences Critical Care. Very few such units existed; there were only two trained Fellows in the country, and this was the only one that actually paid the Fellows a salary. Having just completed my residency in neurology, I was not particularly well prepared for the task ahead, in terms of either knowledge or approach to patient care. I had much to learn not only about the brain but also about how the heart, lungs, kidney, etc. affected the brain. More importantly, I had to learn how to take care of "sick" patients, manage ventilators, insert Swan-Ganz catheters, feed patients, and treat infections. Finally, I had to radically alter how I approached patients. No longer was the adage "time is a neurologist's best friend" an acceptable approach to diagnosis and treatment. No one had even considered writing a textbook on neurocritical care. Most of my peers could not understand why I would want to pursue neurocritical care.

Since then things have changed considerably. Most academic centers have or want a neuro ICU; some have more than thirty beds. There is now board certification for neurointensivists, who are recognized by Leapfrog and have a thriving subspecialty journal and a society with almost a thousand members. Equally important is the growing appreciation by other intensivists of what they can offer to critically ill patients with neurologic conditions. No longer do they see the brain as a "black box" that is best ignored, but rather they are embracing brain-specific monitoring and interventions.

Although growth in the field has been explosive, the educational resources available for trainees have lagged behind. A number of texts are available that emphasize different aspects of neurocritical care. They often delve deeply into the neurologic aspects but give less attention to management of other organ systems. Some are comprehensive and serve best as references; others are designed to be carried around and provide limited depth. What has been missing is a practical guide for decision making that covers all aspects of care, neurologic and systemic.

Neurocritical Care is designed to fill an important niche. It is comprehensive in scope but limited in depth, providing a straightforward practical reference that focuses on clinical decision making and management for critically ill neurologic and neurosurgical patients. The chapters provide practical state-of-the-art guidance for both neuro- and other intensivists caring for these patients and cover all aspects of their management, not just brain-specific ones. I certainly wish this book had been available when I was in training; it would have helped prepare me for the task ahead.

Michael N. Diringer, MD
Immediate Past-President,
Neurocritical Care Society

Introduction

Critically ill neurologic and neurosurgical patients can be difficult to manage, not necessarily owing to significant medical problems but rather as a result of the complexity and vulnerability of the brain vis-à-vis physiologic changes that otherwise would be well tolerated by any other body organ. Hence it is very important to approach these patients in a holistic way, combining the standard critical care approaches with a neuro-focused approach. Most available textbooks in this field have either focused on neurocritical care topics or general critical care topics. The "NICU Book" has been produced to provide all healthcare professionals caring for critically ill neurologic and neurosurgical patients with a straightforward, concise, and practical reference to assist them with management decisions.

The book is intended to be limited in depth but comprehensive in its scope. Emphasis has been placed on selecting well-renowned contributors to provide a logical approach to the diagnosis and management of a wide range of common conditions seen in the neurointensive care unit.

On completing the book the reader should be able to understand the nuances in neurocritical care patients and determine the most effective therapy to limit secondary brain injury.

I am indebted to my wife and children, to the authors, neurocritical nurses, families, and particularly the patients who continue to stimulate my passion for neurocritical care.

Michel T. Torbey, MD, MPH, FAHA, FCCM

1 Cerebral Blood Flow Physiology and Metabolism

Marc Malkoff, MD

The brain comprises only 2% of total body weight; however, under normal conditions, it receives 15–20% of the cardiac output and accounts for 20% of total body oxygen consumption.[1] Because energy reserves within the brain are negligible, adequate blood flow is essential for the provision of a continuous supply of energy-producing substrates and for the removal of the byproducts of cellular metabolism.[1]

NORMAL PHYSIOLOGY OF CEREBRAL BLOOD FLOW

Cerebral blood flow (CBF) is normally approximately 50 mL/100 g per minute.[2] Regionally it is greater for gray matter than for white matter, 70 mL/100 g per minute versus 20 mL/100 g per minute, respectively. This rate is slightly increased in youth, and decreases with age.[3–5]

- CBF less than 30 mL/100 g per minute can produce neurologic symptoms.[2,3]
- CBF between 15 and 20 mL/100 g per minute will cause reversible damage or "electrical failure"[1,6,7]
- CBF rates of 10–15 mL/100 g per minute cause irreversible neuronal damage.[6,7]

CBF is determined by blood viscosity, cerebral perfusion pressure (CPP), and vessel radius. This relationship is expressed with the Hagen–Poiselle formula:

$$Q = P * P_i * r^4 / 8 * n * L$$

where P is CPP, r is the cumulative radii of cerebral regulatory resistance vessels, n is whole blood

viscosity, L is cerebral vessel length, and Q is CBF. Vessel length is not a physiologic variable that changes or can be manipulated. The brain has no significant storage capacity, so metabolism and CBF are tightly coupled, and this is called metabolic-flow coupling. This relationship can be expressed with Fick's equation:

$$CMRo_2 = CBF * AVDo_2.$$

- $AVDo_2$ is the arteriovenous difference in oxygen and $CMRo_2$ is the central nervous system metabolic rate of oxygen consumption.
- Under normal conditions the brain maintains normal $AVDo_2$ by responding to changes in metabolism, CPP, and blood viscosity with changes in cerebral vessel caliber, that is, autoregulation.[2,8,9]
- As demonstrated with the Hagen–Poiselle formula, vessel radius is the largest determinant of CBF.

AUTOREGULATION

- The differentiation between the terms cerebral autoregulation and regulation of CBF is often confusing. The latter term broadly encompasses a variety of vasomotor regulatory mechanisms, of which cerebral autoregulation is one type.[10] Cerebral autoregulation describes the intrinsic ability of the cerebral circulation to maintain a constant blood flow in the face of changing perfusion pressure.[11] This is purely a pressure-related phenomenon. The changes are subserved mainly by precapillary resistance vessels.[12] Arteries dilate in response to

1

decreased perfusion and constrict in response to increased perfusion. The exact mechanism of autoregulation is unknown. Proposed mechanisms include the myogenic hypothesis, the endothelial hypothesis, and the neurogenic hypothesis. The myogenic theory is the most widely accepted explanation for the mechanism of autoregulation.

■ A metabolic hypothesis has also been described, but is better suited as a description of metabolic-flow coupling rather than autoregulation.

Bayliss first proposed the myogenic theory in 1902 after he observed the direct constriction and relaxation of canine arteries in response to changes in intravascular pressure. The myogenic theory assumes that there is a basal tone of vascular smooth muscle, which is affected by changes in transmural pressure.[1,13] This results in constriction of precapillary arterioles to rising intravascular pressure and dilatation to falling intravascular pressure.[8,11] Studies suggest that there may be two myogenic mechanisms involved in cerebral autoregulation: a rapid fast reaction to pressure pulsations and a slower reaction to change in mean arterial pressure (MAP).[14]

Important evidence supporting the myogenic theory is the existence of stretch-activated cation channels (SACCs) in myocytes.[10,15] SACC activation is associated with an influx of cations, especially calcium and sodium, leading to cellular depolarization. This, in turn, results in the opening of membrane voltage-gated calcium channels (VGCCs) with the end result of smooth muscle contraction.[10,16] The neurogenic hypothesis states that alterations in transmural pressure trigger changes in neurotransmitter release from perivascular nerve fibers.[10] The hypothesis is supported by several facts:

■ First, both intracranial and extracranial arteries are endowed with a rich and active network of nerves located throughout the adventitial space as demonstrated by anatomic studies.[10,17] There is innervation from both extrinsic (remote) and intrinsic (local) neurons. Origins of the extrinsic neurons supplying blood vessels are the sympathetics from the superior cervical ganglion, parasympathetics from the pterygopalatine, sphenopalatine, and otic ganglion, trigeminal connections from the gasserian ganglion, and serotonergic neurons from the raphe nuclei.[18]

There are also intrinsic peptidergic neurons from local adventitial neurons.[18]

■ Second, the presence of specific neurotransmitter receptors has been demonstrated on vascular endothelial and smooth muscle cells.[10,18]

■ Third, nerve stimulation studies demonstrated a correlation between altered vasomotor tone after electrical stimulation of deendothelialized arteries.[10]

Current literature suggests that some neurogenic control comes into play only under conditions of cerebrovascular stress.[18–20] It may be that neurogenic mechanisms lead to very fine-tuned modulation or that they protect cerebral vessels during acute, severe stress.[20]

The endothelial hypothesis suggests that the cerebral arterial endothelial cells may act as a mechanoreceptor that senses and transduces variations in mechanical factors such as stretch and flow velocity into altered vascular tone.[10,21,22] It is known that the endothelium releases substances that are vasoactive such as endothelium-derived relaxing factors, nitric oxide, endothelium-derived hyperpolarizing factor, thromboxane, and endothelin-1.[22,23] Observations that increasing flow rate and shear stress without increasing transmural pressure can induce endothelial vasodilatation suggest endothelial dependence of vasomotor activity.[10,23] It is thought that the changes in vasomotor tone are brought about by a change in the endothelium's liberation of relaxing or contracting factors.[22,23] This is corroborated by an experiment wherein changes in vascular smooth muscle tone were observed after smooth muscle cells were exposed to perfusate from normal endothelium that had been exposed to changes in transmural pressure.[23]

The metabolic theory argues that autoregulation is determined by the release of vasoactive substances that regulate the resistance of the cerebral vessels keeping CBF constant. This assumes that the primary determinant of regional blood flow is local cerebral metabolic activity, that is, metabolic-flow coupling. Although no specific agent has been identified as the primary determinant of flow adenosine, potassium, prostaglandins, and nitric oxide have been proposed as metabolic coupling agents.

■ Adenosine is of particular interest, as it is known to be a potent vasodilator. It is formed by the breakdown of ATP, and is abundant when oxygen supply is not sufficient to meet metabolic demands, that is, anaerobic metabolism.[14]

- Adenosine binds to A1 and A2 receptors located on neurons and vascular smooth muscle cells respectively.
  - The A1 receptors inhibit neuronal activity, and the A2 receptors activate a second messenger cascade mediated by adenylate cyclase. These events together are considered protective when there is a flow-metabolism mismatch.

Potassium (K) is released during neuronal excitation. During periods of hypoxia, electrical stimulation, and seizures, increases in perivascular K coincide with increases in CBF.[13] In the range of 2-10 mM, extracellular K causes vasodilatation due to hyperpolarization of the vascular smooth muscle cells and decreased cytosolic calcium ion levels.[10] At concentrations above 10 mM, K acts as a vasoconstrictor.

Arachidonic acid metabolites, or eicosanoids, affect cerebral arterial vasomotor tone, and likely play a role in modulating CBF.[10] Eicosanoids are generated from three major enzyme systems: cyclooxygenase (COX), lipoxygenase (LOX), and epoxygenase (EPOX). Some are vasodilators such as prostacyclin (PGI_2) and others are vasoconstrictors such as thromboxane (TXA_2). Also suggesting the importance of prostaglandins is the fact that the use of the nonsteroidal anti-inflammatory drug (NSAID) indomethacin can block the ability of the brain to maintain constant cerebral perfusion during arterial hypotension.[13]

Nitric oxide (NO) is a freely diffusible molecule that regulates CBF. NO has a short half-life of approximately 6 seconds, and is produced from L-arginine by a group of enzymes designated NO synthases (NOS). NO usually works via a second messenger pathway to stimulate vascular smooth muscle relaxation. Two constitutive forms of NOS, nNOS and eNOS, and one inducible form, iNOS, are present in the brain. The constitutive forms have a role in physiologic regulation of blood flow.

- nNos is found in glia and neurons near the vasculature, and eNOS in the endothelial layers of large vessels and astrocytes in contact with blood vessels.[10,24]
- nNOS has an important role in the regulation of CBF in response to metabolism, hypercapnia, and ischemia.[13]

- eNOS is believed to play a role in blood flow during ischemia. This is supported by the observation that elevated levels of eNOS were detected 4-6 hours after global ischemic insult.[13]

Limits of Autoregulation

In a normotensive individual, the brain is able to keep CBF stable between MAPs of 60-150 mm Hg. This is sometimes called the autoregulatory plateau. Below this level, vasodilation becomes insufficient, and ischemia results. Above this level, increased intraluminal pressure forcefully dilates the arterioles, causing luxury perfusion.[2] This breakthrough of autoregulation is accompanied by damage to the endothelium, and disruption of the blood–brain barrier. This results in extravasation of plasma proteins into the brain, neuronal dysfunction and damage, and development of edema.[2,23]

Autoregulation can be impaired by many pathologic insults including hypoxia, ischemia, head injury, and aneurysmal subarachnoid hemorrhage. Then CBF passively follows changes in arterial pressure. Loss of autoregulation can be a global, focal, or multifocal process.

CO_2 Regulation of CBF

Carbon dioxide has long been known to have an effect on CBF. Between a $PaCO_2$ range of 25-60 mm Hg, a 1 mm Hg change in $PaCO_2$ changes CBF by 3-4%.[1,2,5] Decreases in $PaCO_2$ cause increased in vasoconstriction, and increases in $PaCO_2$ cause vasodilatation. CO_2 is a rapidly diffusible gas that readily crosses the blood–brain barrier into the perivascular space and to the cerebral vascular smooth muscle cells.[14] CO_2 is then broken down by carbonic anhydrase into bicarbonate and hydrogen ions. The change in CBF is not mediated by a direct effect of carbon dioxide. Instead, the change is mediated through one of two different mechanisms: either pH changes in the extracellular fluid around microvessels or the H^+ ions affect vessels directly. Effects occur within seconds after $PaCO_2$ is changed, and complete equilibration occurs within 2 minutes.[14] Decreased responsiveness to $PaCO_2$ variability is seen in severe carotid stenosis, head injury, subarachnoid hemorrhage, cardiac failure, or where vascular response is already exhausted. Carbon dioxide–dependent vasoconstriction of arterioles is also impaired at reduced hematocrit.[25,26]

Oxygen

In the normal physiologic range for PaO_2, 60–100 mm Hg, fluctuations in PaO_2 do not affect CBF. However, CBF does dramatically increase when PaO_2 drops below 50 mm Hg. Important mediators for this enhanced blood flow may be increases in adenosine concentration and/or developing extracellular acidosis related to the anaerobic metabolism of glucose.[27] Molecular oxygen has been shown to directly affect vascular smooth muscle tone, and may be a mediator of the flow response to changes in PaO_2.[1,28]

Shifts in CBF

Chronic hypertension shifts the limits of autoregulation toward higher MAPs, that is, the lowest and highest blood pressures tolerated are higher. This inhibits the ability of chronically hypertensive patients to maintain CBF and $CMRo_2$ during acute hypotensive stimuli. Pressures that would be tolerated in a nonhypertensive individual can be symptomatic in a hypertensive individual.[29,30] Thickening of the tunica media of arterial walls has been seen in chronically hypertensive rats.[31] Hypertrophy of the vessel wall results in a decreased ability of the vasculature to dilate in response to a lower perfusion pressure, and an increased ability to vasoconstrict at higher perfusion pressures. These changes are thought to protect the vascular tissue from increased perfusion pressure.[30–32] Experimental evidence suggests that these adaptive changes are reversible, and that with effective treatment of the hypertension one can shift the autoregulatory limits back toward normal.[30,33]

BLOOD RHEOLOGY

The viscosity of blood refers to its consistency or "thickness," and determines its internal frictional resistance. This constitutes a determinant of flow. The Hagen–Poiselle equation demonstrates that blood flow is inversely related to blood viscosity. Under normal conditions viscosity has little effect on CBF, but in areas of the brain where autoregulation is depressed or completely lost it assumes a greater role.[34,35] Factors that affect whole blood viscosity are erythrocyte aggregation, deformability, shear rate, plasma viscosity, and hematocrit.[34]

Hematocrit is the most important element influencing whole blood viscosity.[36] Increases in CBF are known to occur during anemia. The increase is attributable to both reduced arterial oxygen content and blood viscosity.[25]

- Studies in animals and humans have demonstrated an increase in CBF between 19% and 50% when hematocrit was reduced by 7–14%.[36] The mechanism by which decreased hematocrit changes CBF is not completely clear.
- Studies evaluating changes in CBF under conditions of low CPP show no change in CBF. This suggests that decreasing the hematocrit has a direct vasodilatory effect, likely from the decreased availability of oxygen.[36,37] This implies that in areas of decreased oxygen availability, that is, ischemia, hemodilution would have no effect in increasing blood flow.
- Plasma viscosity has also been shown to affect CBF, and under conditions of increased CBF this role is increased.[38] Changes in CBF due to hemodilution are attributed to both improved rheology of the blood as well as a compensatory response to decreased oxygen delivery.[14,25,38]

Intracranial Pressure

The intracranial space contains three incompressible elements: brain (80%), blood (10%), and CSF (10%). The Monro–Kellie doctrine states that if one changes the volume of any of those three elements there must be a compensatory change in the other spaces to keep intracranial pressure (ICP) the same. In pathologic states, when ICP increases there is initially little change due to small volumes of CSF shifting into distensible spinal subarachnoid spaces. However, the exhaustion of this compensatory mechanism causes increases in ICP. The cerebral perfusion pressure (CPP) is defined as mean arterial pressure (MAP) – ICP, and is maintained in healthy individuals. However, as ICP rises, CPP will decrease if MAP is not changed. Thus, changes in ICP can have tremendous effects on CBF through changes in CPP.

TECHNIQUES FOR MEASUREMENT

KETY–SCHMIDT METHOD. Kety and Schmidt first described their method in 1945.[39] This process assumes that the quantity of any inert substance taken up by brain tissue is equal to the amount of substance carried to the brain in the arteries minus the amount removed by the venous system: the Fick principle. This method requires the inhalation of a highly diffusable inert gas, nitrous oxide. Jugular and arterial concentrations are then monitored to determine the quantity taken up by brain tissue.[39]

■ This method has the advantage of proven reliability and easy repeatability. The Kety–Schmidt method also allows measurement of arteriovenous differences in oxygen, glucose, and lactate useful for determining cerebral metabolic rate.
■ Disadvantages include invasiveness, inability to provide regional information, and the variability of venous drainage.[1]

NONINVASIVE XENON-133. The noninvasive xenon-133 clearance technique is also predicated upon the Fick principle utilizing xenon-133 as the inert substance. Xenon-133 is administrated either intravenously or via inhalation. Detectors positioned against the head monitor clearance of the isotope, and arterial concentrations are estimated from the analysis of end-tidal expired air. The elimination of isotope can be divided into a fast compartment, representing flow to the gray matter, and a slow compartment, representing flow to the white matter.

■ This method has the advantage of not being invasive, and may be performed at the bedside.
■ The disadvantages of this method are the inability to obtain information about deep structures, such as cerebellum or brain stem, and because the method assumes a normal blood–brain barrier.[1,40]

STABLE XENON COMPUTED TOMOGRAPHY. Stable xenon computed tomography relies on the fact that xenon is a radiodense, lipid-soluble gas that acts as a contrast agent during computed tomography. The patient breathes a mixture of oxygen and 30–35% stable xenon. Arterial levels of xenon can be calculated from end-tidal expiratory concentrations. The relatively slow diffusion rate of xenon allows high-resolution imaging from serial tomograms separated by approximately 1 minute.

■ The advantage of this technique is that it provides excellent anatomic resolution and the blood–brain barrier partition coefficient can be determined for discrete regions.
■ The disadvantages are that the patient must remain still for the full study, 20–30 minutes and must inhale high concentrations of xenon. Xenon has been shown to function as a mild anesthetic agent, and has been shown to directly increase CBF.[1,41]

POSITRON EMISSION TOMOGRAPHY. Positron emission tomography requires the intravenous or inhalation administration of positron-emitting isotopes of carbon, fluorine, or oxygen. In the body, the positrons combine with electrons, thus emitting γ photons that are recorded by detectors surrounding the body. The detectors are able to precisely locate the source of the γ-ray emission with very good resolution.

■ This technique allows for ascertainment of the metabolic rate of glucose, oxygen, protein synthesis, and CBF. ^{15}O-labeled water is the most common tracer, and is used because it is inert, stable, has a short half-life, and has few physiologic side effects.
■ The major drawback to this technique is cost.[42]

TRANSCRANIAL DOPPLER ULTRASOUND. Transcranial Doppler ultrasound (TCD) is a relatively inexpensive and noninvasive method that allows repeated measurements and continuous monitoring of CBF. It has a high temporal resolution, making it ideal to study rapid changes in cerebral hemodynamics.[43] Estimates of global CBF can be made using TCD if the amount of flow through all vessels is measured simultaneously. It has more common applications for estimating regional CBF by analyzing the CBF velocity, resistance index, or pulsatility index of intracranial or extracranial arteries such as the middle cerebral artery. Increased flow velocities in both the contralateral and ipsilateral middle cerebral arteries during motor tasks have been demonstrated.[24] Other uses of this tool include monitoring the development of vasospasm after subarachnoid hemorrhage; pattern of collateral flow through the circle of Willis; and state of artery patency before, during, or after thrombolytic therapy.

CEREBRAL METABOLISM

Cerebral metabolism is a term used to denote the multitude of biochemical pathways in the brain collectively geared toward enzyme-mediated use of substrate to carry out cellular work.[10] Because there is no significant source of energy storage, the brain is highly dependent on a continuous supply of energy. As noted previously, the brain receives 15–20% of the total cardiac output, and CBF is meticulously maintained across a wide variety of pressures. This ensures adequate substrate delivery. The main energy substrates are high-energy triphosphates, that is, adenosine triphosphate (ATP). The central nervous system has small stores of glycogen, and is almost entirely dependent on the glucose for production of energy.[3,12] As in other tissues, glucose can be either anaerobically degraded to lactic acid through glycolysis, or oxidized, aerobically degraded, to CO_2 and water via oxidative phosphorylation.[12] Because the energy yield of glycolysis is small compared to that with oxidative phosphorylation, the brain relies for its continuing function on oxidative metabolism.[12] Oxygen is delivered to the tissue where it is involved in a variety of reactions in the cell, but the majority of oxygen is used in the generation of energy by the aerobic metabolism of glucose. In view of the fact that the need for energy is dependent on oxygen, it is not surprising that the brain's metabolic rate of oxygen ($CMRo_2$) in a normal conscious human is approximately 150–160 µmol/100 g per minute or approximately 20% of the resting body oxygen consumption.[13] The global rate of glucose utilization, also known as the cerebral metabolic rate of glucose (CMRGlu), is 35–30 µmol/100 g per minute. If one assumes normal CBF, then the extraction fraction (i.e., the proportion of substance extracted by the brain relative to the amount delivered to it in arterial blood) is 50% for oxygen and 10% for glucose.[3,34] Most of the brain's energy is used for the maintenance and restoration of ion gradients across the cell membrane. However, rapid synthesis, degradation, molecular transport, and synaptic transmission are also significant energy-consuming processes.[1,3,12]

Oxidative Phosphorylation

Glucose is transported into the cells of the central nervous system through two different glucose transports, GLUT-1 and 3. GLUT-1 is located on glia and endothelial cells and GLUT-3, on neuronal surfaces.

- Glucose is brought into the cell, and then phosphorylated by the enzyme hexokinase into glucose-6-phosphate. Through the initial steps of the glycolytic pathway, the glucose is metabolized into pyruvate.
- Another critical enzyme and site of regulation is phosphofructokinase (PFK). This enzyme is inhibited in high-energy states, that is, excess ATP, and activated in low-energy states. In the presence of oxygen, the newly generated pyruvate then enters the citric acid cycle, or Krebs cycle. The pyruvate is completely oxidized, with the products being the reduced forms of nicotinamide-adenine dinucleotide (NADH), guanosine triphosphate (GTP), and flavin adenine dinucleotide ($FADH_2$).
- For pyruvate to enter the Krebs cycle it is irreversibly decarboxylated into acetyl-coenzyme A (acetyl-CoA) by the enzyme pyruvate dehydrogenase (PDH). This is another major regulation point. The PDH is inhibited by NADH and ATP, both indicators of a high-energy state.
- The reduced NADH and $FADH_2$ then act as electron donors within the mitochondria to a series of proton pump complexes designated the electron transport chain. The final electron donor is oxygen, which is converted to water. The proton gradient that is made by the electron transport chain is used to generate ATP. This final step is termed oxidative phosphorylation.
- This entire process is summarized by the equation: $Glucose + 6\ O_2 + 38\ ADP + 38\ P_i$ yields $6\ CO_2 + 44\ H_2O + 38\ ATP$. In conclusion, 1 mole of glucose yields 38 moles of ATP though oxidative metabolism.

Glycolysis

In the absence of oxygen, anaerobic glycolysis occurs. During periods of ischemic stress, experimental evidence shows the upregulation of the GLUT glucose transporters so that more glucose is imported into the cell for energy production.[3,34,44] Glucose is metabolized into pyruvate, as occurs in the steps before entry into the citric acid cycle.

- In a low oxygen state, there is depletion of NADH, and the enzyme PDH is inhibited, impairing the ability of pyruvate to enter the Krebs cycle. Pyruvate is then transformed into lactate through a reversible reaction catalyzed by lactate dehydrogenase.
- The end result of glycolysis is the production of lactate and ATP summarized by this equation: Glucose + 2 ADP + 2 P_i yields 2 lactate + 2 ATP. In summary, through glycolysis 1 mole of glucose yields 2 moles of ATP. The accumulation of lactate is potentially neurotoxic from lactic acidosis.

Pentose Shunt Pathway

The main role of the pentose shunt pathway is to maintain the production of ribose 5-phosphate and reduced nicotinamide adenine dinucleotide phosphate. This is achieved through the use of phosphorylated glucose. The ribose 5-phosphate and its derivatives are incorporated into many biomolecules including ATP, NAD, FAD, RNA, and DNA. This metabolic shunt pathway is critical for maintaining their synthesis. Of the total amount of glucose entering the glycolytic pathway under normal conditions, about 85% enters the Krebs cycle, 5–10% is converted to lactate through anaerobic glycolysis, and the last 5% is metabolized in the pentose shunt pathway.

Ketosis

Metabolism utilizing ketone bodies occurs in circumstances such as starvation or diabetes when glucose is not available for use by the cell. Adipose tissue is catabolized, and the products are brought to the liver. There β-hydroxybutyrate and acetoacetate are generated and transported in the plasma to the brain. In the brain they are metabolized into 2 molecules of acetyl-CoA, which are able to enter the citric acid cycle. Under conditions of hypoglycemia, oxidation of ketone bodies may provide up to 75% of the total cerebral energy supply.[45]

Metabolic Contributions

NEURONS
Gray matter has a metabolic rate that is 3–4 times greater than that of white matter, and is closely linked to the functional activity of neurons.[3] Most of the brain's energy is used for the maintenance and restoration of ion gradients across cell membrane.[1,12] Neurons are the major site of ATP utilization mainly for maintenance of large numbers of Na^+, K^+-ATPase pumps located on axonal membranes as noted above. ATP production is also used for neurotransmitter metabolism and biosynthetic work such as protein chaperoning and axonal transport. Neurons are also involved in ATP production through oxidative metabolism of glucose, and under certain conditions through ketone body metabolism. Byproducts of neuronal metabolism are responsible for the flow-metabolic coupling between brain metabolism and CBF.

ASTROCYTES
Glial cells occupy almost half of the volume of the brain, and there are 20–50 times as many glial cells as neurons.[3,12] However, they consume less than 10% of total cerebral energy due to low metabolic demands.[12] They are instrumental in regulating the composition of the perineuronal fluid environment. This occurs in three important ways:

1. Buffering extracellular potassium concentrations
2. The glutamate-glutamine cycle
3. The lactate shuttle.

After neuronal activity the extracellular fluid (ECF) has an increased concentration of potassium ions (K^+). The K^+ enters astrocytes through both passive and active means. The K^+ continues to spread along osmotic gradients within the astrocytes through gap junctions. This is called K spatial buffering, and is important because excessive accumulation of K^+ in the ECF can affect membrane polarity.

Glutamate can also accumulate in the ECF after neuronal activity. In addition to reuptake by neurons, glutamate is also sequestered by astrocytes. The glutamate is enzymatically changed to glutamine through glutamine synthase, and is subsequently released into the ECF, where it can be taken up by neurons. This is important for limiting the action of this excitatory neurotransmitter through decreasing its presence in the synaptic cleft, and the transfer of glutamine across the ECF from astrocytes to neurons has the advantage of being a non-neuroexcitatory process.[46] This is termed the glutamate-glutamine cycle.

Glucose is also taken up by astrocytes, and can be shunted into one of two pathways:

1. It may enter anaerobic glycolysis, and is metabolized into lactate.
2. It may be converted into glycogen.[47]

Lactate produced by astrocytes can then be transported to neurons, where it enters the Krebs cycle and subsequent oxidative phosphorylation. Energy production from oxidative metabolism of lactate is about half as effective when compared with glucose.[47]

BLOOD–BRAIN BARRIER

The blood–brain barrier (BBB) isolates the brain from variations in body fluid composition, thereby providing a stable environment for neural–neural and neural–glial interactions.[10] It does this by first acting as an ionic and molecular sieve through its involvement in ionic transport and selective transport of small molecules and proteins.[26] Large molecules, polar molecules are generally excluded by the BBB except for metabolically important molecules such as glucose, amino acids, lactate, and neurotransmitter precursors. The movement of these molecules into the CBF depends on special transport mechanisms.[10,26] For example, the movement of glucose depends on the transporter GLUT-1. During times of stress, such as hypoglycemia, the BBB has been shown to have adaptive responses to a changing metabolic environment by increasing the transport of lactate and ketone bodies into the CBF.[48] Second, the endothelial cells contain a host of enzymes that protect the brain from circulating neurochemicals and toxins. For example, amino acid decarboxylase (MAO), pseudocholinesterase, γ-aminobutyric acid (GABA) transaminase, aminopeptidases, and alkaline phosphatase are present in the brain capillaries.[10] This prevents the unrestricted entry of potential toxins into the brain .

Effects of Temperature on Metabolism

In hypothermic conditions, the flux of glucose going through glycolysis and the Krebs cycle declines. The energy state of the brain, as measured by the ATP/P_i ratio, increases, suggesting that energy-consuming reactions are reduced more than ATP synthesis.[49] Measurements of the brain's metabolic rate, for example, $CMRo_2$, is reduced 2-to 4-fold by a 10-degree decrease in temperature.[49] On the other hand, in the setting of hyperthermia several studies using different animal models have observed a rise in $CMRO_2$, supporting the idea that hyperthermia itself leads to a rise in whole brain energy turnover.[50]

SUGGESTED READINGS

Bryan RM. Cerebral blood flow and metabolism during stress. *Am J Physiol Heart Circ Physiol* 1990; **259**: H269–80.

Chillon JM, Baumbach GL. Autoregulation of cerebral blood flow. In Welch KMA, Caplan LR, Reis DJ, et al. (eds), *Primer on Cerebrovascular Diseases*. San Diego: Academic Press, 1997, pp 51–4.

Gonzalez C, Estrada C. Nitric oxide mediates the neurogenic vasodilation of bovine cerebral arteries. *J Cereb Blood Flow Metab* 1991; **11**(3): 366–70.

Harrison MJ, Pollock S, Thomas D, Marshall J. Haematocrit, hypertension and smoking in patients with transient ischaemic attacks and in age and sex matched controls. *J Neurol Neurosurg Psychiatry* 1982; **45**(6): 550–1.

Khurana VG, Smith LA, Weiler DA, et al. Adenovirus-mediated gene transfer to human cerebral arteries. *J Cereb Blood Flow Metab* 2000; **20**(9): 1360–71.

Rebel A, Ulatowski JA, Kwansa H, Bucci E, Koehler RC. Cerebrovascular response to decreased hematocrit: effect of cell-free hemoglobin, plasma viscosity, and CO_2. *Am J Physiol Heart Circ Physiol* 2003; **285**(4): H1600–8.

Symon L, Branston NM, Strong AJ. Autoregulation in acute focal ischemia. An experimental study. *Stroke* 1976; **7**(6): 547–54.

Wade JP, Taylor DW, Barnett HJ, Hachinski VC. Hemoglobin concentration and prognosis in symptomatic obstructive cerebrovascular disease. *Stroke* 1987; **18**(1): 68–71.

Winn HR. Adenosine and its receptors: Influence on cerebral blood flow. In Welch KMA, Caplan LR, Reis DJ, et al. (eds), *Primer on Cerebrovascular Diseases*. San Diego: Academic Press 1997, pp 77–70.

REFERENCES

1. Torbey M, Bhardwaj A. Cerebral blood flow physiology and monitoring. In Suarez JI, (ed.), *Critical Care Neurology and Neurosurgery*. Totowa, NJ: Humana Press, 2004, pp 23–36.
2. Obrist WD, Langfitt TW, Jaggi JL, Cruz J, Gennarelli TA. Cerebral blood flow and metabolism in comatose patients with acute head injury. Relationship to intracranial hypertension. *J Neurosurg.* 1984;**61**(2):241–53.
3. Meyer CH, Lowe D, Meyer M, Richardson PL, Neil-Dwyer G. Progressive change in cerebral blood flow during the first three weeks after subarachnoid hemorrhage. *Neurosurgery.* 1983;**12**(1):58–76.
4. Melamed E, Lavy S, Bentin S, Cooper G, Rinot Y. Reduction in regional cerebral blood flow during normal aging in man. *Stroke.* 1980;**11**(1):31–5.

5. Davis SM, Ackerman RH, Correia JA, et al. Cerebral blood flow and cerebrovascular CO2 reactivity in stroke-age normal controls. *Neurology*. 1983;**33**(4): 391–9.

6. Astrup J, Siesjö BK, Symon L. Thresholds in cerebral ischemia – the ischemic penumbra. *Stroke*. 1981;**12**(6): 723–5.

7. Hossmann KA. Viability thresholds and the penumbra of focal ischemia. *Ann Neurol*. 1994;**36**(4):557–65.

8. Fog M. Cerebral circulation. The reaction of the pial arteries to a fall in blood pressure. *Arch Neurol Psychiatry*. 1937;**37**:351–64.

9. Lassen N. Cerebral blood flow and oxygen consumption in man. *Physiol Rev*. 1959;**39**:183–238.

10. Khurana VG, Benarroch EE, Katusic ZS, Meyer FB. Cerebral blood flow and metabolism, 1467–94.

11. Symon L, Held K, Dorsch NW. A study of regional autoregulation in the cerebral circulation to increased perfusion pressure in normocapnia and hypercapnia. *Stroke*. 1973;**4**(2):139–47.

12. Siesjö BK. Cerebral circulation and metabolism. *J Neurosurg*. 1984;**60**(5):883–908.

13. Zauner A, Daugherty WP, Bullock MR, Warner DS. Brain oxygenation and energy metabolism: Part I - biological function and pathophysiology. *Neurosurgery*. **51**(2):289–301.

14. Vavilala MS, Lee LA, Lam AM. Cerebral blood flow and vascular physiology. *Anesthesiol Clin North Am*. 2002;**20**(2):247–64, v.

15. Sachs F. Stretch-sensitive ion channels: An update. *Soc Gen Physiol Ser*. 1992;**47**:241–60.

16. Davis MJ, Donovitz JA, Hood JD. Stretch-activated single-channel and whole cell currents in vascular smooth muscle cells. *Am J Physiol*. 1992;**262**(4 Pt 1):C1083–8.

17. Obrist WD, Thompson HK Jr, Wang HS, Wilkinson WE. Regional cerebral blood flow estimated by 133-xenon inhalation. *Stroke*. 1975;**6**(3):245–56.

18. Branston NM. Neurogenic control of the cerebral circulation. *Cereb Brain Metab Rev*. 1995;**7**(4):338–49.

19. Gross PM, Heistad DD, Strait MR, Marcus ML, Brody MJ. Cerebral vascular responses to physiological stimulation of sympathetic pathways in cats. *Circ Res*. 1979;**44**(2):288–94.

20. Heistad DD. Protection of cerebral vessels by sympathetic nerves. *Physiologist*. 1980;**23**(5):44–9.

21. Toda N, Okamura T. Nitroxidergic nerve: Regulation of vascular tone and blood flow in the brain. *J Hypertens*. 1996;**14**(4):423–34.

22. Katusic ZS, Shepherd JT, Vanhoutte PM. Endothelium-dependent contraction to stretch in canine basilar arteries. *Am J Physiol*. 1987;**252**(3 Pt 2):H671–3.

23. Rubanyi GM, Freay AD, Kauser K, Johns A, Harder DR. Mechanoreception by the endothelium: Mediators and mechanisms of pressure- and flow-induced vascular responses. *Blood Vessels*. 1990;**27**(2–5):246–57.

24. Hennerici MG, Meairs SP. Cerebrovascular ultrasound. *Curr Opin Neurol*. 1999;**12**(1):57–63.

25. Rebel A, Ulatowski JA, Kwansa H, Bucci E, Koehler RC. Cerebrovascular response to decreased hematocrit: effect of cell-free hemoglobin, plasma viscosity, and CO2. *Am J Physiol Heart Circ Physiol*. 2003;**285**(4):H1600–8.

26. Partridge WM. Blood brain barrier transport mechanisms. In Welch KMA, Caplan LR, Reis DJ, et al. (eds), *Primer on Cerebrovascular Diseases*. San Diego: Academic Press, 1997, pp 21–5.

27. Edvinsson L, MacKenzie E, McCulloch J. *Cerebral Blood Flow and Metabolism*. New York: Raven Press, 1993, pp 524–52.

28. Carrier O, Walker J, Guton A. Role of oxygen in autoregulation of blood flow in isolated vessels. *Am J Physiol*. 1964;**206**:951.

29. Strandgaard S. Autoregulation of cerebral blood flow in hypertensive patients. The modifying influence of prolonged antihypertensive treatment on the tolerance to acute, drug-induced hypotension. *Circulation*. 1976;**53**(4):720–7.

30. Hoffman WE, Miletich DJ, Albrecht RF. The influence of antihypertensive therapy on cerebral autoregulation in aged hypertensive rats. *Stroke*. 1982;**13**(5):701–4.

31. Nordborg C, Johansson BB. Morphometric study on cerebral vessels in spontaneously hypertensive rats. *Stroke*. 1980;**11**(3):266–70.

32. Strandgaard S, Jones JV, MacKenzie ET, Harper AM. Upper limit of cerebral blood flow autoregulation in experimental renovascular hypertension in the baboon. *Circ Res*. 1975;**37**(2):164–7.

33. Barry DI. Cerebrovascular aspects of antihypertensive treatment. *Am J Cardiol*. 1989;**63**(6):14C–18C.

34. Sakuta S. Blood filtrability in cerebrovascular disorders, with special reference to erythrocyte deformability and ATP content. *Stroke*. 1981;**12**(6):824–8.

35. Grotta J, Ackerman R, Correia J, Fallick G, Chang J. Whole blood viscosity parameters and cerebral blood flow. *Stroke*. 1982;**13**(3):296–301.

36. von Kummer R, Scharf J, Back T, Reich H, Machens HG, Wildemann B. Autoregulatory capacity and the effect of isovolemic hemodilution on local cerebral blood flow. *Stroke*. 1988;**19**(5):594–7.

37. Brown MM, Marshall J. Regulation of cerebral blood flow in response to changes in blood viscosity. *Lancet*. 1985;**1**(8429):604–9.

38. Tomiyama Y, Brian JE Jr, Todd MM. Plasma viscosity and cerebral blood flow. *Am J Physiol Heart Circ Physiol*. 2000;**279**(4):H1949–54.

39. Kety S, Schmidt C. The nitrous oxide method for the quantitative determination of cerebral blood flow in man: Theory, procedure, and normal values. *J Clin Invest*. 1948;**27**:476–83.

40. Obrist WD, Thompson HK, King CH, et al. Determination of regional cerebral blood flow by inhalation of 133-xenon. *Circ Res*. 1967;**20**:124–35.

41. Winkler S, Sacketr JF, Holsten J, et al. Xenon inhalation as an adjunct to computerized tomography of the brain: Preliminary study. *Invest Radiol*. 1977;**12**: 15–18.

42. Leenders KL, Perani D, Lammertsma AA, et al. Cerebral blood flow, flood volume and oxygen utilization. Normal values and effect of age. *Brain*. 1990;**113**(Pt1):27–47.

43. Markdus HS. Transcranial Doppler ultrasound. *J Neurol Neurosurg Psychiatry*. 1999;**67**(2):135–7.

44. Vannucci SJ, Maher F, Simpson IA. Glucose transporter proteins in brain: Delivery of glucose to neurons and glia. *Glia*. 1997;**21**:2–21.

45. Owen OE, Morgan AP, Kemp HG, et al. Brain metabolism during fasting. *J Clin Invest*. 1967;**46**:1589–95.

46. Rebel A, Lenz C, Krieter H, Waschke KF, Van Ackern K, Kuschinsky W. Oxygen delivery at high blood viscosity and decreased arterial oxygen content to brains of conscious rats. *Am J Physiol Heart Circ Physiol*. 2001;**280**(6):H2591–7.

47. Magistretti PJ Coupling of cerebral blood flow and metabolism. In Welch KMA, Caplan LR, Reis DJ, et al. (eds), *Primer on Cerebrovascular Diseases*. San Diego: Academic Press, 1997, pp 70–5.

48. Nehlig A. Cerebral energy metabolism, glucose transport and blood flow: Changes with maturation and adaption to hypoglycemia. *Diab Metab*. 1997;**23**:18–29.

49. Erecinska M, Thoreson M, Silver IA. Effects of hypothermia on energy metabolism in mammalian central nervous system. *J Cereb Blood Flow Metab*. 2003;**23**:513–30.

50. Carlsson C, Hågerdal H, Siesjö BK. The effect of hyperthermia upon oxygen consumption and upon organic phosphate, glycolytic metabolites, citric acid cycle intermediates and associated amino acids in rat cerebral cortex. *J Neurochem*. 1976;**26**:1001–6.

2 Cerebral Edema and Intracranial Pressure

Ahmed Raslan, MD, and Anish Bhardwaj, MD, FAHA, FCCM

Cerebral edema is a frequent and challenging problem in the clinical setting and is a major cause of morbidity and mortality in patients with acute brain injury. It is simply defined as an increase in brain water content (normal brain water content is approximately 80%) and is invariably a consequence of a primary brain insult. Etiologies of these neurologic injuries that cause cerebral edema are diverse and commonly include:

- Traumatic brain injury (TBI)
- Subarachnoid hemorrhage (SAH)
- Ischemic stroke
- Intracerebral hemorrhage (ICH)
- Neoplasms (primary and metastatic)
- Inflammatory diseases (meningitis, ventriculitis, cerebral abscess, encephalitis)
- Toxic–metabolic derangements (hyponatremia, fulminant hepatic encephalopathy)

CEREBRAL EDEMA: CLASSIFICATION

Traditional classification of cerebral edema into cytotoxic, vasogenic, and interstitial (hydrocephalic) is overly simplistic in that it does not reflect the complexity of pathophysiologic and underlying molecular mechanisms. However, it serves as a simple therapeutic guide.

- Cytotoxic edema results from swelling of the cellular elements (neurons, glia, and endothelial cells) because of substrate and energy (Na$^+$, K$^+$

This work was supported by Public Health Service NIH grant NS046379.

pump) failure and affects both gray and white matter. This edema subtype is the initial accompaniment of any brain injury irrespective of etiology and conventionally is thought to be resistant to any known medical treatment.

- Vasogenic edema that predominantly affects white matter, typically encountered in TBI, neoplasms, and inflammatory conditions, results from breakdown of the blood–brain barrier (BBB) due to increased vascular permeability and consequent leakage of plasma components. This edema subtype is responsive to both steroids (notably edema associated with neoplasms) and osmotherapy.
- Interstitial edema, manifested as acute or chronic hydrocephalus, is a consequence of impaired absorption of cerebrospinal fluid (CSF) that leads to increases in transependymal CSF flow due to elevations in hydrostatic pressure gradient. This edema subtype is also not responsive to steroids; its response to osmotherapy remains unproven and debatable.

Cerebral edema may or may not result in elevations in intracranial pressure (ICP; normal, 5–15 mm Hg; 8–18 cm H$_2$O). Most cases of brain injury that result in elevated ICP usually begin as focal cerebral edema. Consistent with the Monroe–Kellie doctrine (see below and Chapter 8) as it applies to altered intracranial vault physiology, the consequences of focal or global cerebral edema, with or without elevations in ICP, can be lethal and include cerebral ischemia from compromised regional or global cerebral blood flow (CBF) and intracranial compartmental shifts due to ICP gradients.

Intracranial compartmental shifts can result in compression of vital brain structures from cerebral "herniation" and may cause death. Prompt recognition of these clinical herniation syndromes warrants institution of targeted therapies that constitute the basis for cerebral resuscitation. Herniation syndromes include:

- *Subfalcine or cingulate*: Usually when the cingulate gyrus herniates under the falx cerebri to cause compression of the ipsilateral anterior cerebral artery, resulting in contralateral lower extremity paresis.
- *Central tentorial*: Downward displacement of one or both cerebral hemispheres, resulting in compression of the diencephalon and midbrain through the tentorial notch and typically caused by centrally located masses. Presents with impaired consciousness and eye movements, elevated ICP, and bilateral flexor or extensor posturing.
- *Lateral transtentorial (uncal)*: Most common form of herniation syndrome observed clinically, resulting from laterally located (hemispheric) masses (tumors and hematomas). There is herniation of the mesial temporal lobe, uncus, and hippocampal gyrus through the tentorial incisura leading to compression of occulomotor nerve, midbrain, and posterior cerebral artery. Clinically, the patient has a depressed level of consciousness, ipsilateral pupillary dilatation and contralateral hemiparesis, decerebrate posturing, central neurogenic hyperventilation, and elevated ICP.
- *Tonsillar*: Herniation of cerebellar tonsils through the foramen magnum, leading to medullary compression, most frequently due to mass lesions in the posterior fossa. Clinically, there are precipitous changes in blood pressure, heart rate, small pupils, ataxic breathing, disturbance of conjugate gaze, and quadriparesis.
- *External*: Due to penetrating injuries to the skull, for example, gunshot wound or skull fractures and has accompanying loss of CSF and brain tissue. ICP may not be elevated because of dural opening.
- *Upward*: Not common and usually iatrogenic after placement of ventricular drain for external CSF drainage in the presence of a space-occupying lesion in the posterior fossa. A "spinning top" appearance of midbrain and protrusion of the cerebellum through the quadrigeminal plate cistern on CT scan is characteristic.

It is imperative to underscore the importance of the presence of a cerebral herniation syndrome without accompanying increments in global ICP, particularly when cerebral edema is focal in distribution.

INTRACRANIAL PRESSURE: BASIC ANATOMY AND CEREBRAL PHYSIOLOGY

In adults, the intracranial contents are encased in a rigid, nondistensible, bony skull. The foramen magnum communicates directly with the spinal subarachnoid space and represents the main exit point from the calvarial fortress. Within the skull, folds of the duramater compartmentalize intracranial contents, such that a tightly packed space (the tentorial incisura) serves as the thruway between the middle and posterior fossa. The intracranial compartment is composed of three main noncompressible components:

- *Brain*, with an estimated volume of approximately 1300–1500 mL
- *CSF*, representing approximately 75 mL (20–25 mL within the ventricular system)
- *Cerebral blood volume (CBV)*, accounting for approximately 75 mL. 70% of blood volume is contained in the cerebral venous sinuses that comprise a low-pressure, high-capacity venous system.

In pathologic conditions, with increased intracranial volume (i.e., a tumor, hemorrhage, or brain edema), compensatory mechanisms play a major role in preventing or minimizing changes in ICP. Initially, CSF is displaced from the intracranial compartment into the spinal thecal sac. Once this compensatory mechanism is exhausted, CBV is decreased, primarily at the expense of its venous component, but also by changes in the diameter of the basal arteries. Ultimately, if the initial insult continues to progress, or if the aforementioned compensatory mechanisms fail to control ICP, brain herniation ensues.

This complementary relationship among brain parenchyma, blood, and CSF has been termed the "Monro–Kellie doctrine" proposed in 1783. The doctrine simply can be interpreted as follows: *Skull is a rigid box that contains elements that are incompressible and an increase in the volume of each of the intracranial components will be at the expense of other*.

CEREBRAL EDEMA AND ICP: DIAGNOSIS AND MONITORING

Determination of definitive contribution of cerebral edema to the deterioration in neurologic status in a critically ill patient can be challenging, as this may result from combination of the primary insult, or evolving secondary injury with accompanying cerebral edema over time.

- Serial and close bedside monitoring of neurologic status with a focus on level of consciousness and new or worsening focal neurologic deficits is critical and frequently requires admission to an intensive care unit.
- Serial neuroimaging studies (computed tomography [CT] and magnetic resonance imaging [MRI] scans) can be particularly useful in confirming clinical herniation syndromes, ischemic brain injury, and exacerbation of cerebral edema (sulcal effacement and obliteration of basal cisterns) and can give valuable insights into the type of edema (focal or global, involvement of gray or white matter).
- ICP monitoring is an important adjunctive tool in patients in whom neurologic status is difficult to ascertain serially, particularly in the setting of pharmacologic sedation and neuromuscular paralysis.
  - ▶ The Brain Trauma Foundation guidelines recommend ICP monitoring in TBI patients with Glasgow Coma Scale (GCS) score of <9 and abnormal CT scan or in patients with GCS <9 and normal CT scan in the presence of two of the following:
    - ▷ Age >40 years
    - ▷ Unilateral or bilateral motor posturing
    - ▷ Systolic blood pressure <90 mm Hg
  - ▶ No guidelines exist for ICP monitoring in other brain injury paradigms (ischemic stroke, ICH, cerebral neoplasms), and decisions made for ICP monitoring in this setting are frequently based on the clinical neurologic status of the patient and data from neuroimaging studies .

MEDICAL MANAGEMENT OF BRAIN EDEMA AND ELEVATED ICP

Medical management of cerebral edema (with or without elevations in ICP) consists of a graded algorithmic approach from *general* measures to *specific* therapeutic interventions (Table 2.1).

Table 2.1. Management of cerebral edema and elevated intracranial pressure

General measures

Optimize head position (30–60 degrees from horizontal)

Neck position (midline)

Normoxia (PaO$_2$ approximately 100 mm Hg); avoidance of hypoxemia

Normocarbia (PaCO$_2$ approximately 35 mm Hg); avoidance of hypercarbia

Normothermia

Normoglycemia

Maintain CPP >60 mm Hg

Adequate nutrition

Seizure prophylaxis in select patients

Specific measures

Hyperventilation (PaCO$_2$ 25–30 mm Hg)

Corticosteroids (dexamethasone) in select patients (e.g., brain neoplasms)

Loop diuretics (furosemide)

Osmotherapy (mannitol versus hypertonic saline)

Pharmacologic coma (barbiturates, propofol)

Analgesia, sedation, and paralysis

Hypothermia

Surgical decompression

General Measures

These measures are focused toward limiting cerebral edema that may or may not be accompanied by elevations in ICP, and the overriding goal of their application is to optimize cerebral perfusion, oxygenation, and venous drainage; minimize cerebral metabolic demands; and avoid interventions that may perturb the ionic or osmolar gradient between the brain and the vascular compartment. These general measures include:

- *Head and neck position*: It has been well documented that in normal uninjured patients as well as in patients with brain injury, head elevation decreases ICP. These observations have led most clinicians to widely incorporate elevation of the head to 30 degrees in patients with poor intracranial compliance. However, head position elevation may be a significant concern in patients with

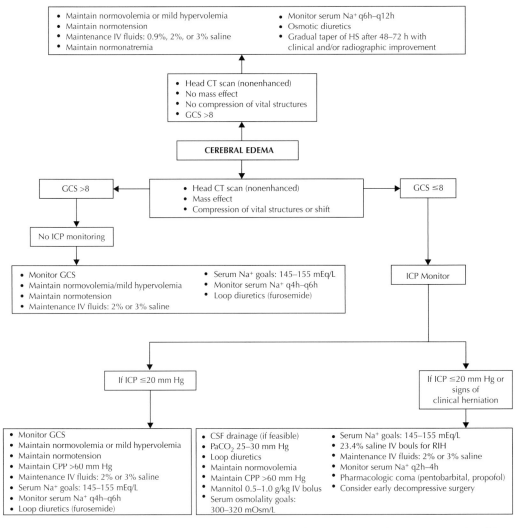

Figure 2.1. Algorithm for the management of cerebral edema and elevated intracranial pressure (Reproduced from Raslan A, Bhardwaj A. *Neurosurg Focus* 2007;22 (5):E12, with permission.).

ischemic stroke, as it may compromise perfusion to ischemic tissue at risk.

- *Ventilation and oxygenation*: As dictated by principles of cerebral physiology, hypoxia and hypercapnia are potent cerebral vasodilators and should be avoided in patients with cerebral edema.
  - $PaCO_2$ should be maintained at levels that support adequate regional CBF (rCBF) to the injured brain, and a value of approximately 35 mm Hg is a generally accepted target in the absence of ICP elevations or clinical herniation syndromes.
  - Avoidance of hypoxemia and maintenance of PaO_2 of approximately 100 mm Hg are recommended.

- *Maintenance of intravascular volume and cerebral perfusion*: Euvolemia or mild hypervolemia with the use of isotonic fluids (0.9% saline) should always be maintained through rigorous monitoring of daily fluid balance, body weight and serum electrolytes.
  - The recommended goal of CPP >60 mm Hg should be adhered to in patients with TBI.
  - Sharp rises and precipitous falls in systemic blood pressure should be avoided.

- *Seizure prophylaxis*: Seizures are deleterious in the setting of acute brain injury. Use of prophylactic anticonvulsants remains controversial in various brain injury paradigms. While use of prophylactic anticonvulsants is recommended in patients with TBI, their utility in a subarachnoid hemorrhage (SAH), ICH, ischemic stroke, and brain neoplasms currently is tailored to the individual patient and is largely dependent on clinical practices.

■ *Management of fever*: Numerous experimental and clinical studies have demonstrated the deleterious effects of fever on outcome after brain injury, which theoretically result from increases in oxygen demand, although the specific effects of fever on cerebral edema have not been elucidated.

▶ Normothermia is strongly recommended in patients with cerebral edema irrespective of underlying etiology.

▶ Acetaminophen (325–650 mg orally or rectally every 4–6 hours) is the most common agent used and recommended to avoid elevations in body temperature.

▶ Some efficacy of other surface and endovascular cooling devices has been demonstrated.

■ *Glycemic control*: Evidence from clinical studies in patients with ischemic stroke, SAH, and TBI suggests a strong correlation between hyperglycemia and adverse clinical outcomes. Hyperglycemia can also exacerbate brain injury and cerebral edema.

▶ Significantly improved outcome has been reported in general ICU patients (including 20% of patients with TBI and post-craniotomy) with adequate but, not tight control.

■ *Nutritional support*: Prompt institution and maintenance of nutritional support is imperative in all patients with acute brain injury. Unless contraindicated, the enteral route of nutrition is preferred. Special attention should be given to the osmotic content of formulations, in order to avoid free water intake that may result in a hypo-osmolar state and worsen cerebral edema.

Specific Measures

■ *Controlled hyperventilation*: Most efficacious therapeutic intervention for cerebral edema, particularly when it is associated with elevations in ICP. Decrease in $PaCO_2$ by 10 mm Hg produces proportional decreases in rCBF (and, in turn, decreases in CBV in the intracranial vault), resulting in rapid and prompt ICP reduction.

▶ Vasoconstrictive effect of respiratory alkalosis on cerebral arterioles lasts only for 10–20 hours, beyond which vascular dilation may result in exacerbation of cerebral edema and rebound elevations in ICP.

▶ Prolonged hyperventilation results in worse outcomes in patients with TBI.

▶ Caution should be exerted in reversing hyperventilation judiciously over 6–24 hours to avoid cerebral hyperemia and rebound elevations in ICP secondary to effects of reequilibration.

■ *Osmotherapy*: The fundamental and simplistic goal of osmotherapy is to create an osmotic gradient to cause egress of water from the brain extracellular (and possibly intracellular) compartment into the vasculature, thereby decreasing intracranial volume and improving intracranial compliance. The goal of osmotherapy for cerebral edema associated with brain injury is to maintain a euvolemic or a slightly hypervolemic state. As a fundamental principle, a hyposmolar state should always be avoided in any patient who has an acute brain injury.

▶ A serum osmolality in the range of 300–320 mOsmol/L has traditionally been recommended for patients with acute brain injury who demonstrate poor intracranial compliance.

▶ Serum osmolality values >320 mOsmol/L can be used with caution, without apparent untoward side effects.

Characteristics of an ideal osmotic gradient include its inertness, being nontoxic, is its exclusion from an intact BBB with minimal systemic side effects. Mannitol and hypertonic saline (HS) solutions are the most studied agents for elevations in ICP.

■ The conventional osmotic agent mannitol, when administered at a dose of 0.25–1.5 g/kg by IV bolus injection, usually lowers ICP, with maximal effects observed 20–40 minutes after its administration. Repeated dosing may be instituted every 6 hours and guided by serum osmolality to a recommended target value of approximately 320 mOsmol/L; higher values result in renal tubular damage. However, this therapeutic goal is based on limited evidence, and higher values can be targeted, provided the patient is not volume depleted.

- Variety of formulations of HS solutions (2%, 3%, 7.5%, 10%, 23%) are utilized in clinical practice for the treatment of cerebral edema with or without elevations in ICP. HS solutions of 2%, 3%, or 7.5% is used as a sodium chloride and sodium acetate mixture (50:50) to avoid hyperchloremic acidosis as continuous IV infusions (via a central venous catheter) at a variable rate to achieve euvolemia or slight hypervolemia (1–2 mL/kg per hour).
  - A 250-mL bolus of HS can be administered cautiously in select patients if more aggressive and rapid resuscitation is warranted.
  - Normovolemic fluid status is maintained, as guided by central venous pressure or pulmonary artery wedge pressure (if available).
  - The goal in using HS is to increase serum sodium concentration to a range of 145–155 mEq/L (serum osmolality approximately 300–320 mOsmol/L), but higher levels can be targeted cautiously. This level of serum sodium is maintained for 48–72 hours, until patients demonstrate clinical improvement, or there is lack of response despite the serum sodium goal being achieved.
  - During withdrawal of therapy, special caution is emphasized owing to the possibility of rebound hyponatremia leading to exacerbation of cerebral edema. Serum sodium and potassium are monitored every 4–6 hours, both during institution and withdrawal of therapy. Other serum electrolytes are monitored daily (particular attention to calcium and magnesium).
  - Chest radiographs are performed at least once every day to look for evidence of pulmonary edema from congestive heart failure, especially in elderly patients with poor cardiovascular reserve.
  - IV bolus injections (30 mL) of 23.4% HS have been utilized in cases of intracranial hypertension refractory to conventional ICP-lowering therapies; repeated injections of 30-mL boluses of 23.4% HS may be given if needed to lower ICP.

SAFETY OF HYPEROSMOLAR THERAPY
- Safety concerns with mannitol include hypotension, hemolysis, hyperkalemia, renal insufficiency, and pulmonary edema.

- No trials have been conducted to investigate safety with HS solutions. However, clinical experience suggests that the side-effect profile of HS is superior to that of mannitol, but some notable theoretical complications are possible with HS therapy, including:
  - CNS changes (encephalopathy, lethargy, seizures, coma)
  - Myelinolysis
  - Congestive heart failure, cardiac stun, cardiac arrhythmias
  - Pulmonary edema
  - Electrolyte derangements (hypokalemia, hypomagnesemia, hypocalcemia)
  - Metabolic academia (hyperchloremic with use of chloride solutions)
  - Potentiation of nontamponaded bleeding
  - Subdural hematomas resulting from shearing of bridging veins due to hyperosmolar contracture of brain
  - Hemolysis with rapid infusions, resulting in sudden osmotic gradients in serum, phlebitis with infusion via the peripheral route
  - Coagulopathy (elevated prothrombin and partial thromboplastin time, platelet dysfunction)
  - Rebound hyponatremia leading to cerebral edema with rapid withdrawal
- *Diuretics*: The use of loop diuretics (commonly furosemide) for the treatment of cerebral edema, particularly when used alone, remains controversial. The combination of furosemide with mannitol produces a profound diuresis; however, the duration of this treatment and its efficacy on cerebral edema remain unknown. If used, rigorous attention to systemic hydration status is advised, as risk of serious volume depletion is substantial, and this may compromise cerebral perfusion.
  - A common strategy to raise serum sodium rapidly is to administer an IV bolus of furosemide (10–20 mg) to enhance free water excretion and to replace it with a 250-mL IV bolus of 2% or 3% HS.
- *Corticosteroids*: The main indication for the use of steroids is for the treatment of vasogenic edema, commonly associated with brain tumors, after brain radiation, and retraction injury from surgical manipulation. While the precise mechanisms of the beneficial effects of steroids in this paradigm are not known, steroids decrease tight-junction permeability and, in turn, stabilize the disrupted BBB. Therapeutic role of steroids in TBI and stroke

has been studied extensively. In TBI, steroids failed to control elevations in ICP or show any benefit in outcome and may even be harmful. In stroke, steroids have failed to show any substantial benefit despite some success in animal models.

▶ Glucocorticoids, especially dexamethasone, are the preferred agents due to its low mineralocorticoid activity.

▶ In light of deleterious side effects (peptic ulcers, hyperglycemia, impairment of wound healing, psychosis, and immunosuppression), until further studies are published, caution is advised in the use of steroids for cerebral edema unless absolutely indicated.

■ Pharmacologic Coma

▶ Barbiturates: Known over several decades from numerous experimental studies that *barbiturates* are neuroprotective and lower elevated ICP via reduction in cerebral metabolic activity that is coupled to reduction in rCBF (and CBV indirectly, thereby decreasing intracranial elastance). Use of barbiturates in clinical practice is not without controversy as experimental studies have not readily translated into clinical paradigms. In patients with TBI, barbiturates are effective in reducing ICP but have failed to show improvement in clinical outcome. Evidence is limited for utility of barbiturates in the setting of cerebral pathologies that include space-occupying lesions (tumor, ICH) and ischemic stroke.

▷ Pentobarbital is the preferred agent over thiopental (short acting; half-life approximately 5 hours) or phenobarbital (long-acting; half-life approximately 72–96 hours) because of its intermediate physiologic half-life (72–96 hours).

▷ The recommended regimen entails a loading IV bolus dose of pentobarbital (3–10 mg/kg), followed by a continuous IV infusion (0.5–3.0 mg/kg per hour; serum levels 3 mg/dL), which is titrated to sustained reduction in ICP or achieving a "burst-suppression pattern" on continuous EEG monitoring.

▷ Barbiturate (pentobarbital) coma should be maintained for 48–72 hour, with gradual tapering by decreasing the hourly infusion by 50% each day.

▷ Several adverse effects of barbiturates that limit their clinical use include sustained vasodepressor effect (hypotension and decrease in CPP), myocardial depression, immunosuppression leading to increased risk of infection, and hypothermia.

▷ The most important limitation with barbiturate coma is the inability to follow subtle changes in clinical neurologic status, which necessitates frequent and serial neuroimaging.

▶ *Propofol*: Because of the potential side effects of barbiturates and relative long half-life, propofol has emerged as an appealing alternative, especially due to its ultra-short half-life. Efficacious in controlling ICP in TBI patients, it also has antiseizure properties and decreases cerebral metabolic rate.

▷ While propofol use continues to become more popular due to these properties, hypotension can be the limiting factor to its use in the clinical setting.

▷ Other adverse effects include hypertriglyceridemia and increased CO_2 production due to the lipid emulsification vehicle.

▷ Careful monitoring of serum triglycerides is recommended with its use.

▷ Cases of "propofol infusion syndrome" that can be fatal have been reported, particularly in children, when propofol is used over a long period of time at high doses.

■ Analgesia, Sedation, and Neuromuscular Blockade

Pain and agitation can exacerbate cerebral edema and raise ICP and compromise CPP significantly. Judicious bolus IV administration of short-acting narcotics such as morphine (2–5 mg) and fentanyl (25–100 μg) or a continuous titratable IV infusion of fentanyl (25–200 μg/h) are preferred agents for analgesia. Special care must be taken for airway protection and not to mask the serial bedside neurologic examination.

Neuromuscular blockade can be a useful adjunct in control of refractory elevations in ICP. Nondepolarizing agents (pancuronium, vecuronium, rocuronium) are the preferred agents, as a depolarizing neuromuscular blocker such as succinylcholine can potentially cause elevations in ICP (usually transient), due to muscle contraction. Other considerations include hepatic and renal insufficiency, as these may significantly prolong metabolism and excretion of these agents. Inability to follow serial neurologic examinations may necessitate frequent and sometimes unwarranted neuroimaging studies.

- *Hypothermia*: Robust data from experimental and a few clinical studies demonstrate that hyperthermia exacerbates brain injury. However, specific effects of hypothermia on brain edema per se remain unclear at present. Further, beneficial effects of therapeutic hypothermia demonstrated in laboratory-based studies have not translated in all brain injury paradigms as dictated by beneficial effects on neurologic outcomes.
  - Therapeutic hypothermia has several accompanying adverse side effects including pneumonia, thrombocytopenia, severe coagulopathy, hemodynamic instability (cardiac arrhythmias, hypotension, cardiac failure), and pancreatitis.
  - Recent trials of therapeutic mild hypothermia (32°C) following out-of-hospital cardiac arrest, accomplished within 8 hours and maintained for 12–24 hours, improved mortality and functional outcomes. Based on these trials, mild hypothermia is quickly becoming a standard of care globally in management of patients after cardiac arrest.
  - The role of hypothermia in the setting of TBI is less clear and previous clinical trials have not demonstrated efficacy. Nevertheless, achieving and maintaining normothermia is a desirable goal in critically ill patients with brain injury irrespective of etiology.
  - A variety of surface as well as endovascular cooling methods are presently utilized in clinical practice.
- *Surgical decompression:* Surgical decompression via craniectomy with or without brain amputation is an old therapy that is increasingly gaining resurgence as a rescue therapy for malignant cerebral edema that may or may not be accompanied by elevations in ICP. This surgical treatment is applicable in a variety of brain injury paradigms that have space-occupying components in the intracranial vault including malignant ischemic strokes, TBI, ICH, and encephalitis.
  - Timing of surgery, age of the patient, and critical findings on neuroimaging studies are important determinants in decision making.
  - Recent studies, particularly for malignant cerebral infarctions, strongly suggest that mortality is markedly attenuated in younger patients who undergo early decompressive craniectomy. However, debate continues as to long-term functional outcomes, although recent metanalysis is encouraging.
  - An early neurosurgical consult for this intervention is strongly suggested in select few patients with poor neurologic status with severe brain injury and space-occupying pathologies on neuroimaging studies.
  - Technical considerations for hemicraniectomy for malignant ischemic strokes include:
    - Durotomy with duroplasty is recommended.
    - The procedure is performed over entire region of bony decompression.
    - Cruciate or circumferential durotomy is acceptable.
    - Dural grafting is recommended.
    - The bone flap is saved in a bone bank or peritoneal cavity and replaced within 3 months
    - Noncompression dressing should be applied.
    - Ventriculostomy is not recommended.
    - Brain amputation is not recommended.

SUMMARY AND CONCLUSIONS

Cerebral edema is frequently encountered in clinical practice and is a major cause of morbidity and mortality in critically ill neurology and neurosurgical patients with acute brain injury. Consequences of cerebral edema can be catastrophic and include cerebral ischemia from compromised regional or global CBF and intracranial compartmental shifts due to ICP gradients in the intracranial vault that result in compression of vital brain structures. Management of cerebral edema entails a timely, systematic, and algorithmic approach with an overarching goal of maintaining regional and global CBF to meet the metabolic requirements of the brain and prevent secondary neuronal injury from cerebral ischemia. Early surgical decompression should be considered in some brain injury paradigms.

REFERENCES

Bernstein A. Treatment of brain edema. *Neurologist.* 2006; **12**:59–73.

Bhardwaj A. Cerebral edema and intracranial hypertension. In Bhardwaj A, Mirski MA, Ulatowski JA (eds),

Handbook of Neurocritical Care. Totowa, NJ: Humana Press, 2004, pp 63–72.

Bhardwaj A, Ulatowski JA. Cerebral edema: hypertonic saline solutions. *Curr Treat Options Neurol.* 1999;**1**:179–88.

Bhardwaj A, Ulatowski JA. Hypertonic saline solutions in brain injury. *Curr Opin Crit Care.* 2004;**10**:126–31.

Brain Trauma Foundation, American Association of Neurological Surgeons, Joint Section on Neurotrauma and Critical Care. Guidelines for cerebral perfusion pressure. *J Neurotrauma.* 2000;**17**:507–11.

Bruno A, Williams LS, Kent TA. How important is hyperglycemia during acute brain infarction? *Neurologist.* 2004;**10**:195–200.

Cremer OL, Moons KG, Bouman EA, Kruijswijk JE, de Smet AM, Kalkman CJ. Long-term propofol infusion and cardiac failure in adult head-injured patients. *Lancet.* 2001;**357**:117–8.

Dearden NM, Gibson JS, McDowall DG, Gibson RM, Cameron MM. Effect of high-dose dexamethasone on outcome from severe head injury. *J Neurosurg.* 1986;**64**:81–8.

Diringer MN, Zazulia AR. Osmotic therapy: fact or fiction? *Neurocrit Care.* 2004;**1**:219–34.

Eccher M, Suarez JI. Cerebral edema and intracranial pressure. Monitoring and intracranial dynamics. In Suarez JI (ed), *Critical Care Neurology and Neurosurgery.* Totowa, NJ: Humana Press, 2004, pp 47–100.

Frank JI. Management of intracranial hypertension. *Med Clin North Am.* **77**:61–76, 1993.

Harukuni I, Kirsch J, Bhardwaj A. Cerebral resuscitation: role of osmotherapy. *J Anesth.* 2002;**16**:229–37.

Hypothermia After Cardiac Arrest Study Group. Mild therapeutic hypothermia to improve the neurologic outcome after cardiac arrest. *N Engl J Med.* 2002;**346**:549–56.

Knapp JM. Hyperosmolar therapy in the treatment of severe head injury in children. Mannitol and hypertonic saline. *AACN Clin Issues.* 2005;**16**:199–211.

Muizelaar JP, Marmarou A, Ward JD, et al. Adverse effects of prolonged hyperventilation in patients with severe head injury: A randomized clinical trial. *J Neurosurg.* 1991;**75**:731–9.

Paczynski RP. Osmotherapy. Basic concepts and controversies. *Crit Care Clin.* 1997;**13**:105–29.

Qureshi AI, Suarez JI. Use of hypertonic saline solutions in treatment of cerebral edema and intracranial hypertension. *Crit Care Med.* 2000;**28**:3301–13.

Rabinstein AA. Found Comatose. In Rabinstein AA, Wijdicks EFM (Eds): *Tough Calls in Acute Neurology.* Philadelphia: Elsevier, 2004, pp 3–18.

Raslan A, Bhardwaj A. Medical management of cerebral edema. *Neurosurg Focus.* 2007;**22**(5):E12.

Ropper AH, Diringer MN, Green DM, Mayer SA, Bleck TP. Management of intracranial hypertension and mass effect. In *Neurological and Neurosurgical Intensive Care.* Philadelphia: Lippincott Williams and Wilkins, 2004, pp 26–51.

Rosner MJ, Coley IB. Cerebral perfusion pressure, intracranial pressure, and head elevation. *J Neurosurg.* 1986;**65**: 636–41.

Schell RM, Applegate RL II, Cole DJ. Salt, starch, and water on the brain. *J Neurosurg Anesth.* 1996;**8**:178–82.

Schwarz S, Georgiadis D, Aschoff A, Schwab S. Effects of hypertonic (10%) saline in patients with raised intracranial pressure after stroke. *Stroke.* 2002;**33**:136–40.

Vahedi K, Hofmeijer J, Juettler E, et al.; DECIMAL, DESTINY, and HAMLET investigators. Early decompressive surgery in malignant infarction of the middle cerebral artery: a pooled analysis of three randomised controlled trials. *Lancet Neurol.* 2007;**6**(3):215–22.

Zornow MH. Hypertonic saline as a safe and efficacious treatment of intracranial hypertension. *J Neurosurg Anesth.* 1996;**8**:175–7.

3 Vasoactive Therapy

Santiago Ortega-Gutierrez, MD, Kristin Santa, PharmD,
Marta Lopez-Vicente, MD, and Michel T. Torbey, MD, MPH, FAHA, FCCM

The brain is highly vulnerable to the effects of hypotension and untreated hypertension, both of which are important risk factors for continued cerebral ischemia, intracranial hemorrhage (ICH), and to a lesser extent, subarachnoid hemorrhage (SAH).

The brain plays an important role in the modulation and control of blood pressure (BP) through the baroreceptor reflex, the brain stem pressor and depressor center, and the interaction between the bulbospinal pressor and depressor center. Further, activation and/or dysfunction of these structures may occur during acute neurologic insults triggered by direct injury or, more commonly, by neurohumoral stimulation as a protective response to further neurologic damage.

BLOOD PRESSURE THERAPEUTICS

After a neurologic emergency, it is often desirable to maintain mean arterial pressure (MAP) or cerebral perfusion pressure (CPP) within a relatively narrow range because a patient's autoregulation at the site of injury may not be intact. Excessive hypertension can compromise the brain's ability to autoregulate cerebral blood flow (CBF) and may aggravate elevated intracranial pressure (ICP) and cerebral edema. In contrast, hypotension may worsen ischemic damage in marginally perfused tissue and can trigger cerebral vasodilation and ICP plateau waves.

Initial interventions for elevated blood pressure should begin with antihypertensive medication injections, such as labetalol, hydralazine, or enalaprilat. However, once these medications have been maximized, a short-acting continuous IV infusion with a predictable dose–response relationship

and favorable safety profile should be initiated. The agents of choice in neurologic injury include esmolol, labetalol, and nicardipine. Sodium nitroprusside should typically be avoided in neurologically unstable patients because it may increase ICPs and cause toxicity with prolonged infusion times.

To elevate blood pressure, the preferred vasopressor agents include phenylephrine, norepinephrine, and dopamine. Various agents used to either elevate or lower blood pressure are discussed in more detail, focusing on each agent's mechanism of action, pharmacokinetic parameters, and adverse effect profile.

Vasopressor Therapy

Optimizing blood pressure in patients with neurologic injury may require intervention to reduce the pressure to avoid risk of hemorrhage. However, clinical situations may necessitate inducing hypertension to preserve adequate cerebral perfusion and avoid further injury. Ischemic stroke is an example in which either intervention may be warranted depending on the patient's clinical status.

- Cerebral blood flow may be compromised poststroke, requiring blood pressure elevation to optimize cerebral perfusion and minimize further damage to the ischemic penumbra.
- Induced hypertension is also recommended for the prevention and treatment of ischemic complications in SAH patients experiencing vasospasms.

Despite initiating aggressive fluid resuscitation and volume expansion as means of elevating pressure, often a vasopressor agent must be added. When utilizing these agents, the goal is to maximize MAP, which increases organ perfusion pressure and preserves distribution of cardiac output (CO) to the vital organs. Maintenance of an adequate systemic pressure is essential for tissue perfusion and sufficient CBF, which may improve neurologic outcomes. Vasopressor agents also improve CO and oxygen delivery by augmenting venous return. This is achieved by decreasing the compliance of the venous compartment. Although vasopressors improve tissue perfusion pressure by increasing the MAP, they also carry the risk of producing damaging regional vasoconstriction. The choice of vasopressor must be made after consideration of the desired therapeutic endpoints as well as each agent's mechanism of action and regional perfusion effects.

Close monitoring is required when utilizing vasopressor drips, as typical side effects include severe hypertension and dysrhythmias. Multiple dosage titrations are often required, demanding frequent calculations of drip rates and adjustments in admixture concentrations. Many agents require administration through a central venous line to avoid extravasation and tissue damage.

- If extravasation is noted, 5 mg of phentolamine (an adrenergic blocking agent) mixed with 9 mL of 0.9% sodium chloride solution may be injected into the affected area to help prevent necrosis.

DOBUTAMINE

Dobutamine is primarily a β_1-agonist with positive inotropic and chronotropic effects with some additional stimulation of α_1- and β_2-receptors. The counterbalance of vasoconstriction with α_1 stimulation and vasodilation due to β_2 activity allows dobutamine to have minimal peripheral vascular effects.

- Dobutamine achieves its increase in MAP and blood pressure by increasing CO, stroke volume, and oxygen distribution.
- Treatment with dobutamine should be tailored toward achieving goal endpoints, as its pharmacokinetic profile is inconsistent in critically ill patients.
- Dobutamine is optimally used for low CO states with high filling pressures or in cardiogenic shock.
- Additional vasopressors may be required to counteract arterial vasodilation.

In hypovolemic patients, dobutamine tends to result in hypotension and reflex tachycardia. When utilized in surgical or trauma patients with septic shock, the effects on hemodynamics and oxygen transport variables are less significant. Theories set forth to explain this blunted effect include potential receptor desensitization and late initiation of the drug in the course of therapy when irreversible organ failure has already occurred. Another factor identified as a potential cause is the increased oxygen extraction ratio noted with concurrent dopamine treatment. This can negate the beneficial effects of dobutamine on oxygen distribution and delivery. If dobutamine is utilized for more than 24–72 hours, patients may develop tolerance to its effects, requiring the addition of or transition to another vasopressor.

DOSING
- IV infusions should be initiated at rates of 2.5–5 µg/kg per minute.
- Evidence suggests that doses >5 µg/kg per minute provide only limited improvement in hemodynamic parameters, while doses >20 µg/kg per minute result in no added benefit.
- High doses may actually worsen the oxygen extraction ratio as well as increase the risk of adverse effects such as tachydysrhythmias and cardiac ischemia.

DOPAMINE

Dopamine (DA), the immediate precursor of epinephrine and norepinephrine (NE), increases MAP through increasing CO and stroke volume, thus increasing cardiac index (CI). In healthy subjects DA displays dose-dependent pharmacologic effects, with the predominant dopamine receptor sites changing as the dose is increased. However, this receptor interaction is not as predictable in critically ill patients due to alterations in receptor density. Approximately 25% of DA is metabolized to NE within the adrenergic nerve terminals, which adds to its cardiac effects. Caution should be used when utilizing DA in patients with an elevated preload, as it may worsen pulmonary edema.

The literature has shown varying results when assessing the effects of dopamine on the splanchnic and gastric regions. At low doses, DA increases splanchnic oxygen delivery by 65% but oxygen consumption by only 16%. The drug's effects on cellular oxygen supply in the gut remain unclear, although gastric motility is often impaired. However, DA may decrease the pH_i (gastric intramucosal pH) through direct effects on the gastric mucosal cells.

DOSING

- Low doses (0–5 µg/kg per minute) have historically been referred to as renal-dose dopamine since the dopaminergic (DA_1) receptor activation leads to vasodilation of the renal and mesenteric vascular beds.
  - This increases blood flow to the kidneys and therefore glomerular filtration rate, urine output (UO), and sodium excretion.
  - In the past, many clinicians believed low-dose DA therapy to be renally protective. However, literature has proven this theory invalid and the drug should not be used for this purpose.
- Midrange doses (5–10 µg/kg per minute) activate β-receptors, leading to positive inotropic and chronotropic effects.
- At higher doses (10–20 µg/kg per minute) the predominant receptor interaction changes to the α-adrenergic subtype, which produces systemic vasoconstriction.
- Little improvement in hemodynamic and oxygen transport is seen with DA doses
- >20 µg/kg per minute.
  - High infusion rates can cause increases in right atrial and ventricular pressures and tachycardia, potentially warranting the addition of or conversion to another agent.

EPINEPHRINE

Epinephrine has a mixed mechanism of action utilizing β-receptor stimulation ($β_1$ and $β_2$ subtypes) coupled with some α-mediated effects to produce blood pressure elevation. Through increases in stroke volume and CI, epinephrine can increase MAPs in patients that are refractory to fluid administration and other vasopressors. Infusions produce consistent elevations in MAP, CO, and oxygen delivery; varying effects on heart rate (HR), systemic vascular resistance (SVR), and oxygen consumption; and no change in the pulmonary capillary wedge pressure (PCWP).

Epinephrine alters oxygen supply in the splanchnic circulation by decreasing splanchnic blood flow, increasing gastric mucosal P_{CO_2} production, and decreasing pH_i. Serum lactate levels rise significantly during initiation of epinephrine therapy but return to baseline within 24 hours. This may be attributed to a reduced oxygen delivery to the splanchnic circulation or to a direct effect on gluconeogenesis and glycolysis resulting in lactate production. Due to its indiscriminate stimulation of all sympathetic receptor subtypes and resultant detrimental cardiac and regional perfusion effects, epinephrine should be reserved as last-line therapy.

DOSING

- Typical infusion rates range from 0.04 to 1 µg/kg per minute.
- Small doses are sufficient in catecholamine "näive" patients. However, higher infusion rates are needed for patients with concomitant vasopressor drips due to receptor desensitization.

NOREPINEPHRINE

The blood pressure elevating effects of NE are a result of its combination of $β_1$-agonist and potent vasoconstrictive α-agonist properties. Depending on concomitant catecholamine use, NE increases systemic oxygen delivery without precipitating a change in the oxygen extraction ratio. Urine output may increase with NE due to improved renal perfusion and a greater vasoconstrictive effect on the efferent arteriole of the kidney. By causing increased myocardial oxygen demand and risk of tachydysrhythmias, the inotropic and chronotropic effects of β stimulation can potentially be detrimental.

In patients remaining hypotensive despite adequate volume resuscitation, NE is superior to high-dose DA for reducing end-organ damage and improving survival. Historically, NE has fallen out of favor due to reports of negative effects on splanchnic and renal vascular beds, resulting in ischemic damage. However, recent experience suggests that NE effectively increases blood pressure without causing deleterious effects on these organs, sparking renewed interest in this agent. In a randomized, controlled trial NE was found to be superior to DA in achieving and maintaining predetermined hemodynamic, metabolic, and oxygen transport parameters in septic shock. This may have been due to the drug's ability to correct splanchnic ischemia or to optimize regional oxygen extraction by preferentially increasing oxygen delivery to the areas with the greatest demand.

DOSING

- Doses of 0.01–2 µg/kg per minute predictably elevate MAP mainly through increasing PVR. In addition, NE triggers minimal change in CO and HR and no alteration in the PCWP.

PHENYLEPHRINE

Phenylephrine, a selective α_1-agonist, increases blood pressure by peripheral vasoconstriction and carries a decreased risk of tachydysrhythmias due to its negligible β-receptor activity. A pure α-agonist is a desirable treatment option in patients requiring increased MAP or blood pressure with marked reductions in SVR. Due to the low volume of α_1-receptors in cerebral vessels, phenylephrine has minimal direct cerebral vasoconstrictive effects. The effects of phenylephrine on CO and HR vary depending on the patient's underlying conditions. Similarly, effects on oxygen transport are also variable but generally positive with an increase in oxygen distribution and consumption. This is perhaps due to the restoration of adequate perfusion pressure and redistribution of blood flow to previously underperfused organs. Because of its selective α-activity, this agent is less likely to cause direct cerebral vasoconstriction, β-receptor-mediated tachydysrhythmias, and elevated myocardial oxygen demand, making it the best choice for elevating blood pressure after ischemic stroke.

DOSING

- Dosing can begin at 0.5 µg/kg per minute and be quickly titrated upward to achieve goal hemodynamic endpoints.

VASOPRESSIN

Vasopressin is an endogenously released stress hormone, which normally has no pressor effects. However, it may play a role in treating patient's with vasodilatory shock, which is associated with a vasopressin deficiency. Exogenously administered vasopressin restores vascular tone lost in shock states due to impaired baroreflex-mediated secretion. Vasopressin binds to vasopressin type 1 (V_1) receptors, resulting in profound vasoconstriction with no significant alterations in CO, PCWP, or HR. Whether the elevations in MAP are due to

the vasoconstrictive actions of the drug or are only an enhancement of the effects of endogenous catecholamines remains undetermined. Utilizing vasopressin in patients with distributive shock syndromes refractory to other catecholamines may be clinically warranted.

DOSING. Vasopressin drips can be infused at rates of 0.03–0.1 units/min.

SUMMARY

When selecting a specific vasopressor agent, the most important considerations include the patient's clinical condition, underlying cardiovascular state, and therapeutic goals. If blood pressure elevation is required in a tachycardic patient, the α_1-receptor agonist phenylephrine would be the preferred agent because it does not directly stimulate the heart and may often cause a mild reflex bradycardia. In patients who develop bradycardia or if blood pressure and CO augmentation is desired, the combined α_1- and β_1-stimulating effects of high-dose dopamine or norepinephrine would be preferred. Dobutamine, a pure β_1- and β_2-agonist, is most useful for augmenting CO in patients who are already hypertensive. It is not a strong vasopressor due to its β_2-mediated vasodilation, which counteract any blood pressure increasing effects. Vasopressin and epinephrine may be utilized as last-line medications in patients who have not tolerated or responded to other vasopressor infusions. (See Tables 3.1 and 3.2.)

ANTIHYPERTENSIVE AGENTS

The maintenance of adequate cerebral perfusion is vital in all patients, but is of particular importance in the neurologic or neurosurgical populations. The treatment of elevated blood pressure is vital in preventing devastating events such as hemorrhage or edema. Therefore, the utilization of antihypertensive medications is common practice in the neuro-ICU. This section discusses only treatment with intravenous agents because care for the hypertensive patient in the ICU setting often requires immediate action. A review of the mechanism of action, dosing, side effects, and other pertinent clinical information of various IV blood pressure agents is provided in the text that follows. Please refer to the table following this section for a concise comparison of these agents.

Table 3.1. Comparison of vasopressor agents

| | Pharmacokinetic parameters | | | | Dosing | | Administration |
	Onset (min)	Duration (min)	Half-life (min)	Metabolism	Usual (µg/kg per minute)	Max* (µg/kg per minute)	Required intravenous access
Dobutamine	1–10	10–15	2	Tissues and liver	2.5–10	40	Central line
Dopamine	5	<10	2	Plasma, liver, and kidneys by MAO	5–20	50**	Central line
Epinephrine	1–2	Short	1–2	Liver; COMT and MAO	0.03–0.5	10–20 µg/min***	Central line
Norepinephrine	1–2	1–2	1–2	COMT and MAO	0.01–0.5	30 µg/min	Central line
Phenylephrine	Immediate	15–30	150	To phenolic conjugates in liver and intestine by MAO	0.5–8	360 µg/min	Central line or peripheral line
Vasopressin	Immediate	30–60	10–20	Liver and kidneys	0.03–0.1 units/min	0.1 units/min	Peripheral line

COMT = catechol-O-methyltransferase; MAO = monoamine oxidase.

* Maximum dosages are not routinely recommended.

** Should consider changing vasopressor or adding a second agent if rates reach 20–30 µg/kg per minute.

*** Severe cardiac dysfunction may require dosages higher than typical ranges (up to 0.1 µg/kg per minute).

Table 3.2. Comparison of vasopressor pharmacokinetic parameters

	Receptor activity					Hemodynamic effects					
	α_1	β_1	β_2	DA_1	V_1	CO	HR	MAP	PCWP	SVR	CI
Dobutamine	1/0	3	2	0	0	↑	↑	↑	↓	↓↔	↑
Dopamine											
1–5 µg/kg per minute	0	1	0	2	0	↑	↔	↔	↔	↔	↔
5–10 µg/kg per minute	1	2	0	2	0	↑	↑	↑	↑↔	↓↔	↑
10–20 µg/kg per minute	2	2	0	2	0	↑↑	↑↑	↑	↑	↑	↑
Epinephrine	3	3	2	0	0	↑↑↑	↑↑	↑↑	↑	↑↑	↑↑
Norepinephrine	3	2	0	0	0	↓↔	↑↔	↑↑↑	↑↑	↑↑↑	↑↓↔
Phenylephrine	3	0	0	0	0	↑↓	↓↔	↑	↑	↑	↑↓↔
Vasopressin	0	0	0	0	2	↔	↔	↑↑	↑	↑↑	↓↔

CO = cardiac output; HR = heart rate; MAP = mean arterial pressure; PCWP = pulmonary capillary wedge pressure; SVR = systemic vascular resistance.
3 = strong effect; 2 = moderate effect; 1 = weak effect; 0 = no effect.

Intravenous Agents

Acute cases of hypertension (HTN) often necessitate immediate correction, which may require the administration of an intravenous antihypertensive agent. The ideal agent should have a rapid, smooth, and predictable onset as well as a short duration of action to allow for careful dosage adjustments and quick termination of effect. Minimal effects on the HR, cardiac function, and myocardial oxygen demand along with a benign side effect profile are also desirable characteristics. Unfortunately, no single agent fulfills all of these criteria. Therefore, the drug of choice is dependent on the patient's clinical presentation and characteristics, the properties of the drug, and the prescribing clinician's experience. Continuous infusions of esmolol, labetalol, nicardipine, and sodium nitroprusside in addition to intermittent IV injections of enalaprilat, hydralazine, and labetalol are some of the options for the treatment of acute HTN.

ENALAPRILAT

HEMODYNAMIC EFFECTS. Enalaprilat is the only angiotensin-converting enzyme inhibitor available in the IV form. Its hemodynamic effects, primarily caused by vasodilation, include a reduction in mean MAP, systolic and diastolic blood pressure, and preload. Enalaprilat causes a decreased sympathetic response, renal efferent arteriolar vasodilation, and sodium retention. Bradykinin may also contribute to this medication's vasodilatory effects. Reflex tachycardia and arterial oxygenation changes are not seen with this agent. However, it does cause variable effects on CO. The overall response rate to enalaprilat is lower than that for other agents and does not appear to be dose-dependent.

DOSING
- Initial IV injection dosing is 0.625–1.25 mg administered slowly over 5 minutes.
- Doses can be repeated in 20–30 minutes, but typical dosing frequency is q6h as needed to achieve desired blood pressure parameters.
- Maximum dosage is 5 mg q6h.

SIDE EFFECTS AND PRECAUTIONS. Side effects include potentially prolonged hypotension, decreased renal function, hyperkalemia, and rare cases of angioedema. Special attention must be paid to patients' volume status, as those with intravascular volume depletion are more likely to experience hypotension and renal effects. Enalaprilat is contraindicated in pregnant women and in patients with bilateral renal artery stenosis.

Angiotensin-converting enzyme inhibitors should also be held for 24 hours before any plasmapheresis or plasma exchange procedure. This is due to the increased bradykinin production, which is believed to be the cause of the angioedema reported with this drug class.

ESMOLOL

HEMODYNAMIC EFFECTS. Esmolol is a cardioselective β-receptor antagonist that causes reductions in systolic blood pressure (SBP), MAP, HR, CO, and stroke volume. Other hemodynamic effects include slight increases in preload and SVR and a significant reduction in left ventricular stroke work (an indicator of myocardial oxygen demand). By reducing cardiac function and causing minimal effects on vascular resistance, esmolol produces opposite effects when compared to sodium nitroprusside. Esmolol and labetalol have shown equivalent efficacy.

DOSING

- Dosing is initiated with an IV bolus of 0.5 mg/kg (500 µg/kg) over 1 minute followed by a continuous infusion starting at a rate of 50 µg/kg per minute.
- A bolus dose can be repeated every 5 minutes and the infusion rate increased by 25–50 µg/kg per minute every 10–20 minutes until the goal blood pressure is achieved.
- The maximum infusion rate for esmolol is 300 µg/kg per minute.

SIDE EFFECTS AND PRECAUTIONS. The most common side effects include hypotension, bradycardia, conduction delays, left ventricular dysfunction, and bronchospasms. Patients with impaired left ventricular function should receive a different agent. Close monitoring is required if esmolol is administered to patients with bronchospastic lung conditions such as asthma and chronic obstructive pulmonary disease (COPD), impaired cardiac conduction, or preexisting bradycardia. If possible, a different agent should be initiated in these patient populations.

HYDRALAZINE

HEMODYNAMIC EFFECTS. Hydralazine causes direct relaxation of arteriolar smooth muscle, causing a reduction in arteriolar vascular resistance with no effect on venous smooth muscle or epicardial coronary arteries. Its main hemodynamic effects include decreases in MAP, SBP, and diastolic blood pressure (DBP) and increases in HR, CO, and myocardial contractility. After the administration of IV hydralazine, a baroreceptor-mediated increase in sympathetic activity is noted. Hydralazine can also cause the release of norepinephrine from sympathetic nerve terminals as well as directly increase cardiac contractility. Due to its negative effects on myocardial metabolism, elevations in HR and contractility, lack of effect on epicardial blood flow, and potential to cause coronary steal syndrome, hydralazine may precipitate acute cardiac ischemia and infarction.

DOSING

- IV injections begin at 5–10 mg administered over 2 minutes and are usually repeated every 6 hours due to the long duration of action.
- The dose and frequency required to achieve goal parameters can be quite variable.

SIDE EFFECTS AND PRECAUTIONS. Hydralazine is contraindicated in patients with known CAD or evidence of cardiac ischemia.

LABETALOL

HEMODYNAMIC EFFECTS. Labetalol utilizes a combination of α_1-receptor and β-receptor antagonism to enact its antihypertensive effect. This agent also exhibits some β_2-receptor blockade, which may contribute to its vasodilation and inhibition of the neuronal uptake of NE. The α-blocking activity accounts for some of the vasodilatory effects while β-blockade prevents reflex tachycardia. After IV administration, the potency of the β-receptor blockade is about 5–10 times higher than the α_1-receptor antagonism. The main hemodynamic effects of labetalol include reductions in SBP, MAP, HR, and CO with no significant alterations in SVR. Right ventricular filling pressure is either slightly increased or remains unchanged. Cerebral, renal, and coronary blood flows are maintained, which may make labetalol a preferred agent for suspected or documented myocardial ischemia. Labetalol is also the agent of choice in neurosurgical patients because it has no effect on ICP and cerebral blood flow.

DOSING

- Labetalol is administered by intermittent IV bolus injections, continuous IV infusion, or both depending on clinical necessity.
  - ‣ Intermittent bolus injections are recommended as initial therapy due to the drug's duration of action.
- Initial doses of 10–20 mg may be administered over 2 minutes followed by sequentially increasing doses every ten minutes until the desired blood pressure has been attained.
- The continuous infusion may be started at 0.5–2 mg/min and titrated upward.
  - ‣ Intermittent bolus doses may be given every 10 minutes at the initiation of the continuous infusion to achieve more rapid pressure control.
  - ‣ However, large bolus doses have been associated with significant drops in blood pressure and should therefore be avoided.
- The injections and infusion can be titrated to a maximum total dosage of 300 mg per 24 hours.

SIDE EFFECTS AND PRECAUTIONS. Blood pressure should be carefully monitored during labetalol therapy, but invasive monitoring is generally not required. Patients with impaired left ventricular function (ejection fraction [EF] <40% or CI <2.5 L/min/m^2), severe bronchospastic respiratory conditions such as asthma or COPD, impaired cardiac conduction, or resting bradycardia should be treated with a different agent.

NICARDIPINE

HEMODYNAMIC EFFECTS. Nicardipine, a dihydropyridine calcium-channel blocker, is relatively selective for vascular smooth muscle, exerts little effect on cardiac conduction, and possesses little inotropic activity. Its predominant hemodynamic effects are a reduction in vascular resistance and MAP caused by the vasodilation of arterial vessels. Nicardipine causes small increases in HR and CO and variable effects on preload. Beneficial effects on myocardial metabolism have been noted. Nicardipine has no effect on ICP or CBF, which is beneficial in the neurologic patient. This agent's antihypertensive efficacy is equivalent to sodium nitroprusside. However, nicardipine reduces both cardiac and cerebral ischemia by preserving tissue perfusion. Compared to sodium nitroprusside, nicardipine produces a more consistent and controlled reduction in MAP, requiring fewer dosage adjustments.

DOSING

- The continuous infusion can be initiated at a rate of 5 mg/h. However, the initial dosing rate for patients with renal insufficiency is 3 mg/h.
- Adjustments of 1–2.5 mg/h can be made every 15 minutes until the desired blood pressure parameters have been achieved (maximum infusion rate = 15 mg/h).
- For a more rapid effect, the infusion may be increased every 5 minutes.
- Once the goal blood pressure has been reached, the infusion should be decreased to its maintenance rate of 3 mg/h.

SIDE EFFECTS AND PRECAUTIONS. Side effects, most commonly hypotension, sinus tachycardia, and nausea and vomiting, were reported in 7–17% of trial patients. Most were transient and less common than those reported from sodium nitroprusside.

SODIUM NITROPRUSSIDE

HEMODYNAMIC EFFECTS. Sodium nitroprusside is a direct-acting, potent vasodilator that affects the arterial and venous vasculature, reducing both preload and afterload. Nitroprusside reacts with cysteine to form nitrocysteine, which ultimately relaxes smooth muscle by stimulating the formation of cyclic guanosine monophosphate. The hemodynamic effects of nitroprusside include reductions in SVR, MAP, pulmonary vascular resistance, and left ventricular filling pressure. Cardiac output and stroke volume are either maintained or increased. A mild to moderate (10–15%) increase in HR is observed but there is an overall improvement in myocardial oxygen balance. The advantages of nitroprusside include its rapid onset of action, short duration of action, minimal HR effects, and lack of damaging changes in cardiac function. The utilization of nitroprusside requires careful consideration and close monitoring, as its significant side effect profile may outweigh any potential benefits.

DOSING

- To prevent possible adverse effects, it is recommended that nitroprusside be continued for only a short duration and be maintained at the lowest effective rate.
- The infusion is typically initiated at 0.25–5µg/kg per minute, which can be increased by 0.5–1 µg/kg per minute every 5–10 minutes until the desired blood pressure is reached.
- The maximum recommended infusion rate as stated by the manufacturer is 10 µg/kg per minute. However, the rate should not be increased >5 µg/kg per minute for more than a few minutes due to the risk of cyanide toxicity.
  - Data have shown toxic cyanide levels in as little as 2–3 hours after infusion rates of >4 µg/kg per minute.
- Once the infusion is stopped, blood pressure begins to rise immediately and returns to pretreatment levels within 1–10 minutes.
  - To avoid the risk of rebound hypertension, the infusion should not be abruptly discontinued.

SIDE EFFECTS AND PRECAUTIONS. The most common side effects of nitroprusside are excessive hypotension, tachycardia, myocardial ischemia, cyanide and thiocyanate toxicity, and worsening of hypoxemia. The potent and labile blood pressure reductions associated with this agent require continuous pressure monitoring, ideally utilizing an arterial catheter. Excessive blood pressure reduction with a loss of coronary perfusion pressure and reflex tachycardia may cause myocardial ischemia. This results in an increased myocardial oxygen demand and redistribution of coronary blood flow away from the ischemic areas, which is termed the coronary steal syndrome.

Increased hypoxemia may occur with nitroprusside, as the agent can reverse pulmonary hypoxic vasoconstriction and worsen ventilation-to-perfusion matching. Therefore, sodium nitroprusside should be used with caution in patients with compromised oxygenation due to chronic lung diseases, acute respiratory distress syndrome, or severe pneumonia.

Nitroprusside administration causes a dose-dependent reduction in CBF and can cause acute ICP increases in patients already exhibiting elevated intracranial pressure. Therefore, it should not be used in this patient population. Concentration and time-dependent ototoxicity has also been observed.

CYANIDE TOXICITY. Sodium nitroprusside is metabolized nonenzymatically via the guanyl cyclase-cyclic guanosine monophosphate (GMP) pathway. One molecule of sodium nitroprusside is metabolized by combining with hemoglobin, which produces one molecule of cyanmethemoglobin and four cyanide radicals. Cyanide radicals are detoxified in the liver by reacting with thiosulfate to form thiocyanate, which is 100 times less toxic than cyanide. Thiocyanate is excreted in the urine with a 3-day half-life of elimination. Cyanide removal, therefore, requires adequate liver and kidney function, making the use of sodium nitroprusside unfavorable in patients with hepatic or renal insufficiency. Acutely ill patients often have a reduced red blood cell mass and a depletion of sulfur donors, which allows for a more rapid onset of cyanide accumulation with lower infusion rates.

The signs and symptoms of acute cyanide toxicity include progressive centra nervous system (CNS) dysfunction characterized by headache, anxiety, confusion, lethargy, convulsions, and coma. Administration of nitroprusside to already neurologically impaired patients makes monitoring for cyanide toxicity much more challenging, as it is often difficult to detect new onset CNS depression. Other signs and symptoms of cyanide toxicity include:

- Cardiovascular instability with ischemia, dysrhythmias, atrioventricular block, and cardiovascular collapse
- Changes in oxygenation and pH with venous hyperoxemia and lactic acidosis
- Nausea and vomiting, abdominal pain, increased salivation, and tachyphylaxis to the drug's effects

Cyanide toxicity can be prevented by the administration of sodium thiosulfate in the same infusion, typically in a 10:1 ratio of nitroprusside to sodium thiosulfate. This acts as a sulfur donor and provides the substrate necessary to detoxify cyanide without interfering with the agent's antihypertensive effects. A prophylactic infusion of hydroxocobalamin (vitamin B_{12}) at a rate of 25 mg/h has also successfully reduced cyanide concentrations and tissue hypoxia by combining with cyanide to form cyanocobalamin. However, this agent is not routinely available. Cyanocobalamin (vitamin B_{12}) has not been found to be effective in preventing cyanide toxicity. Thiocyanate may be removed through hemodialysis.

SUMMARY

In neurologic patients requiring intravenous blood pressure reduction, esmolol and labetalol are preferred in the presence of preexisting tachycardia. The peripheral vasodilator, nicardipine, is desirable in patients with bradycardia, congestive heart failure, or a history of bronchospastic lung disease. None of these agents appear to have an effect on ICPs. Nitroprusside can dilate the cerebral vasculature, increase ICPs, impair autoregulation, and produce acute cyanide toxicity, making this agent undesirable in neurologically injured patients. Initial treatment with intravenous bolus injections of enalaprilat, hydralazine, and labetalol allow practitioners to reduce blood pressure quickly while preparing to initiate a continuous infusion. (See Table 3.3.)

BLOOD PRESSURE MANAGEMENT IN ACUTE NEUROLOGIC EMERGENCIES

INTRACEREBRAL HEMORRHAGE AND ISCHEMIC STROKE

Hypertension is not uncommon in the acute stages of ICH and ischemic stroke. The immediate approach to blood pressure management can certainly have long-term implications on neurologic outcome. In ICH hematoma expansion is an important consideration, whereas in ischemic stroke hemorrhagic transformation or worsening of stroke should be prevented. The management of blood pressure on both ICH and ischemic stroke is discussed in detail in Section III of the book.

TRAUMATIC BRAIN INJURY

Hypertension and tachycardia are frequently encountered in patients with traumatic brain injury (TBI). These findings are usually the result of a hyperadrenergic states. However, they may be related to pain, agitation, or the result of Cushing's reflex when ICP is elevated. ß-Adrenergic blocking agents are the agents of choice after head injury especially in patients with hyperadrenergic conditions however;

treatment priority should focus on CPP and ICP optimization.

Hypotension may be neurogenic, resulting from processes such as spinal shock or neurogenic-stunned myocardium, but more frequently as a result of other complications of severe trauma such as blood loss, pneumothorax, cardiac tamponade, or sepsis. Acute hypotension (SBP <90 mm Hg) is an important factor associated with poor outcome in TBI and its reversal should be a priority.

SPINAL CORD INJURY

There are two syndromes that can present with markedly abnormal BP unique to spinal cord injury (SCI): neurogenic shock as a result of inhibition of resting sympathetic peripheral vasomotor tone and autonomic dysreflexia, in which BP is labile and extreme HTN can be triggered by minor stimulation below the level of injury. Both syndromes are usually the result of a cervical or upper thoracic cord injury. Several uncontrolled studies show that hypotension is associated with increases in mortality and morbidity. Current guidelines recommend that MAP should be maintained above 85–90 mm Hg during the first week after injury.

In acute spinal cord infarction, induced hypertension combined with aggressive lumbar cerebrospinal fluid (CSF) drainage to maximize spinal perfusion pressure is the evolving treatment. Despite the lack of guidelines, experts recommend periodic lumbar drainage to maintain CSF pressure below 10 cm of H_2O with or without vasoactive drugs to maintain MAP >95 mm Hg.

SUBARACHNOID HEMORRHAGE

Aneurysmal subarachnoid hemorrhage (SAH) carries a high rate of mortality and morbidity, most of which is related to the direct effects of the hemorrhage and aneurysm rebleeding. If left untreated, rebleeding occurs in 4% of patients within the first 24 hours, which significantly increases mortality. Hence, early aneurysm surgical or endovascular treatment is a priority. HTN is often present immediately after aneurysm rupture but may not require treatment in all patients. HTN in the setting of SAH may represent a hyperadrenergic state or a Cushing's reflex as well. Thus it is essential to recognize if BP elevation is associated with increase ICP. Even though clear guidelines have not been

Table 3.3. Comparison of intravenous antihypertensive agents

Agent	Mechanism of action	Initial dose	Dose titration	Maximum dosage	Onset of action	Duration of action	Half-life	Comments
Enalaprilat	ACE inhibitor	0.625–1.25 mg injection over 5 minutes	Can repeat in 20–30 minutes Typically redose q6h Titrate by increments of 1.25 mg q12 or 24h.	5 mg q6h	15 minutes	Approximately 6 hours	Approximately 11 hours	• Close attention to volume status • Contraindicated in patients with bilateral renal artery stenosis and pregnancy
Esmolol	Cardioselective β₁ receptor antagonist	Bolus: 500 µg/kg IV injection over 1 min Continuous IV infusion: 50 µg/kg per minute	Bolus may be repeated every 5 min and infusion ↑ by 25–50 µg/kg per minute	300 µg/kg per minute	1–2 minutes	10–30 minutes	Approximately 9 minutes	• Short duration of action • Caution in patients with impaired left ventricular function and bronchospastic respiratory diseases • Not dependent on renal or hepatic function for metabolism
Hydralazine	Vasodilator	Injection: 5–10 mg over 2 minutes	Typically redose q6h as needed	40 mg	5–20 minutes	2–12 hours	Elimination: 2–8 hours (7–16 hours in end-stage renal disease)	• Risk of coronary steal syndrome • Contraindicated in CAD or evidence of cardiac ischemia

Drug	Class	Dose	Titration	Maximum	Onset	Duration	Elimination	Comments
Labetalol	α_1-, β_1-, β_2- receptor antagonist	Injection: 10–20 mg over 2 minutes Continuous IV infusion: 1–2 mg/min	Injection: repeat q10 min in sequentially increasing doses Infusion: may give 10–20 mg bolus doses q10 min during start of infusion.	Up to 300 mg total dose in 24 hours	2–5 minutes	3–6 hours	Elimination: 2.5–8 hours	• Caution in patients with impaired left ventricular function and bronchospastic respiratory disease • Does not affect ICPs or CBF
Nicardipine	Dihydropyridine calcium-channel antagonist	Continuous IV infusion: 5 mg/h (Start infusion at 3 mg/h in patients with renal insufficiency)	Titrate by 2.5 mg/h q15 min (q5 min for more rapid control); once goal BP reached ↓ rate to 3 mg/h	15 mg/h	5–10 minutes	1–4 hours	2–4 hours	• No effect on ICPs • Smooth reduction in pressure • Entire IV line must be changed q12h if given peripherally

(continued)

Table 3.3 (continued)

Agent	Mechanism of action	Initial dose	Dose titration	Maximum dosage	Onset of action	Duration of action	Half-life	Comments
Sodium Nitroprusside	Direct-acting vasodilator	Continuous IV infusion: 0.25 µg/kg per minute	↑ every 5 min by 0.5–1 µg/kg per minute	5 µg/kg per minute (due to risk of cyanide toxicity)*	Within 30 seconds	1–10 minutes	Plasma: 3–4 minutes	• Potent and labile BP reductions • Do not abruptly discontinue • ↑ICPs and ↓ CBF • Risk of cyanide toxicity • Coronary steal syndrome may occur • Use with caution in patients with hypoxemia, renal, and hepatic insufficiency

* The manufacturer states a maximum dose of 10 µg/kg per minute; however, clinically unsafe and should not be increased beyond 5 µg/kg per minute.

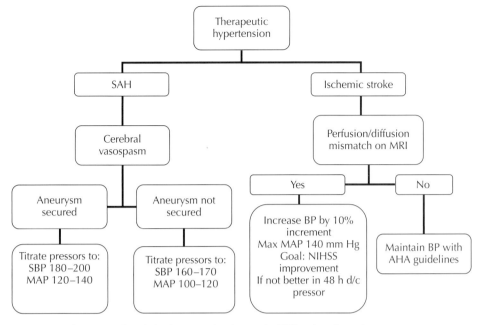

Figure 3.1. Permissive hypertensive therapy in SAH and stroke patients.

established, in our center we maintain an SBP <140. Agents with minimal cardiovascular side effects and ICP effects are preferred. In our institution labetalol, esmolol and nicardipine are the most frequently used.

In patients with poor grade subarachnoid hemorrhage (Hunt-Hess grade IV or V), the overriding concern is maintenance of adequate CPP in the face of elevated ICP. Aggressive volume resuscitation with isotonic volume is also indicated to minimize hypovolemia from excessive natriuresis.

Finally, delayed cerebral ischemia from vasospasm may occur in 60–75% of patients with SAH. It characteristically occurs between days 4 and 21 and it is associated with significant morbidity and mortality. In addition to nimodipine, sympathetic vasospasm begins with "triple H therapy": hypertension, hypervolemia, and hemodilution achieved by colloid or crystalloid infusion and vasopressors with a target CVP >8 and pulmonary artery pressure >14. Phenylephrine is the first-line agent because tachycardia often complicates the use of dopamine and norepinephrine. Dobutamine is often useful for cardiac output augmentation in the face of medically refractory spasm. CHF and myocardial ischemia are the most common side effects and therefore frequent

EKGs, chest radiograph, and cardiac enzymes should be performed (Figs. 3.1 and 3.2).

POSTCAROTID ENDARTERECTOMY

Some degree of hemodynamic instability (hypertension, hypotension, or bradycardia) commonly develops after carotid endarterectomy (CEA). Postoperative arterial hypertension is significantly associated with stroke or death. In addition, patients with preoperative high-grade stenosis may be at higher risk of cerebral hyperperfusion postoperatively because of defective vascular autoregulation. Hence these patients should be treated aggressively to lower their MAP to 80–100 mm Hg. Our experience indicates that these patients have an exaggerated bradycardic response with β-blockers and hence nicardipine, hydralazine, or enalaprilat might be a better choice agent.

Patients with Intracranial Mass

Total volume of intracranial contents (brain, CSF, and blood volume) in the rigid skull must remain constant. Increase in any of these three components without increase of ICP is possible only under simultaneous reduction of the other two components.

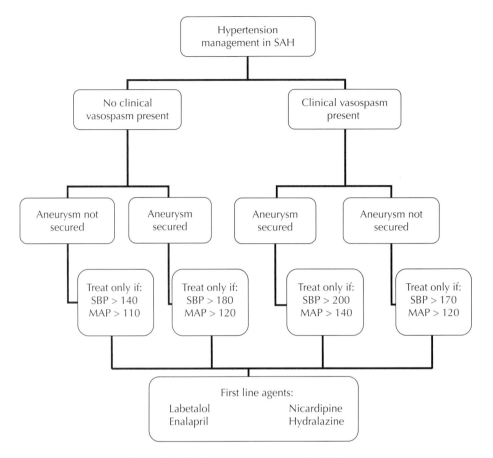

Figure 3.2. Blood pressure management in SAH.

With the exhaustion of compensatory mechanisms (CSF displacement from cerebral ventricles and subarachnoid space), even a slight increase in intracranial volume induces a dramatic increase in ICP. ICP monitoring is highly desirable in this subset of patients because hypertension may be a manifestation of Cushing's reflex.

A short-acting agent such as labetalol is recommended for BP control. However, CPP must be maintained greater than 70 mm Hg and hypotension must be avoided. Extreme caution should be taken to avoid reduction of CPP below 70 mm Hg, which can trigger reflex vasodilatation and ICP elevation. If CPP is below 70 mm Hg and ICP is above 20 mm Hg, elevation of MAP (and thus CPP) with a vasopressor may lead to a reflex reduction of ICP by reducing cerebral vasodilatation (and thus cerebral blood volume) that occurs in response to inadequate perfusion. Hydralazine and other

vasodilators should be avoided due to its adverse effect on ICP.

GUILLAIN-BARRÉ SYNDROME
Dysautonomia occurs frequently and is an important cause of death in severe Guillain-Barré syndrome (GBS). In a series of 169 patients with GBS, 65% of all patients had some evidence of autonomic dysfunction. Frequent manifestations are sinus tachycardia, hypertension, and labile blood pressure. Hypertension developed in 13.5% of the control patients in the American plasma exchange trial and systolic BP varied by more than 40 mm Hg in 36% of the control patients in the French plasma exchange trial. In GBS, hypertension and tachycardia are best left untreated because they are only transient, and β-blockade and antihypertensive treatment may aggravate incipient bradycardia or hypotension. However, older patient with coronary

heart disease must be treated. Any use of vasoactive medications should be done with caution, and preferably with only those medications with a short half-life. If there is evidence of cardiac decompensation, or other end-organ injury or the MAP exceeds 120 mm Hg, then sodium nitroprusside should be administered cautiously.

HYPERTENSIVE ENCEPHALOPATHY

Hypertensive encephalopathy (HE) is a manifestation of hypertensive emergency. Hypertensive emergency is defined as a severe elevation of BP that precipitates end-organ damage. In addition to HE, other complications include acute pulmonary edema, acute ischemic coronary disease, hypertensive retinopathy, aortic dissection, and acute renal failure. Successful therapy relies on appropriate and prompt diagnosis in the setting of global central dysfunction with concomitant severe elevation of BP and confirmatory imaging studies. The mortality rate in patients appropriately treated is <5%. Survivors generally have a complete recovery of neurologic function and imaging abnormalities.

The Joint Committee on Detection, Evaluation and Treatment of High Blood Pressure recommends that BP should be lowered within minutes to decrease mortality. In general, the goal is to gradually decrease the MAP no more than 20–25% or to reduce the DBP approximately 100 mm Hg during the first 1–2 hours. Evidence suggests that autoregulation set points for BP begin to change within hours after the onset of hypertension. Thus, aggressive lowering of BP can precipitate an ischemic event.

The best therapeutic agent to use, and the degree to which the BP should be acutely reduced, depends on several variables, including the patient's premorbid BP, the duration of the hypertensive emergency, concomitant medical diseases, and the extent of neurologic involvement. Also, it should be considered, almost by definition, that patients with HE are at risk for developing ICP.

Labetalol is usually the preferred agent for its favorable pharmacokinetics and lack of side effects in intracranial vessels, although it should be avoided in patients with congestive heart failure or AV block.

Nicardipine is also a reasonable first line agent. It is easy to titrate and demonstrated unusual effects on ICP. Sodium nitroprusside is still one of the most common drugs used in the medical ICU for the treatment of hypertensive crisis. However, its vasodilatory effect can potentially increase the ICP. For this reason and its longer half-life, it should be used with discretion in the treatment of hypertensive encephalopathy.

Nitroglycerin will also increase ICP but it is probably a useful option in patients with concomitant myocardial ischemia. Phentolamine should be considered in patients with HE as a result of pheochromocytoma. Trimethaphan is often used in patients with aortic dissection, but it can complicate the neurologic examination in patients with altered mental status due to its mydriatic effect. Fenoldopam also can be a reasonable option in patients with concomitant renal failure.

Clonidine should be avoided because of its potential for CNS depression. Finally, bed rest, sedation and analgesia may further help BP control.

ECLAMPSIA

Eclampsia refers to a particular form of HE that occurs in the setting of pregnancy-induced hypertension. BP management is more complex than in routine HE since the physiology of pregnancy can alter drug metabolism and certain classes of medications such as angiotensin-converting enzyme (ACE) inhibitors and angiotensin receptor blockers are strictly contraindicated.

Early detection, followed by delivery is the mainstay of treatment follow by delivery. If delivery is not possible, BP control should be started. As a consensus, MAP in eclampsia should be maintained between 105 and 125 mm Hg. As in other neurologic emergencies, control of BP in the ICU setting with an easily titratable agent such as labetalol and nicardipine is advised. Nitroprusside is commonly used. In patients with associated seizures, magnesium remains the drug of choice. A 4–6 g IV bolus in 5 minutes followed by a 1–2 g/h IV infusion for at least 48 hours postpartum is commonly the protocol used. If the treatment is used prophylactically in preeclampsia, it can be stopped after 24 hours. In addition, magnesium also will reduce BP. Dosage should be lowered in half in patients with creatinine >1.3.

In conclusion, during the acute phase of many neurologic emergencies it is often desirable to maintain MAP and CPP within a relatively narrow range because it cannot be assumed that autoregulation is intact at the site of injury. The basic principles of

BP management in critically ill neurologic patients include: (1) ameliorate systemic hypertension; (2) avoid systemic hypotension; (3) maintain adequate BP and perfusion pressure, thereby avoiding secondary brain and spinal cord injury; and (4) utilize agents that have minimal effects on ICP and CBF autoregulation.

REFERENCES

Adams HP, Jr, Brott TG, Crowell RM, et al. Guidelines for the management of patients with acute ischemic stroke. A statement for healthcare professionals from a special writing group of the Stroke Council, American Heart Association [see comments]. *Stroke.* 1994;**25**(9):1901–14.

Adams HP Jr, Brott TG, Furlan AJ, et al. Guidelines for thrombolytic therapy for acute stroke: a supplement to the guidelines for the management of patients with acute ischemic stroke. A statement for healthcare professionals from a Special Writing Group of the Stroke Council, American Heart Association. *Circulation.* 1996;**94**(5):1167–74.

Beale RJ, Hollenberg SM, Vincent JL, Parillo JE. Vasopressor and inotropic support in septic shock: An evidence-based review. *Crit Care Med.* 2004;**32**[Suppl]:S455–65.

Bridges E, Dukes MS. Cardiovascular aspects of septic shock: pathophysiology, monitoring, and treatment. *Critical Care Nurse.* 2005;**25**:32–3.

Britton M, Carlsson A. Very high blood pressure in acute stroke. *J Intern Med.* 1990;**228**(6):611–5.

Broderick JP, Adams HP Jr, Barsan W et al. Guidelines for the management of spontaneous intracerebral hemorrhage: a statement for healthcare professionals from a special writing group of the Stroke Council, American Heart Association. *Stroke.* 1999;**30**(4):905–15.

Brott, Broderick J, Kothari R et al. Early hemorrhage growth in patients with intracerebral hemorrhage. *Stroke.* 1997;**28**(1):1–5.

Clifton GL, Robertson CS, Kyper K et al. Cardiovascular response to severe head injury. *J Neurosurg.* 1983;**59**(3):447–54.

Fagan SC, Bowes MP, Lyden PD, et al. Acute hypertension promotes hemorrhagic transformation in a rabbit embolic stroke model: effect of labetalol. *Exp Neurol.* 1998;**150**(1):153–8.

Fenves AZ, Ram VS. Drug treatment of hypertensive urgencies and emergencies. *Semin Nephrol.* 2005;**25**:272–80.

French Cooperative Group on Plasma Exchange in Guillain-Barre syndrome. Efficiency of plasma exchange in Guillain-Barre syndrome: role of replacement fluids. *Ann Neurol.* 1987;**22**(6):753–61.

Fulgham JR, Wijdicks EF. Guillain-Barré syndrome. *Crit Care Clin.* 1997;**13**(1):1–15.

Guillain-Barré Syndrome Study Group. Plasmapheresis and acute Guillain-Barré syndrome. *Neurology.* 1985;**35**(8):1096–104.

Haas CE, LeBlanc JM. Acute postoperative hypertension: a review of therapeutic options. *Am J Health-Syst Pharm.* 2004;**61**:1661–75.

Holmes, Cheryl. Vasoactive drugs in the intensive care unit. *Curr Opin Crit Care.* Lippincott Williams & Wilkins. 2005;**11**:413–17.

Jorgensen LG, Schroeder TV. Defective cerebrovascular autoregulation after carotid endarterectomy. *Eur J Vasc Surg.* 1993;**7**(4):370–9.

Karlsson AK. Autonomic dysreflexia [see comments]. *Spinal Cord.* 1999;**37**(6):383–91.

Kassell NF, Peerless SJ, Durward QJ, et al. Treatment of ischemic deficits from vasospasm with intravascular volume expansion and induced arterial hypertension. *Neurosurgery.* 1982;**11**(3):337–43.

Kassell NF, Torner JC, Haley EC Jr, et al. The International Cooperative Study on the Timing of Aneurysm Surgery. Part 1: Overall management results. *J Neurosurg.* 1990;**73**(1):18–36.

Kazui S, Naritomi H, Yamamoto H et al. Enlargement of spontaneous intracerebral hemorrhage. Incidence and time course. *Stroke.* 1996;**27**(10):1783–7.

Lindan R, Leffler EJ, Kedia KR. A comparison of the efficacy of an alpha-I-adrenergic blocker in the slow calcium channel blocker in the control of autonomic dysreflexia. *Paraplegia.* 1985;**23**(1):34–8.

Mistri AK, Robinson RG, Potter JF. Pressor therapy in acute ischemic stroke. *Stroke.* 2006;**37**:1565–71.

Mueller BA, Chant C, Rudis M, et al. Pharmacotherapy self-assessment program: critical care urgent care. American College of Clinical Pharmacy. 4th ed. 2002;**6**:18–21.

NINDS t-PA Stroke Study Group. Intracerebral hemorrhage after intravenous t-PA therapy for ischemic stroke. *Stroke.* 1997;**28**(11):2109–18.

Oppenheimer SM, Hachinski VC. The cardiac consequences of stroke. *Neurol Clin.* 1992;**10**(1):167–76.

Passerini L. Indications for intensive care unit care after carotid endarterectomy [see comments]. *Can J Surg.* 1996;**39**(2):99–104.

Paulson OB, Waldemar G, Schmidt JF, Strandgaard S. Cerebral circulation under normal and pathologic conditions. *Am J Cardiol.* 1989;**63**:2C–5C.

Powers WJ. Acute hypertension after stroke: the scientific basis for treatment decisions [editorial]. *Neurology.* 1993;**43**(3 Pt 1):461–7.

Powers WJ, Adams RE, Yundt KD, et al. Acute pharmacological hypotension after intracerebral hemorrhage does not change cerebral blood flow. *Stroke.* 1999;**30**(1):64.

Robertson CS, Clifton GL, Taylor AA, et al. Treatment of hypertension associated with head injury. *J Neurosurg.* 1983;**59**(3):455–60.

Rordorf G, Cramer SC, Efrid JT, et al. Pharmacological elevation of blood pressure in acute stroke. Clinical effects and safety. *Stroke.* 1997;**28**(11): 2133–8.

Rose JC, Mayer SA. Optimizing blood pressure in neurological emergencies. *Neurocritical Care.* 2004;**3**:287–300.

Rosner MJ, Rosner SD, Johnson AH. Cerebral perfusion pressure: Management protocol and clinical results [see comments]. *J Neurosurg.* 1995;**83**(6):949–62.

Schulte Esch J, Murday H, Pfeifer G. Haemodynamic changes in patients with severe head injury. *Acta Neurochir.* 1980;**54**(3–4):243–50.

Schwartz RB, Mulkern RV, Gudbjartsson H, et al. Diffusion-weighted MR imaging in hypertensive encephalopathy: clues to pathogenesis. *AJNR.* 1998;**19**(5):859–62.

Shimoda M, Oda S, Tsugane R et al. Intracranial complications of hypervolemic therapy in patients with a delayed ischemic deficit attributed to vasospasm [see comments]. *J Neurosurg.* 1993;**78**(3):423–9.

Skinhoj E, Strandgaard S. Pathogenesis of hypertensive encephalopathy. *Lancet.* 1973;1(7801):461–2.

Teasell RW, Arnold JM, Krassioukov A, Delaney GA. Cardiovascular consequences of loss of supraspinal control of the sympathetic nervous system after spinal cord injury. *Arch Phys Med Rehabil.* 2000;**81**(4):506–16.

Tietjen CS, Hurn PD, Ulatowski JA, Kirsch JR. Treatment modalities for hypertensive patients with intracranial pathology: options and risks. *Crit Care Med.* 1996;**24**(2): 311–22.

Truax BT. Autonomic disturbances in the Guillain-Barré syndrome. *Semin Neurol.* 1984;**4**:462–8.

Vaidyanathan S, Soni BM, Sett P, Watt JW, Oo T, Bingley J. Pathophysiology of autonomic dysreflexia: long-term treatment with terazosin in adult and paediatric spinal cord injury patients manifesting recurrent dysreflexic episodes. *Spinal Cord.* 1998;**36**(11):761–70.

Varon J, Marik PE. The diagnosis and management of hypertensive crisis. *Chest.* 2000;**118**:214–27.

Wise G, Sutter R, Burkholder J. The treatment of brain ischemia with vasopressor drugs. *Stroke.* 1972;**3**(2): 135–40.

Wong JH, Findlay JM, Suarez-Almazor ME. Hemodynamic instability after carotid endarterectomy: risk factors and associations with operative complications. *Neurosurgery.* 1997;**41**(1):35–41; discussion 41–3.

Zazulia AR, Diringer MN, Videen TO, et al. Acute intracerebral hemorrhage does not produce per-clot cerebral ischemia. *Neurology.* 2000;**54**(7):A261–2.

Zochodne DW. Autonomic involvement in Guillain-Barré syndrome: a review. *Muscle Nerve.* 1994;**17**(10): 1145–55.

4 Hypothermia: Physiology and Applications

Carmelo Graffagnino, MD FRCPC

By the time that a patient with an acute neurologic injury is admitted to the neurocritical care unit, the primary damage has already occurred and the major focus of intervention shifts to that of preventing secondary injury. The brain accounts for only 2% of the body's mass, yet it utilizes 25% of the body's energy stores and receives 15–20% of the total cardiac output. It is exquisitely sensitive to even the briefest period of anoxia, with the latter frequently resulting in dire consequences.

Brain temperature plays a major role in modulating the effects of ischemia and anoxia. The potential life-saving effects of hypothermia have been evident ever since early people first noted that individuals who became immersed in ice-cold water and drowned were able to be revived with no apparent neurologic injury. Cold-water immersion was recognized as having life-preserving effects; however, the mechanisms by which this occurred remained largely unknown. Although early physicians such as Hippocrates understood that cold water or ice had tissue-preserving and anti-inflammatory effects, its application to preserving the brain tissue took severalcenturies of medical advancement to be realized.

Induced hypothermia was first used as a modern neurologic therapeutic tool by Dr. Temple Fay, who reported cooling 124 patients with severe head injury in the 1940s.[1] This then led Bigelow et al. to use hypothermia as a neuroprotective agent during cardiac surgery that required cardiac arrest (CA), causing global cerebral ischemia.[2] The robustness of hypothermia neuroprotection was elegantly demonstrated by Busto et al. in preclinical models of cerebral ischemia when they showed that as little

as a 2–5°C drop in brain temperature resulted in marked protection against global ischemia.[3]

MECHANISMS OF HYPOTHERMIA NEUROPROTECTION

Induced therapeutic hypothermia's appears to exert its neuroprotective mechanism of action via multiple pathways.

- Hypothermia has been shown to alter metabolic rate[4] by decreasing cellular metabolism by retarding high-energy phosphate depletion and facilitating postischemic glucose utilization.
- Hypothermia attenuates the cytotoxic cascade by suppressing elevations of intracellular calcium, thus inhibiting the release of excitotoxic amino acids and reducing intracellular acidosis.[5-7]
- Hypothermia suppresses the breakdown of the blood–brain barrier[8,9] and reduces free radical formation.[7,10]
- Hypothermia may even protect the injured neurovascular tissues against the toxic effects of tissue plasminogen activator (t-PA) while still allowing the lytic effect to function.[11]
- Hypothermia also prevents cell injury from leading to apoptosis[12] by inhibition of caspase activation.[12-14]

THERAPEUTIC HYPOTHERMIA IN PRECLINICAL MODELS OF BRAIN INJURY

Global Ischemia

The potential benefits of induced hypothermia as a protective strategy for global ischemic injury were first evaluated in an intraischemic rat model.

- Cooling to 33–34°C markedly reduced brain damage after 20 minutes of forebrain ischemia.[3]
- Subsequent studies demonstrated that global ischemic damage could also be reduced by selective brain cooling even after prolonged (30 minutes) ischemia.[15]

Once intraischemic hypothermia was demonstrated to be neuroprotective, the effectiveness of postischemic induction of hypothermia was explored.

- Three hours of hypothermia (30°C), started 5 minutes after a 10-minute period of global forebrain ischemia, was able to reduce ischemic injury by 50%[16] but the effect was lost if cooling was delayed by 30 minutes after the ischemic insult.
- It was subsequently demonstrated that longer periods of postischemic hypothermia resulted in more extensive neuroprotection.[17-19]

Although intraischemic hypothermia seemed to provide permanent neuroprotection, other studies suggested that postischemic neuroprotection might be transient and cell death was not prevented but rather delayed.[20,21] Longer periods of ischemia or delays in initiating treatment seemed to require prolonged periods of hypothermia in order to demonstrate permanent and effective neuroprotection.

- Chopp et al. showed that 2 hours of moderate hypothermia (34°C) protected against 8 minutes of ischemia but not 12.[22]
- Using a similar experimental paradigm, 12 hours of hypothermia started 1 hour postischemia protected totally against 3 minutes but only partially against 5 minutes of global ischemia.[23]
- Extending the period of cooling to 24 hours protected completely.[23] Even if hypothermia was started as late as 6 hours postischemia it was protective as long as it was extended.[24]
- Hypothermia started 6 hours after 10 minutes of global ischemia and extended for 48 hours, reduced neuronal loss to 14% in a 28-day survival model.[24] The benefit of this treatment (32°C for 24 hours) was as effective in older animals as it was in younger ones even when evaluated out to 30 days post-treatment.[25]

If these experimental results were to be translated to the case of the post-CA patient it would suggest that:

1. The longer the period of ischemia and the greater the latency between the ischemic insult and the onset of therapy, the longer the period of hypothermia that would be required to obtain permanent and effective neuroprotection.
2. As of the present time, only 12 hours and 24 hours of hypothermia have been evaluated clincally.[26,27]

Focal Ischemia

Although the human condition of global ischemia after CA is represented well by existing animal models of transient global ischemia, the same cannot be said for focal ischemia (ischemic stroke). Focal ischemic stroke in humans is a heterogeneous condition with similar clinical syndromes being produced by different pathophysiologic mechanisms including embolic as well as locally thrombotic processes. The location and caliber of the occluded vessels vary considerably, as does the collateral flow within a particular vascular distribution. Animal studies attempting to model ischemic stroke utilize either transient or complete occlusion of large vessels. The middle cerebral artery occlusion model using either an intraluminal suture or direct ligation or clipping the vessel has been most commonly utilized[28,29] and produce strokes that resemble human large-vessel infarctions (middle cerebral artery [MCA] strokes). Outcome variables of interest include histopathology, neurotransmitter studies, and functional assessments measured early (hours to days) in some studies and late in others (days to weeks).

Direct comparison of outcomes between studies has been difficult. The treatment paradigms utilized have been highly variable. Some studies induced hypothermia before or immediately after the onset of ischemia[30-37] while others delayed the treatment from minutes up to 6 hours after the ischemia.[32,34,35,38]

- Given the variability in experimental designs, the degree of neuroprotection demonstrated ranges markedly (0–65% reduction in infarct volume).[32,34,35,38]

- Brief periods of hypothermia (30°C) have been shown to provide transient neuroprotection while prolonging it for up to 24 hours results in sustained neuroprotection (48% reduction in infarct volume seen at 3 weeks).[30]

There is no experimental evidence that if the ischemia is permanent hypothermia can be delayed beyond 1 hour and still be protective.[32] The situation is different in the case of transient cerebral ischemia, where the potential benefits of immediate and delayed hypothermia have been evaluated more extensively and with more consistent results than with permanent occlusion models. Most of the reported studies use 2 hours of ischemia (range from 30 minutes to 6 hours) and report outcomes analyzed immediately as well as delayed (1–2 months postinfarct).

Intraischemic hypothermia has demonstrated neuroprotection (30–92% reduction in infarct volume) with exposures from as little as 1 hour up to 24 hours in duration.[36,37,39-46] Although intrasischemic induction of hypothermia is associated with the best protection, it has also been found to be effective even when applied postischemia although to a lesser extent.[37,40-42,45] There is a limit, however, to how long this can be postponed, as delays of greater than 6 hours have not been shown to be effective in focal ischemia compared to global ischemia, where prolonged periods of hypothermia may still be beneficial.

- The longer the delay from the onset of ischemia to hypothermia, the longer hypothermia needs to be applied to produce a benefit.[12,41,42,44,45,47]
- While increasing the length of cooling seems to improve outcomes, deeper cooling (27°C vs. 32°C) has not been shown to be superior to moderate cooling,[41] thus supporting moderate hypothermia (32–34°C) as the temperature of choice for neuroprotection.
- The optimal duration of cooling has not been clearly worked out and may depend on the length of the ischemic period and the time delay to onset of therapy.
- Further studies are needed to support specific time-dependent cooling paradigms.

Traumatic Brain Injury

Posttraumatic hypothermia has been reported to improve histopathological and functional outcome in several models of traumatic brain injury (TBI).[48-51] The benefits of hypothermia in TBI are mediated through the same pathways seen in ischemic injury including modulation of excitotoxicity, free radical production, reduction in metabolism, membrane stabilization, and apoptosis.[52]

Spinal Cord Injury

Selective spinal cord cooling with cold saline infused into isolated aortic segments has been shown to reduce the neurologic damage of spinal cord ischemia in an animal model of aortic ischemic injury.

- Models simulating physical injury have shown that directly applied cooling of the spinal cord to 19°C was able to provide neuroprotection after a mild to moderate injury but not in severely injured animals.[54]
- Systemically applied hypothermia (32°C) after spinal cord contusional injury has also been shown to be neuroprotective but only if the injury was of moderate severity.[55]

CLINICAL STUDIES OF THERAPEUTIC HYPOTHERMIA

Cardiac Arrest

Several small pilot studies of hypothermia after CA showing great promise led to two randomized controlled studies that proved the effectiveness of moderate hypothermia for anoxic encephalopathy. Both of these studies limited enrollment to patients with anoxic injury after out-of-hospital CA from ventricular fibrillation or ventricular tachycardia (VT/VF).[26,27]

- The study of Bernard et al.[27] randomized 77 patients (43 to hypothermia and 34 to normothermia), with the hypothermia started in the ambulance and then maintained at 33°C for 12 hours.
  - The study was limited in that only outcomes at hospital discharge were reported.
  - At the time of discharge from the hospital, 21 of the 43 (49%) hypothermia-treated patients had a good outcome compared to 9 of the 34 (26%) in the control group ($p = 0.46$).

- The larger Hypothermia After Cardiac Arrest (H.A.C.A.)[26] study randomized 273 patients (136 to hypothermia and 137 to normothermia) with the hypothermia group cooled to 33°C for 24 hours.
  - This study had long-term follow-up, with Cerebral Performance Category (CPC) scores reported at 6 months.
  - Good outcomes were seen in 55% of the hypothermia-treated patients compared to 39% of the normothermia controls (CPC 1 or 2).
- Although both of these studies limited entry to patients with VT/VF, hypothermia may also be effective even in other cardiac rhythms (asystole).[60]
- Current recommendations by the American Heart Association (AHA) and International Liaison Committee on Resuscitation (ILCOR) are that unconscious patients with spontaneous circulation after out-of-hospital CA due to VF/VT be treated with moderate hypothermia (32–34°C) for 12–24 hours and that such cooling may be beneficial for other rhythms or in-hospital arrest [61,62]

Focal Ischemic Stroke

Unlike the positive outcomes reported for patients after CA, the evidence that hypothermia is clinically effective for the treatment of acute ischemic stroke remains to be definitively proven. Several small feasibility studies have been published showing that the induction and maintenance of hypothermia is possible and may even improve outcome after focal ischemic stroke.[63-66]

- A small prospective study from Copenhagen[63] compared 17 patients, presenting within 12 hours of symptom onset and cooled with an air-forced cooling blanket for 6 hours, to 56 historical controls.
  - Core body temperature was decreased from 36.8°C to 35.5°C, with shivering suppressed by the use of meperidine.
  - Although there was no difference between groups based on the Scandinavian stroke scale score at 6 months, all-cause mortality was lower in the hypothermia group than in the controls (12% vs. 23% respectively).[63]

Most of the hypothermia stroke studies have excluded patients treated with recombinant tissue type plasminogen activator (rt-PA). The safety of inducing hypothermia after thrombolytic therapy

for ischemic stroke was assessed in a small pilot study by Krieger et al. in which 10 patients presenting with symptoms of an MCA stroke and an NIHSS score of >15 within 6 hours of onset were cooled to 32°C using topical cooling blankets for a period of 12–72 hours depending on vessel patency.[67] Nine concurrent control patients were chosen for comparison. Three of the hypothermia patients died. The surviving patients had a mean modified Rankin score at 3 months of 3.1 ± 2.3.

- Overall hypothermia was well tolerated and appeared safe in the setting of thrombolysis.
- The results of this small study are consistent with other preclinical as well as small clinical studies that suggest hypothermia is safe and may be protective when added to thrombolytic therapy.[67-69]

While surface cooling methods were used in all of the aforementioned studies, newer intravascular catheter–based cooling methods became available in the late 1990s. Intravascular induced hypothermia for ischemic stroke was fist reported by Georgiadis et al.,[70] who cooled six patients with severe acute ischemic stroke using this technique. The procedure was well tolerated with minimal side effects.[70] The largest reported study utilizing intravascular cooling randomized 40 patients to receive either hypothermia at 33°C for 24 hours or best medical care.[71] Eighteen patients were cooled. All had magnetic resonance imaging (MRI) scans at 3–5 days and then again at 30–37 days. Unfortunately, the study failed to show any difference in MRI lesion size or clinical outcomes between groups. Caution is advised in interpreting this study because the number of patients treated was small and the study may have been underpowered to show a clinical benefit.

- Based on the available published literature there is insufficient evidence support routine use of induced hypothermia for neuroprotection in patients with acute ischemic stroke.

Hypothermia has, however, been shown to be able to reduce cerebral edema in the setting of malignant ischemic strokes,[64-66] although it is not as effective at preventing death as hemicraniectomy.[72] This was demonstrated in a study of 36 patients with severe acute ischemic stroke (17 randomized to hemicraniectomy and 19 to moderate hypothermia).

- The hypothermia-treated patients had a significantly higher mortality compared to the hemicraniectomy group (47% vs. 12%, respectively).[73]
- Hypothermia seems to be able to control ICP in most studies of malignant MCA stroke[64-66] yet uncontrolled rebound ICP during rewarming frequently leads to death. The key to solving this problem is in controlling the rewarming rate which reduces the degree of rebound ICP and a reduction in death.[74]

TRAUMATIC BRAIN INJURY

In spite of hundreds of animal studies demonstrating a beneficial effect of induced moderate hypothermia following TBI, the evidence supporting its routine use in humans with TBI remains controversial. Since the early 1990s, at least 14 clinical studies have been completed[75-88] and 3 meta-analyses published on the efficacy of moderate hypothermia (32–34°C) for TBI.[89-91] Some of the published studies were not included in the meta-analyses because they were not all randomized and some were published after the meta-analyses.

- The largest study conducted in the United States included 392 patients with Glasgow Coma Score (GCS) of 3–8 and randomized to hypothermia or normothermia within 8 hours of injury.[92]
  - Hypothermia was maintained for 48 hours and then the patients were actively rewarmed.
  - A poor outcome (GCS of 1–3) was seen in 57% of patients in both groups and mortality was also equal (28% in hypothermic group vs. 26% in controls).[92]
- Contradicting these findings were the results of the Chinese single center study by Zhi et al.[88] in which 396 patients with TBI were randomized to hypothermia or normothermia within 24 hours of trauma.
  - This study differed from the Clifton et al.[92] trial in that patients were kept hypothermic until ICP had remained normal for 24 hours.
  - Mortality was 36.4% in the normothermic patients compared to 25.7% in the hypothermic group.[92]
  - The study[88] results have come into question as little information is provided in the published report regarding randomization, blinding and medical management of the patients.

In an effort to coalesce the results of the many published studies into a single assessment, three meta-analyses have been carried out and published. In spite of evaluating essentially the same studies, the three meta-analyses have come to slightly different conclusions. The published studies vary considerably in method of blinding, randomization and management of ICP as well as the care of control subjects.

- The Cochrane Review included 10 trials with 771 patients and did not find any evidence of benefit with respect to death or severe disability although hypothermia seemed to be associated with an increased risk for pneumonia.[89]
- Henderson et al.[91] likewise failed to find evidence of benefit in favor of hypothermia. They only included 8 trials in their analysis with a total of 748 patients.
- MacIntyre and his colleagues[93] included the largest number of studies in their work with 12 trials and 1069 patients. Of note, two of the studies included were published in Asian journals and included 300 patients whom the other 2 meta-analysis did not include.
  - The authors concluded[93] that hypothermia following TBI was associated with a reduction in death (Relative Risk [RR] of 0.81 (95% confidence interval [CI] 0.69-0.96) as well as improved neurologic outcome (RR was 0.78 for Glasgow Outcome Scale [GOS] 1–3 [95% CI 0.63-0.98]).
  - Subgroup analysis also suggested that cooling for a longer period of time (>48 hours) had an even greater beneficial effect.
- In spite of the optimistic assessment of the literature by McIntyre et al.,[93] the use of hypothermia in all patients with acute TBI cannot be advised at this time. Clinical trials in this area continue with the expectation that their results will more clearly guide the management of patients in the future.

IMPLEMENTING THERAPEUTIC HYPOTHERMIA IN THE NEUROCRITICAL CARE UNIT

Based on the literature reviewed in the preceding text, the only definitively proven indication for the use induced therapeutic hypothermia is for patients with post arrest ischemic encephalopathy. Although the two pivotal studies[26,27] of induced hypothermia after CA both concluded that the treatment was clinically effective, they used significantly different protocols to induce and maintain hypothermia, different duration of cooling, and different rewarming techniques and rates. Significant clinical and technical advances have occurred since the studies above were published. Some of these are reviewed in the text that follows.

Induction and Maintenance of Hypothermia

CRANIAL COOLING

Although directly cooling the brain would be most desirable, the effectiveness of surface cooling has been less than desirable. Surface cranial cooling with ice during ACLS has been shown to be ineffective in reducing brain temperature.[94]

- One small study demonstrated the effectiveness of a novel cooling helmets when used to induce cooling after CA.[95]
  - They were able to reduce core temperature to 34°C in a median time of 180 minutes (0.6°C per hour) after return of spontaneous circulation (ROSC) in CA patients with pulseless electrical activity (PEA) and asystole.
  - No long-term outcome-based studies using this methodology are available.

The induction of systemic hypothermia may also have protective effects on other organs suffering from postischemic injury, thus potentially favoring whole body cooling.

EXTERNAL SURFACE COOLING

External surface cooling depends on conductive loss of heat from the skin surface. Various methods can be used including the direct application of ice, cold water, forced cold air, cold water containing blanket, or cooled gel containing surface pads.

- Cold ice packs can reduce core temperature by 0.9°C per hour[27,56]; however, this is a labor-intensive method and may result in damage to the skin if prolonged periods of direct ice to skin contact occur.
- Cold air cooling is even slower at a rate of 0.3–0.5°C per hour.[96,97]
- Cold water containing blankets have been compared to forced cold air cooling and no significant advantages have been found for either method.[98]

INTRAVENOUS COLD SALINE

Iced normal saline infusions have been shown to be effective at rapidly reducing core temperatures.[99-104]

- Healthy volunteers can be cooled by 2.5°C within an hour of starting a 30-minute infusion of 4°C saline (40 mL/kg) after neuromuscular block with vecuronium and general anesthesia.[101]
- Bernard et al. cooled 22 resuscitated CA patients by 1.7°C using 30 mL/kg of 4°C lactated Ringer's solution given over 30 minutes.[99] All of these patients received neuromuscular blocking agents.
- In a similar study Kim et al.[102] gave 2 L of 4°C saline over 20–30 minutes following ROSCR after CA. This resulted in a mean drop of 1.4°C 30 minutes after initiation of infusion. This did not affect the left ventricular ejection fraction, vital signs, or coagulation parameters.
- Virkkunen et al. recently studied the feasibility of inducing hypothermia in a prehospital setting using an infusion of 30 mL/kg of ice-cold Ringer's solution given at a rate of 100 mL/min to comatose patients with out of hospital CA. They were able to reduce core temperature from 35.8°C at the onset of infusion to 34°C on arrival to hospital.[103]

Together, these studies demonstrate that the use if intravenous cold saline is a safe, easy to use, and effective method of inducing systemic hypothermia.

ENDOVASCULAR COOLING

Al-Senani et al.[105] showed that a closed loop endovascular system placed in the inferior vena cava could reduce core body temperature by 0.8°C per hour after ROSC in patients with VF. Similarly, Georgiadis[70] studied the feasibility of inducing and maintaining moderate hypothermia with the use of endovascular cooling. Six patients with severe acute ischemic stroke were treated with moderate hypothermia. They were able to cool patients at a rate of 1.4°C per hour and reached target temperature after 3 hours (range, 2–4.5 hours). None of the patients experience significant complications in either of these studies.

EXTRACORPOREAL COOLING

This technique is by far the most invasive of the methods listed. Rapid core cooling using an extracorporeal heat exchanger has been reported in a small study in which eight patients were cooled down to 32°C within a mean time of 113 minutes.[106]

Measuring Temperature

Although target organ for hypothermia is the brain, several other sites requiring less invasive measures have been evaluated. Direct brain temperature measurements are possible by using a thermistor in a ventriculostomy catheter; however, this is not always possible or desirable and therefore surrogate sites are frequently utilized. Several studies have compared bladder, tympanic membrane, esophageal, and pulmonary artery temperatures with brain temperature and found them to correlate closely.[107-109] Although rectal temperatures have been shown to correlate with brain temperatures in some studies, they are considered less accurate than the other modalities.

Complications of Hypothermia

ARRHYTHMIAS

While ventricular ectopy many occur in the setting of induced mild to moderate hypothermia, ventricular fibrillation is very rare. Even in the setting in which patients present with VT/VF, therapeutic hypothermia is very rare as seen in the H.A.C.A. study.[26] Bradycardia is the most common arrhythmia seen at temperatures from 32°C to 36.5°C.[26]

ELECTROLYTE ABNORMALITIES

Most common is transient hypokalemia. Caution must be noted as this is mostly due to intracellular shift of K^+ and overcorrection may result in life-threatening rebound hyperkalemia during rewarming.[79]

IMMUNE SYSTEM

Hypothermia may suppress the immune system including T-cell-mediated antibody production,[110] predisposing the patients to infection. Schwab et al. reported that 7 of 25 stroke patients undergoing hypothermia suffered a septic syndrome.[66] In contradistinction to the experience by Schwab et al., the H.A.C.A. investigators did not find a significant difference in infections between the control and hypothermia treated groups.[26]

COAGULOPATHY

Hypothermia may cause coagulation abnormalities including prolongation of bleeding time and inhibition of the enzymatic reactions of the coagulation cascade.[110-113]

CONCLUSIONS

In spite of decades of clinical trials costing millions of dollars and involving thousands of patients, a proven neuroprotective agent is not yet available for use in patients with ischemic or traumatic brain damage. Most of the agents that have been tested thus far have targeted single mechanisms in the pathophysiologic process leading to cell death after ischemia. Hypothermia, conversely, exerts its influence via multiple mechanisms making it the ideal neuroprotective therapy. Preclinical studies have proven that it provides the most effective neuroprotection. The challenge for the clinician now is to translate this to an effective form of therapy for patients with brain injury. We have come a long way toward that goal. Randomized controlled studies have proven that induced moderate hypothermia can reduce cerebral ischemic injury after global ischemia. Much work is left to be done in the areas of focal stroke and TBI as well as spinal cord injury. Only with well designed and executed studies can this promising therapy be translated into effective clinical practice.

REFERENCES

1. Fay T. Observation on generalized refrigeration in cases of severe cerebral trauma. *Assoc Res Nerv Ment Dis Proc.* 1943;**24**:611–9.
2. Bigelow W, Lindsay W, Greenwood W. Hypothermia. Its possible role in cardiac surgery: an investigation of factors governing survival in dogs at low body temperatures. *Ann Surg.* 1950;**132**:849–66.
3. Busto R, Dietrich W, Globus M-T, et al. Small differences in intraischemic brain temperature critically determine the extent of ischemic neuronal injury. *J Cereb Blood Flow Metab.* 1987;**7**:729–38.
4. Chopp M, Knight R, Tidwell C, et al. The metabolic effects of mild hypothermia on global cerebral ischemia and recirculation in the cat: comparison to normothermia and hypothermia. *J Cereb Blood Flow Metab.* 1989;**9**:141–8.
5. Busto R, Globus M, Dietrich D, et al. Effect of mild hypothermia on ischemia induced release of neurotransmitters and free fatty acids in rat brain. *Stroke.* 1989;**20**:904–10.

6. Globus M, Busto R, Dietrich W, et al. Intra-ischemic extracellular release of dopamine and glutamate is associated with striatal vulnerability to ischemia. *Neurosci Lett.* 1988;**91**:36–40.

7. Globus M, Busto R, Lin B, et al. Detection of free radical activity during transient global ischemia and recirculation: effects of intraischemic brain temperature modulation. *J Neurochem.* 1995;**65**:1250–6.

8. Smith S, Hall E. Mild pre-and posttraumatic hypothermia attenuates blood-brain barrier damage following controlled cortical impact injury in the rat. *J Neurotrauma.* 1996;**13**:1–9.

9. Ishikawa M, Sekizuka E, Sata S, et al. Effects of moderate hypothermia on leukocyte-endothelium interaction in the rat pial microvasculature after transient middle cerebral artery occlusion. *Stroke.* 1999;**30**:1679–86.

10. Globus M, Alonson O, Dietrich D, et al. Glutamate release and free radical production following brain injury; effects of post-traumatic hypothermia. *J Neurochem.* 1995;**65**:1704–11.

11. Yenari M, Palmer J, Bracci P, et al. Thrombolysis with tissue plasminogen activator (tPA) is temperature dependent. *Thromb Res.* 1995;**77**:475–81.

12. Xu L, Yenari M, Steinberg G, et al. Mild hypothermia reduces apoptosis of mouse neurons in vitro early in the cascade. *J Cereb Blood Flow Metab.* 2002;**22**:21–8.

13. Povlishock J, Buki A, Koiziumi H, et al. Initiating mechanisms involved in the pathophysiology of traumatically induced axonal injury and interventions targeted at blunting their progression. *Acta Neurochir. Suppl (Wien).* 1999;**73**:15–20.

14. Ning X, CHen S, Xu C, et al. Hypothermic protection of the ischemic heart via alterations in apoptotic pathways as assessed by gene array analysis. *J Appl Physiol.* 2002;**92**:2200–7.

15. Kuluz J, Gregory G, Yu A, et al. Selective brain cooling during and after prolonged global ischemia reduces cortical damage in rats. *Stroke.* 1992;**23**:1792–6.

16. Busto R, Dietrich D, Globus M, et al. Postischemic moderate hypothermia inhibits CA1 hippocampal ischemic neuronal injury. *Neurosci Lett.* 1989;**101**:299–304.

17. Carroll M, Beek O. Protection against hippocampal CA1 cell loss by post-ischemic hypothermia is dependent on delay of initiation and duration. *Metab Brain Dis.* 1992;**7**:45–50.

18. Coimbra C, Wieloch T. Moderate hypothermia mitigates neuronal damage in the rat brain when initiated several hours following transient cerebral ischemia. *Acta Neuropathol.* 1994;**87**:325–31.

19. Corbett D, Nurse S, Colbourne F. Hypothermic neuroprotection; a global ischemia study using 18- to 20-month old gerbils. *Stroke.* 1997;**28**:2238–43.

20. Welsh F, Harris V. Postischemic hypothermia fails to reduce ischemic injury in gerbil hippocampus. *J Cereb Blood Flow Metab.* 1991;**11**:617–20.

21. Dietrich W, Busto R, Alonso O, et al. Intraischemic but not postischemic brain hypothermia protects chronically following global forebrain ischemia in rats. *J Cereb Blood Flow Metab.* 1993;**13**:541–9.

22. Chopp M, Chen H, Dereski M, et al. Mild hypothermic intervention after graded ischemic stress in rats. *Stroke.* 1991;**22**(1):37–43.

23. Colbourne F, Corbett D. Delayed and prolonged post-ischemic hypothermia is neuroprotective in the gerbil. *Brain Res.* 1994;**654**:265–72.

24. Colbourne F, Li H, Buchan AM. Indefatigable CA1 sector neuroprotection with mild hypothermia induced 6 hours after severe forebrain ischemia in rats. *J Cereb Blood Flow Metab.* 1999;**19**(7):742–9.

25. Colbourne F, Sutherland G, Corbett D. Postischemic hypothermia: a critical appraisal with implications for clinical treatment. *Mol Neurol.* 1997;**14**:171–201.

26. The Hypothermia after Cardiac Arrest Study. Mild therapeutic hypothermia to improve the neurologic outcome after cardiac arrest. *N Engl J Med.* 2002;**346**(8):549–56.

27. Bernard S, Gray T, Buist M, et al. Treatment of comatose survivors of out-of-hospital cardiac arrest with induced hypothermia. *N Engl J Med.* 2002;**346**:557–63.

28. Ginsberg M, Busto R. Rodent models of cerebral ischemia. *Stroke.* 1989;**20**:1627–42.

29. McAuley M. Rodent models of focal ischemia. *Cerebrovasc Brain Metab Rev.* 1995;**7**:153–80.

30. Yanamoto H, Nagata I, Niitsu Y, et al. Prolonged mild hypothermia therapy protects the brain against permanent focal ischemia. *Stroke.* 2001;**32**:232–9.

31. Baker C, Onesti S, Barth K, et al. Hypothermic protection following middle cerebral artery occlusion in the rat. *Surg Neurol.* 1991;**36**:175–80.

32. Baker C, Onesti S, Solomon R. Reduction by delayed hypothermia of cerebral infarction following middle cerebral artery occlusion in the rat: a time-course study. *J Neurosurg.* 1992;**77**:438–44.

33. Onesti S, Baker C, Sun P, et al. Transient hypothermia reduces focal ischemic brain injury in the rat. *Neurosurgery.* 1991;**29**:369–73.

34. Kader A, Brisman MH, Maraire N, et al. The effect of mild hypothermia on permanent focal ischemia in the rat. *Neurosurgery.* 1992;**31**(6):1056–61.

35. Moyer D, Welsh F, Zager E. Spontaneous cerebral hypothermia diminishes focal infarction in rat brain. *Stroke.* 1992;**23**:1812–6.

36. Ridenour T, Warner D, Todd M, et al. Mild hypothermia reduces infarct size resulting from temporary but not permanent focal ischemia in rats. *Stroke.* 1992;**23**:733–8.

37. Xue D, Huang Z, Smith K, et al. Immediate or delayed mild hypothermia prevents focal cerebral infarction. *Brain Res.* 1992;**587**:66–72.

38. Doerfler A, Schwab S, Hoffmann T, et al. Combination of decompressive craniectomy and mild hypothermia ameliorates infarction volume after permanent focal ischemia in rats. *Stroke.* 2001;**32**:2675–81.

39. Chen H, Chopp M, Zhang Z, et al. The effect of hypothermia on transient middle cerebral artery occlusion in the rat. *J Cereb Blood Flow Metab.* 1992;**12**:621–8.

40. Karibe H, Chen H, Zarow G, et al. Delayed induction of mild hypothermia to reduce infarct volume after temporary middle cerebral artery occlusion in rats. *J Neurosurg.* 1994;**80**:112–9.

41. Huh P, Belayev L, Zhao W, et al. Comparative neuroprotective efficacy of prolonged intraischemic and postischemic hypothermia in focal cerebral ischemia. *J Neurosurg*. 2000;**92**:91–9.

42. Maier C, Sun G, Kunis D, et al. Delayed induction and long-term effects of mild hypothermia in focal model of transient cerebral ischemia: neurological outcome and infarct size. *J Neurosurg*. 2001;**94**:90–6.

43. Morikawa E, Ginsberg M, Dietrich W, et al. The significance of brain temperature in focal cerebral ischemia: histopathological consequences of middle cerebral artery occlusion in the rat. *J Cereb Blood Flow Metab*. 1992;**12**:380–9.

44. Schmid-Elsaesser R, Hungerhuber E, Zausinger S, et al. Combination drug therapy and mild hypothermia: a promising treatment strategy for reversible, focal cerebral ischemia. *Stroke*. 1999;**30**:1891–9.

45. Yanamoto H, Nagata I, Nakahara I, et al. Combination of intraischemic and postischemic hypothermia provides potent and persistent neuroprotection against temporary focal ischemia in rats. *Stroke*. 1999;**30**: 2720–6.

46. Zausinger S, Hungerhuber E, Baethmann A, et al. Neurological impairment in rats after transient middle cerebral artery occlusion: a comparative study under various treatment paradigms. *Brain Res*. 2000;**863**:94–105.

47. Corbett D, Hamilton M, Colbourne F. Persistent neuroprotection with prolonged postischemic hypothermia in adult rats subjected to transient middle cerebral artery occlusion. *Exp Neurol*. 2000;**163**:200–6.

48. Smith S, Hall E. Mild pre- and post-traumatic hypothermia attenuates blood-brain barrier damage following controlled cortical impact injury in the rat. *J Neurotrauma*. 1996;**13**:1–9.

49. Jiang J, Lyeth B, Kapasi M, et al. Moderate hypothermia reduces blood-brain barrier disruption following traumatic brain injury in the rat. *Acta Neuropathol*. 1992;**84**:495–500.

50. Dietrich W, Alonso O, Busto R, et al. Post-traumatic brain hypothermia reduces histopathological damage following concussive brain injury in the rat. *Acta Neuropathol*. 1994;**87**:250–8.

51. Clifton G, Jiang J, Lyeth B, et al. Marked protection by moderate hypothermia in after experimental traumatic brain injury. *J Cereb Blood Flow Metab*. 1991;**11**:114–21.

52. Dietrich W, Busto R, Globus M, et al. Brain damage and temperature: cellular and molecular mechanisms. *Adv Neurol*. 1996;**7**:177–94.

53. Mitsuhiro I, Kumagai H, Sugawara Y, et al. Cold spinoplegia and transvertebral cooling pad reduce spinal cord injury during thoracoabdominal aortic surgery. *J Vasc Surg*. 2006;**43**:1257–62.

54. Dimar J, Shields C, Zhang Y, et al. The role of directly applied hypothermia in spinal cord injury. *Spine*. 2000;**25**:2294–302.

55. Inamasu J, Nakamura Y, Ichikizaki K. Induced hypothermia in experimental traumatic spinal cord injury: an update. *J Neurol Sci*. 2002;**209**:55–60.

56. Bernard S, Jones B, Horne M. Clinical trial of induced hypothermia in comatose survivors of out-of-hospital cardiac arrest. *Ann Emerg Med*. 1997;**30**:146–53.

57. Yanagawa Y, Ishihara S, Norio H, et al. Preliminary clinical outcome study of mild resuscitative hypothermia after out-of-hospital cardiopulmonary arrest. *Resuscitation*. 1998;**39**(1–2):61–6.

58. Nagao K, Hayashi N, Kanmatsuse K, et al. Cardiopulmonary cerebral resuscitation using emergency cardiopulmonary bypass, coronary reperfusion therapy and mild hypothermia in patients with cardiac arrest outside the hospital. *J Am Coll Card*. 2000;**36**:776–83.

59. Zeiner A, Holzer M, Sterz F, et al. Mild resuscitative hypothermia to improve neurological outcome after cardiac arrest. A clinical feasibility trial. Hypothermia After Cardiac Arrest (HACA) Study Group. *Stroke*. 2000;**31**(1):86–94.

60. Polderman K, Stertz F, van Zanten A, et al. Induced hypothermia improves neurological outcome in asystolic patients with out-of-hospital cardiac arrest. *Circulation*. 2003;**108**:IV-581 (Abstr).

61. Nolan JP, Morley PT, Vanden Hoek TL, et al. Therapeutic hypothermia after cardiac arrest: an advisory statement by the advanced life support task force of the International Liaison Committee on Resuscitation. *Circulation*. 2003;**108**:118–21.

62. Anonymous. Part 7.5: Postresuscitation support. *Circulation*. 2005;**112**(24_Suppl):IV-84–8.

63. Kammersgaard L, Rasmussen B, Jorgensen H, et al. Feasibility and safety of inducing modest hypothermia in awake patients with acute stroke through surface cooling: a case-control study. The Copenhagen Stroke Study. *Stroke*. 2000;**31**:2251–6.

64. Schwab S, Schwarz S, Aschoff A, et al. Moderate hypothermia and brain temperature in patients with severe middle cerebral artery infarction. *Acta Neurochir Suppl*. 1998;**71**:131–4.

65. Schwab S, Schwartz S, Spranger M, et al. Moderate hypothermia in the treatment of patients with severe middle cerebral artery infarction. *Stroke*. 1998;**29**:2461–6.

66. Schwab S, Georgiadis D, Berrouschot J, et al. Feasibility and safety of moderate hypothermia after massive hemispheric infarction. *Stroke*. 2001;**32**(9):2033–5.

67. Krieger DW, De Georgia MA, Abou-Chebl A, et al. Cooling for acute ischemic brain damage (COOL AID): An open pilot study of induced hypothermia in acute ischemic stroke. *Stroke*. 2001;**32**(8):1847–54.

68. Naritomi H, Shimizu T, Oe H, et al. Mild hypothermia in acute embolic stroke: A pilot study. *J Stroke Cereb Dis*. 1996;**6**:193–6.

69. Shimizu T, Naritomi H, Kakud W, et al. Mild hypothermia is effective for the treatment of acute embolic stroke if induced within 24 hours after onset but not in the latter phase. *J Cereb Blood Flow Metab*. 1997;**17**:42.

70. Georgiadis D, Schwarz S, Kollmar R, et al. Endovascular cooling for moderate hypothermia in patients with acute stroke: first results of a novel approach. *Stroke*. 2001;**32**(11):2550–3.

71. De Georgia M, Krieger D, Abou-Chebl A, et al. Cooling for acute ischemic brain damage (COOL AID). A feasibility trial of endovascular cooling. *Neurology.* 2004;**63**:312–7.

72. Geogiadis D, Schwarz S, Aschoff A, et al. Hemicraniectomy and moderate hypothermia in patients with severe ischemic stroke. *Stroke.* 2002;**33**:1584–8.

73. Georgiadis D, Schwarz S, Aschoff A, et al. Hemicraniectomy and moderate hypothermia in patients with severe ischemic stroke. *Stroke.* 2002;**33**:1584–8.

74. Steiner T, Friede T, Aschoff A, et al. Effect and feasibility of controlled rewarming after moderate hypothermia in stroke patients with malignant infarction. *Stroke.* 2001;**32**:2833–5.

75. Marion D, Obrist W, Carlier P, et al. The use of moderate therapeutic hypothermia for patients with severe head injuries: a preliminary report. *J Neurosurg.* 1993;**79**:354–62.

76. Clifton GL, Allen S, Barrodale P, et al. A Phase-II study of moderate hypothermia in severe brain injury. *J Neurotrauma.* 1993;**10**(3):263–71.

77. Shiozaki T, Sugimoto H, Mamoru T, et al. Effect of mild hypothermia on uncontrollable intracranial hypertension after severe head injury. *J Neurosurg.* 1993;**79**:263–71.

78. Hirayama T, Katayama Y, Kano T, et al. Impact of moderate hypothermia on therapies for intracranial pressure control in severe traumatic brain injury. Paper presented at Intracranial Pressure IX. Tokyo International Symposium, Tokyo, 1994.

79. Marion D, Penrod L, Kelsey S, et al. Treatment of traumatic brain injury with moderate hypothermia. *N Engl J Med.* 1997;**336**:540–6.

80. Shiozaki T, Kato A, Taneda M, et al. Little benefit from mild hypothermia therapy for severely head injured patients with low intracranial pressure. *J Neurosurg.* 1999;**91**:185–91.

81. Aibiki M, Maekawa S, Yokono S. Moderate hypothermia improves imbalance of thromboxane A2 and prostaglandin 12 production after traumatic brain injury in humans. *Crit Care Med.* 2000;**28**:3902–6.

82. Jiang J, Ming-Kun Y, Zhu C. Effect of long term mild hypothermia therapy in patients with severe traumatic brain injury: 1-year follow up review of 87 cases. *J Neurosurg.* 2000;**93**:546–9.

83. Jiang JY, Xu W, Li WP, et al. Effect of long-term mild hypothermia or short-term mild hypothermia on outcome of patients with severe traumatic brain injury. *J Cereb Blood Flow Metab.* 2006;**26**(6):771–6.

84. Clifton G, Miller E, Sung C, et al. Lack of effect of induction of hypothermia after acute brain injury. *N Engl J Med.* 2001;**344**:556–63.

85. Shiozaki T, Hayakata T, Taneda M, et al. A multi-center prospective randomized controlled trial of the efficacy of mild hypothermia for severely head injured patients with low intracranial pressure. *J Neurosurg.* 2001;**94**:50–4.

86. Yan Y, Tang W. Changes of evoked potential and evaluation of mild hypothermia for treatment of severe brain injury. *Chinese J Traunatol.* 2001;**4**:8–13.

87. Polderman K, Joe R, Peerdeman S, et al. Effects of therapeutic hypothermia on intracranial pressure and outcomes in patients with severe head injury. *Intens Care Med.* 2002;**28**:1563–73.

88. Zhi D, Zhang S, Lin X. Study on therapeutic mechanism and clinical effect of mild hypothermia in patients with severe head injury. *Surg Neurol.* 2003;**59**:381–5.

89. Gadkary C, Alderson P, Signori D. Therapeutic hypothermia for head injury (Chochrane Review). *Cochrane Library.* 2003(4).

90. McIntyre LA, Fergusson DA, Hebert PC, et al. Prolonged therapeutic hypothermia after traumatic brain injury in adults: a systematic review. *JAMA.* 2003;**289**(22):2992–9.

91. Henderson W, Dhingra V, Chittock D, et al. Hypothermia in the management of traumatic brain injury. A systematic review and meta-analysis. *Intens Care Med.* 2003;**29**(10):1637–44.

92. Clifton GL, Miller ER, Choi SC, et al. Lack of effect of induction of hypothermia after acute brain injury. *N Engl J Med.* 2001;**344**(8):556–63.

93. MacIntyre NR. Evidence-based ventilator weaning and discontinuation. *Respir Care.* 2004;**49**(7):830–6.

94. Callaway C, Tadler S, Katz L, et al. Feasibility of external cranial cooling during out-of-hospital cardiac arrest. *Resuscitation.* 2002;**52**:159–65.

95. Hachimi-Idrissi S, Corne L, Ebinger G, et al. Mild hypothermia induced by a helmet device: A clinical feasibility study. *Resuscitation.* 2001;**51**:275–81.

96. Dong P, Guan Y, He M, et al. Clinical application of retrograde cerebral perfusion for brain protection during surgery of ascending aortic aneurysm—a report of 50 cases. *J Extra Corpor Technol.* 2002;**34**(2):101–6.

97. Felberg R, Krieger D, Chuang R, et al. Hypothermia after cardiac arrest: feasibility and safety of an external cooling protocol. *Circulation.* 2001;**104**:1799–804.

98. Theard M, Temelhoff R, et al. Convection versus conduction cooling for induction of mild hypothermia during neurovascular procedures in adults. *J Neurosurg Anesthesiol.* 1997;**9**:250–5.

99. Bernard S, Buist M, Monteiro O, et al. Induced hypothermia using large volume, ice-cold intravenous fluid in comatose survivors of out-of-hospital cardiac arrest: a preliminary report. *Resuscitation.* 2003;**56**:9–13.

100. Rijnsburger E, Girbes A, Spijkstra J, et al. Induction of hypothermia using large volumes of ice-cold intravenous fluid: A feasibility study. *Intens Care Med.* 2004;**30** (Suppl 1):S143 (Abstr).

101. Rajek A, Greif R, Sessler DI, et al. Core cooling by central venous infusion of ice-cold (40°C and 200°C) fluid. *Anesthesiology.* 2000;**93**(3):629–37.

102. Kim F, Olsufka M, Carlbom D, et al. Pilot study of rapid infusion of 2 L of 40°C normal saline for induction of mild hypothermia in hospitalized, comatose survivors of out-of-hospital cardiac arrest. *Circulation.* 2005;**112**:715–9.

103. Virkkunen I, Yli-Hankala A, Silfvast T. Induction of therapeutic hypothermia after cardica arrest in prehospital patients using ice-cold Ringer's solution: a pilot study. *Resuscitation.* 2004;**62**:299–302.

104. Sunde K. Therapeutic hypothermia with endovascular cooling. *Scand J Trauma Resusc Emerg Med*. 2004;**12**:23–5.

105. Al-Senani F, Graffagnino C, Grotta J, et al. A prospective, multicenter pilot study to evaluate the feasibility and safety of using the CoolGard system and icy catheter following cardiac arrest. *Resuscitation*. 2004;**62**:143–50.

106. Piepgras A, Roth H, Schurer L, et al. Rapid active internal core cooling for induction of moderate hypothermia in head injury by use of an extracorporeal heat exchanger. *Neurosurgery*. 1998;**42**:317–8.

107. Veerloy J, Heytens L, Veeckmans G, et al. Intracerebral temperature monitoring in severely head injured patients. *Acta Neurochir (Wien)*. 1995;**134**:76–8.

108. Henker R, Brown D, Marion M. Comparison of brain temperature with core (rectal and bladder) temperatures in head injured adults. *Crit Care Med*. 1997;**25**:A73.

109. Stone J, Goodman R, Baker K, et al. Direct intraoperative measurement of human brain temperature. *Neurosurgery*. 1977;**41**:20–4.

110. Saririan K, Nickerson D. Enhancement of murine in vitro antibody formation by hyperthermia. *Cell Immunol*. 1982;**74**:306–12.

111. Reed Rn, Johnson T, Hudson J, et al. The disparity between hypothermic coagulopathy and clotting studies. *J Trauma*. 1992;**33**:465–70.

112. Valeri C, Feingold H, Cassidy G, et al. Hypothermia-induced reversible platelet dysfunction. *Ann Surg*. 1987;**205**:175–81.

113. Rohrer M, Natale A. Effect of hypothermia on the coagulation cascade. *Crit Care Med*. 1992;**20**:1402–5.

5 Analgesia, Sedation, and Paralysis

Wendy C. Ziai, MD, MPH and Rehan Sajjad, MD

The recent evolution of critical care management has emphasized the need to minimize continuous deep sedation and paralysis to improve outcome and decrease length of stay in the intensive care unit (ICU). This recommendation is especially important in patients with neurologic dysfunction.

In this sense, sedative regimens in the neurologic ICU have been well ahead of general ICU doctrine. One of the primary tenets of care of these patients is the capacity to perform repeated neurologic exams as the optimal means of assessing the patients' condition. With respect to bedside evaluation and titration of sedation, the neurologically injured patient may indeed be the most difficult ICU population to manage. Cognitive dysfunction leads to increased fear, restlessness, and agitation from the inability to understand one's predicament. Yet even modest sedation may mask subtle neurologic deterioration, hence the need for close nursing and physician support and observation, and titrating medications as needed without impairing neurologic evaluation.

Patients with traumatic brain injury (TBI) constitute the hallmark brain disorder when discussing difficult sedation paradigms. They are often agitated and at risk of injury to self or the medical staff caring for them. Many TBI patients are also withdrawing from chronic alcohol and drug use, and this must be factored into the choice and duration of sedation.

SEDATION

Indications for Sedation

Before initiation of sedation in any ICU patient, it is imperative to exclude all alternative explanations for agitation, confusion, or sympathetic hyperactivity.

- Hypoxemia or hypercarbia related to decreased respiratory drive or poor airway protection must be detected and treated appropriately.
- Metabolic disturbances, including acidosis, hyponatremia, hypoglycemia, hypercalcemia, hyperamylasemia, hyperammonemia, or hepatic or renal insufficiency may contribute to behavioral changes in critically ill patients.
- Infection is also a frequent trigger of delirium in hospitalized and critically ill patients.
- Cardiac ischemia, hypotension, and associated cerebral hypoperfusion may also contribute to mental status changes, and must be ruled out as a cause of delirium in critically ill neurologic patients.
- Concomitant administration of other psychoactive medications such as antidepressants, anticonvulsants, peptic ulcer prophylactics and interactions with promotility agents, corticosteroids, or even antibiotics and antiretroviral, may adversely affect cognition and behavior.

Goals of sedation in the neurocritical care patient:

- Treat anxiety and pain.
- Facilitate mechanical ventilation.
- Facilitate neurologic exams.
- Avoid deleterious change in intracranial pressure and cerebral perfusion pressure.

Sedation consists of anxiolysis, hypnosis, and amnesia. In neurologically ill patients, an ideal sedation regimen will either preserve the neurologic examination as required for constant clinical monitoring or has the potential to be discontinued with rapid return of an uncompromised examination. Preferred agents therefore should have rapid onset, short duration of action, and a large therapeutic window without significant hemodynamic effects. Periodic interruption of sedative infusions and titration to the lowest effective dose are associated with shorter duration on mechanical ventilation, fewer tracheostomies, and shortened ICU stay.

Sedation Assessment

SUBJECTIVE ASSESSMENT OF SEDATION AND AGITATION

Frequent assessment of the degree of sedation or agitation may facilitate the titration of sedatives to predetermined endpoints. An ideal sedation scale should provide data that are simple to compute and record, accurately describe the degree of sedation or agitation within well defined categories, guide the titration of therapy, and have validity and reliability in ICU patients (see Fig. 5.1).

A sedation goal or endpoint should be established and regularly redefined for each patient. Regular assessment and response to therapy should be systematically documented. The use of a validated sedation assessment scale (SAS, MAAS, or VICS) is recommended (Table 5.1). Objective measures of sedation using, for example, a Bispectral Index (BIS) monitor have not been completely evaluated and are not yet proven useful in the ICU.

PATIENT CLASSIFICATION SEDATION GOAL

Acutely ill (weaning not a goal): 5–9
Ventilated patient being weaned: 7–10
Chronic ventilated patient: 6–9 (weaning not a goal)
Nonventilated patient: 7–9

PHARMACOLOGY OF SELECTED SEDATIVES

Benzodiazepines and propofol are currently the sedative agents most commonly administered in the Neuro ICU.

Benzodiazepines

- Mechanism of action: Interacts at specific binding sites on neuronal γ-aminobutyric acid (GABA) receptors.
- Sedative, hypnotic, but lacks intrinsic analgesic benefits.

- Potentiates effects of narcotics.
- Induces anterograde amnesia, not retrograde.
- CNS advantages: Anticonvulsant, decreases cerebral blood flow (CBF), decreases cerebral metabolic rate of oxygen demand ($CMRo_2$), no change in intracranial pressure (ICP), central muscle relaxation.
- Reversible with flumazenil (0.2–1.0 mg; maximum dose 3 mg), a benzodiazepine (BZ) antagonist which acts at the BZ binding site on the GABA receptor with
  - ▸ Onset of action: 5 minutes
  - ▸ Elimination half-life: 60 minutes
  - ▸ Duration of action: 0.5–3.5 hours
  - ▸ May require continuous infusion or alternative airway support
  - ▸ Precipitates withdrawal in benzodiazepine-dependent patients
  - ▸ May precipitate seizures or status epilepticus
  - ▸ With prolonged use: Tachyphylaxis, reversible encephalopathy
  - ▸ Withdrawal syndrome, possible seizures on acute cessation
  - ▸ Paradoxical reactions causing increased agitation and delirium in patients with preexisting CNS pathology can occur due to altered sensory perception
  - ▸ Decrease tidal volume, compensated by increase in respiratory rate
  - ▸ Blunts response to hypoxia and hypercarbia

MIDAZOLAM (VERSED)

- Drug of choice for acute and short-term sedation; 3–4 times more potent than diazepam, shortest half life of all BZs, no significant active metabolites, water soluble.
- Highly lipophilic; therefore, crosses the blood–brain barrier quickly, resulting in a rapid onset of action, 2–5 minutes
- Prescribed dose for maintenance of sedation in critically ill adult patients: 2–5 mg/h (0.02–0.1 mg/kg per hour)
- Short duration of action (2–6 hours) due to rapid metabolism by the liver to an inactive metabolite
  - ▸ Distribution half-life: 7–10 minutes
  - ▸ Elimination half-life: 2–2.5 hours
- Half-life (time for drug plasma concentration to decrease by 50% after cessation of a continuous infusion) depends on infusion duration.

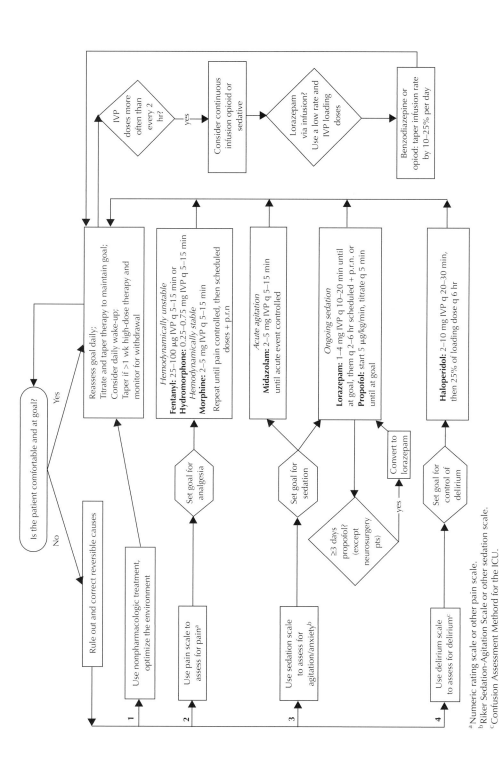

Figure 5.1. Algorithm for the sedation and analgesia of mechanically ventilated patients. This algorithm is a general guideline for the use of analgesics and sedatives. Refer to the text for clinical and pharmacologic issues that dictate optimal drug selection, recommended assessment scales, and precautions for patient monitoring. Doses are approximate for a 70-kg adult. IVP = intravenous push.

[a]Numeric rating scale or other pain scale.
[b]Riker Sedation–Agitation Scale or other sedation scale.
[c]Confusion Assessment Method for the ICU.

Is the patient comfortable and at goal?

No

Yes

Rule out and correct reversible causes

Reassess goal daily;
Titrate and taper therapy to maintain goal;
Consider daily wake-up;
Taper if >1 wk high-dose therapy and monitor for withdrawal

1 Use nonpharmacologic treatment, optimize the environment

Set goal for analgesia

Hemodynamically unstable
Fentanyl: 25–100 µg IVP q 5–15 min or
Hydromorphone: 0.25–0.75 mg IVP q 5–15 min
Hemodynamically stable
Morphine: 2–5 mg IVP q 5–15 min
Repeat until pain controlled, then scheduled doses + p.r.n

2 Use pain scale to assess for pain[a]

Acute agitation
Midazolam: 2–5 mg IVP q 5–15 min until acute event controlled

Set goal for sedation

Ongoing sedation
Lorazepam: 1–4 mg IVP q 10–20 min until at goal, them q 2–6 hr scheduled + p.r.n. or
Propofol: start 5 µg/kg/min, titrate q 5 min until at goal

≥3 days propofol? (except neurosurgery pts)

yes

Convert to lorazepam

3 Use sedation scale to assess for agitation/anxiety[b]

Set goal for control of delirium

Haloperidol: 2–10 mg IVP q 20–30 min, then 25% of loading dose q 6 hr

4 Use delirium scale to assess to delirium[c]

IVP doses more often than every 2 hr?

yes

Consider continuous infusion opioid or sedative

Lorazepam via infusion?
Use a low rate and IVP loading doses

Benzodiazepine or opiod: taper infusion rate by 10–25% per day

Table 5.1. Sedation assessment scales

Score	Description	Definition
Riker Sedation–Agitation Scale (SAS)		
7	Dangerous agitation	Pulling at endotracheal tube (ETT); trying to remove catheters; climbing over bed rail; striking at staff; thrashing side-to-side.
6	Very agitated	Does not calm despite frequent verbal reminding of limits; requires physical restraints, biting ETT.
5	Agitated	Anxious or mildly agitated; attempts to sit up; calms down to verbal instructions.
4	Calm and cooperative	Calm, awakens easily; follows commands.
3	Sedated	Difficult to arouse; awakens to verbal stimuli or gentle shaking but drifts off again; follows simple commands
2	Very sedated	Arouses to physical stimuli but does not communicate or follow commands; may move spontaneously.
1	Unarousable	Minimal or no response to noxious stimuli; does not communicate or follow commands.
Motor Activity Assessment Scale (MAAS)		
6	Dangerously agitated	No external stimulus is required to elicit movement and patient is uncooperative, pulling at tubes or catheters or thrashing side to side or striking at staff or trying to climb out of bed and does not calm down when asked.
5	Agitated	No external stimulus is required to elicit movement and attempting to sit up or moves limbs out of bed and does not consistently follow commands (e.g., will lie down when asked but soon reverts back to attempts to sit up or move limbs out of bed).
4	Restless and cooperative	No external stimulus is required to elicit movement and patient is picking at sheets or tubes or uncovering self and follows commands.
3	Calm and cooperative	No external stimulus is required to elicit movement and patient is adjusting sheets or clothes purposefully and follows commands.
2	Responsive to touch or name	Opens eyes or raises eyebrows or turns head toward stimulus or moves limbs when touched or name is loudly spoken.
1	Responsive only to noxious stimulus	Opens eyes or raises eyebrows or turns head toward stimulus or moves limbs with noxious stimulus.
0	Unresponsive	Does not move with noxious stimulus.

Ramsay Scale

1 Awake patient anxious and agitated or restless or both.
2 Patient cooperative, oriented and tranquil.
3 Patient responds to commands only.

Score	Description	Definition
4	Asleep; a brisk response to a light glabellar tap or loud auditory stimulus.	
5	A sluggish response to a light glabellar tap or loud auditory stimulus.	
6	No response to a light glabellar tap or loud auditory stimulus.	

AVRIPAS – Revised Sedation Scale

Agitation Alertness

1	Unresponsive to command/1 difficult to arouse, eyes remain closed physical stimulation.	
2	Appropriate response to physical 2 mostly sleeping, eyes closed stimuli/calm.	
3	Mild anxiety/delirium/agitation 3 dozing intermittently, arouses easily (calms easily).	
4	Moderate anxiety/delirium/agitation 4 awake, calm.	
5	Severe anxiety/delirium/agitation 5 wide awake, hyperalert.	

Respiration

1	Intubated, no spontaneous effort.	
2	Respirations even, synchronized with ventilator.	
3	Mild dyspnea/tachypnea; occasional asynchrony.	
4	Frequent dyspnea/tachypnea; ventilator asynchrony.	
5	Sustained, severe dyspnea/tachypnea.	

- Special precautions:
  - Elderly and patients with liver disease: Increased volume of distribution and decreased elimination
  - Increased effect in patients with renal failure due to increase in active unbound portion
- Repeated doses or continuous IV can lead to prolonged sedation because of sequestration in fat stores although respiratory and cardiovascular depression are minimal with continuous infusion due to lower peak plasma concentration than with bolus dosing.

LORAZEPAM (ATIVAN)
- Five to six times more potent than Diazepam; most potent BZ in ICU

- Slower onset of action, 5–10 minutes due to lower lipid solubility; therefore, less appealing for acute agitation
- Prescribed dose: 0.044 mg/kg every 2–4 hours; infusion rates up to 10 mg/h safe and effective in ICU patients
- Greater water solubility which prolongs its serum half-life
  - Distribution half-life: 3–10 minutes
  - Context sensitive half-life: 12–14 hours
  - Elimination half-life: 10–20 hours
- No active metabolite; therefore resistant to drug interactions except valproic acid, which inhibits lorazepam metabolism
- Solvent used (propylene glycol) may cause acute but reversible renal tubular necrosis.

DIAZEPAM (VALIUM)

- Rapid onset, 2–5 minutes, but long-acting lipophilic benzodiazepine
- Prescribed dose: 0.1–0.2 mg/kg every 2–4 hours
- Distribution half life: 50–120 minutes
- Elimination half-life: 20–40 hours. Active metabolite, desmethyl-diazepam, with elimination half-life of 96 hours, results in accumulation of both the parent diazepam and metabolite with repeated doses; further converted to oxazepam ($t_{1/2}$ 10 hours).
- Limited use in ICU due to potent active metabolites that depend on renal excretion
- Resedation occurs after reversal with flumazenil because of its long duration of action.
- Formulated in sterile fat emulsion (previously in propylene glycol) which has reduced complications (thrombophlebitis, thrombosis, metabolic acidosis)
- Minimal cardiovascular depressant effects on blood pressure and respiratory drive

Synergistic Sedation Regimens with Benzodiazepines

- Haloperidol + BZ
  - Decreases dose of BZ required to produce sedation; therefore less potential for impaired respiratory drive.
  - Decreased risk of extrapyramidal symptoms caused by haloperidol
- Propofol + BZ
  - Better homodynamic stability and faster weaning from ventilator with lower total doses of both drugs

PROPOFOL (2,6-DIISOPROPYL PHENOL)

- Mechanism of action: Enhances γ-aminobutyric acid transmission; antagonist at N-methyl-D-aspartate receptors.
- Pure sedative–hypnotic, little analgesic action, some antegrade amnesia.
- Useful for sedation in neuro-intensive care due to titratability facilitating serial neurologic exams.
- Also used to treat status epilepticus and raised intracranial pressure.
- No intrinsic anticonvulsant property.
- Implicated as a cause of peri-operative seizures and seizure like events: Nonictal myoclonus,

pseudoseizures; potential for proconvulsant activity at low doses although not common.
- Usual dosage in ICU: 1–3 mg/kg per hour.
- CNS: Decreases CBF, $CMRo_2$, ICP, and potentially cerebral perfusion pressure (CPP); may impair autoregulation in traumatic brain injured patients; pressors often required to maintain mean arterial pressure (MAP) and CPP.
- Laboratory evidence of neuroprotection has not been substantiated in human studies
- CVS: Decreases MAP, systemic vascular resistance (SVR), central venous pressure (CVP), cardiac output (CO), and heart rate (HR).
- In general sedative infusion doses of propofol cause minimal hemodynamic alteration without compromising CPP.
- Produces general anesthesia at induction dose of 2 mg/kg.
- Onset of action: 1–2 minutes.
- Ultra-short-acting due to:
  - Highly lipophilic structure and extensive tissue redistribution
  - Extrahepatic metabolism
- After cessation of continuous infusion, recovery from unconsciousness to awake, responsive state occurs within 10–15 minutes without withdrawal or tolerance; more reliable weaning from mechanical ventilation than midazolam infusion.
- Predictable kinetics even in presence of hepatic and renal failure
- Three half-lives:
  - Distribution half-life: 2–4 minutes
  - Elimination half-life: 30–60 minutes
  - Terminal half-life, during which propofol is eliminated from tissue fat, 300–700 minutes
- Unfavorable characteristics:
  - *Hypotension,* especially in hypovolemic patients; however, better cardiovascular stability compared with barbiturate therapy
  - *Respiratory depressant;* infusions increase respiratory rate and reduce ventilation response to hypercarbia; impair upper airway reflexes; bronchodilator effects in patients with reactive airways disease; increases CO_2 production – requires increased minute ventilation to maintain normal acid–base status
  - *Hypertriglyceridemia and pancreatitis* because it is mixed as an emulsion in a phospholipid vehicle

▶ Potential for *infection and drug incompatibility* requiring a dedicated IV catheter

▶ *Pain with peripheral injection* necessitating central access; consider lidocaine before administration

▶ Tonic–clonic *seizures* when abruptly stopped after days of infusion

▶ Rarely, urine, hair, and nail beds turn green

PROPOFOL INFUSION SYNDROME (PRIS)

■ Syndrome of metabolic acidosis, rhabdomyolysis, elevated creatine kinase, renal failure, myocardial failure, cardiac arrhythmias, and hyperlipidemia

■ Pathogenesis related to propofol-induced blockade of mitochondrial fatty oxidation and accumulation of free fatty acids with proarrhythmic effects

■ Most cases reported in children, resulting in part from reduced energy stores and higher sympathetic tone

■ Approximately 20 adult cases reported, usually in setting of head injury or other brain injury including status epilepticus

■ Recommended to avoid prolonged propofol infusion (>18 hours) at rates >5 mg/kg per hour in adults

■ Patients on long-term propofol infusions (>72 hours) should be monitored for hypertriglyceridemia.

α_2-Agonists

DEXMEDETOMIDINE (PRECEDEX)

■ Mechanism of action: Highly selective α_2-adrenergic agonist, decreases sympathetic activity

■ Unique properties: Sedative, analgesic, not a respiratory depressant or amnestic agent, easy arousability

■ Recommended for short term sedation <24 hours

■ Shown to provide adequate sedation without affecting respiratory drive and facilitates neurologic exams in patients with neurosurgical conditions without clinically significant changes in ICP or CPP

■ Decrease in ICP reported in experimental studies and may be due to α_2-receptor-induced arteriolar vasoconstriction causing decreased CBV

■ Usual dosage: Load at 0.1 µg/kg IV for 10 minutes, then 0.2–0.7 µg/kg per hour; avoid bolus dose to minimize hypotension

■ Elimination half-life: 2 hours; duration of action: 2–6 hours

■ Route of elimination: 95% renal

■ Side effects: Hypotension and bradycardia, agitation

■ Multicenter studies revealed that dexmedetomidine recipients required no additional supplements for sedation; however, due to lack of amnestic properties, benzodiazepines and narcotics may be required to improve amnesia and analgesia.

CLONIDINE (CATAPRES)

■ Mechanism of action: Central α_2-agonist

■ Uses: Sedative, analgesic, hypertension, blunt manifestations of substance abuse withdrawal, postoperative shivering

■ CNS: Decrease CBF; decrease CPP, no clear effect on $CMRo_2$

■ Distribution half-life: 6–14 minutes

■ Elimination half-life: 7–10 hours

■ Side effects: Sedation, dry mouth, rebound HTN approximately 18 hours after clonidine is discontinued, decrease MAP

■ Usual dose: 0.1 mg q8–24h; up to 0.6 mg/day; duration of action: 12–48 hours

■ Studied as adjuvant to morphine PCA: bolus of clonidine at end of operation improved analgesia for first 12 hours postoperatively and addition of clonidine to PCA (20 µg; 5 minutes LI) significantly reduced nausea and vomiting in females undergoing lower abdominal surgery

Neuroleptics

HALOPERIDOL (BUTYROPHENONE)

■ Mechanism of action: Central postsynaptic dopamine antagonist

■ Not recommended as first-line drug for sedation

■ Sedative and antipsychotic; no analgesic or amnestic properties

■ Usual dose (for delirium): 1–5 mg increments IV, q hourly; infusions of approximately 300 mg/24 h shown to provide sedation without respiratory depression

■ Distribution half-life: 5–17 minutes

■ Elimination half-life: 10–19 hours

■ Metabolized by liver and excreted by kidneys

■ Contraindication: Allergy to droperidol, Parkinson's disease, pregnancy, seizure (decreases seizure threshold)

- Complications:
  - Extrapyramidal symptoms (acute dystonic reaction) treated with diphenhydramine
  - Hypotension due to α blocking property
  - Neuroleptic malignant syndrome (NMS)
    - Symptoms and signs: Hyperthermia, muscle rigidity, autonomic instability, increased CPK, granulocytosis, hyperglycemia
    - Pathophysiology: Dysautonomia due to dopamine antagonism
    - Treatment: Dantrolene and/or bromocriptine
- Prolongation of QT interval – potentially lethal torsades de pointes

DROPERIDOL (INAPSINE)

- Mechanism of action: Central postsynaptic dopamine antagonist
- Like haloperidol, useful for decreasing anxiety associated with psychosis, but less effective for situational anxiety; antiemetic effect
- Usual sedative dose: 0.625–2.5 mg IV q4–24 h; up to 5 mg in 24 hours
- Duration of action: 2–12 hours
- Side effects: Extrapyramidal reactions, hypotension, dysphoria, akathisia, depressed carotid body drive to ventilate

Other Sedatives

ETOMIDATE

- Mechanism of action: Pharmacologically active component is dextroisomer, which produces sedation through stimulation of GABA receptor
- Nonanalgesic sedative and drug of choice for emergent intubation
- Usual dose for induction of anesthesia: 0.3 mg/kg
- Elimination half-life: Approximately 30 minutes
- Metabolized by liver to inactive carboxylic acid ester
- CNS: Decreases CBF, decreases $CMRO_2$, decreases ICP, increases CPP
- CVS: No hypotension, unchanged CO and HR; therefore useful in patients with limited cardiovascular reserve
- Side effects: Nausea, vomiting, thrombophlebitis (due to propylene glycol formulation), generalized seizures, myoclonus, adrenal suppression in repeated doses, increase IOP
- Contraindications: Acute intermittent porphyria, seizures
- Prolonged infusions for sedation in critically ill patients associated with increased mortality,

likely resulting from suppression of adrenal steroid synthesis

KETAMINE

- Mechanism of action: Phencyclidine (angel dust) derivative; interacts with the following receptors: N-methyl-D-aspartate (NMDA), opioid, monoaminergic, and muscarinic and voltage-sensitive calcium channels and sodium channels
- Short-acting IV anesthetic, hypnotic, profound amnestic, excellent analgesic
- Stimulates the limbic system, such as the hippocampus and suppresses thalamocortical region, leading to a dissociative state.
- Most useful in ICU to facilitate brief, but painful procedures
- Usual dose: sub anesthetic: 0.2–0.5 mg/kg IV or 1.5–2.0 mg/kg IM; induction of anesthesia: 1–2 mg/kg IV or 5–10 mg/kg IM
- Elimination half-life: 2–3 hours
- Metabolized by hepatic microsomal enzymes to active metabolite norketamine, then hydrolyzed to inactive glucuronide metabolite
- Beneficial effects of ketamine include patients ability to maintain spontaneous ventilation, bronchodilation and cardiovascular stimulation by activation of the sympathetic nervous system; potentially useful for induction of anesthesia in patients with acute hypovolemia and asthma
- CNS: Increase CBF, increase CMRO2, increase ICP, and decrease CPP
- CVS: Increase MAP, increase SVR, and increase HR, unchanged CO
- Contraindication: Increase ICP, seizure disorder, ischemic heart disease
- Side effects: Epileptogenic, nightmares and hallucination (attenuated by cotreatment with benzodiazepines), delirium, excessive salivation and lacrimation (limited by use of anticholinergic – glycopyrrolate), increased ICP; rapid tolerance

BARBITURATES

- Mechanism of action: Interacts at specific barbiturate receptor on neuronal GABA receptor complex; also acts on chloride channels at high concentrations
- Generally not used for sedation in ICU patients
- Primary uses in the ICU: treatment of seizures and intractable intracranial hypertension
- Progressive increase in dose results in sedation, hypnosis, and then anesthesia

- Thiopental (Pentothal):
  - Usual dose: Induction of anesthesia – thiopental: 5 mg/kg IV; rapid short-term treatment for increased ICP: 25–50 mg IV, while awaiting effect of longer acting agents; significant hypotension may occur
  - Elimination half-life: 5–12 hours, but duration of action short (after single bolus injection) due to rapid diffusion from brain back to inactive peripheral sites
- Phenobarbitol (Luminal):
  - Usual dose (sedation): Phenobarbital: 1–3 mg/kg IV or IM; up to 200 mg in 24 hours
  - Duration of action: 10–24 hours (elimination may take up to 120 hours)
- Pentobarbital (Nembutal):
  - Usual dose (drug-induced coma): Pentobarbital: 10 mg/kg IV loading dose, followed by infusion of 1–2 mg/kg per hour; thiopental (less often used for this indication): 5–11 mg/kg loading dose, followed by infusion of 4–6 mg/kg per hour
  - Metabolism: Hepatic; enzyme inducer; affects metabolism of other drugs
  - CNS: Decreases CBF, decreases $CMRo_2$, decreases ICP, decreases CPP
  - CVS: Decreases MAP, decreases SVR, tachycardia in hypovolemic patients with hypotension
  - Side effects: Central respiratory depression, apnea, hyper salivation, bronchospasm, laryngeal spasm, renal artery constriction and decreased urine output; potential lethal withdrawal syndrome; allergic reaction in 2%; depression of gastrointestinal motility; cardiac contractility and white blood cell function
  - Patients in barbiturate coma require mechanical ventilation, vasoactive agents, nasogastric decompression often with parenteral nutrition, and surveillance cultures due to high risk of infection.
  - EEG monitoring recommended to ensure optimal dosing.

DIPHENHYDRAMINE (BENADRYL)
- Mechanism of action: First-generation H-1 receptor antagonist
- Extensive hepatic metabolism
- Clinical ICU uses: Sedation (insomnia), treatment for haloperidol/droperidol-induced extrapyramidal reactions, allergic dermatitis (pruritis, urticaria)

- Usual sedative dose: 25–50 mg IV q6–8 h; up to 400 mg in 24 hours
- Duration of action: 6–24 hours
- Side effects: Overdose can produce flushed face, fever, mydriasis, and seizures

Recommendations:

- Midazolam or diazepam should be used for rapid sedation of acutely agitated patients.
- Propofol is the preferred sedative when rapid awakening (e.g., for neurologic assessment or extubation) is important.
- Midazolam is recommended for short-term use only, as it produces unpredictable awakening and time to extubation when infusions continue longer than 48–72 hours.
- Lorazepam is recommended for the sedation of most patients via intermittent IV administration or continuous infusion.
- The titration of the sedative dose to a defined endpoint is recommended with systematic tapering of the dose or daily interruption with retitration to minimize prolonged sedative effects.
- Triglyceride concentrations should be monitored after 2 days of propofol infusion, and total caloric intake from lipids should be included in the nutrition support prescription.
- The use of sedation guidelines, an algorithm, or a protocol is recommended.

DELIRIUM

As many as 80% of ICU patients have delirium, characterized by an acutely changing or fluctuating mental status, inattention, disorganized thinking, and an altered level of consciousness that may or may not be accompanied by agitation.

Confusion Assessment Method for the Diagnosis of Delirium in the ICU (Cam-Icu)

FEATURE ASSESSMENT VARIABLES
1. Acute onset of mental status changes or fluctuating course
2. Inattention
3. Disorganized thinking

For those still on the ventilator, can the patient answer the following four questions correctly?

1. Will a stone float on water?
2. Are there fish in the sea?

3. Does one pound weigh more than two pounds?
4. Can you use a hammer to pound a nail?

Was the patient able to follow questions and commands throughout the assessment?

1. "Are you having any unclear thinking?"
2. "Hold up this many fingers." (Examiner holds two fingers in front of patient.)
3. "Now do the same thing with the other hand." (Not repeating the number of fingers)
4. Altered level of consciousness (any level of consciousness other than alert, e.g., vigilant, lethargic, stupor, or coma)

Patients are diagnosed with delirium if they have both Features 1 and 2 and either
Feature 3 or 4.

Treatment of Delirium

Haloperidol is the preferred agent for the treatment of delirium in critically ill patients. Patients should be monitored for electrocardiographic changes (QT interval prolongation and arrhythmias) when receiving haloperidol.

SLEEP

Sleep is believed to be important to recover from an illness. Sleep deprivation may impair tissue repair and overall cellular immune function Similar to pain assessment, the patient's own report is the best measure of sleep adequacy.

Nonpharmacologic Strategies

Titrating environmental stimulation:

- *Noise* in critical care settings is an environmental hazard that disrupts sleep.
- *Lighting* mimicking the 24- hour day helps patients achieve normal sleep patterns, so bright lights should be avoided at night.
- *Relaxation.* Head-to-toe relaxation may benefit anxious critically ill patients who can follow directions. Relaxation will lead to a parasympathetic response and a decrease in respiratory rate, heart rate, jaw tension, and blood pressure. Relaxation techniques include deep breathing followed by the sequential relaxation of each muscle group.

- *Music therapy.* Music therapy relaxes patients and decreases their pain. When selecting music, a patient's personal preference should be considered.
- *Massage.* Back massage is an alternative or adjunct to pharmacologic therapy in critically ill patients.
- Sleep occurs best below 35 decibels.
- *Earplugs* effectively decreased noise and increased REM sleep.

Pharmacologic Therapy to Promote Sleep

Sleep promotion should include optimization of the environment and nonpharmacologic methods to promote relaxation with adjunctive use of hypnotics.

ANALGESIA

Pain control in the neurocritical care unit is important in the management of postoperative neurosurgical conditions and critical conditions where concern that opioids will adversely affect the neurologic examination may lead to inadequate treatment. After craniotomy, moderate to severe pain occurs in 60–84% of patients. Frontal craniotomy appears to be associated with lower pain scores and posterior fossa procedures, with the greatest percentage of patients reporting moderate and severe pain (85%) and the highest use of analgesics. Procedures involving greater degrees of muscle and tissue damage are associated with a higher incidence of severe pain. This includes subtemporal and suboccipital approaches.

Pain Assessment

Studies of pain in the critically ill indicate the importance of systematic and consistent assessment and documentation. The most reliable and valid indicator of pain is the patient's self-report. The location, characteristics, aggravating and alleviating factors, and intensity of pain should be evaluated.

Pain assessment and response to therapy should be performed regularly by using a scale appropriate to patient population. It should also be systematically documented. The level of pain reported by the patient must be considered the current standard for assessment of pain and response to analgesia whenever possible. Use of the numeric rating scale (NRS) is recommended to assess pain.

Patients who cannot communicate should be assessed through subjective observation of pain-related behaviors (movement, facial expression) and physiologic indicators (heart rate, blood pressure, and respiratory rate) and the change in these parameters after analgesic therapy.

Assessment of pain intensity may be performed with unidimensional tools, such as a verbal rating scale (VRS), visual analogue scale (VAS), and numeric rating scale (NRS).

- VAS comprises a 10-cm horizontal line with descriptive phrases at either end, from "no pain" to "severe pain" or "worst pain ever." Variations include vertical divisions or numeric markings.
- NRS is a 0–10-point scale and patients choose a number that describes the pain, with 10 representing the worst pain.
- Multidimensional tools, such as the McGill Pain Questionnaire (MPQ) and the Wisconsin Brief Pain Questionnaire (BPQ), measure pain intensity and the sensory, affective, and behavioral components of that pain but take longer to administer and may not be practical for the ICU environment
- Wong–Baker Faces Pain Rating Scale.

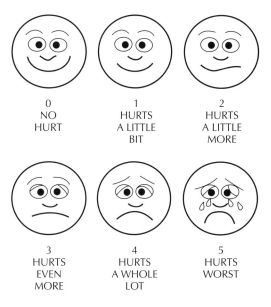

| 0 NO HURT | 1 HURTS A LITTLE BIT | 2 HURTS A LITTLE MORE |
| 3 HURTS EVEN MORE | 4 HURTS A WHOLE LOT | 5 HURTS WORST |

- Family members or other surrogates have been evaluated for their ability to assess the amount of pain experienced by noncommunicative ICU patients. While surrogates could estimate the presence or absence of pain in 73.5% of patients, they less accurately described the degree of pain (53%).

The most appropriate pain assessment tool will depend on the patient involved, his/her ability to communicate, and the caregiver's skill in interpreting pain behaviors or physiologic indicators.

Analgesic Agents

While codeine is widely used for post neurosurgical pain control, its association with moderate to severe pain in three-quarters of patients argues for more potent analgesics after craniotomy. A pediatric study of patient-controlled analgesia (PCA) with fentanyl and midazolam for postoperative neurosurgical pain demonstrated efficacy in controlling both pain and anxiety in this subset of patients without major side effects. Comparison of morphine PCA, tramadol PCA and intramuscular codeine in adults after craniotomy reported better analgesia and reduced nausea and vomiting with morphine PCA. The addition of scheduled atypical analgesics such as cyclo-oxygenase-2 (COX-2) inhibitors to narcotic regimens for postoperative craniotomy patients has been associated with better pain control, decreased narcotic use, earlier walking, and lower total hospitalization costs. Other approaches to pain control include cranial nerve block with agents such as bupivacaine (with or without adrenalin) or ropivacaine which have been shown to improve pain assessment, reduce requirement for morphine, and reduce nausea and vomiting after supratentorial craniotomy.

For management of non–surgery-related pain in acute neurologic conditions, reasonable options include acetaminophen, codeine, oxycodone, and low-dose fentanyl. The ability to monitor the patient is of prime importance when narcotics are used both to prevent opioid-related complications and unnecessary neuroimaging for medication induced changes in mental status.

OPIATES

- Mechanism of action: Interact at opioid μ-receptors
- Primarily analgesic, sedative, anxiolytic but no appreciable amnesia
- CNS: Decreases CBF, $CMRo_2$, ICP, Centrally mediated thoracoabdominal (wooden chest syndrome)/laryngeal/pharyngeal, muscle rigidity attributed to rapid administration, attenuated by neuromuscular blockers
- CVS: Decreases MAP due to venodilation, decrease sympathetic tone and histamine release,

dose-dependent vagal-mediated bradycardia attenuated by atropine

■ Respiratory: Depresses ventilation; hence, any increase in $PaCO_2$ can lead to increase CBF and ICP. Exercise caution in nonmechanically ventilated patients with impaired intracranial pressure dynamics.

■ Other effects: Delayed gastric emptying, ileus, sphincter of Odi spasm, urinary retention

■ Metabolized by the liver, excreted renally

■ Reversible with use of a pure opioid antagonist, naloxone, and agonist-antagonist, nalbuphine

  ▸ Naloxone: Onset time 1–2 minutes, elimination half-life 60 minutes, short duration of action results to renarcotization which is be prevented by repeated boluses. Pain, hypertension, dysrhythmias, pulmonary edema, cardiac arrest or withdrawal in opioid-dependent patients are some complications to be kept in mind.

FENTANYL (SUBLIMAZE)

■ A synthetic opiate with 75–100 times the potency of morphine

■ Single dose of fentanyl has more rapid onset and shorter duration than morphine because of its greater solubility and rapid redistribution.

■ With continuous infusion, fentanyl accumulates in fat stores, resulting in markedly prolonged duration.

■ The elimination half-life of fentanyl, 5 hours, is longer than that of morphine, 4 hours, due to its large volume of distribution, 4 L/kg.

■ Does not cause histamine release like morphine; hence, less hemodynamic instability, making it suitable in patients in shock.

■ Metabolized to norfentanyl in liver, which has its own analgesic power

■ Usual dose: PCA: demand: 10–50 μg; lockout interval (LI): 5–10 minutes; basal rate: ≤50 μg/h

■ Usual dose: Sedation: 25–50 μg/hf with or without bolus; up to 200–300 μg/h

■ Duration of action: 30–60 minutes (increases with higher cumulative doses)

■ Sufentanil: Analogue of fentanyl with 5–10 times the potency of fentanyl

  ▸ Not often used for PCA. Dose: demand: 4–6 μg; LI: 5–10 minutes; basal rate: ≤5 μg/h

REMIFENTANIL (ULTIVA)

■ Selective μ-receptor agonist; analgesic potency similar to fentanyl

■ Rapid clearance because it is rapidly hydrolyzed by the nonspecific esterases in tissue and blood, does not accumulate and rapid recovery after discontinuation.

■ Not a good analgesic for postoperative use, but used commonly for analgesia for craniotomy due to these properties.

■ Usual dose (sedation): Bolus 0.5–1.0 μg/kg IV; infusion: 0.025–0.2 μg/kg per minute

■ Duration of action: 5–10 minutes after discontinuation of infusion

MORPHINE SULFATE

■ Least lipid solubility causing slow CNS entry

■ Has a long distribution half-life, 4–11 minutes, because it is relatively water soluble

■ Metabolized by conjugation with glucuronic acid in hepatic and extrahepatic sites, especially kidneys. Morphine 6-glucuronide, a hepatic metabolite excreted in the urine, can accumulate in renal failure.

■ Releases histamine

■ Usual dose (analgesia): 2–10 mg IV q4h; PCA: demand: 1–2 mg; LI: 5–10 minutes; basal rate: ≤0.5 mg/h

■ Duration of action: 4–12 hours

HYDROMORPHONE (DILAUDID)

■ Morphine derivative

■ 6–8 times the potency of morphine (1.3 mg of dilaudid = 10 mg IM morphine)

■ Metabolized as inactive glucuronide; no active metabolite; therefore good choice for patients with renal dysfunction.

■ Used for moderate-to-severe pain in opioid-tolerant patients who require larger than usual doses of opioids to provide adequate pain relief; especially useful in spinal surgery patients with history of narcotic use.

■ Available in IV, IM, and SC preparations.

■ Usual PCA dose: demand: 0.20–0.5 mg; LI: 5–10 minutes; basal infusion rate: ≤0.4 mg/h

OXYCODONE (PERCOCET, PERCODAN)

■ Mechanism of action: Semisynthetic narcotic with multiple actions qualitatively similar to those of morphine

■ Used for moderate to moderately severe postoperative pain

■ Usual dose: 10–30 mg PO q4–6 h

- Side effects: Constipation, dry mouth, confusion, sedation, light-headedness, respiratory depression, nausea, vomiting, headache, sweating

CODEINE (EMPIRIN #2,3,4; TYLENOL #2,3,4)

- Mechanism of action: acts on μ-opiate receptors predominantly via its metabolite morphine.
- Metabolized by the highly polymorphic enzyme cytochrome P450 (CYP)2D6. Patients with different CYP2D6 genotypes may respond differently in terms of pain relief and adverse events (poor metabolizers and ultrafast metabolizers).
- Available alone or in combination with aspirin or acetaminophen
- Usual dose: 15–60 mg PO/IM q4 h
- Compared to morphine, codeine produces less analgesia, sedation, and respiratory depression

TRAMADOL (ULTRAM)

- Synthetic opioid; aminocyclohexanol group
- Opioid mechanism: Acts centrally; weak opioid receptor agonist
- Binding to μ-receptor 6000-fold less than morphine; weaker affinity for δ- and κ-receptors
- Nonopioid mechanism: Inhibits central uptake of monoamines: norepinephrine and serotonin
- Metabolized by O- and N-demethylation; O-demethyltramadol is active metabolite.
- Slow metabolism in humans with large amount of unchanged renal excretion
- High oral bioavailability of 70%
- Oral form available in United States; intravenous PCA available in Europe
- Used for moderate to moderately severe chronic pain not requiring rapid onset of analgesic effect
- Oral dosing: 50–100 mg PO q4–6h, up to 400 mg/day; start at 25 mg/day dose and titrate up by 25 mg/day over 3 days to 100 mg, then by 50 mg/day over 3 days to 200 mg/day.
- PCA dosing: Demand dose: 10–20 mg; 5–10 minutes LI; 4-hour limit.
- Side effects: Sweating, dry mouth, drowsiness, nausea, vomiting, headache, dizziness
- Tramadol is a less effective analgesic than opioids.

Narcotics with active metabolites:

1. Codeine – Morphine
2. Hydrocodone – Hydromorphone
3. Morphine sulfate – Morphine 3-glucuronide, morphine 6-glucuronide
4. Oxycodone – weak metabolites, oxymorphone and noroxycodone

- Significance: Active metabolites accumulate in renal and liver disease, further extending the duration of action of narcotics.

NONOPIATES

KETAMINE

- Potent NMDA receptor antagonist
- Counteracts development of tolerance in perioperative pain management
- Studies of systemic combination of ketamine and morphine PCA suggest no clear benefit due to psychomimetic effects and cognitive impairment.

LOCAL ANESTHETICS (LIDOCAINE, BUPIVACAINE, OTHERS)

- Local anesthetic: Produces reversible conduction block of impulses along central and peripheral nerves after regional anesthesia; reduces inflammatory mediators and pain perception
- Central effects: Modifies neuronal responses in dorsal horn
- Little evidence for postoperative morphine sparing analgesic effect when lidocaine used systemically with morphine PCA
- Intercostals or thoracic paravertebral nerve block with long-acting local anesthetics can be used to control postoperative pain after thoracotomy for certain spine procedure and for managing pain in patients with lumbar spine injury and multiple rib fractures.
- Scalp nerve block after cranial surgery provides analgesia similar to morphine for first 24 hours.

ACETAMINOPHEN (TYLENOL)

- Nonopiate, nonsalicylate analgesic and antipyretic
- Effective for moderate pain, but no anti-inflammatory action
- Present in many oral analgesics used for postoperative pain: Percocet, Vicodin (hydrocodone bitartrate and acetaminophen), and Darvocet (propoxyphene napsylate)
- Usual dose: 325, 500 and 650 mg PO, 1–2 tablets q4–6h
- Hepatic metabolism

NONSTEROIDAL ANTI-INFLAMMATORY DRUGS (NSAIDS)

- Mechanism of action: Inhibit production of prostanoids via reduced activity of two cyclo-oxygenases (COX-1 and COX-2). COX-2 is an isoform predominantly expressed during the inflammatory process. With exception of selective COX-2 inhibitors, all other NSAIDs have few or no selective properties.

■ Primary effect is pain relief, but also has antipyretic and anti-inflammatory effects.
■ The major advantage is lack of respiratory depression.
■ Risk of hemorrhage in patients undergoing intracranial or spinal surgery due to platelet inhibition limits use in this population, although current exposure to NSAIDs is not a risk factor for intracerebral hemorrhage or subarachnoid hemorrhage.

Ketoralac (Toradol):

■ Hepatic metabolism (with renal clearance)
■ Usual dose: 15–60 mg IV or IM q6h; up to 120 mg/day; decrease dose by one-half in patients >65 years
■ Duration of action: 4–12 hours

Ibuprofen (Motrin):

■ Renal metabolism
■ Usual dose: 400–800 mg PO q6-8h; up to 1200–3200 mg/day
■ Higher doses have increased risk of bleeding.
■ Duration of action: 6–8 hours
  ▸ Side effects: Symptomatic gastroduodenal ulcers, digestive bleeding, perforation and renal damage are the most common serious adverse effects.

SELECTIVE COX-2 INHIBITORS

■ Mechanism of action: Selective COX-2 inhibition
■ Major advantage over other NSAIDs is no adverse effect on platelet function (COX-2 is not expressed by platelets).
■ Celecoxib (Celebrex)
■ Hepatic metabolism
■ Usual dose: 100–200 mg PO q12-24h; up to 400 mg in 24 hours
■ Duration of action: 12–33 hours

Rofecoxib (Vioxx) Not currently available
    Lumiracoxib Available in United Kingdom; awaiting FDA approval in United States

---

NEUROMUSCULAR BLOCKADE

Commonly cited reasons for the use of neuromuscular blocking agents (NMBA) in the ICU are to facilitate mechanical ventilation or in certain cases for control of intracranial pressure. Independent of the reasons for using NMBAs, all other modalities to improve the clinical situation must be tried, using NMBAs only as a last resort.

■ NMBAs should be used for an adult patient in an ICU to manage ventilation, manage increased ICP, treat muscle spasms, and decrease oxygen consumption only when all other means have been tried without success.
■ The majority of patients in an ICU who are prescribed an NMBA can be managed effectively with pancuronium.
■ For patients for whom vagolysis is contraindicated (e.g., those with cardiovascular disease), NMBAs other than pancuronium may be used.
■ Because of their unique metabolism, cisatracurium or atracurium is recommended for patients with significant hepatic or renal disease.
■ Patients receiving NMBAs should be assessed both clinically and by train of four (TOF) monitoring with a goal of adjusting the degree of neuromuscular blockade to achieve one or two twitches.
■ Before initiating neuromuscular blockade, patients should be medicated with sedative and analgesic drugs to provide adequate sedation and analgesia in accordance with the physician's clinical judgment to optimize therapy.
■ For patients receiving NMBAs and corticosteroids, every effort should be made to discontinue NMBAs as soon as possible.
■ Drug holidays (i.e., stopping NMBAs daily until forced to restart them based on the patient's condition) may decrease the incidence of acute quadriplegic myopathy syndrome (AQMS).
■ Patients receiving NMBAs should have prophylactic eye care therapy and deep venous thrombosis (DVT) prophylaxis.
■ Patients who develop tachyphylaxis to one NMBA should try another drug if neuromuscular blockade is still required.
■ Institutions should perform an economic analysis using their own data when choosing NMBAs for use in an ICU.

Indications

The most common indications for long-term administration of NMBAs include facilitation of mechanical ventilation, control of ICP, ablation of muscle spasms associated with tetanus, and decreasing oxygen consumption. NMBAs are often used to facilitate ventilation and ablate muscular activity in patients with elevated ICP or seizures but have no direct effect on either condition. Patients who are being treated for seizures who also take NMBAs should have electroencephalographic monitoring to ensure that they are not actively seizing while paralyzed.

- Facilitate mechanical ventilation: NMBAs are given to prevent respiratory dyssynchrony, stop spontaneous respiratory efforts and muscle movement, improve gas exchange, and facilitate inverse ratio ventilation.
- Manage increased ICP: No adverse events were reported. Patients could undergo a neurologic examination within minutes after discontinuing atracurium. There have been no controlled studies evaluating the role of NMBAs in the routine management of increased ICP.
- Treat muscle spasms: In the treatment of muscle contractures associated with tetanus, drug overdoses, and seizures.
- Decrease oxygen consumption.

PHARMACOLOGY OF NEUROMUSCULAR-RECEPTOR BLOCKERS

Aminosteroidal Compounds

The aminosteroidal compounds include pancuronium, pipecuronium, vecuronium, and rocuronium.

PANCURONIUM
- A long-acting, nondepolarizing compound
- Intravenous bolus dose of 0.06–0.1 mg/kg for up to 90 minutes; continuous infusion by adjusting the dose to the degree of neuromuscular blockade that is desired.
- Side effects
  ▸ Vagolytic (more than 90% of ICU patients will have an increase in heart rate of 10 beats/min).
  ▸ In patients with renal failure or cirrhosis, the neuromuscular blocking effects of pancuronium are prolonged because of its increased elimination half-life and the decreased clearance of its 3-hydroxypancuronium metabolite that has one-third to one-half the activity of pancuronium.

PIPECURONIUM
- Long-acting NMBA with an elimination half-life of about 2 h.
- The administration of 8 mg of either drug followed by intermittent boluses of 4–6 mg when needed resulted in optimal paralysis.

VECURONIUM
- Vecuronium is an intermediate-acting NMBA that is a structural analogue of pancuronium and is not vagolytic.
- An IV bolus dose of vecuronium 0.08–0.1 mg/kg, produces blockade within 60–90 seconds that typically lasts 25–30 minutes. After an IV bolus dose, vecuronium is given as a 0.8–1.2 μg/kg per minute of continuous infusion, adjusting the rate to the degree of blockade desired.
- 35% of a dose is renally excreted, patients with renal failure will have decreased drug requirements.
- 50% of an injected dose is excreted in bile, patients with hepatic insufficiency will also have decreased drug requirements to maintain adequate blockade.
- Vecuronium has been reported to be more commonly associated with prolonged blockade once discontinued, compared with other NMBAs.
- Recovery time averaged 1–2 hours but ranged from 30 minutes to more than 48 hours.

ROCURONIUM
- Rocuronium is a newer nondepolarizing NMBA with a monoquaternary steroidal chemistry that has an intermediate duration of action and a very rapid onset.
- When given as a bolus dose of 0.6–1.0 mg/kg, blockade is almost always achieved within 2 minutes, with maximum blockade occurring within 3 minutes. Continuous infusions are begun at 10 mg/kg per minute.
- The rocuronium metabolite 17-desacetylrocuronium has only 5–10% activity compared with the parent compound.

RAPACURONIUM
- Rapacuronium, a propionate analogue of vecuronium, was marketed as a nondepolarizing NMBA as an alternative to succinylcholine.
- It was withdrawn from the market on March 27, 2001 because of reports of morbidity (bronchospasm) and mortality associated with its use.

Benzylisoquinolinium Compounds

The benzylisoquinolinium compounds include D-tubocuranine, atracurium, cisatracurium, doxacurium, and mivacurium.

D-TUBOCURARINE
- Tubocurarine was the first nondepolarizing NMBA to gain acceptance and usage in the ICU.
- It induces histamine release and autonomic ganglionic blockade. Hypotension is rare, however, when the agent is administered slowly in appropriate dosages (e.g., 0.1–0.2 mg/kg). Metabolism and elimination are affected by both renal and hepatic dysfunction.

ATRACURIUM
- Atracurium is an intermediate-acting NMBA with minimal cardiovascular adverse effects and is associated with histamine release at higher doses.
- It is inactivated in plasma by ester hydrolysis and Hofmann elimination so that renal or hepatic dysfunction does not affect the duration of blockade.
- Laudanosine is a breakdown product of Hofmann elimination of atracurium and has been associated with central nervous system excitation.
- Seizures in patients who have received extremely high doses of atracurium or who are in hepatic failure
- 10–20 g/kg per minute with doses adjusted to clinical endpoints or by train-of-four (TOF) monitoring. Infusion durations ranged from 24 hours to 200 hours. Recovery of normal neuromuscular activity usually occurred within 1–2 hours after stopping the infusions and was independent of organ function.
- Long-term infusions have been associated with the development of tolerance, necessitating significant dose increases or conversion to other NMBAs.
- Atracurium has been associated with persistent neuromuscular weakness as have other NMBAs.

CISATRACURIUM
- Cisatracurium, an isomer of atracurium, is an intermediate-acting NMBA that is increasingly used in lieu of atracurium.
- It produces few, if any, cardiovascular effects and has a lesser tendency to produce mast cell degranulation than atracurium.
- Bolus doses of 0.1–0.2 mg/kg result in paralysis in an average of 2.5 minutes, and recovery begins at approximately 25 minutes; maintenance infusions should be started at 2.5–3 μg/kg per minute.
- Cisatracurium is also metabolized by ester hydrolysis and Hofmann elimination, so the duration of blockade should not be affected by renal or hepatic dysfunction.
- Prolonged weakness has been reported after the use of cisatracurium.

DOXACURIUM
- Doxacurium, a long-acting agent, is the most potent NMBA currently available.
- Doxacurium is essentially free of hemodynamic adverse effects.
- Initial doses of doxacurium 0.05–0.1 mg/kg may be given with maintenance infusions of 0.3–0.5 μg/kg per minute and adjusted to the degree of blockade desired. An initial bolus dose lasts an average of 60–80 minutes.
- Doxacurium is primarily eliminated by renal excretion. In elderly patients and patients with renal dysfunction, a significant prolongation of effect may occur.

MIVACURIUM
- Mivacurium is one of the shortest-acting NMBAs currently available.
- It consists of multiple stereoisomers and has a half-life of approximately 2 minutes, allowing for rapid reversal of the blockade.

Recommendations for Monitoring Degree of Blockade

Even though the patient may appear quiet and "comfortable," experienced clinicians understand the indications and therapeutic limits of NMBAs. Despite multiple admonitions that NMBAs have no analgesic or amnestic effects, it is not uncommon to find a patient's degree of sedation or comfort significantly overestimated or even ignored. It is difficult to assess pain and sedation in the patient receiving NMBAs, but patients must be medicated for pain and anxiety, despite the lack of obvious symptoms or signs. In common practice, sedative and analgesic drugs are adjusted until the patient does not appear to be conscious and then NMBAs are administered.

- Monitoring neuromuscular blockade is recommended. Monitoring the depth of neuromuscular blockade may allow use of the lowest NMBA dose and may minimize adverse events.
- Visual, tactile, or electronic assessment of the patient's muscle tone or some combination of these three is commonly used to monitor the depth of neuromuscular blockade.
- Observation of skeletal muscle movement and respiratory effort forms the foundation of clinical assessment; electronic methods include the use of ventilator software allowing plethysmographic recording of pulmonary function to detect spontaneous ventilatory efforts and "twitch monitoring," i.e., the assessment of the muscular response by visual, tactile, or electronic means to a transcutaneous delivery of electric current meant to induce peripheral nerve stimulation (PNS).
- TOF monitoring (with a goal of three of four twitches).
- Implementation of a protocol using PNS to monitor the level of blockade in patients receiving a variety of NMBAs found a reduction in the incidence of persistent neuromuscular weakness.

Currently, there is no universal standard for twitch monitoring. The choice of the number of twitches necessary for "optimal" blockade is influenced by the patient's overall condition and level of sedation. The choice of the "best" nerve for monitoring may be influenced by site accessibility, risk of false positives, considerations for the effect of stimulation on patient visitors, and whether faint twitches should be included in the assessment of blockade. The low correlation of blockade measured peripherally compared with that of the phrenic nerve and diaphragm underscores the importance of three issues:

1. More than one method of monitoring should be utilized,
2. Poor technique in using any device will invariably produce inaccurate results.
3. More clinical studies are necessary to determine the best techniques.
   ▶ Patients receiving NMBAs should be assessed both clinically and by TOF monitoring with a goal of adjusting the degree of neuromuscular blockade to achieve one or two twitches.

▶ Before initiating neuromuscular blockade, patients should be medicated with sedative and analgesic drugs to provide adequate sedation and analgesia in accordance with the physician's clinical judgment to optimize therapy.

Potential complications of neuromuscular blockade use in the ICU:

- Complications and contraindications of succinylcholine in the ICU
- General complications associated with NMBAs in the ICU
- Loss of airway awake, paralyzed patient anxiety and panic
- Hyperkalemia risk of ventilator disconnect or airway mishap
- Plasma pseudocholinesterase Autonomic and cardiovascular effects (i.e., vagolytic)
- Decreased lymphatic flow
- Risk of generalized deconditioning
- Skin breakdown
- Peripheral nerve injury
- Corneal abrasion, conjunctivitis
- Myositis ossificans
- Risk of prolonged muscle weakness, AQMS
- Potential central nervous system toxicity

Skeletal muscle weakness in ICU patients is multifactorial, producing a confusing list of names and syndromes, including acute quadriplegic myopathy syndrome (AQMS), floppy man syndrome, critical illness polyneuropathy (CIP), acute myopathy of intensive care, rapidly evolving myopathy, acute myopathy with selective lysis of myosin filaments, acute steroid myopathy, and prolonged neurogenic weakness.

Prolonged Recovery from NMBAs

- The steroid-based NMBAs are associated with reports of prolonged recovery and myopathy. This association may reflect an increased risk inferred by these NMBAs or may reflect past practice patterns in which these drugs may have been more commonly used.
- Steroid based NMBAs undergo extensive hepatic metabolism, producing active drug metabolites.
- The 3-desacetyl vecuronium metabolite is poorly dialyzed, minimally ultrafiltrated, and accumulates in patients with renal failure because

hepatic elimination is decreased in patients with uremia. Thus, the accumulation of both 3-de-sacetyl vecuronium and its parent compound, vecuronium, in patients with renal failure contributes to a prolonged recovery by this ICU subpopulation.

Acute Quadriplegic Myopathy Syndrome

Acute quadriplegic myopathy syndrome (AQMS) consists of clinical triad of:

1. Acute paresis.
2. Myonecrosis with increased creatine phosphokinase (CPK) concentration.
3. Abnormal electromyography (EMG). The latter is characterized by severely reduced compound motor action potential (CMAP) amplitudes and evidence of acute denervation.

- AQMS, also referred to as postparalytic quadriparesis, is one of the most devastating complications of NMBA therapy and one of the reasons that indiscriminate use of NMBAs is discouraged.
- Neurologic examination reveals a global motor deficit affecting muscles in both the upper and lower extremities and decreased motor reflexes. However, extraocular muscle function is usually preserved. This myopathy is characterized by low amplitude CMAPs, and muscle fibrillations but normal (or nearly normal) sensory nerve conduction studies.
- Muscle biopsy shows prominent vacuolization of muscle fibers without inflammatory infiltrate, patchy type 2 muscle fiber atrophy, and sporadic myofiber necrosis .
- Modest CPK increases (0 to 15-fold above normal range) are noted in approximately 50% of patients and are probably dependent on the timing of enzyme measurements and the initiation of the myopathic process. Thus, there may be some justification in screening patients with serial CPK determinations during infusion of NMBAs, particularly if the patients are concurrently treated with corticosteroids.
- Also, since AQMS develops after prolonged exposure to NMBAs, there may be some rationale to daily "drug holidays."
- Other factors that may contribute to the development of the syndrome include nutritional deficiencies, concurrent drug administration with aminoglycosides or cyclosporine, hyperglycemia,

renal and hepatic dysfunction, fever, and severe metabolic or electrolyte disorders.
- The incidence of myopathy may be as high as 30% in patients who receive corticosteroids and NMBAs.
- Acute myopathy in ICU patients is also reported after administration of the benzylisoquinolinium NMBAs (i.e., atracurium, cisatracurium, doxacurium).

Critical Illness Polyneuropathy

Critical illness polyneuropathy (CIP) is a sensory and motor polyneuropathy identified in elderly, septic patients or those with MODS . EMG testing reveals decreased CMAP, fibrillation potentials, and positive sharp waves. CIP is primarily an axonopathy and may be related to microvascular ischemia of the nerve but is not directly related to the use of NMBAs.

- As for any critically ill patient, particularly immobilized patients, deep venous thrombosis (DVT) prophylaxis and physical therapy to maintain joint mobility are important.
- Patients receiving NMBAs are also at risk of developing keratitis and corneal abrasion. Prophylactic eye care is highly variable and recommendations may include methylcellulose drops, ophthalmic ointment, taping the eyelids shut to ensure complete closure, or eye patches

Myositis Ossificans (Heterotopic Ossification)

- Ossification that occurs within the connective tissue of muscle but may also be seen in ligaments, tendons, fascia, aponeuroses, and joint capsules.
- The acquired form of the disease may occur at any age in either sex, especially around the elbows, thighs, and buttocks.
- The basic defect is the inappropriate differentiation of fibroblasts into osteoblasts and is usually triggered by trauma and muscle injury, paraplegia or quadriplegia, tetanus, and burns.
- Treatment consists of promoting an active range of motion around the affected joint and surgery when necessary.

Tachyphylaxis

- Tachyphylaxis to NMBAs can and does develop, which prompted discontinuation of NMBAs.

Drug–Drug Interactions of NMBAs

- Drugs that potentiate the action of nondepolarizing NMBAs
- Drugs that antagonize the actions of nondepolarizing NMBAs
- Local anesthetics: phenytoin, lidocaine, carbamazepine
- Antimicrobials: aminoglycosides, polymyxin B, clindamycin, tetracycline, theophylline
- Antiarrhythmics: (procainamide, quinidine), ranitidine magnesium
- Calcium channel blockers
- Adrenergic blockers
- Immunosuppressive agents (cyclophosphamide, cyclosporine)
- Dantrolene
- Diuretics
- Lithium carbonate

REFERENCES

Angelini G, Ketzler JT, Coursin DB. Use of propofol and other nonbenzodiazepine sedatives in the intensive care unit. *Crit Care Clin.* 2001;**17**(4):863–80.

Aryan HE, Box KW, Ibrahim D, Desiraju U, Ames CP. Safety and efficacy of dexmedetomidine in neurosurgical patients. *Brain Inj.* 2006;**20**(8):791–8.

Ayoub C, Girard F, Boudreault D, Chouinard P, Ruel M, Moumdjian R. A comparison between scalp nerve block and morphine for transitional analgesia after remifentanil-based anesthesia in neurosurgery. *Anesth Analg.* 2006;**103**(5):1237–40.

Bala I, Gupta B, Bhardwaj N, Ghai B, Khosla VK. Effect of scalp block on postoperative pain relief in craniotomy patients. *Anaesth Intens Care.*2006;**34**(2):224–7.

Chiaretti A, Genovese O, Antonelli A, Tortorolo L, Ruggiero A, Focarelli B, Di Rocco C. Patient-controlled analgesia with fentanil and midazolam in children with postoperative neurosurgical pain. *Childs Nerv Syst.* 2008;**24**(1):119–24.

De Benedittis G, Lorenzetti A, Migliore M, Spagnoli D, Tiberio F, Villani RM. Postoperative pain in neurosurgery: A pilot study in brain surgery. *Neurosurgery.* 1996;**38**:466–70.

Giuditta Angelini MD, Jonathan T, Ketzler MD, Douglas B, Coursin MD. Use of propofol and other nonbenzodiazepine sedatives in the intensive care unit. *Crit Care Clin.* 2001;**17**(4):863–80.

Gottschalk A, Berkow LC, Stevens RD, et al. Prospective evaluation of pain and analgesic use following major elective intracranial surgery. *J Neurosurg* 2007;**106**(2):210–6.

Hernandez Palazon J, Domenech Asensi P, Burguillos Lopez S, Perez Bautista F, Sanchez Amador A, Clavel Claver N. Cranial nerve block with bupivacaine for postoperative analgesia following supratentorial craniotomy. *Rev Esp Anestesiol Reanim.* 2007;**54**(5):274–8.

Hutchens MP, Memtsoudis S, Sadovnikoff N. Propofol for sedation in neuro-intensive care. *Neurocrit Care.* 2006;**4**(1):54–62.

Jacobi J. Clinical practice guidelines for the sustained use of sedatives and analgesics in the critically ill adult. *Crit Care Med.* 2002;**30**(1).

Jirarattanaphochai K, Jung S, Thienthong S, Krisanaprakornkit W, Sumananont C. Peridural methylprednisolone and wound infiltration with bupivacaine for postoperative pain control after posterior lumbar spine surgery: a randomized double-blinded placebo-controlled trial. *Spine.* 2007;**32**(6):609–16.

Kirchheiner J, Schmidt H, Tzvetkov M, Keulen JT, Lötsch J, Roots I, Brockmöller J. Pharmacokinetics of codeine and its metabolite morphine in ultra-rapid metabolizers due to CYP2D6 duplication. *Pharmacogenom J.* 2007;**7**(4):257–65.

Kress JP, Pohlman AS, O'Connor MF, et al. Daily interruption of sedative infusions in critically ill patients undergoing mechanical ventilation. *N Engl J Med.* 2000;**342**:1471–7.

Kumar MA, Urrutia VC, Thomas CE, Abou-Khaled KJ, Schwartzman RJ. The syndrome of irreversible acidosis after prolonged propofol infusion. *Neurocrit Care.* 2005;**3**(3):257–9.

Law-Koune JD, Szekely B, Fermanian C, Peuch C, Liu N, Fischler M. Scalp infiltration with bupivacaine plus epinephrine or plain ropivacaine reduces postoperative pain after supratentorial craniotomy. *J Neurosurg Anesthesiol.* 2005;**17**(3):139–43.

Mirski MA, Hemstreet MK. Critical care sedation for neuroscience patients. *J Neurol Sci.* 2007;**261**:16–34.

Murray MJ. Clinical practice guidelines for sustained neuromuscular blockade in the adult critically ill patient. *Crit Care Med.* 2002;**30**(1).

Nguyen A, Girard F, Boudreault D, et al. Scalp nerve blocks decreases the severity of pain after craniotomy. *Anesth Analg.* 2001;**93**:1272–6.

Quiney N, Cooper R, Stoneham M, Walters F. Pain after craniotomy. A time for reappraisal? *Br J Neurosurg.* 1996;**10**:295–9.

Rahimi SY, Vender JR, Macomson SD, French A, Smith JR, Alleyne CH Jr. Postoperative pain management after craniotomy: evaluation and cost analysis. *Neurosurgery.* 2006;**59**(4):852–7.

RxList: The Internet Drug Index. http://www.rxlist.com/script/main/hp.as

Sudheer PS, Logan SW, Terblanche C, Ateleanu B, Hall JE. Comparison of the analgesic efficacy and respiratory effects of morphine, tramadol and codeine after craniotomy. *Anaesthesia.* 2007;**62**(6):555–60.

Thibault M, Girard F, Moumdjian R, Chouinard P, Boudreault D, Ruel M. Craniotomy site influences postoperative pain following neurosurgical procedures: a retrospective study. *Can J Anaesth.* 2007;**54**(7):544–8

Young CC, Prielipp RC. Benzodiazepines in the intensive care unit. *Crit Care Clin.* 2001;**4**:843–862.

Zarovnaya EL, Jobst BC, Harris BT. Propofol-associated fatal myocardial failure and rhabdomyolysis in an adult with status epilepticus. *Epilepsia.* 2007;**48**(5):1002–6.

6 Mechanical Ventilation and Airway Management

Rahul Nanchal, MD, and Ahmed J. Khan, MD

Airway management and mechanical ventilation represent the cornerstones of ICU care for critically ill patients. In this chapter we deal with basic concepts and focus on the practical considerations that confront critical care practitioners on a daily basis.

AIRWAY MANAGEMENT

It is essential for critical care specialists to be proficient in securing an airway in a variety of patients and clinical scenarios. Critically ill patients often have hypoxia, acidosis, or hemodynamic instability and poorly tolerate delays in placing an airway. Further, underlying conditions such as intracranial hypertension and myocardial ischemia may be exacerbated by the attempt to secure an airway itself. Compounding the problem are the myriad of comorbid and associated conditions such as vascular disease, cervical fractures, facial trauma, laryngeal edema, and patient combativeness associated with the critically ill that complicate the situation .

Criteria for Intubation

Although never validated, the decision to establish a definitive airway is based on three general criteria:

1. Failure to protect or maintain airway, e.g., loss of protective airway reflexes in brain injured patients
2. Failure to oxygenate or ventilate, e.g., during cardiopulmonary arrest, acute respiratory distress syndrome (ARDS), septic shock, neuromuscular disease

3. Anticipation of a deteriorating clinical course, e.g., anatomical airway distortion. Serial clinical assessment is requisite to determine the ability of patients to protect their airway.

- The gag reflex does not correlate well with airway protection and is of no clinical value when assessing the need for intubation.
- Arterial blood gases are rarely helpful in the decision to intubate and may lead to faulty decision making.
- The Glasgow Coma Scale (GCS) has been traditionally used in a variety of traumatic and nontraumatic neurologic conditions as a simple tool to gauge airway compromise on serial examinations.
  - ▶ A GCS of <8 is associated with severe brain injury and these patients typically require intubation due to loss of protective reflexes.
  - ▶ However, the GCS has several limitations and was recently reported to have only moderate degree of interrater reliability in the emergency department.
- Standard pulmonary function testing parameters such as NIF and vital capacity are frequently used to follow the clinical course in patients with neuromuscular disease such as myasthenia gravis and Guillain-Barré syndrome to discern respiratory muscle weakness and the need for intubation.
  - ▶ However, abnormalities are frequently subtle and patients may not manifest the usual signs and symptoms of respiratory failure.
  - ▶ One retrospective study found that vital capacity is a poor predictor of the need for mechanical ventilation in myasthenia gravis secondary to the erratic nature of the disease.

Sound judgment and clinical decision making are imperative as failure to recognize impending respiratory failure may have life-threatening consequences. If the anticipated clinical course if one of deterioration, it is prudent to err on the side of intubation rather than confronting a disastrous situation of not being able to intubate, oxygenate, or ventilate.

Rapid Sequence Intubation

Rapid sequence intubation (RSI) is the cornerstone of emergency airway management. It entails using a specific sequence of drug therapy for rapid induction and paralysis to facilitate placement of an endotracheal tube. The administration of drugs is preceded by preoxygenation. Intubation is ideally performed without bag mask ventilation to limit gastric distension and aspiration. Cricoid pressure (Sellick's maneuver) is applied to occlude the esophagus. The National Emergency Airway Registry demonstrated that RSI is the most commonly performed intubation technique, with a success rate of greater than 98.5%. Several studies have now demonstrated increased success rates and fewer complications with protocols utilizing RSI compared to traditional intubating techniques. However, one should be aware that not all critically ill patients are candidates for RSI. The most common contraindication to RSI is the predicted difficult airway

RSI SEQUENCE

- Preparation: Suction, Tubes, Oxygen, pharmacology, IV access, Connections, Blades, Alternatives, Rescue, Surgery (STOPIC BARS)
- Preoxygenation: Administration of 100% oxygen prior to paralysis to replace FRC with oxygen to allow for prolonged apnea without desaturation. It is important to remember that the time to desaturation from 90% to 0% is dramatically less than that from 100% to 90% (Fig. 6.1).
- Pretreatment: Agents given to reduce the adverse physiologic effects of laryngoscopy
  ‣ Lidocaine: Suppresses cough reflex and mitigates increase in intracranial pressure (ICP) in response to intubation
  ‣ Opioids: Fentanyl is generally used to attenuate the sympathetic response and prevent blood pressure increases associated with intubation. Also provides analgesia and sedation.
  ‣ Atropine: Used to prevent vagal response in children
  ‣ Defasciculating dose of neuromuscular blockers: Used to prevent fasciculations associated with succinylcholine and prevent associated rises in ICP but the use of this is controversial.
- Paralysis with induction: Induction is immediately followed by paralysis. Knowledge of airway pharmacology is paramount (see later).

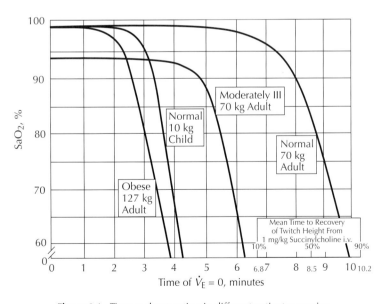

Figure 6.1. Time to desaturation in different patient scenarios.

- Protection and positioning: Sellick's maneuver- (cricoid pressure to occlude esophagus) to prevent passive aspiration and optimal positioning
- Placement with proof: Confirmation of placement with end-tidal CO_2
- Postintubation management: Securing the tube, sedation, and mechanical ventilation

RSI is the method of choice to intubate patients with brain injury and raised intracranial pressure as it minimizes the adverse effects associated with intubation.

Airway Pharmacology

Familiarity with the various preinduction, induction, and neuromuscular blocking agents facilitates proper drug selection for the particular clinical situation. Appropriate selection not only increases the likelihood of successful intubation but also decreases the complication rate.

- Induction agents (Table 6.1)
- Neuromuscular blocking agents (Table 6.2)
  - Depolarizing, e.g., succinylcholine
  - Nondepolarizing, e.g., vecuronium, rocuronium

Assessment of the Difficult Airway

The American Society of Anesthesiology defines a difficult airway as either difficult to intubate or difficult to ventilate.

- Difficult intubation: More than three attempts by an experienced operator or attempts that last more than 10 minutes. The mnemonic LEMON is a useful guide to quickly assess the patients in whom a difficulty airway would be predicted. The elements of this mnemonic are currently being validated by the investigators of the National Emergency Airway Registry project.
  - Look externally: External evidence that bag mask ventilation or laryngoscopy would be difficult
  - Evaluate the 3–3–2 rule: 3 fingers in the patient's mouth, 3 fingers from the mentum to hyoid, and 2 fingers from the floor of the mouth to the thyroid notch. These evaluations relate to geometric considerations that predict likelihood of successful laryngoscopy and intubation

  - Mallampati score: Although not validated for the ICU population, this scoring system predicts difficulty with laryngoscopy on the basis of visualization of posterior pharyngeal elements
  - Obstruction: Signs and symptoms of upper airway obstruction are a hallmark for difficulty with laryngoscopy
  - Neck mobility: Limited neck mobility, e.g., with cervical spine trauma will limit an optimum view of the larynx on attempted intubation.
- Difficult ventilation: Inability to maintain oxygen saturation above 90% using a face mask for ventilation and 100% inspired oxygen by a trained operator. The various indicators that predict difficult ventilation can be recalled by the mnemonic MOANS:
  - Mask seal: Beards and facial trauma are some examples of situations were it is difficult to obtain a good mask seal.
  - Obesity/obstruction: For example, pregnant women and patients who have a BMI >26
  - Age: Age >55 is associated with a higher risk of difficult ventilation due to loss of upper airway muscle tone.
  - No teeth
  - Stiffness: Patients who require high ventilation pressure, e.g., ARDS are often difficult to bag mask ventilate.

There is a paucity of studies validating these airway assessment techniques in the ICU population; nevertheless a quick examination of these elements frequently assists in preintubation planning. However, a recent retrospective study indicated that performing an airway assessment in critically ill patients was not possible in approximately 70% of patients presenting to the emergency department. In addition, absence of these features does not guarantee that one will not encounter a difficult airway. So, it is imperative to be prepared for a difficult airway.

Failed Airway

A failed airway is defined as either failure to intubate despite three attempts by an experienced operator or failure to maintain acceptable oxygen saturation during one or more failed attempts at laryngoscopy. If one is unable to intubate and oxygenate, cricothyrotomy should be performed in the vast majority of circumstances.

Table 6.1. Induction agents

Agent and dosage	Pros	Cons	Contraindications
Thiopental 1.5–5 mg/kg IV push	Rapid onset Brief duration Decreases ICP Anticonvulsant	Decreases blood pressure Myocardial depression Respiratory depression Histamine release No analgesic effect	Hypotensive patient Asthmatic patient Porphyria
Methohexital 1.5 mg/kg IV	Very rapid onset Very short duration Decreases ICP	Decreases blood pressure Respiratory depression Seizures (rare) Hypertonus/hiccuping Laryngospasm No analgesic effect	Hypotensive patient Seizure disorder Porphyria
Etomidate 0.3 mg/kg IV	No deleterious effect on blood pressure Minimal depression of respiration Decreases ICP and IOP	Myoclonic movements Seizures Hiccups Nausea/vomiting Decreases steroid synthesis Minor pain on injection No analgesic effect	Focal seizure disorder (use with caution) Adrenal insufficiency Should not be used as a continuous IV sedating agent because it depresses steroid synthesis
Propofol 0.5–2 mg/kg IV	Decreases ICP Titratable – useful for maintenance sedation Antiemetic Anticonvulsant	Decreases blood pressure Myocardial depression Respiratory depression Myoclonic movements Minor pain on injection Rare bronchospasm No analgesic effect	Hypotensive patient Asthmatic patient (use with caution)
Ketamine 2 mg/kg IV	"Dissociative" anesthesia without impairing airway reflexes Analgesia Amnesia Bronchodilator No decrease in blood pressure – useful in hypotensive patients No significant respiratory depression	Increases ICP Minimally increases IOP Increases airway secretions Laryngospasm Increases blood pressure Increases heart rate Increases muscle tone Nausea/vomiting Emergence reactions	Uncontrolled hypertension Increased ICP Penetrating eye injury Glaucoma Acute URI CAD/CHF History of psychosis Thyroid storm
Midazolam 0.1–0.3 mg/kg IV	Amnesia anticonvulsant	Delayed onset Inconsistent effect Respiratory depression Hypotension – variable and dose-dependent	Hypotensive patient

Table 6.2. Neuromuscular blocking agents

Agent	Dosage	Indications	Contraindications
Succinylcholine	1.5 mg/kg IV push	Default paralytic unless contraindications exist	Difficult airway and insecurity about the ability to successfully bag mask ventilate Family or personal history of malignant hyperthermia
			Known hyperkalemia
			Certain chronic muscle dystrophies, prior spinal cord injury, prior strokes, any demyelinating diseases
			Preexisting tissue injury >3 days prior to RSI Burns >24 hours prior to RSI
			Renal failure with hyperkalemia Renal failure without hyperkalemia (relative)
Rocuronium	1 mg/kg IV push	If succinylcholine is contraindicated	Difficult airway and insecurity about the ability to sucessfully bag mask ventilateAllergy to neuromuscular blocking drugs

Airway Management with Increased Intracranial Pressure

Patients with known or suspected increased ICP represent a special population and prevention of secondary brain injury is paramount.

- The process of laryngoscopy and intubation can increase ICP.
- Hypotension from sedative administration or hypovolemia is common.
- Hypoxia can occur during attempts to intubate.
- Cervical spine injuries are found concomitantly with TBI and manipulation of the spine should be avoided.

Careful consideration has to be given to drug selection and technique. RSI is the technique of choice so that the patient is sedated, paralyzed, and the total time taken to intubate is as short as possible. Preinduction medication as described in the preceding text can be given. Induction and paralysis are generally performed with etomidate and succinylcholine, respectively. Difficult airway equipment should always be at hand.

Approach to the ICU Patient

An algorithmic protocol approach to airway management, though never validated in the ICU, has been associated with improved outcomes in the emergency departments as well as field intubations. These algorithms, developed by Wall et al., classify intubation attempts as (1) universal (Fig. 6.2), (2) crash (Fig. 6.3), (3) difficult (Fig. 6.4), and (4) failed (Fig. 6.5). The starting point for every intubation is the universal airway algorithm. The intensivist first determines if the patient is near death or a difficult airway is anticipated. The crash airway or difficult airway algorithms are respectively initiated depending on the circumstance. Failure to oxygenate and intubate leads to the activation of the failed airway algorithm.

Proficiency with handling an airway is an obligatory skill for all intensivists. Extrapolation of the emergency room data supports the practice of adopting an algorithmic approach to airway management and RSI should be the technique of choice for intubation in a vast majority of cases.

MECHANICAL VENTILATION

Mechanical ventilation has been revolutionized by the arrival of sophisticated new technology that now offer a plethora of modes, alarms and monitoring capabilities that facilitate patient safety and patient ventilator synchrony. One should, however, keep in mind that no mode of mechanical ventilation has ever

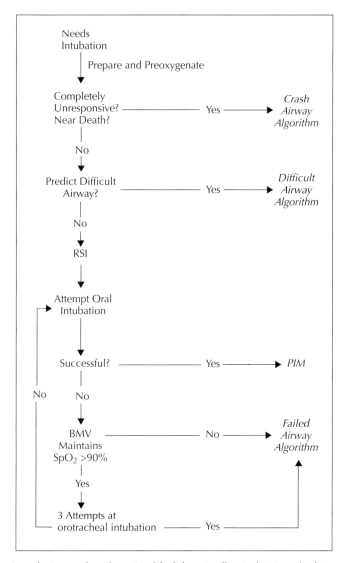

Figure 6.2. Universal airway algorithm. (Modified from Walls et al: *Manual of Emergency Airway Management*. Philadelphia: Lippincott Williams and Wilkins, 2004, p. 9.)

been shown to be superior to the other in terms of patient outcomes. Most of these studies have looked at oxygenation as an endpoint. In fact, the largest trial to date comparing low versus high tidal volume for ARDS, showed a mortality benefit for patients that were ventilated with low tidal volumes (6 mL/kg). This group of patients had worse oxygenation parameters compared to the group with high tidal volumes.

It is not as important to remember all the modes and variables available on modern ventilators as it is essential to grasp the basic physiologic concepts. There are however nuances, especially when dealing with brain-injured patients and hyperventilation that the intensivist should be familiar with.

- Mechanical ventilation can be delivered invasively of noninvasively.
- There are two basic formats of mechanical ventilation: pressure driven and volume driven. The various modes available generally utilize either of these two formats for breath delivery.
- Each breath in a particular mode then has three phase variables of inspiration: trigger, target, and cycling off criteria.

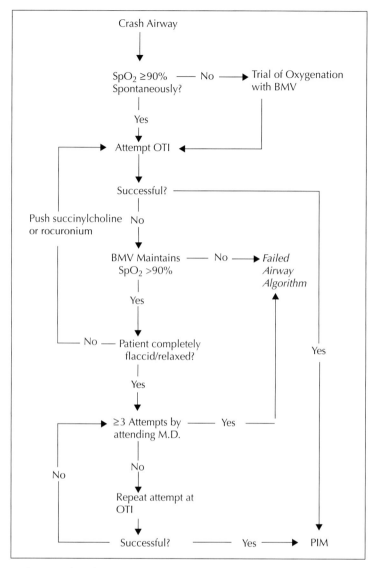

Figure 6.3. Crash airway algorithm. (Modified from Walls et al: *Manual of Emergency Airway Management.* Philadelphia: Lippincott Williams and Wilkins, 2004, p. 13.)

■ Breaths can either be mandatory or spontaneous.
■ Expiration is almost always passive except with specialized modes like high frequency oscillatory ventilation.

Modes of Mechanical Ventilation

CONTROLLED MECHANICAL VENTILATION

■ All delivered breaths totally controlled by the machine and patient triggering is not possible.
■ Breath delivery is in the volume or pressure format.

ASSIST CONTROL VENTILATION

■ Breath delivery in either the volume or pressure format
■ Patient can trigger the ventilator but each breath delivers the set tidal volume or pressure.
■ Ventilator senses patient effort by either pressure or flow triggering mechanisms.
  ▶ Volume assist control: Breaths are time or patient triggered, flow targeted, and volume cycled (see Fig. 6.6).
    ▷ The physician sets respiratory rate, flow rate and tidal volume.

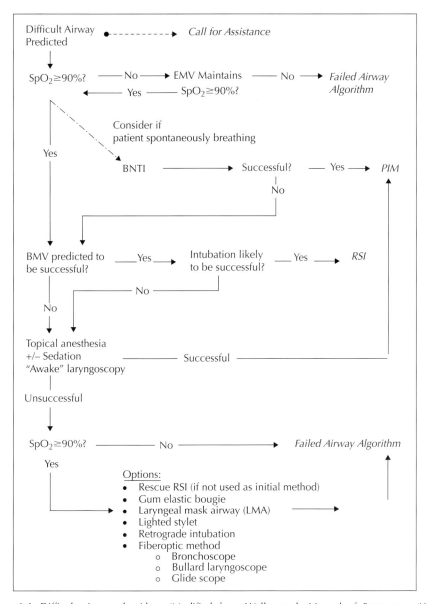

Figure 6.4. Difficult airway algorithm. (Modified from Walls et al: *Manual of Emergency Airway Management*. Philadelphia: Lippincott Williams and Wilkins, 2004, p. 15.)

▷ Pressures in the system are variable depending on the resistance and compliance of the lungs as well as patient effort.

▶ Pressure assist control: Breaths are time or patient triggered, pressure targeted, and time cycled (see Fig. 6.7).

▷ The physician sets the respiratory rate, inspiratory pressure, and inspiratory time.

▷ Flow in the system is variable depending on the resistance and compliance of the lung and patient effort. Due to this variability of flow, tidal volumes are variable.

SYNCHRONIZED INTERMITTENT MANDATORY VENTILATION

■ CMV breaths are delivered in either the pressure or volume format.

■ In between breaths the patient can breathe spontaneously from either a demand valve or continuous flow of gas.

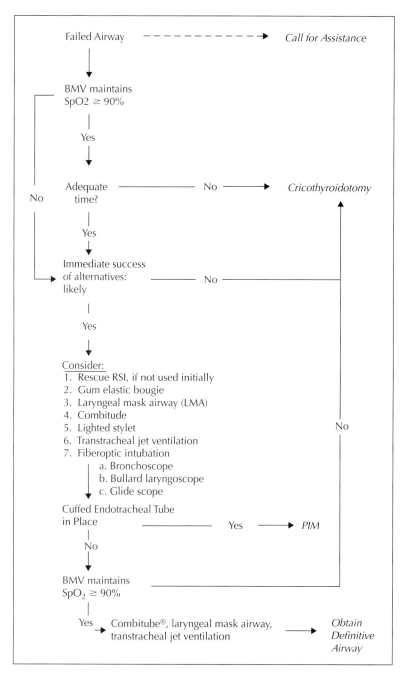

Figure 6.5. Failed airway algorithm. (Modified from Walls et al: *Manual of Emergency Airway Management*. Philadelphia: Lippincott Williams & Wilkins, 2004, p. 18.)

■ Mandatory breaths delivered in synchrony with the patient's efforts, i.e., the unit functions in the assist control mode only during a window of time established by the manufacturer.

■ Synchronized intermittent mandatory ventilation (SIMV) may be combined with pressure support, so each spontaneous effort not falling within the specified window is assisted with a

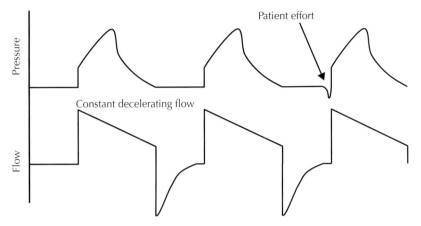

Figure 6.6. Assist control (volume format).

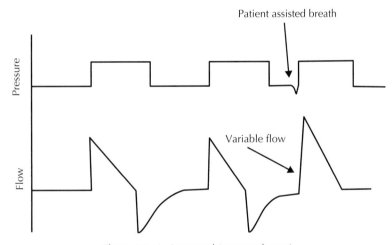

Figure 6.7. Assist control (pressure format).

set pressure applied at the airway opening (see Fig. 6.8).

PRESSURE SUPPORT

- Breaths are triggered by patient effort only; there are no mandatory breaths.
- Each breath is patient triggered, pressure targeted, and flow cycled.
- Inspiration is terminated when flow falls to a preset level (usually 25% of peak flow; see Fig. 6.9).
- The physician sets the inspiratory pressure and on the newer generation of ventilators the rise time and termination criteria can be adjusted.
  - ▶ Rise time refers to the rate of initial pressurization of the airway.

- ▶ Termination criteria can be manipulated by changing the flow at which the breath terminates.

DUAL-BREATH MECHANICAL VENTILATION

- Closed loop mechanical ventilation that combines both formats to usually guarantee a tidal volume
- Most commonly the physician sets a tidal volume, the inspiratory time, and a maximum pressure.
- Gas delivery for these breaths is in the pressure format.
- The ventilator then by feedback enhancement of breaths tries to deliver the set tidal volume in the specified time at the lowest possible pressure.

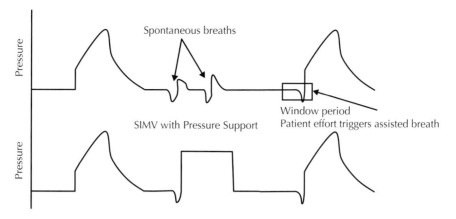

Figure 6.8. SIMV without pressure support.

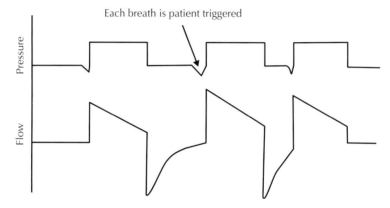

Figure 6.9. Pressure support ventilation.

- For example, VC+ on the Puritan Bennett 840 ventilator or PRVC on the Servo series of ventilators by Siemens

Positive End-Expiratory Pressure

High levels of positive end-expiratory pressure (PEEP) are routinely used to treat ARDS/ALI. However, its effect on brain injured patients remains controversial for the following reasons:

- By increasing mean airway pressure, PEEP may decrease cerebral venous outflow and raise ICP.
- By reducing venous return, PEEP leads to a drop in mean arterial pressure and thereby cerebral perfusion pressure.
- By causing alveolar recruitment, PEEP improves lung compliance and oxygenation leading to beneficial effects.

However, a recent study explored cerebropulmonary interactions and concluded that PEEP leading to alveolar recruitment did not increase ICP but patients with normal respiratory system compliance had an increase in $Paco_2$, cerebral blood flow, and ICP. A thought provoking editorial accompanied this study and explored the beneficial effect of PEEP in traumatic brain injury. Overall it seems that as long as euvolemia is maintained, moderate levels of PEEP are safe in brain-injured patients. Therapy should be tailored to each individual patient with a careful vigil over the ICP, $Paco_2$, and neurologic status.

Hyperventilation

From the standpoint of mechanical ventilation the intensivist should keep the following few things in mind:

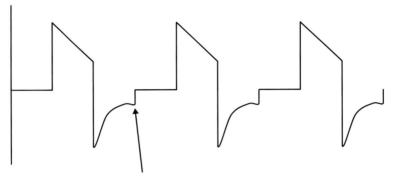

Flow does not return to baseline

Figure 6.10. Dynamic hyperinflation.

- If hyperventilation leads to dynamic hyperinflation secondary to insufficient expiratory time, mean airway pressure will increase which may lead to adverse effects on the ICP secondary to impaired venous sinus drainage. $PaCO_2$ may actually rise secondary to the hyperinflation (see Fig. 6.10).
- Using faster flow rates will permit more time for exhalation and will lower the mean airway pressure.

Before beginning hyperventilation careful consideration should be given to factors that can improve CO_2 clearance, such as removing unnecessary excessive dead space in the form of ventilator circuitry, improving respiratory system compliance by draining pleural effusions and ascites, achieving optimum patient ventilator synchrony, and ensuring an unobstructed endotracheal tube.

Noninvasive Ventilation

With dramatic improvements in the patient ventilator interface, noninvasive ventilation (NIV) has become very sophisticated with a variety of modes at the intensivist's disposal. Bilevel positive airway pressure ventilation (BIPAP) is the most commonly used.

- The ventilator cycles between two different set levels of pressure and the breaths are patient initiated.
- The unique advantage of NIV is the avoidance of complications associated with invasive ventilation.

- When used properly in the right patient population, NIV lowers the risk of infection including nosocomial pneumonia and sinusitis, preserves upper airway defenses, and allows patients to vocalize and eat normally.

However, patient selection is the key. NIV should be used as a bridge in patients where the primary process is expected to improve relatively quickly.

- Patients with an inability to handle secretion, loss of upper airway function, hemodynamic instability, and upper gastrointestinal bleeding are better managed with invasive mechanical ventilation.
- The data is most extensive in chronic obstructive pulmonary disease (COPD) exacerbations where the use of NIV has been shown to benefit morbidity and mortality and shorten hospital length of stay, thereby leading to a reduction in associated cost.
- NIV theoretically should benefit patients with neuromuscular disease. However, there is a paucity of data and there have been only two small published trials. The most recent retrospective study examined 9 patients with 11 episodes of acute respiratory failure due to myasthenic crisis. The use of NIV prevented intubation in 7 out of the 11 episodes.

Respiratory failure in the ICU is an exceedingly common entity and patients often require ventilatory support in one form or the other. Familiarity with the physiologic principles underpinning mechanical ventilation will allow the intensivist better manage the patients on mechanical ventilation and troubleshoot the common bedside problems that arise.

REFERENCES

American Society of Anesthesiologists. Practice guidelines for management of the difficult airway: A report by the American Society of Anesthesiologists Task Force on Management of the Difficult Airway. *Anesthesiology.* 1993;**78**:597–602.

Andrews PJ. Pressure, flow and Occam's razor: a matter of 'steal'? *Intens Care Med.* 2005; **31**:323–4.

Bair AE, Filbin MR, Kulkarni RG, et al. The failed intubation attempt in the emergency department: analysis of prevalence, rescue techniques, and personnel. *J Emerg Med.* 2002;**23**:131–40.

Branson RD, Davis K Jr. Dual control modes: combining volume and pressure breaths. *Respir Care Clin N Am.* 2001;**7**(3):397–408.

Davis DP, Ochs M, Hoyt DB, et al. Paramedic-administered neuromuscular blockade improves prehospital intubation success in severely head-injured patients. *J Trauma.* 2003;**55**:713–9.

Dearden NM. Mechanisms and prevention of secondary brain damage during intensive care. *Clin Neuropathol.* 1998;**17**:221–8.

Dunham CM, Barraco RD, Clark DE, et al. Guidelines for emergency tracheal intubation immediately after traumatic injury. *J Trauma.* 2003;**55**:162–79.

Gill MR, Reiley DG, Green SM. Interrater reliability of Glasgow Coma Scale scores in the emergency department. *Ann Emerg Med.* 2004;**43**:215–23.

Girou E, Schortgen F, Delclaux C, et al: Association of noninvasive ventilation with nosocomial infections and survival in critically ill patients. *JAMA.* 2000;**284**:2361–7.

Jones JH, Weaver CS, Rusyniak DE, et al. Impact of emergency medicine faculty and an airway protocol on airway management. *Acad Emerg Med.* 2002;**9**,1452–6.

Ko SH, Kim DC, Han YJ, Song HS. Small-dose fentanyl: optimal time of injection for blunting the circulatory responses to tracheal intubation. *Anesth Analg.* 1998;**86**:658–61.

Levitan RM, Everett WW, Ochroch EA. Limitations of difficult airway prediction in patients intubated in the emergency department. *Ann Emerg Med.* 2004;**44**(4):307–13.

Mascia L, Grasso S, Fiore T, et al. Cerebro-pulmonary interactions during the application of low levels of positive end-expiratory pressure. *Intens Care Med.* 2005; **31**:373–9.

Nava S, Ambrosino N, Clini E, et al: Noninvasive mechanical ventilation in the weaning of patients with respiratory failure due to chronic obstructive pulmonary disease: a randomized, controlled trial. *Ann Intern Med.* 1998;**128**:721–8.

Pierson DJ. Indications for mechanical ventilation in adults with acute respiratory failure. *Respir Care.* 2002;**47**:249–62, discussion 262–5.

Rabinstein A, Wijdicks EF. BiPAP in acute respiratory failure due to myasthenic crisis may prevent intubation. *Neurology.* 2002;**59**(10):1647–9.

Rieder P, Louis M, Jolliet P, Chevrolet JC. The repeated measurement of vital capacity is a poor predictor of the need for mechanical ventilation in myasthenia gravis. *Intens Care Med.* 1995;**21**:663–8.

Sakles, JC, Laurin, EG, Rantapaa, AA, et al. Airway management in the emergency department: a one-year study of 610 tracheal intubations. *Ann Emerg Med.* 1998;**31**:325–32.

Schwartz DE, Matthay MA, Cohen NH. Death and other complications of emergency airway management in critically ill adults: a prospective investigation of 297 tracheal intubations. *Anesthesiology.* 1995;**82**:367–76.

Tayal VS, Riggs RW, Marx JA, et al. Rapid-sequence intubation at an emergency medicine residency: success rate and adverse events during a two-year period. *Acad Emerg Med.* 1999;**6**:31–7.

The Acute Respiratory Distress Syndrome Network. Ventilation with lower tidal volumes as compared with traditional tidal volumes for acute lung injury and the acute respiratory distress syndrome. *N Engl J Med.* 2000;**342**:1301–8.

Ward NS, Hill NS. Pulmonary function testing in neuromuscular disease. *Clin Chest Med.* 2001;**22**:769–81.

Yukioka H, Hayashi M, Terai T, Fujimori M. Intravenous lidocaine as a suppressant of coughing during tracheal intubation in elderly patients. *Anesth Analg.* 1993;**77**:309–31.

7 Neuropharmacology

Kristin Santa, PharmD and Rebecca Schuman, PharmD

This chapter focuses on selected pharmacologic topics that play an important role in patient care in the neurointensive care unit. The role of a clinical pharmacist in maximizing patient care in the ICU is discussed. Medication classes that are reviewed include antiplatelet and antithrombotic agents, and antiepileptics. The pharmacologic properties of these agents, including mechanism of action, dosing, side effects, drug interactions, and pharmacokinetic parameters, are discussed in this chapter. More detailed information and in-depth discussion regarding use of these medication classes in specific neurologic and neurosurgical situations is provided in other chapters within this text.

THE PHARMACIST'S ROLE IN THE ICU

As health care evolves and becomes more varied and complex, so must the roles of its professionals. The focus of a pharmacist's place in health care is shifting from the more reactionary established activities of preparation and dispensing to more proactive and influential participation in total patient care. Although physicians are educated in the fundamentals of medication therapy, the specialized training and education of clinical pharmacists allows them to serve as medication experts who are better equipped to recognize, understand, and prevent medication errors. While assuming an increasing responsibility for pharmacotherapeutic outcomes, pharmacists are well suited to aid physicians in drug therapy selection, monitoring, and decision making. Including pharmacists as proactive members of the multidisciplinary healthcare team can maximize drug selection in many ways, including:

- Prevention and monitoring of drug interactions and/or adverse drug events (ADEs)
- Medication dose adjustments for renal and/or hepatic dysfunction, age, or obesity
- Selection of appropriate medication route of administration
- Determination of intravenous fluid, medication, and IV line compatibility
- Identification and recommendation of cost-effective therapeutic options

Medication Safety and Error Prevention

Reviewing error prevention data is one of the most straightforward ways to quantify a pharmacist's impact as a more active member in the healthcare team. Studies have shown that nearly half of all preventable ADEs occur during the prescribing process. Errors during this first phase of care can cause a cascade effect, allowing for potential errors in the dispensing and administration steps of care as well. Since pharmacist retrospective review of medication orders has proven to prevent errors, including the pharmacist in the decision-making process at the time of prescribing can have an even more substantial impact on the prevention and identification of medication errors.

One of the most effective strategies in promoting medication safety is the incorporation of pharmacists into daily patient care rounds. Studies have proven that the inclusion of a pharmacist on rounds reduces the incidence of medication errors and the duration an error persists once it has occurred. Rounding provides the pharmacist with a more comprehensive understanding of a patient's clinical picture. This allows medication regimens to be tailored to each individual. Utilizing this patient-specific knowledge, pharmacists can analyze drug regimens while keeping in mind important safety factors, including:

• Current disease state	• Organ function
• Past medical history	• Laboratory abnormalities
• Potential adverse effects	• Drug–food interactions
• Drug–drug interactions	• Drug contraindications

One study, completed in a large teaching hospital, measured the impact of pharmacist participation in medical rounds on the rate of preventable ADEs due to ordering errors by comparing a 17-bed medical ICU (study unit) to a 15-bed coronary care unit (control unit). The study was completed in two phases, the first without pharmacist involvement in the study unit and the second after addition of a clinical pharmacist to daily rounds.

■ The rate of preventable ordering ADEs per 1000 patient days decreased in the study unit by 66% (10.4 vs. 3.5, $p < 0.001$).

■ Comparison between the control unit (no pharmacist on rounds) and the study unit found 72% fewer ordering ADEs in the intervention unit (3.5 vs. 12.4 per 1000 patient days, $p < 0.001$).

■ The estimated financial savings due to the 66% reduction in ADEs (58 ADEs prevented during the study) was $270,000 per year in the 17-bed medical ICU. Extrapolated to the entire hospital, the financial ramifications of the pharmacist interventions are even more substantial.

■ Mean length of stay, cost, and mortality are nearly doubled in patients who suffer an adverse drug event.

Another study by Scarsi et al. performed in a 600-bed academic medical center analyzed pharmacist impact when added to daily rounds for 30 days on one general medicine service. The study organizers concluded that the reduction in medication errors at the time of prescribing may have been due to the pharmacist gaining a more thorough clinical picture of the patient by participating in rounds. Medication errors were reduced by 51% ($p < 0.05$) after inclusion of the pharmacist. The number of patients without a medication error during their hospitalization increased by 22.9% in the control group versus 40% in the intervention group ($p < 0.05$).

In addition to preventing a large number of errors before their occurrence, the pharmacist was also able to more quickly identify and rectify errors that had already taken place. The amount of time an error persisted after it had occurred was less than 1 day and one dose of medication given in the intervention group compared to 2.4 days and two doses of medication in the control group. Other data from this study that support the vital impact of a clinical pharmacist include the positive effects on the total number of errors in the intervention group (46) versus the control group (96) as well as the mean number of errors per patient (1.3 in the intervention group and 2.6 in the control group).

In addition to the numeric data captured by various studies, several other factors that provide a positive impact became apparent when the pharmacist played a more active role on daily rounds.

■ Immediate education was provided to nurses and physicians by answering questions at the time they arise.

■ Pharmacists were able to reduce nursing errors by providing timely consultations and medication safety information before drug administration.

■ Administration errors were eliminated by adjustments of inappropriate food–drug related dosage times, drug–drug interactions, and encouragement of timely medication dosing for time-dependent drugs.

■ Barriers to communication between the healthcare team members were also reduced with more frequent interactions.

Cost Savings

Critical care pharmacist involvement has the potential to save between $25,140 and $318,891 annually depending on the type of unit and institution, number of interventions, number of beds monitored, and pharmaceutical services provided. Despite these variables, the presence of a pharmacist has consistently demonstrated a significant economic advantage. Quantifying actual dollar savings is sometimes difficult, as one must account for both cost savings and cost avoidance. However, numerous studies have confirmed the significant financial impact of pharmacist interventions.

A review of 104 articles published between 1988 and 1995 that evaluated the economic impact of clinical pharmacy services registered a positive financial benefit in 89% of cases. However, many of those evaluations were not performed in an ICU setting. Pharmacy charges comprise approximately 14% of a patient's ICU costs and rank as the fourth highest ICU charge. Expensive and frequently used drug therapies can be targeted by the pharmacist to promote cost savings while optimizing patient care.

A study conducted by Katona et al. in a medical ICU recorded 345 pharmacist interventions including the discontinuation of unnecessary medications and dosage changes (mostly associated with antimicrobials). The interventions accounted for cost savings of $95,972 annually. When extrapolated to all ICUs in that particular institution, the potential savings soared to $551,563. A study by Miyagawa et al. in a surgical ICU counted 332 interventions, which were related to duplicate therapy; inappropriate therapy adjustments; discontinuation of adequate courses of therapy; and medication dosage, route, and frequency changes. These 332 interventions accounted for $72,122 annual cost savings for that intensive care unit.

Summary

Pharmacist education, training, and experience have proven to undoubtedly improve the outcomes and overall quality of pharmaceutical care provided to patients. The addition of a pharmacist to daily patient care rounds improves both the safety and efficacy of drug therapy and promotes more effective communication with physicians and nurses. As healthcare practices continue to change, the activities of the pharmacist will evolve as well, continuing to redefine and prove their role as a vital member of the healthcare team.

ANTIPLATELET AGENTS

Antiplatelet therapy has been established as the treatment of choice for secondary prevention of strokes and transient ischemic attacks (TIAs). Numerous clinical trials have shown a significant relative risk reduction in the incidence of further cerebrovascular ischemia through use of various antiplatelet agents. Currently, four agents have shown efficacy for preventing stroke and/or other vascular events in patients with a history of cerebrovascular disease: aspirin, clopidogrel, ticlopidine, and dipyridamole/aspirin.

In 2004, the Seventh ACCP Conference on Antithrombotic and Thrombolytic Therapy for Ischemic Stroke developed recommendations to help guide practitioners in appropriate management of patients with ischemic stroke.

- In patients who have experienced a noncardio-embolic stroke or TIA, acceptable initial therapy options include:
  ▸ Acetylsalicylic acid (ASA, aspirin) 50–325 mg daily
  ▸ ASA 25 mg in combination with extended-release dipyridamole 200 mg twice daily
  ▸ Clopidogrel 75 mg daily
- For secondary prevention in patients who have previously experienced a noncardio-embolic stroke or TIA, the combination of ASA/dipyridamole 25/200 mg twice daily or clopidogrel 75 mg/day are recommended.

Acetylsalicylic Acid (Aspirin)

Due to its low cost, broad availability, and safety profile, ASA has continued to be the most commonly used antiplatelet medication. Although its efficacy has been proven and its use widely accepted in daily practice, controversy still exists over the appropriate dosing regimen.

MECHANISM OF ACTION

In stimulated platelets, phospholipase A_2 is activated to generate arachidonic acid. Through a series of reactions, arachidonic acid ultimately produces thromboxane A_2, which is a potent vasoconstrictor and stimulator of platelet aggregation. The initial step in this conversion is mediated by the enzyme cyclooxygenase (COX).

- Three isoforms of COX have been identified, with COX-1 being the major isoform expressed in platelets.
- ASA inhibits platelet COX-1 production of thromboxane A_2, preventing platelet aggregation lasting for the entire life of the platelet, 7–10 days.

ASA also exerts antiplatelet effects by inhibiting prostacyclin activity in the smooth muscle of vascular walls, although this has been found to be dose and duration related.

After oral ingestion, ASA is rapidly absorbed in the proximal gastrointestinal (GI) tract (stomach and duodenum), achieving peak serum levels in 15–20 minutes and antithrombotic effects within 40–60 minutes. Owing to the decreased absorption of enteric coated (EC) formulations, platelet inhibition is seen in 60–90 minutes. Since the body replenishes its entire pool of platelets every 10 days, a single dose of ASA can be expected to sustain its effects for more than a week.

DOSING

Owing to its enhanced selectivity against COX-1 as opposed to COX-2 activity, which is expressed in tissues during inflammation, lower doses of ASA are required to achieve its antiplatelet effects than are needed for its anti-inflammatory indications. Recommendations from the Seventh ACCP Conference on Antithrombotic and Thrombolytic Therapy for Ischemic Stroke include early aspirin therapy for patients with ischemic stroke utilizing doses of 160–325 mg/day.

- ASA should be initiated within 48 hours of stroke symptom onset, utilizing nonenteric coated formulations to avoid impaired absorption.
- ASA doses ranging from 25 mg twice daily to 325 mg four times daily have been shown to be efficacious for secondary stroke prevention after TIA.
- Controversy still exists as to whether higher doses offer greater protection. Numerous studies have been completed in an attempt to identify the safest and most efficacious dosing regimen, but to date none have emerged as superior.
- Currently, the approved dosing of ASA for the secondary prevention of stroke is 50–325 mg/day.

The question of the most appropriate ASA dosage for patients that experience an ischemic event while taking ASA still persists. Evidence has not pointed toward enhanced benefit from increasing the dose of ASA as opposed to continuing the same regimen. Physicians may empirically add a second agent or discontinue ASA and initiate therapy with a different antiplatelet medication.

SIDE EFFECTS AND PRECAUTIONS

Side effects from ASA appear to be dose and duration related, with most patients tolerating the drug

in doses ≤325 mg/day for a brief time (6–8 weeks). Side effects include epigastric pain, heartburn, bleeding, nausea, tinnitus, and rash.

- The GI toxicity is dose related, but even low doses increase the risk for developing hemorrhages, especially GI bleeds.
- Conflicting reports exist as to whether enteric coated ASA significantly reduces the risk for major bleeding.
- Minor dyspepsia has also been reported, but often can be attenuated by dosing with meals or reducing the ASA dose.
  - ▸ Patients with a history of or current GI erosions should be prescribed a proton pump inhibitor (PPI) for further GI protection.
- Doses of >2 g/day have been associated with ototoxicity and toxic hepatitis.
- ASA is contraindicated in patients with active GI bleeding or those with an allergy to ASA and should not be given to children due to the risk of Reye's syndrome.

DRUG INTERACTIONS

ASA exhibits interactions with drugs that can increase the risk of bleeding. Increased patient education and monitoring should accompany the concomitant use of any of these medications. These interacting agents include but are not limited to heparin, low molecular weight heparins, warfarin, and nonsteroidal anti-inflammatory drugs (NSAIDs).

- Coadministration with NSAIDs may interfere with the irreversible inactivation of COX-1 due to competition for receptor binding sites on the platelet surface, thus reducing platelet inhibition.
  - ▸ This competition is not seen with COX-2 selective NSAIDs such as diclofenac.
- Owing to aspirin's COX-1 inhibition, the antihypertensive effects of angiotensin converting enzyme inhibitors (ACE-I) may be blunted when administered with doses of ASA >100 mg. Patients in whom this decreased effect is noted may be changed to clopidogrel or an angiotensin II receptor antagonist.

ASA RESISTANCE

ASA resistance is a topic that has started to receive more attention, as the drug's clinical benefit may be blunted in up to 35% of patients. It is important to separate the concepts of ASA resistance (insufficient platelet inhibition seen through laboratory tests) and ASA failure (patients that have recurrent vascular events despite ASA therapy). Some of the hypotheses attempting to explain the etiology of ASA resistance include:

- Poor compliance
- Drug interactions
- Inadequate absorption
- Subtherapeutic dosing
- Genetic factors

Other mechanisms that may add to ASA resistance include:

- Cigarette smoking
- Diabetes mellitus
- Stress
- Elevated serum cholesterol

A study of 129 patients taking ASA attempted to quantify the incidence of ASA resistance and identify possible associations between dosage, drug formulation, and resistance. This study utilized the PFA-100, a laboratory assessment tool used to analyze platelet function. Overall, the PFA-100 was more likely to show therapeutic antiplatelet effects with higher doses and uncoated formulations of ASA. Other results noted in this study included:

- 37% percent of patients on any ASA dose had a normal PFA-100, which indicates no antiplatelet effect despite ASA therapy.
- 56% of patients taking 81 mg/day had insufficient antiplatelet effects compared to 28% of patients taking 325 mg/day ($p = 0.001$).
- There was a 65% resistance rate for EC ASA versus 25% for non-EC ASA ($p < 0.001$).
- Patients >63 years of age showed reduced response to ASA independent of dose or formulation.
- Approximately 7% of patients never achieved therapeutic values even with doses of 650 mg twice daily of non-enteric coated ASA.

Clopidogrel

Clopidogrel represents an alternative to ASA therapy with a better safety profile and at least equivalent efficacy in the secondary prevention of cerebrovascular ischemic events. The use of clopidogrel in clinical practice has steadily increased owing to its proven efficacy and improved safety profile compared to other antiplatelet agents.

The Clopidogrel versus Aspirin in Patients at Risk of Ischemic Events (CAPRIE) trial assessed the efficacy of 75 mg/day of clopidogrel and 325 mg/day of ASA in reducing ischemic events in patients with recent ischemic stroke or myocardial infarction (MI).

- In the intention-to-treat analysis, clopidogrel showed a statistically significant 8.7% relative risk reduction in the incidence of ischemic stroke, MI, and vascular death compared to ASA.
- In the stroke subgroup, the 7.3% relative risk reduction in favor of clopidogrel was not statistically significant.
- Although clopidogrel was slightly more efficacious in reducing the cluster of ischemic events, the benefit was small (0.5% absolute annual risk reduction) and no significant benefit was seen in patients with a recent stroke.

MECHANISM OF ACTION

Clopidogrel is a prodrug that inhibits platelet aggregation by interfering with adenosine diphosphate (ADP)-induced membrane mediated platelet-fibrinogen binding. By directly blocking the binding of ADP to its receptor site, clopidogrel halts the subsequent ADP-mediated activation of the glycoprotein IIb/IIIa complex, thereby inhibiting platelet aggregation. The effect on platelet function is irreversible for the life of the platelet.

In vitro, clopidogrel fails to exert any activity on ADP-induced platelet activation, indicating the necessity of in vivo hepatic transformation of the parent compound into an active metabolite. The metabolite responsible for the clinical effects of clopidogrel has not yet been isolated. With typical daily dosing, approximately 25% inhibition is seen within 48 hours and a response of 40–50% is noted after 3–4 days of regular administration. Full inhibition of platelet aggregation is seen within 2 hours after a single loading dose of ≥525 mg.

DOSING

Typical dosing of clopidogrel is 75 mg once daily.

SIDE EFFECTS AND PRECAUTIONS

The safety profile of clopidogrel, as seen through results of clinical trials, is at least as good as that of

ASA, with only diarrhea and rash occurring more frequently.

- The incidence of GI disturbance and hemorrhage was more significant with ASA.
- Clopidogrel is contraindicated in patients with active bleeding, coagulation disorders, or in those with hypersensitivity reactions to the drug.

DRUG INTERACTIONS

Drug interactions with clopidogrel include medications that increase the risk of bleeding, including other antiplatelet medications, NSAIDs, and warfarin. Lipophilic 3-hydroxy-3-methylglutaryl coenzyme A (HMG-CoA) reductase inhibitors or "statins" may interfere with the therapeutic effects of clopidogrel through inhibition of CYP3A4 enzymes. This reduces the activity of clopidogrel by decreasing the breakdown of the drug to its active metabolite.

- An in vitro study with clopidogrel plus atorvastatin showed the metabolism of the antiplatelet agent was inhibited by >90%.
- However, post hoc analyses of statins and clopidogrel failed to detect any significant interaction.

Other 3A4 substrates such as cyclosporine or erythromycin may have similar interactions due to a decrease in the bioavailability of the active metabolite. CYP3A4 inducers such as rifampin may enhance the effects of clopidogrel by increasing hepatic transformation of the prodrug to its active metabolite.

Recent studies have demonstrated a new and potentially clinically significant drug interaction between clopidogrel and the PPIs. The main interacting medication identified has been omeprazole, which has shown that concomitant therapy increases the risk of thrombosis and adverse outcomes and may decrease the ability of clopidogrel to prevent acute myocardial events.

- Studies have shown omeprazole significantly reduces clopidogrel's effect on platelet activity.
- Case-controlled and cohort studies have demonstrated an increased risk of recurrent myocardial infarction or rehospitalization for acute coronary syndrome.
- However, an observational study with esomeprazole and pantoprazole demonstrated no effect on platelet activity, posing the question of whether the interaction is truly consistent throughout the PPI drug class or applies solely to omeprazole.

The true clinical implications of this interaction have yet to be determined. However, it may be prudent for practitioners to reassess patients that are on these medications concomitantly. Points of consideration include:

- Clinical necessity of acid-lowering therapy with a PPI.
- Opportunity to utilize an alternative class of acid-reducing medications such as the histamine-2 receptor antagonists.

Potentially choosing to utilize pantoprazole or esomeprazole instead of omeprazole if a PPI is required.

Combination Therapy

Combination antiplatelet therapy with clopidogrel and ASA is being utilized more readily in clinical practice. Since the two agents enact their platelet inhibition through different mechanisms, their combined use would theoretically provide enhanced antiplatelet effects. Multiple studies have analyzed this combination compared to each agent alone.

The Management of Atherothrombosis with Clopidogrel in High-risk patients (MATCH) trial assessed clopidogrel (75 mg/day) plus ASA (75 mg/day) versus clopidogrel alone (75 mg/day) over 18 months in patients with a recent TIA or ischemic stroke.

- Combination therapy provided no significant benefit over clopidogrel alone (absolute risk reduction 1%).
- However, this study was completed on a high-risk patient population and may not necessarily be extrapolated to the stroke population as a whole.
- There was a statistically significant increase in life-threatening bleeding seen in the dual agent group (2.6% vs. 1.3%).

In contrast, results of the Clopidogrel and Aspirin for the Reduction of Emboli in Symptomatic Carotid Stenosis (CARESS) trial showed greater efficacy with dual antiplatelet agents in the reduction of the incidence of silent microemboli (an independent predictor of subsequent cerebrovascular events in patients with recent symptomatic carotid stenosis).

- In comparison to ASA alone, treatment with a 300-mg loading dose of clopidogrel on day 1 with 75 mg/day thereafter in addition to 75 mg/day of ASA provided a 25% reduction in the incidence of cerebral microemboli present on Doppler ultrasonography on day 1 and a reduction of 37% after 7 days of dual therapy.

■ No reports of life-threatening bleeding episodes were seen with dual therapy.

The Plavix Use for Treatment of Stroke (PLUTO-Stroke) trial was designed to determine if clopidogrel with ASA was more effective than ASA alone in patients with a recent ischemic stroke. After 30 days of treatment, the addition of clopidogrel resulted in statistically significant decreases in various platelet activities including platelet aggregation.

Ticlopidine

Ticlopidine hydrochloride, which is chemically related to clopidogrel, also prevents platelet aggregation induced by ADP and is approved in the United States for the prevention of stroke in patients with a prior TIA or minor stroke. Although ticlopidine has been proven efficacious for this indication, its use is limited by its poor side effect profile, typically reserving its use for patients intolerant to ASA or those who have experienced subsequent ischemic events despite aspirin therapy.

The results of two large, randomized, multicenter trials serve as the major clinical evidence supporting the efficacy of ticlopidine in stroke prevention. The Canadian American Ticlopidine Study (CATS) assessed the efficacy of ticlopidine in reducing the incidence of vascular events such as stroke, MI, or vascular death in patients with a recent stroke. Patients that had experienced a stroke in the past week to 4 months were randomized to receive either ticlopidine 250 mg twice daily or placebo.

■ The relative risk reduction in vascular events associated with the use of ticlopidine was 23.3% ($p = 0.02$).

■ Ticlopidine reduced the relative risk of ischemic stroke by 33.5% ($p = 0.008$).

The Ticlopidine Aspirin Stroke Study (TASS) compared the efficacy of ticlopidine 250 mg twice daily to 650 mg twice daily of aspirin therapy in the reduction of stroke incidence and death from all causes in patients with ischemic symptoms in the preceding 3 months.

■ The overall risk reduction of fatal and nonfatal stroke by ticlopidine at 3 years was 21%.

■ Ticlopidine exhibited a 9% reduction in the endpoints of stroke, MI, and vascular death.

■ When compared to ASA, ticlopidine exhibited a 12% reduction in the risk of stroke and all causes of death.

■ A subgroup analysis revealed that ticlopidine was particularly effective in patients that had been taking ASA or anticoagulant therapy at the time of their qualifying cerebral ischemic event.

MECHANISM OF ACTION

Similar to clopidogrel, ticlopidine exerts its inhibition of platelet aggregation by blocking ADP-mediated platelet binding. By inhibiting the ADP pathway, the platelet membrane is affected and the membrane-fibrinogenic interaction is altered, resulting in the blocking of the platelet glycoprotein IIb/IIIa receptor. Unlike ASA, ticlopidine alters the first and second phases of platelet aggregation by altering epinephrine, arachidonic acid, and collagen-mediated platelet aggregation to varying degrees.

The inhibition of platelet function by ticlopidine lasts for the lifetime of the platelet. Optimal antiplatelet effects are not seen for 8–11 days, however. During treatment, bleeding time is prolonged up to 5 times normal and returns to baseline 14 days after discontinuation of the drug. Platelet inhibiting effects persist for 72 hours after discontinuation of the drug and progressively decline over the next 4–8 days.

DOSING

The recommended dosing regimen for ticlopidine is 250 mg twice daily with food.

SIDE EFFECTS AND PRECAUTIONS

Diarrhea (12.5%) was the most frequently reported side effect of ticlopidine, but others include rash, nausea, vomiting, dyspepsia, and GI pain. The most severe side effects associated with ticlopidine are hematologic in nature, including neutropenia (2.4%), thrombotic thrombocytopenic purpura (TTP), bone marrow suppression, and agranulocytosis.

■ Severe neutropenia (approximately 1%) usually occurs within the first 90 days of therapy, requiring additional monitoring during the initiation of ticlopidine treatment.

▷ Recommendations include obtaining a complete blood count with differential every 2 weeks for the first 3 months of therapy.

- Although the neutropenia is reversible on discontinuation of the drug, the potential severity of the effect limits the clinical use of ticlopidine.
- Since the severe hematologic side effects typically emerge within the first 90 days of therapy, patients that have safely tolerated the medication through this initial phase can probably continue taking the drug.

DRUG INTERACTIONS

Ticlopidine has the potential to interact with other medications metabolized in the liver. These medications can increase or decrease the effects of ticlopidine depending on their inhibiting or inducing properties.

- Case reports have shown that serum levels of carbamazepine and phenytoin may be increased with concomitant ticlopidine administration due to protein binding interactions.
- Antacids reduce the absorption and bioavailability of ticlopidine and should be administered 2 hours before or after ticlopidine.
- Other interactions include medications that increase the bleeding risk such as antiplatelet agents and anticoagulants such as warfarin.

Dipyridamole

Dipyridamole, a phosphodiesterase inhibitor, paired with ASA theoretically provides an advantage over each agent alone. Used as a single agent, dipyridamole has no role for stroke prevention. When used in combination with ASA, reduction in stroke risk was actually greater than that reported with clopidogrel, although no direct comparisons have been studied.

The main trial that gained dipyridamole its approval for stroke prevention was the second European Stroke Prevention Study (ESPS-2), which was designed to assess the efficacy of extended-release dipyridamole in combination with ASA for the prevention of stroke or death. The ESPS-2 also attempted to determine whether the drug combination was superior to each agent individually.

- Compared with placebo, stroke risk was reduced by 18% with ASA monotherapy ($p = 0.013$), 16% with dipyridamole alone ($p = 0.039$), and 37% with the ASA dipyridamole combination ($p < 0.001$).
- Risk of stroke or death was reduced by 13% with ASA, 15% with dipyridamole, and 24% with combination therapy, although the treatment had no statistically significant effect on death rate alone.

MECHANISM OF ACTION

Dipyridamole is a pyrimidopyrimidine derivative with both vasodilatory and antiplatelet properties. The exact means by which dipyridamole affects platelet aggregation is unknown, but several suggested mechanisms include:

- Inhibition of cyclic nucleotide phosphodiesterase (the enzyme that degrades cAMP), resulting in intraplatelet accumulation of cAMP
- Blockade of adenosine uptake into the platelet at adenosine A_2 receptors, which increases cAMP
- Direct stimulation of prostacyclin (PGI_2) synthesis and protection against its degradation

DOSING

The recommended dosing for ASA/dipyridamole is 25/200 mg twice daily.

SIDE EFFECTS AND PRECAUTIONS

The most commonly reported side effects of dipyridamole-containing products are headache, epigastric pain, nausea, diarrhea, vomiting, and fatigue. When combined with ASA, bleeding episodes are more frequent and severe.

Summary

Over the years, ASA has consistently proven beneficial for ischemic indications and is commonly prescribed today. However, as clinical trial and practical experience with alternative antiplatelet agents such as clopidogrel and dipyridamole/ASA have increased, the utilization of these agents has become a standard of care incorporated into the treatment of patients with acute ischemic events. The choice of medication should be considered carefully to ensure patients experience optimal antiplatelet effects while avoiding potentially severe side effects. Table 7.1 reviews the different antiplatelets used in clinical practice.

Table 7.1. Comparison of antiplatelet agents

Medication	Mechanism of action	Dosing	Peak serum concentration	Half-life	Duration of action	Metabolism	Elimination
Aspirin	Inhibits COX-1 production of thromboxane A_2 and inhibits prostacyclin activity in smooth muscle of vascular walls	50–325 mg once daily	Approximately 1–2 hours	Parent Compound: 15–20 minutes Metabolite: 3–10 hours (dose dependent)	4–6 hours	Hydrolyzed to salicylate (active) by esterases in the GI mucosa, red blood cells, synovial fluid, and blood; metabolism of salicylate primarily hepatic	Follows zero order kinetics. Renal elimination of unchanged drug depends upon urine pH (pH > 6.5 significantly increases renal clearance)
Acetylsalicylic acid (aspirin)/ dipyridamole	Additive effects with aspirin. Dipyridamole inhibits uptake of adenosine into platelets, endothelial cells, and erythrocytes. Inhibits phosphodiesterase, increasing cAMP levels in platelets.	25/200 mg twice daily	Dipyridamole: within 2 hours	Dipyridamole: initial phase 40–80 min, terminal phase 10–12 hrs.	Dipyridamole: no data	Hepatic	Approximately 95% of the metabolite excreted via bile into the feces, with some enterohepatic circulation
Clopidogrel	Blocks ADP binding to its receptor site, preventing subsequent ADP-mediated activation of the glycoprotein IIb/IIIa complex	75 mg daily	Within 2 hours (main circulating metabolite)	8 hours (main circulating metabolite)	72 hours after single 400-mg dose; 5 days after multiple doses	Hepatic CYP 3A4/5 (required for transformation into active metabolite)	Renal
Ticlopidine	Blocks ADP binding to its receptor site, preventing subsequent ADP-mediated activation of the glycoprotein IIb/IIIa complex	250 mg twice daily with food	2 hours (serum levels do not correlate with antiplatelet activity)	4–5 days (variable due to nonlinear pharmacokinetic profile)	Bleeding time returned to baseline within 4–10 days	Hepatic (required for transformation into active metabolite)	Renal

ANTITHROMBOTIC THERAPY

The use of antithrombotic therapy is a delicate science requiring a fine balance between the need for these agents versus the high risk they can often carry. The optimal method of clot prevention without causing bleeding episodes is not always straightforward and varies from patient to patient. Therefore, a thorough understanding of the mechanisms of action, dosing, safety, and efficacy of the various antithrombotic agents is essential. Medications indicated for the prevention of venous thromboembolism (VTE) and the treatment of heparin-induced thrombocytopenia are evaluated in more detail to aid clinicians in determining the safest and most effective options for each patient.

Prevention of Venous Thromboembolism

Venous thromboembolism (VTE) including deep venous thrombosis (DVT) and pulmonary embolism (PE) represent a life-threatening problem that can be a silent but preventable killer. Strategies for preventing DVT and PE are aimed at preventing stasis and reversing coagulation changes, which allow thrombi to form.

Pharmacologic techniques counteract the propensity for thrombus formation by dampening the coagulation cascade. The American College of Chest Physicians (ACCP) guidelines recommend routine prophylaxis with low molecular weight heparin (LMWH) or low-dose unfractionated heparin (UFH) for moderate to high-risk patients.

Appropriately selected pharmacologic therapy can dramatically decrease the incidence of VTE. The choice of drug depends on the relative risk of developing VTE and bleeding complications from therapy. Low-dose subcutaneous (SQ) heparin is the most widely used and studied pharmacologic method for prevention of VTE. It has been shown to be effective in reducing the incidence of DVT and PE in general, abdominal, thoracic, urologic, and some orthopedic surgery patients as well as bedridden patients after MI and stroke.

LMWHs appear to be slightly more effective in preventing VTE when compared to UFH in higher risk patient populations. However, UFH is a highly cost-effective choice for many patients and is effective when dosed properly.

- Routine lab monitoring is not required for preventative UFH therapy.
- The recommended dosage of UFH is 5000 units SQ q8–12h, with the q8h frequency required for high-risk patients but possibly possessing a slightly higher bleeding risk.

Low-dose heparin therapy is not sufficient, however, for preventing VTE in high-risk surgical patients. In this patient population, LMWH is a better option and the combination of pharmacologic and mechanical methods may be prudent. LMWH was found to be equally effective as UFH in DVT prophylaxis in general surgery patients but to a much lower degree in wound hematoma.

No differences in efficacy have been found between the various LMWH products, but they cannot be considered interchangeable because of their pharmacologic differences. No specific guidelines delineate a clear duration of therapy, but prophylaxis should be continued throughout the period of risk. As long as no other risk factors are present, prophylaxis for general surgical procedures and medical conditions may be discontinued once the patient is able to ambulate regularly.

Multiple clinical trials have been completed to assess the safety and efficacy of the various pharmacologic methods of VTE prophylaxis. The MEDENOX (prophylaxis in medical patients with enoxaparin) trial was conducted using the LMWH enoxaparin 20 mg or 40 mg once daily compared to placebo to analyze the incidence of VTE in both groups.

- After 14 days, the incidence of total, proximal, and distal DVT was significantly reduced in the group receiving enoxaparin 40 mg.
- The incidence of VTE in the treatment group was 5.5% compared to 14.9% in the placebo group, representing a 63% relative risk reduction ($p = 0.0002$).
- Outcomes in the 20 mg enoxaparin group were not different from placebo.
- There was also a nonstatistically significant trend toward mortality reduction in the higher dose enoxaparin group.
- The incidences of hemorrhage, thrombocytopenia, or other adverse events were similar in both groups.

The first prospective head-to-head investigation of heparin versus LMWH was the THE-PRINCE

(Thromboembolism-Prevention in Cardiac or Respiratory Disease with Enoxaparin) study. This was the first study to determine that enoxaparin 40 mg SQ daily was equally as effective as heparin 5000 units SQ administered three times daily.

- The enoxaparin group experienced fewer bleeding events, adverse effects, and deaths.
- Thromboembolic events were seen in 8.4% of enoxaparin patients and 10.4% of heparin patients, indicating that enoxaparin was at least as effective as heparin.

A second multicenter, randomized, double-blinded comparison study of enoxaparin 40 mg daily and heparin 5000 units three times daily, the PRIME study group, showed similar results with equivalent efficacy and an improved safety profile in the enoxaparin group.

VTE prophylaxis with LMWH is a cost-effective option in high-risk patients owing to its effectiveness and positive safety profile. There is a stronger risk-to-benefit ratio when using LMWH over UFH for VTE prophylaxis, which supports its utilization in clinical practice. LMWH also carries the advantage of outpatient usage, secondary to its lack of monitoring and convenient dosing and administration. This improves the cost-to-benefit ratio as well.

Heparin

Unfractionated heparin (UFH) is one of the most widely known and utilized anticoagulant medications in clinical practice today. Heparin prevents the growth and propagation of a formed thrombus, allowing the patient's intrinsic thrombolytic system to degrade the clot. However, heparin cannot inhibit thrombin that is fibrin bound, which becomes problematic when thrombolytic therapy is administered. Despite the presence of heparin, fibrin-bound thrombin is released after fibrinolysis and is available to convert fibrinogen to fibrin, which may lead to rethrombosis.

MECHANISM OF ACTION

The anticoagulant effect of heparin is mediated through a specific pentasaccharide sequence on the heparin molecule that binds to antithrombin III, provoking a conformational change. Antithrombin III then binds with factors Xa and thrombin (IIa), causing their inactivation and inhibition of the clotting cascade. The UFH-antithrombin complex is 100–1000 times more potent as an anticoagulant than antithrombin alone. Antithrombin III inactivates multiple factors in the clotting cascade, including factors IXa, Xa, XI, XIIa, and antithrombin (IIa).

Heparin has a strong affinity for platelet factor 4, which is exposed on the surface of activated platelets, but binds nonspecifically to a variety of cells and plasma proteins including antithrombin, macrophages, platelets, fibrinogen, von Willebrand factor, and others. This allows for dose-dependent absorption from subcutaneous injection sites and variability in plasma levels depending on the endogenous concentration of heparin-binding proteins.

MONITORING

Although routine laboratory monitoring is not required when utilizing SO heparin as prophylaxis, it is warranted when utilizing therapeutic IV heparin. This is due to its unpredictable anticoagulant effects, variable, half-life, and utility in dosage titration to maintain a balance between clot prevention and bleeding.

- Heparin causes prolongation of the activated partial thromboplastin time (aPTT), prothrombin time (PT), and thrombin time.
- The most sensitive marker to evaluate heparin therapy is the aPTT.
  - Initial aPTT levels should be drawn 6 hours after initiation of the heparin infusion. Levels drawn any earlier may be misleading and cause inappropriate dosage adjustments.

DOSING

UFH must be given parenterally, with IV and SQ routes being preferred. Intramuscular administration is associated with erratic absorption and is discouraged due to the risk of developing large hematomas. Because the bioavailability after SQ injection is low, <30%, continuous IV administration is more effective than intermittent bolus dosing when rapid anticoagulation is desired, as in the case of DVT or PE. Continuous intravenous administration allows for a more constant plasma level, reducing the risk of bleeding that is associated with high peaks in anticoagulant activity seen with intermittent dosing.

Table 7.2. Heparin Continuous Infusion: Weight Based Protocol*

Initial Dose: 80 units/kg bolus followed by 18 units/kg per hour continuous IV infusion
Dosage Rate Adjustments Based on aPTT levels:

<1.2 times control**	80 unit/kg bolus and increase infusion rate by 4 units/kg per hour
1.2–1.5 times control	40 unit/kg bolus and increase infusion rate by 2 units/kg/per hour
>1.5–2.3 times control	No change
>2.3–3 times control	Decrease infusion rate by 2 units/kg per hour
>3 times control	Hold infusion for 1 hour, then decrease infusion rate by 3 units/kg per hour

*Recommended protocol for treatment of VTE; other protocols are available for differing diagnoses.
**Actual aPTT values may be institution/laboratory specific due to varying laboratory aPTT reagents; goal PTT ranges may need to be decreased in patients at higher risk for hemorrhagic side effects.

- VTE Prophylaxis: 5000 units SQ q8h or q12h
- VTE Treatment: Dosing should be initiated with a bolus of 70–100 units/kg followed by a continuous infusion starting at 15–25 units/kg per hour.
  ▶ If the heparin infusion is held for more than 1 hour, a bolus dose of 25–50 units/kg may be required once restarted.
- Obesity: Doses are based on actual body weight (Table 7.2) but require adjustment for obese patients (>130% of ideal body weight).

SIDE EFFECTS AND PRECAUTIONS

The two most severe side effects of UFH are bleeding and thrombocytopenia. Heparin-induced thrombocytopenia (HIT), a rare but severe drug-induced autoimmune reaction, requires immediate intervention and is discussed in further detail later in this chapter.

- Bleeding risk is dose and duration dependent with a reported 7-day risk of 3.4–9.1%. Low-dose, prophylactic SQ heparin does not carry a high bleeding risk.
  ▶ The most common bleeding sites are GI, genitourinary, and soft tissues.
  ▶ Symptoms include headache, joint pain, chest pain, abdominal pain, swelling, tarry stools, hematuria, and bright red blood per rectum.
- Many factors can increase a patient's bleeding risk, including gender (women > men), age, dose, concurrent ASA use, heavy ethanol use, and comorbid conditions such as liver or kidney failure, cancer, or severe anemia.

If bleeding occurs, heparin should be stopped immediately and protamine sulfate can be given as a reversal agent. Protamine is indicated for the treatment of heparin toxicity in the presence of hemorrhage or an increased risk of hemorrhage. It is not indicated in cases of minor bleeding as withdrawal of heparin will generally result in correction of bleeding within several hours. Protamine combines with heparin to form salts devoid of any anticoagulant effect. Since IV heparin has a short half-life, its concentration declines rapidly after discontinuation of the infusion, requiring lower protamine doses as the heparin is metabolized. Protamine sulfate itself can exhibit anticoagulant properties if given in excessive doses so it is extremely important to appropriately calculate the reversal dose. Dosing can be determined by using the following recommendations:

- Heparin prophylactic 5000 unit SQ doses:
  ▶ <2 hours since last heparin dose: administer 25 mg of protamine
  ▶ > 2 hours since last heparin dose: administered 12.5 mg of protamine
  ▶ A portion of the protamine dose can be given as a slow IV infusion over 10 minutes followed by the remainder administered as a continuous IV infusion over 8–16 hours, which represents the expected absorption time of the SQ heparin dose
- Heparin treatment IV doses: 1 mg of protamine can be expected to neutralize 100 units of heparin. Practitioners should calculate the total amount of

heparin administered to the patient based upon time intervals. The maximum protamine dosage is 50 mg.

Time elapsed since previous heparin dose	Protamine dose per 100 units of heparin administered
30 minutes	1 mg
30–60 minutes	0.5–0.75 mg
60–120 minutes	0.375–0.5 mg
>120 minutes	0.25–0.375 mg

Protamine injections have been associated with the occurrence of hypotension and anaphylactoid-like symptoms such as dyspnea, bradycardia, and flushing. In order to avoid these side effects the administration of protamine should be over 10 minutes and should never exceed 50 mg in any 10 minute time period. Coagulation tests can be performed 5–15 minutes after the protamine dose has been given.

Other side effects of heparin include local irritation at the administration site with mild pain, erythema, histamine-like reactions, and hematomas. Patients may also experience hypersensitivity reactions characterized by chills, fever, urticaria, and rarely bronchospasm, nausea, vomiting, and shock. Long-term UFH use has been reported to case alopecia, priapism, hyperkalemia, and osteoporosis.

Contraindications to UFH include hypersensitivity to the drug, active bleeding, hemophilia, severe liver disease with an elevated PT, severe thrombocytopenia, malignant hypertension, and inability to monitor therapy. Due to the hemorrhagic risk, patients with bacterial endocarditis, active tuberculosis, and visceral carcinoma should not receive heparin as well as those undergoing a lumbar puncture or regional anesthetic block.

Low Molecular Weight Heparins

Low molecular weight heparins (LMWH), which are prepared by depolymerization of porcine heparin, are being utilized more frequently because of their safety profile and minimal monitoring requirements. The mean molecular weight of LMWH (5000 daltons) is one-third of the molecular weight of UFH. LMWH has been shown to be at least as effective or superior to UFH in the treatment of DVT with or without PE with an overall reduction in major bleeding episodes and mortality. It is also an alternative to warfarin when international normalized ratio (INR) monitoring is unavailable. Advantages of LMWH over UFH include:

- More predictable anticoagulation dose response
- Improved SQ bioavailability
- Dose-independent clearance
- Longer half-life
- Lower incidence of thrombocytopenia
- Less need for routine laboratory monitoring

MECHANISM OF ACTION

LMWH prevents the growth and propagation of a formed thrombus by binding to antithrombin III, thus enhancing and accelerating its activity. The LMWH/antithrombin complex binds to factor Xa and thrombin, causing their inactivation and disruption of the clotting cascade. Similar to UFH, LMWH is unable to inhibit fibrin-bound thrombin.

- Fewer than half of the LMWH chains are long enough to bind thrombin (IIa). Therefore, the LMWH–antithrombin complex has weak antithrombin activity but retains the ability to inactivate factor Xa.
  - This preferential binding is apparent when reviewing the ratio of anti-Xa to anti-IIa activity, which varies from 2:1 to 4:1 depending on the LMWH product.
  - Because of its weak effect on thrombin, LMWH prolongs the aPTT only when present in very high concentrations.

MONITORING

Due to its lack of protein binding, LMWH has a high rate of absorption and more predictable plasma levels than heparin, making routine lab monitoring usually unnecessary. Before initiation of therapy, a baseline PT/INR, aPTT, complete blood count (CBC), platelet count, and serum creatinine (SCr) should be obtained. Periodic monitoring of the CBC, platelet count, and presence of fecal blood is recommended.

It is recommended, however, that plasma anti-Xa levels be checked in patients in whom higher levels may be anticipated, such as:

- Adults <50 kg or >110 kg
- Pregnant women (dose may change as weight changes during pregnancy)

- Patients with a high bleeding risk
- Patients with renal insufficiency (LMWH is largely excreted through the kidneys)

LMWH anti-Xa levels should be drawn after the third or fourth dose approximately 4 hours after the dose has been given. Acceptable levels for LMWH differ based on dosing frequency and indication (may be institution/lab specific):

- Treatment: 0.6–1 international units/mL in patients receiving LMWH twice daily or 1–2 international units/mL for once daily administration
- Prophylaxis: 0.2–0.5 international units/mL regardless of dosing frequency

LMWH Products

Several different LMWH products are currently available, each with a different manufacturing process and slightly altered pharmacologic properties including plasma clearance, bioavailability, and inhibitory activities against factor Xa. Therefore, dosing regimens are different for each product. All are highly bioavailable, however, allowing for SQ administration based off of total body weight. Two LMWH products, enoxaparin and dalteparin, are currently approved by the U.S. Food and Drug Administration (FDA) for VTE prophylaxis and treatment.

Enoxaparin

DOSING

- VTE prophylaxis: 30 mg SQ q12h or 40 mg SQ daily, based off of actual body weight
- VTE treatment: 1 mg/kg SQ q12h or 1.5 mg/kg daily
  - Each 1 mg of enoxaparin = approximately 100 international units of anti-Xa activity
- Renal insufficiency: The manufacturer recommends reducing the daily dose by 50% in patients with a creatinine clearance (CrCl) <30 mL/min achieved by adjusting the frequency from q12h to q24h.
- Obesity: Enoxaparin dosing in obese patients may also require adjustments.
  - Prophylaxis: It is reasonable to increase the dose by 25% to 40 mg SQ twice daily. Prophylactic doses can be adjusted based upon a patient's body mass index (BMI).
  - Treatment: It is still acceptable to utilize total body weight for treatment dosing; however, no studies for enoxaparin have been completed

on patients >140 kg. Therefore, caution must be taken if practitioners choose to prescribe doses >140 mg and checking LWMH anti-Xa levels to ensure the regimen is appropriate is recommended.
  - Twice daily dosing is recommended for obese patients instead of 1.5 mg/kg daily.

Dalteparin

DOSING

- VTE prophylaxis: 2500 units SQ q12h or 5000 units SQ daily
- VTE treatment: 100 units/kg SQ q12h or 200 units/kg SQ daily
- Renal insufficiency: Total clearance is lower with delayed elimination in severe renal failure. Dosage adjustment is required due to an increased risk for bleeding. However, no specific dosage recommendations have been developed.

SIDE EFFECTS AND PRECAUTIONS

The major side effect of any LMWH product is bleeding, including gastrointestinal, genitourinary, intracerebral, and retroperitoneal hemorrhages. The incidence of bleeding is lower with LMWH as compared to UFH and most commonly occurs at the site of injection.

- Bleeding may occur at sites of trauma, the most worrisome being epidural bleeding and spinal hematoma after epidural catheter insertion for anesthetic administration.
- Bleeding rates are increased in patients with low body weight, increased age (>70 years), recent surgery or trauma, and patients with concomitant medications that can affect homeostasis (ASA, NSAIDs, etc.).

Protamine can be utilized to aid in the reversal of bleeding caused by LMWH. Protamine completely reverses factor IIa but only partially affects factor Xa, which makes it less effective when used after bleeding from LMWH compared to UFH.

- Recommended dosing:
  - Dalteparin: 1 mg of protamine per 100 anti-Xa units of dalteparin given in the previous 8 hours. If the dalteparin dose was given 8–12 hours

prior, the dose should be reduced by 50%. The maximum neutralization of anti-Xa activity is approximately 60–75%.

▶ Enoxaparin: 1 mg of protamine per 1 mg of enoxaparin given in the previous 8 hours. If the enoxaparin dose was given 8–12 hours prior, the dose should be reduced by 50%. The maximum neutralization of anti-Xa acitivity is approximately 60%.

▶ aPTT levels can be measured 2–4 hours after the protamine infusion. If the aPTT remains prolonged prescribers may consider administering a second protamine infusion with a dose reduction of 50% from the first infusion. Despite a second dose, aPTT results may continue to be prolonged.

■ Protamine is not recommended if the LMWH dose was administered >12 hours prior to the bleeding event.

Injection site reactions characterized by urticaria, pain, and hematoma as well as elevated serum transaminase levels are also seen with LMWH therapy. Thrombocytopenia is rarely seen with LMWH. However, antibodies against platelet factor 4 can be detected in some patients. Therefore, patients that have experienced HIT with UFH should not be changed to LMWH, as cross-reactivity and the risk of developing this severe reaction are likely.

Heparin-induced Thrombocytopenia

The anticoagulant effect of heparin is neutralized when it binds to platelet factor 4. The immune system may then produce antibodies against the platelet factor 4/heparin complex, leading to platelet activation and aggregation. This may lead to a paradoxical effect of a low platelet count but a procoagulant state. Two different types of thrombocytopenia related to heparin use have been described, heparin-associated thrombocytopenia (HAT, sometimes termed heparin-induced thrombocytopenia type 1) and heparin-induced thrombocytopenia (HIT or type 2). It is important to distinguish between the two phenomena because they require different clinical interventions.

HEPARIN-ASSOCIATED THROMBOCYTOPENIA

Heparin-associated thrombocytopenia (HAT) is a benign, transient, mild reaction that occurs within the first 5 days of treatment. This reaction is most likely due to the temporary sequestration of platelets secondary to the mild platelet aggregating effects of heparin. The platelet count rarely drops below $100,000/mm^3$ and will rebound to normal values during continued heparin therapy. Therefore, heparin therapy need not be discontinued.

HEPARIN-INDUCED THROMBOCYTOPENIA

Heparin-induced thrombocytopenia is a serious reaction that requires immediate discontinuation of all heparin products and initiation of an alternative anticoagulant. HIT is associated with a 25–50% incidence of venous and arterial thromboembolic events with a 20–30% mortality rate. This immune-mediated reaction is dose and route independent and can occur with IV and SQ forms of heparin as well as with heparin flushes administered through IV lines.

During normal heparin therapy, platelet counts should be monitored at least every 2–3 days and a diagnosis of HIT should be suspected if the platelet count drops by >50% or to $<100,000/mm^3$. Platelet counts typically begin to decrease after 5–14 days of heparin use and can drop as low as $20,000/mm^3$. The immune-mediated platelet activation and thrombin generation seen in HIT can lead to severe thrombotic complications in arteries or veins including limb artery occlusions, stroke, MI, DVT, and PE. Skin lesions occur in 10–20% of patients with HIT and vary from painful, localized, erythematous plaques to widespread dermal necrosis that may require amputation. Table 7.3 summarizes the difference between HAT and HIT.

HIT Treatment

When the diagnosis of HIT is made, patients should not be switched to LMWH because there is a high risk of cross-reactivity. Rather, therapy should be initiated with one of the direct thrombin inhibitors lepirudin or argatroban, which are FDA approved for the treatment of HIT. Fondaparinux has also been used off-label for HIT but is not ideal due to its long half-life and renal elimination. Alternate anticoagulation therapy should be continued until the platelet count has rebounded to near normal levels ($>100,000/mm^3$) and no new thromboses have emerged. Transitioning to an oral

Table 7.3. Difference between heparin-associated thrombocytopenia and heparin induced thrombocytopenia

Heparin-associated thrombocytopenia	Heparin-induced thrombocytopenia
Benign reaction	Severe reaction
Platelet count rarely falls to <100,000/mm³ (up to 30% from baseline)	Platelet count falls below 100,000/mm³ (50% from baseline)
Occurs during first 5 days of therapy	Occurs during days 5–14 of therapy
Heparin may be continued	Heparin must be immediately discontinued
Not associated with ↑ risk of thrombosis	Associated with ↑ risk of thrombosis
Not autoimmune mediated	Autoimmune mediated
Resolves spontaneously	Resolves only after heparin discontinued

anticoagulant such as warfarin can then cautiously be undertaken.

Direct Thrombin Inhibitors

Direct thrombin inhibitors (DTIs) are capable of inhibiting both circulating and clot-bound thrombin, which is a potential advantage over UFH and LMWH. These agents have no cross-reactivity with HIT antibodies and lack immune-mediated thrombocytopenia, which makes them ideal alternatives for prophylaxis or treatment of thrombosis in patients currently exhibiting or previously experiencing HIT. Currently, three DTIs are commercially available, with only two, argatroban and lepirudin, carrying the FDA indication for the prophylaxis and treatment of thrombosis in patients with HIT. Argatroban is usually avoided in patients with hepatic impairment due to drug accumulation and increased risk for hemorrhagic side effects, but is preferred over lepirudin for patients with renal insufficiency.

Although not FDA approved for the treatment of HIT, the third DTI, bivalirudin, a recombinant analog of hirudin, has also been successfully employed off-label for thrombosis. The incidence of bleeding and antibody production may be lower with bivalirudin than with lepirudin. Bivalirudin also represents an alternative option to argatroban and lepirudin in patients with both renal and hepatic dysfunction.

MONITORING
- DTIs alter PT and INR levels but the aPTT is utilized as the main monitoring parameter.

- A CBC should be obtained at baseline and periodically thereafter to detect potential bleeding complications.
- After baseline coagulation studies are obtained, the dose should be titrated to achieve specified aPTT ratios compared to the control value.
  - ▹ Patients with aPTT levels elevated to 2.5 times greater than control before initiation of therapy with a DTI should probably not be started on the medication until lab normalization occurs.
- Close monitoring of the aPTT and INR is required when transitioning patients from a direct thrombin inhibitor to warfarin, as the INR may be falsely elevated.

Argatroban

MECHANISM OF ACTION. Argatroban is a synthetic agent derived from L-arginine that reversibly binds to the active catalytic site of thrombin. As with all DTIs, argatroban is able to bind to both clot-bound and free thrombin, thus inhibiting fibrin formation and activation of coagulation factors V, VIII, XIII, protein C, and platelet aggregation.

DOSING
- The recommended dosage for HIT is 2 µg/kg per minute by continuous IV infusion. Doses can be made using patient's actual body weight up to a maximum of 140 kg.
- Renal insufficiency: No adjustments are required because elimination is primarily through hepatobiliary excretion.

- Hepatic insufficiency: Significant dosing reductions to 0.5 µg/kg per minute are necessary.
- The first aPTT should be obtained 2–4 hours after initiation of the infusion.
- Dose adjustments should be made until the aPTT has reached 1.5–3 times baseline with a maximum rate of 10 µg/kg per minute.
  - No standards or guidelines exist for dosage titrations.
  - aPTT levels should be checked 2–3 hours after each dosage adjustment. Once the PTT has stabilized for two measurements, levels can be check daily, unless another dosage change occurs.

SIDE EFFECTS AND PRECAUTIONS

Since no specific agent is available to reverse bleeding due to argatroban, treatment should be supportive after discontinuation of the drug. Reversal of the anticoagulant effects will take longer in patients with reduced hepatic function. Dyspnea, hypotension, and fever have also been reported.

DRUG INTERACTIONS

The main drug interactions are those with medications such as NSAIDs, warfarin, thrombolytics, and antiplatelet agents that increase the incidence of hemorrhage.

TRANSITIONING TO WARFARIN

Conversion of argatroban to warfarin can be difficult and requires close monitoring due to the combined effects of both medications on the INR. If conversion to warfarin is indicated, therapy should not be initiated until after the platelet count has reached >100,000/mm³. Overlap of argatroban with warfarin is required for 4–5 days with daily monitoring of the INR. No loading dose is necessary with warfarin initiation but a baseline INR should be obtained. Transitioning from argatroban to warfarin can be completed as follows:

- Patients receiving <2 µg/kg per minute of argatroban:
  - Administer warfarin dose.
  - INR measurement should be repeated in 4–6 hours.
  - Argatroban therapy can be stopped once INR on both medications is >4.
  - If the INR is <4, argatroban should be restarted and the sequence should be repeated daily

until the desired INR is achieved on warfarin alone.
- Patients maintained on argatroban doses >2 µg/kg per minute:
  - Decrease argatroban infusion rate to 2 µg/kg per minute when warfarin is started.
  - Check INR in 4–6 hours after the argatroban dose reduction.
  - Argatroban therapy can be stopped once INR on both agents is >4.
  - After discontinuation of the argatroban drip, a second INR should be obtained in 4–6 hours. If the level is <4 then argatroban should be restarted at the previous infusion rate and this sequence repeated daily until the goal INR is achieved.

Lepirudin

MECHANISM OF ACTION. Lepirudin is a recombinant hirudin analog derived from leech saliva that binds irreversibly and with high specificity to thrombin.

DOSING

- Recommended dosing for HIT is 0.4 mg/kg (max 44 mg) slow IV bolus followed by 0.15 mg/kg per hour of continuous IV infusion based on total body weight (max rate 16.5 mg/h).
- Renal insufficiency: The recommended dose adjustment for CrCl <60 mL/min or SCr >1.5 mg/dL is a bolus of 0.2 mg/kg followed by a decreased infusion rate. Lepirudin should be avoided in patients on hemodialysis.
- Hepatic insufficiency: No adjustment required.

The dosage should be adjusted based upon the aPTT levels with the goal range of 1.5–2.5 times the baseline result. The first aPTT should be obtained 4 hours after the start of the infusion and repeat checks are recommended 4 hours after any rate change. Once the aPTT level stabilizes, repeat checks can be completed on a daily basis with more frequent assessments in patients with renal or hepatic impairment. Dose modifications based on the aPTT results can be made as follows:

- aPTT ratio > goal range: hold infusion for 2 hours, then restart at 50% of prior rate.
  - Recheck aPTT 4 hours after restarting infusion.

- aPTT ratio < goal range: increase the infusion rate in increments of 20%.
  - Recheck aPTT 4 hours after increasing infusion rate.

SIDE EFFECTS AND PRECAUTIONS
Approximately 40% of patients treated with lepirudin for 10 days develop antihirudin antibodies, which reduce its renal clearance rate and may increase its anticoagulant effect. Therefore, monitoring of the aPTT is required to assess the need for dose adjustments as clearance is altered.

As with all anticoagulants, the major side effect of lepirudin is bleeding. Bleeding can occur at virtually any site. No antidote is available to counteract bleeding, but the drug should be discontinued immediately if bleeding is noted. Case reports have suggested that hemofiltration or hemodialysis may be useful. Anemia has also been reported with lepirudin use.

DRUG INTERACTIONS
Drug interactions include medications that increase the risk of hemorrhage such as aspirin, warfarin, and NSAIDs. Some cephalosporin and parenteral penicillin antibiotics may enhance the bleeding risk. Contraindications are similar to those for other anticoagulants.

TRANSITIONING TO WARFARIN
When transitioning patients from lepirudin to warfarin, the dose of lepirudin should be gradually reduced to reach an aPTT ratio slightly above 1.5 times control before beginning oral anticoagulation. An overlap of lepirudin with warfarin of 4–5 days is recommended. Loading doses of warfarin are not required. Once the INR is ≥2 lepirudin can be discontinued.

Summary
The prevention and treatment of VTE can be a difficult area to navigate, as the medications for these indications can carry a high risk. Therapy with UFH or LMWH is effective but requires close attention owing to the severity of their potential side effects. If the immune-mediated adverse effect of HIT is noted, then the utilization of a direct thrombin inhibitor is warranted. Although practitioners may be starting to become more familiar with argatroban

and lepirudin, caution is needed in certain patient populations. Therefore, a thorough understanding of the dosing, side effects, and pharmacokinetic parameters of these medications is essential.

ANTIEPILEPTIC MEDICATIONS
With multiple drug entities on the market, choosing an antiepileptic drug (AED) for a patient can be a daunting task. Patient specific characteristics, administration idiosyncrasies, and side effect profiles must all be considered to select the medication with the best patient-specific fit. After an AED is initiated, monitoring must be performed to ensure efficacy and tolerability, as well as prevent toxicities (or minimize them should they arise). Specially trained to evaluate drug interactions, detect subtle side effects, and interpret lab data regarding medications, pharmacists can be a powerful ally in this drug selection process.

Outlined below are several of the AEDs frequently used to treat seizures in the ICU. Specific FDA-approved indications, mechanisms of action (MOA), drug interactions, and adverse effects are discussed for each medication individually.

Carbamazepine (Tegretol, Carbatrol)
Carbamazepine is an AED indicated for the treatment of complex partial seizures, generalized seizures, and mixed seizure types including those listed above. Use in patients with absence seizures is not indicated.

MECHANISM OF ACTION
While the postulated mechanism of action involves the inhibition of voltage-gated sodium channels, the exact mechanism of action of carbamazepine remains unknown.

ADVERSE EFFECTS
The FDA has placed a black-box warning on the prescribing of this medication for the risk of agranulocytosis and aplastic anemia. These hematologic abnormalities occur 6–8 times more frequently in patients on carbamazepine therapy than those in the general public, but the overall risk remains quite low. Nevertheless, it is recommended that a baseline check and periodic monitoring of complete blood counts (CBC) be performed. Potentially

Table 7.4. Antithrombotics used in clinical practice

Medication	Mechanism of action	Dosing	Onset	Half-life	Reversal agent	Monitoring	Other considerations
Heparin (UFH)	Binds to antithrombin III causing a conformational change and inhibition of clotting cascade. Inactivates coagulation factors IXa, Xa, XI, XIIa, and IIa and prevents conversion of fibrinogen to fibrin.	*Treatment:* continuous IV infusion – weight based protocol *Prophylaxis:* 5000 units SQ q8–12h	*IV:* immediate *SQ:* 20–30 minutes	Averages 90 minutes (Dose-dependent)	Protamine sulfate	aPTT levels	*MOA:* Unable to inhibit fibrin-bound thrombin *Side effect:* Rare but severe thrombocytopenia (HIT) *Other:* The mean molecular weight of UFH is 15,000 daltons.
Low molecular weight heparins	Binds to antithrombin III and inactivates factors Xa and thrombin. Possess a higher affinity for coagulation factor Xa.	Enoxaparin* *Treatment:* 1 mg/kg SQ q12h or 1.5 mg/kg daily *Prophylaxis:* 30 mg q12h or 40 mg SQ daily Dalteparin *Treatment:* 100 units/kg q12h or 200 units/kg SQ daily *Prophylaxis:* 2500 units q12h or 5000 units SQ daily	3–5 hours	Enoxaparin 4.5 hours Dalteparin 3.5 hours	Protamine sulfate (less effective than with UFH)	Anti-Xa level (Not routinely needed)	*MOA:* Unable to inhibit fibrin-bound thrombin *Side effect:* Cross-reactivity possible with risk of thrombocytopenia

(continued)

Table 7.4. (continued)

Medication	Mechanism of action	Dosing	Onset	Half-life	Reversal agent	Monitoring	Other considerations
Argatroban	Reversibly binds to active catalytic site of thrombin. Inhibits fibrin formation and activation of coagulation factors V, VIII, XIII, protein C, and platelet aggregation.	*Standard dose:* 2 µg/kg per minute continuous infusion *Hepatic impairment:* 0.5 µg/kg per minute *Maximum dosage:* 10 µg/kg per minute	30 minutes	39–51 minutes (Up to 181 minutes in severe hepatic insufficiency)	None	aPTT Levels	*MOA:* Able to inhibit fibrin-bound thrombin *Side effect:* No cross-reactivity with UFH for HIT *Other:* Platelet counts returned to normal after day 3 in 53% of patients with HIT
Lepirudin	Binds irreversibly and with high specificity to thrombin.	*Standard dose:* 0.4 mg/kg (max 44 mg) slow IV bolus followed by 0.15 mg/kg per hour continuous IV infusion (max 16.5 mg/h) *Renal impairment:* 0.2 mg/kg IV bolus followed by continuous infusion started at a lower rate	*Bolus:* 10 minutes *Infusion:* 40 minutes	1.3 hours (Up to 2 days in severe renal insufficiency)	None	aPTT Levels	*MOA:* Able to inhibit fibrin-bound thrombin *Side effect:* No cross-reactivity with UFH for thrombocytopenia

*Requires 50% dose reduction in patients with renal insufficiency (CrCl <50 mL/min); dosing choice based on clinical indication.

dangerous dermatological reactions (including Stevens–Johnson syndrome) have been reported, though rarely, with carbamazepine therapy. More commonly reported but less severe side effects include dizziness, drowsiness, unsteadiness, nausea, and vomiting. These lesser side effects can be minimized by initiating therapy at the lowest doses and increasing gradually to the therapeutic range.

DRUG–DRUG INTERACTIONS

Many drug–drug interactions can occur with carbamazepine. Carbamazepine is a substrate and inducer for the CYP 450 hepatic enzyme system, and has an active metabolite, the 10, 11-epoxide. While it is agreed that this metabolite does have antiepileptic activity, the clinical significance of this has yet to be determined. Medications which induce the CYP 450 isoenzyme 3A4 will decrease the serum concentrations of carbamazepine by increasing the metabolism of the drug. Examples of these inducers include, but are not limited to, theophylline, rifampin, and other AEDs such as phenobarbital, primidone, phenytoin, and felbamate. With felbamate, however, research has shown an increase in the presence of the active 10, 11-epoxide metabolite, but the clinical significance of this is unknown.

Inhibitors of CYP 450 3A4 will increase the circulating levels of carbamazepine in the body by decreasing its metabolism. These inhibitor medications include, but are not limited to macrolide antibiotics, "azole" antifungals, nondihydropyridine calcium channel blockers, loratadine, cimetidine, and acetazolamide. Valproic acid is also included in this list, but with its addition, increased levels of the active 10, 11-epoxide metabolite are seen.

As an inducer of the CYP 450 enzyme system, carbamazepine can decrease the effectiveness of other medications by increasing their metabolism. These medications include oral contraceptives, corticosteroids, dihydropyridine calcium channel blockers, tricyclic antidepressants, warfarin, and other AEDs (including ethosuximide, lamotrigine, phenytoin, tiagabine, topiramate, valproic acid, and zonisamide). The list of medications that carbamazepine affects is extensive and only partially listed here.

Gabapentin (Neurontin)

Though indicated for only adjunctive use in patients with partial seizures (with or without secondary generalization), its lack of drug interactions makes gabapentin a choice agent in patients with multiple AEDs or other drug therapies.

MECHANISM OF ACTION

Though structurally similar to gamma-aminobutyric acid (GABA), an inhibitory neurotransmitter, gabapentin appears to lack activity at GABA binding sites, is not metabolized to GABA or a GABA analogue, and does not appear to alter the uptake or release of GABA or other neurotransmitters. Further, gabapentin does not appear to bind to other common neuronal binding sites, which may explain its activity. In vitro studies have shown high binding affinity of gabapentin to voltage-gated calcium channels in animal brain tissue, but the clinical significance is unknown.

ADVERSE EFFECTS

Generally, gabapentin is a very well tolerated medication, even when doses are escalated to the high end of the therapeutic dosing range. Neurologic side effects such as emotional lability, hostility, thought disorders, and hyperkinesias seen in patients younger than 12 years of age are not appreciably noted in adult patients. Dizziness, somnolence, ataxia, fatigue, and nystagmus were the most frequently reported side effects in adults, all occurring in >10% of the treatment population.

DRUG–DRUG INTERACTIONS

As gabapentin is excreted unchanged in the urine and is not highly bound to plasma proteins, the incidence of drug-drug interactions is negligible.

Levetiracetam (Keppra)

Without the need to monitor drug levels, and with no clinically significant drug–drug interactions, levetiracetam, FDA approved for the treatment of partial seizures, is gaining popularity in use.

MECHANISM OF ACTION

The exact mechanism of levetiracetam is unknown. In animal models, a neuronal binding site for levetiracetam has been elucidated and may explain antiepileptic activity.

ADVERSE EFFECTS

Overall, levetiracetam is a very well tolerated medication. One relatively unique side effect described with levetiracetam therapy, however, is behavioral abnormalities. Increased prevalence of agitation, aggression, irritability, depression, etc. was noted. Because of this, it may be prudent to use caution when considering levetiracetam therapy in patients with a psychiatric history. Somnolence, asthenia, infection, and dizziness were also reported in >10% of the treated population.

DRUG–DRUG INTERACTIONS

At this time, levetiracetam appears devoid of clinically significant drug–drug interactions.

Oxcarbazepine (Trileptal)

Oxcarbazepine, through the effects of its active metabolite 10-monohydroxy (MHD), is clinically indicated for the treatment of partial seizures as both adjunctive and monotherapy for adults.

MECHANISM OF ACTION

While the full mechanism by which oxcarbazepine and MHD achieve their antiepileptic effects is unknown, research has shown activity at receptor sites that may account for at least some of its activity. Through the inhibition of voltage-gated sodium channels, as seen in in vitro studies, MHD and oxcarbazepine cause a stabilization of neural membranes, inhibition of neuronal firing, and thereby a decrease in the propagation of neuronal signals. There is also an increase in potassium conductance accompanying this medication, which may additionally play a role in its therapeutic activity.

ADVERSE EFFECTS

One of the most prevalent and potentially harmful side effects seen with oxcarbazepine therapy is clinically significant hyponatremia. Sodium levels of <125 mmol/L, occurring predominantly within the first 3 months of oxcarbazepine therapy, have been noted in 2.5% of patients in clinical trials. As hyponatremia can occur without clinical symptoms, patients should have routine sodium monitoring performed while treated with oxcarbazepine.

Occurring in >5% of the treated population, the most frequently reported side effects of oxcarbazepine therapy include dizziness, diplopia, ataxia, vomiting, nausea, somnolence, headache, fatigue, abnormal vision, abdominal pain, tremor, dyspepsia, and abnormal gait. While there is much lower incidence of dermatologic side effects noted with oxcarbazepine than with carbamazepine, there have been reports of potentially life-threatening rashes, including Stevens–Johnson syndrome, occurring during oxcarbazepine therapy. For patients experiencing a hypersensitivity reaction to carbamazepine, oxcarbazepine should be utilized for treatment only if the benefit of use clearly outweighs its risk, as cross-reactivity between the two agents will occur in approximately 25–30% of patients.

DRUG–DRUG INTERACTIONS

Clinical studies have shown that oxcarbazepine and high concentrations of MHD are responsible for both induction and inhibition of the CYP 450 hepatic enzyme system, potentially affecting the metabolism of many other medications. Thankfully, in practice this has not been proven clinically relevant, with the following exceptions: potential increases in phenytoin and phenobarbital serum concentrations, decreased concentrations of hormonal contraceptives and felodipine. Oxcarbazepine and MHD are affected by the administration of other medications, altering the serum levels of either of these molecular entities, which can affect clinical response. The coadministration of carbamazepine, phenobarbital, phenytoin, valproic acid, or other competent inducers of the CYP 450 system decreases MHD concentrations. Similarly, the administration of verapamil decreases MHD concentrations by 20%.

Barbiturates

As one of the oldest classes of AEDs, the barbiturates as a family of medications have proven greatly effective in the suppression of seizures. With many available medications in this family, as well as many dosage forms that accompany the drugs (including intravenous formulations), there should be a barbiturate available to treat most patients with generalized and partial seizures. With quite an extensive list of potential adverse effects, however, clinical practice is moving away from barbiturates in the chronic management of patients and toward the use of the newer AEDs with more favorable side effect profiles.

MECHANISM OF ACTION

Phenobarbital and all barbiturates are nonspecific central nervous system (CNS) depressants which decrease neuronal postsynaptic excitation. Because of this nonspecific activity, barbiturates are effective against most seizure types.

ADVERSE EFFECTS

Since the advent of the newer generation AEDs, barbiturate usage has significantly decreased. This decrease is not surprisingly due, in part, to their extensive side effect profile. Somnolence, estimated to occur in one-third of all patients treated with phenobarbital, is a major complaint. Other reported side effects include lethargy, vertigo, and hyperexcitability in children.

DRUG–DRUG INTERACTIONS

As inducers and substrates of the hepatic enzyme system, barbiturates interact with many medications, including warfarin, exogenous corticosteroids, oral contraceptives, and many AEDs, which may be concomitant therapy in a treatment-resistant patient. Therapeutic levels of carbamazepine, oxcarbazepine, and phenytoin may decrease when barbiturate therapy is initiated, calling for more vigilant patient monitoring. Valproic acid, being a hepatic enzyme inhibitor, may increase circulating barbiturate levels.

Phenytoin (Dilantin, Phenytek)

Phenytoin has long held its reign as one of the most commonly used AEDs due to broad antiepileptic activity. This medication carries indications for the treatment of generalized seizures (with the exception of absence seizures), complex partial seizures, and prophylaxis of seizures after neurosurgical procedures. Though prescribers are often familiar with this medication, complex pharmacokinetics and pharmacodynamics, requiring the need for therapeutic drug level monitoring, treating patients with this medication has never been simple.

MECHANISM OF ACTION

The action of phenytoin in promoting sodium ion efflux with the resultant stabilization of neuronal cell membranes is its widely accepted antiepileptic mechanism of action.

ADVERSE EFFECTS

Like many of the AEDs, experienced side effects include rash, which is occasionally reported, and rarely Stevens–Johnson syndrome. CBC and hepatic enzyme monitoring may alert prescribers to bone marrow suppression and hepatitis that can also occur with chronic phenytoin therapy.

The most commonly reported but less severe side effects of phenytoin therapy include symptoms of CNS depression such as lethargy, fatigue, blurred vision, and incoordination. As serum drug levels rise above the therapeutic levels, nystagmus, lateral gaze preference, and altered mental status are noted to occur. Side effects associated with chronic therapy include gingival hyperplasia, hirsutism, osteomalacia, hypothyroidism, and peripheral neuropathy.

In addition to side effects associated with phenytoin therapy, there are also adverse effects that must be considered for the administration of the medication.

- With the administration of intravenous (IV) phenytoin, there can be a marked hypotension and cardiac effects. This can be mediated by administering the dose at a slower rate in an adequate volume.
- Extravasation of phenytoin can also be a devastating occurrence, and appropriate dilution of the dose may minimize damage should an extravasation occur.
- In patients with fragile vasculature or pronounced cardiac comorbidities, the prodrug fosphenytoin is available to be administered IV or intramuscularly (IM), and has a much diminished administration risk.

DRUG–DRUG INTERACTIONS

Monitoring of phenytoin therapy can be confusing and complicated for even the most experienced professionals. As a hepatic enzyme inducer and substrate, phenytoin is highly susceptible to drug interactions. The addition of an enzyme-inducing medication (e.g., barbiturates, rifampin, etc.) will dramatically decrease the circulating levels of phenytoin, while the introduction of a hepatic enzyme inhibitor (e.g., valproic acid) will increase those levels. A nonlinear elimination and high affinity for protein binding make the pharmacokinetics of this medication even less predictable. The addition of another highly protein-bound medication (e.g., digoxin, valproic acid) can significantly increase the free or unbound percentage of circulating phenytoin. While the goal serum blood level for the average patient is 10–20 μg/dL, the evaluation of the free percentage of drug will provide a more accurate picture of drug activity.

Topiramate (Topamax)

MECHANISM OF ACTION

While the exact mechanism of action of topiramate is unknown, there are four clinical activities of the drug that may, in part, explain some of its antiepileptic properties. Blockade of voltage-dependent sodium channels, augmentation of GABA at the $GABA_A$ receptor, antagonism of subtypes of the excitatory glutamate receptors, and inhibition of isoenzymes of the carbonic anhydrase enzymes have been seen in preclinical studies.

ADVERSE EFFECTS

Some very serious adverse effects have been associated with topiramate therapy. Nonanion gap metabolic acidosis, due to the disproportionate loss of bicarbonate via the inhibition of carbonic anhydrase, has been reported.

- Periodic monitoring of the serum bicarbonate levels in treated patients is recommended, and if depleted should be treated.
- Treatment may include the reduction of topiramate dose (if clinically possible) or the initiation of alkali therapy.

Acute increases in intraocular pressure have also been noted with topiramate therapy. Therefore, this medication should not be used in patients with known glaucoma. The occurrence of this side effect is a medical emergency, as nontreatment could lead to permanent blindness.

Oligohidrosis, and associated hyperthermia, though seen most commonly in children, are potentially life-threatening adverse effects of topiramate therapy. The incidence of this dangerous state can be elevated when topiramate is given in conjunction with other carbonic anhydrase inhibitors or other medications with anticholinergic effects. Less serious side effects seen in premarketing trials include cognitive dysfunction (confusion, memory impairment, speech or language difficulties, etc.), psychiatric or behavioral disturbances, and somnolence or fatigue. As may be expected with its inhibition of carbonic anhydrase, the development of kidney stones during topiramate therapy occurs approximately 2–4 times more frequently than in the general population. This may be an especially important clinical consideration for patients with a history of renal calculi.

DRUG–DRUG INTERACTIONS

While not shown to affect the CYP450 enzyme system, topiramate does interact with other medications, particularly other AEDs. The addition of topiramate to phenytoin therapy may increase phenytoin concentrations, while its addition to valproic acid therapy will decrease valproic acid levels. When coadministered, carbamazepine, phenytoin, and valproic acid will all decrease topiramate levels, while lamotrigine will increase topiramate levels. In addition to the interactions between valproic acid and topiramate listed above, the coadministration of these AEDs can lead to a hyperammonemia, with or without encephalopathy. Of other medications tested, decreases in the activity of oral contraceptives, lithium, and risperidone were noted when therapies overlapped with topiramate. Studies suggest that the potential exists for interactions between topiramate and metformin, pioglitazone, and hydrochlorothiazide, but the clinical ramifications are not yet clear. Concurrent use of topiramate and other carbonic anhydrase inhibitors should be avoided.

Valproic Acid (Depakote, Depakene, Depacon)

Valproic acid is the only AED proven effective against all seizure types, including generalized, absence, and partial seizures. With an available intravenous formulation, valproic acid is one of the few AEDs available for use in the acute care setting in patients unable to take oral medications.

MECHANISM OF ACTION

Although the exact mechanism of action of valproic acid is not known, activity has been postulated to include potentiation of postsynaptic GABA inhibitory responses, direct membrane stabilizing effects, and alterations in potassium channel functions.

ADVERSE EFFECTS

Hepatic failure and teratogenic effects have been noted with valproate therapy, prompting an FDA-mandated black-box warning. Hepatic failure occurs much less frequently in adults than in children, and will usually appear within the first 6 months of therapy. As a precaution, baseline and routine monitoring of liver function tests (LFTs) are advised. Neural tube defects in children born to mothers treated with valproate are documented. Valproate therapy in any woman with child bearing potential should be undertaken only if its benefits clearly outweigh the potential fetal risks.

Hyperammonemia has also been commonly reported with valproic acid therapy, and may occur in the absence of hepatic injury. While usually mild, benign ammonia elevations occur. If clinical signs signaling hyperammonemia develop during therapy, measurement of serum ammonia and the potential discontinuation of the drug should be considered. Reports of thrombocytopenia related to valproic acid therapy have been documented in 6–40% of treated patients, but this side effect usually responds to a decrease in dose. Other, milder, side effects frequently reported include gastrointestinal disturbances, which can be alleviated through modification in administered dosage form, and adverse effects associated with CNS depression, such as somnolence, dizziness, tremor, and diplopia.

DRUG–DRUG INTERACTIONS

As valproic acid undergoes metabolism via glucuronosyltransferase enzymes in the liver, hepatic enzyme inducers will decrease circulating valproic acid levels. This includes other AEDs such as carbamazepine, phenobarbital, and phenytoin. In contrast, hepatic enzyme inhibitors seem to have little effect on valproic acid metabolism. Valproic acid itself is an inhibitor of hepatic enzymes, including the CYP 450 system, glucuronosyltransferases, and epoxide hydrase. Through this inhibition, the concentrations of the ethosuximide, lamotrigine, phenobarbital, and the active carbamazepine 10, 11-epoxide metabolite were shown to increase in the presence of valproic acid. Through interactions at serum protein binding sites and alterations in metabolism, increased levels of unbound or free phenytoin are seen in patients when both medications are administered. More vigilant monitoring of adverse effects and therapeutic drug levels should be considered when valproic acid and any of the above mentioned AEDs are simultaneously prescribed.

Summary

In conclusion, the panacea for seizures and epilepsy has yet to be found. No single medication has been found to control partial, generalized, and alcohol-induced seizures while eliminating all side effects. The expertise of the pharmacist, however, can guide decisions and monitor outcomes to ensure that the best medication is chosen for the given patient and his or her unique needs.

Table 7.5. Medications for the treatment of epilepsy in adults

AED	Route	Elimination half-life	% Protein Bound	Initial dose	Maintenance dose	Dose adjustments indicated	Comments
Carbamazepine	PO	12–65 hours	76	400 mg in 3–4 divided doses	800–1600 mg in 3–4 divided doses	Hepatic impairment	• Target blood level: 4–12 μg/mL • Active metabolite (10–11 epoxide) • Auto-induction (half-life decreases with longer therapy duration) • Increased rate of absorption with suspension form (approximately 10%)
Gabapentin	PO	5–7 hours	<3	300 mg three times daily	900–3600 mg in 2–3 divided doses	Renal impairment	• Bioavailability is dose dependent (e.g., at high doses divide and dose more frequently)
Levetiracetam	PO/IV	6–8 hours	<10	500 mg twice daily	1000–3000 mg twice daily	Renal impairment	• IV:PO ratio is 1:1 with same dosing frequency
Oxcarbazepine	PO	2 hours (parent) 9 hours (metabolite)	40	300 mg twice daily	1200–2400 mg twice daily	Renal impairment	• Active metabolite (MHD) • Linear kinetics
Phenobarbital	PO/IV	53–118 hours	50	60 mg daily	60–200 mg in 1–3 divided doses	Hepatic impairment	• FDA schedule IV substance • IV:PO ratio is 1:1

Phenytoin	PO/IV	7–42 hours	90–95	10–20 mg/kg load	100 mg three times daily or 4–6 mg/kg in 2–3 divided doses	Hepatic impairment	• Target blood level: 10–20 µg/mL (total) • Free level monitoring may be beneficial • IV:PO ratio is 1:1; total daily PO dose should be divided q8h • Zero-order kinetics • Coadministration of PO form with enteral tube feeds may result in decreased absorption
Valproic acid	PO/IV	9–16 hours (oral dose)	Approximately 80–90	10–15 mg/kg in 2–4 divided doses	<60 mg/kg in 2–4 divided doses	Hepatic impairment	• Target blood level: 50–100 µg/mL • Free level monitoring may be beneficial • IV:PO ratio is 1:1; total PO dose should be divided q8h–q6h • Divide oral doses if dose >250 mg/24 h

REFERENCES

Albers GW, Hart RG, Lutsep HL, Newell DW, Sacco RL. Supplement to the Guidelines for the Management of Transient Ischemic Attacks: a statement from the Ad Hoc Committee on Guidelines for the Management of Transient Ischemic Attacks, Stroke Council, American Heart Association. *Stroke*. 1999;**30**:2502–11.

Albers, GW, Amarenco P, Easton JD, Sacco RL, Teal P. Antithrombotic and thrombolytic therapy for ischemic stroke. The Seventh ACCP Conference on Antithrombotic and Thrombolytic Therapy. *Chest*. 2004;**126**:483S5–12S.

Becker RC, Fintel DJ, Green D. *Antithrombotic Therapy*, 1st ed. West Islip, NY: Professional Communications, pp 27–33, 57–65, 69–79, 83–92.

Dilantin Kapseals (phenytoin) [package insert]. New York, New York. Parke-Davis, Pfizer Inc. February 2003.

Dipiro JT, Talbert RL, Yee GC, Matzke GR, Wells BG, Posey LM. *Pharmacotherapy*. 3rd ed. East Norwalk: Appleton & Lange; pp 406–412, 423–9.

Goldhaber SZ, Tapson VF, Elkayam U, et al. Prophylaxis of venous thromboembolism (VTE) in the hospitalized medical patients: optimizing recognition, assessment, and prophylaxis of at-risk patients. *Hosp Med Consens Rep*. May 1, 2003, pp 1–20.

Graves NM, Garness WR. Epilepsy. In: Dipiro JT, Talbert RL, Yee GC, Matzke GR, Wells BG, Posey LM, eds. *Pharmacotherapy: a pathophysiologic approach*. 4th ed. Stamford, CT: Appleton & Lange, 1999, pp 952–75.

Hawkins D. Limitations of traditional anticoagulants. *Pharmacotherapy*. 2004;**24**(7 Pt 2):62S–65S.

Juurlink DN, Gomes T, Ko DT, et al. A population-based study of the drug interaction between proton pump inhibitors and clopidogrel. *CMA J*. 2009.

Kane SL, Weber RJ, Dasta JF. The impact of critical care pharmacists on enhancing patient outcomes. *Intens Care Med*. 2003;**29**:691–8.

Keppra (levetiracetam) [package insert]. Smyrna, GA. UCB Inc. July 2006.

Lacy CF, Armstrong LL, Goldman MP, Lance LL. *Drug Information Handbook*, 9th ed. Hudson, OH: Lexi-Comp, 2001–2002, pp 96–7, 593–6, 696–9.

Leape LL, Cullen DJ, Dempsey Clapp M, Burdick E, Demonaco HJ, Ives Erickson J, Bates DW. Pharmacist participation on physician rounds and adverse drug events in the intensive care unit. *JAMA*. 1999;**281**(3):267–71.

Merli GJ. Venous thromboembolism prophylaxis guidelines: use by primary care physicians. *Clin Cornerst*. 2005;**7**(4):32–8.

Neurontin (Gabapentin) [package insert]. New York, NY. Parke-Davis, Pfizer Inc. December 2005.

Phenobarbital Elixir [package insert]. Huntsville, AL. Vintage Pharmaceuticals LLC. May 2005.

Scarsi KK, Fotis MA, Noskin GA. Pharmacist participation in medical rounds reduces medication errors. *Am J Health-Syst Pharm*. 2002;**59**:2089–92.

Shargel L, Mutnick AH, Souney PF, Swanson LN. *Comprehensive Pharmacy Review*, 4th ed. Philadelphia: Lippincott Williams & Wilkins, 2001, pp 713–31.

Sibbing D, Morath T, Stegherr J, et al: Impact of proton pump inhibitors on the antiplatelet effects of clopidogrel. *Thromb Haemost*. 2009;**101**(4):714–19.

Siller-Matula JM, Spiel AD, Lang IM, et al: Effects of pantoprazole and esomeprazole on platelet inhibition by clopidogrel. *AM Heart J*. 2009;**157**(1) 148e1–e5.

Tegretol (Carbamazepine) [package insert]. East Hanover, NJ. Novartis Pharmaceuticals Corporation. September 2003.

Thomson Medical Economics. *Antiplatelet & Antithrombotic Prescribing Guide*, 3rd ed, 2003, pp 56–71.

Trileptal (oxcarbazepine) [package insert]. East Hanover, NJ. Novartis Pharmaceuticals Corporation. January 2006.

Wells BG, DiPiro JT, Schwinghammer TL, Hamilton CW. *Pharmacotherapy Handbook*, 5th ed. New York: McGraw-Hill, 2003, pp 145–8.

8 Intracranial Pressure and Cerebral Blood Flow Monitoring

Andrew Beaumont, MD, PhD

Neurocritical care is dependent on the ability to accurately monitor cerebral physiology. One of the most important physiologic variables to consider is cerebral blood flow (CBF) because neuronal survival is directly linked to an appropriate match between metabolic demand and metabolic substrate. CBF depends on cerebral perfusion pressure (CPP), defined as the mean arterial blood pressure (mABP) minus the mean intracranial pressure (ICP).

There are many ways (invasive and noninvasive) to measure CBF and ICP in the ICU setting. This chapter reviews techniques for measuring both these parameters and considers the benefits and pitfalls of the different techniques, along with a basic consideration of their interpretation. The reader is directed to relevant sections elsewhere in this text for a detailed consideration of ICP and CBF physiology.

MEASUREMENT OF INTRACRANIAL PRESSURE

Physical Principles

ICP can be measured in several anatomic spaces:

- Intraventricular
- Intraparenchymal
- Subdural
- Subarachnoid
- Epidural

Intracranial pressure is synonymous with CSF pressure. ICP depends on several parameters:

- Internal (intracranial) volume
- Elastance of the system

- Contribution from the atmosphere
- Orientation of the craniospinal axis relative to the gravitational vector

The traditional reference point for ICP measurement is the foramen of Monro, the location of which is estimated by the external acoustic meatus (EAM). ICP is variably expressed in either mm Hg, or in mm H_2O. Dividing the pressure in mm H_2O by 13.6 yields the equivalent pressure in mm Hg; this constant is based on the ratio of the density of water to mercury.

The intracranial contents that contribute to the ICP are blood, brain, cerebrospinal fluid (CSF), and any pathological masses. Changes in the volume of one component can be compensated for by both the system and by reduction of the volume of another component (Monro–Kellie doctrine). Compliance is defined by the reciprocal of the pressure change per unit of volume change of the intracranial contents.[1] This relationship is not linear across all volumes, and not necessarily constant under all physiologic conditions (see later). Changes in compliance reflect a "tightening" brain that may herald increased or unstable ICP.

The ICP Waveform

The ICP waveform is normally pulsatile and can be divided into systolic and diastolic components along with cardiac and respiratory variation (Fig. 8.1). Normal mean ICP's are typically less than 15 mm Hg under steady-state conditions. This baseline, or average, level is commonly referred to as the ICP, while rhythmic components superimposed on

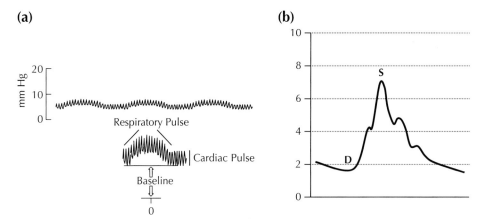

Figure 8.1. Normal intracranial pressure waveform. **(a)** The baseline pressure level is affected by rhythmic components caused by cardiac and respiratory activity. MABP fluctuation with heart rate causes small amplitude rapid pulsation, and respiration causes larger amplitude fluctuations of lower frequency. **(b)** Higher speed recording shows systolic (S) and diastolic (D) variations in ICP along with smaller variations corresponding to dichrotic waves in the arterial pressure waveform. Although clinically ICP is often reported only as a single number, ICP is completely described only by information about both the baseline level and the pulsatile components.

this level are associated with cardiac and respiratory activity. Changes in these components can be one of the earliest signs that the intracranial pressure is beginning to rise, as a reflection of the increased conductance of pressure waves through a "tightening" brain.

Lundberg pioneered the early work on ICP monitoring and he described three additional patterns of ICP waveform variation:[2]

- A waves (plateau waves): Characterized by increases of ICP that are sustained for several minutes and then return spontaneously to a new baseline
- B waves: Short elevations of a modest nature (10–20 mm Hg) that occur at a frequency of 0.5–2 Hz and were thought to relate respiratory fluctuations in $Paco_2$ or vasomotor waves
- C waves: More rapid sinusoidal fluctuations occurring approximately every 10 seconds corresponding to Traube–Hering–Mayer fluctuations in arterial pressure.

Indications for Intracranial Pressure Monitoring

Several published clinical trials show that monitoring ICP, under situations in which ICP may be high, either facilitates outcome or promotes aggressive

management.[3] There is strong clinical evidence that careful control of ICP is important,[4] and maintaining cerebral perfusion pressure under different pathological circumstances is of benefit for outcome.[5] An understanding of the indications for initiating monitoring and the methods by which this can be done is important. The ultimate goal of ICP monitoring should be that of directed therapy and preservation of CBF.

- Intracranial hypertension is found in 40–60% of severe head injuries and is a major factor in 50% of all fatalities.
- There is no uniform agreement about the critical level of ICP beyond which treatment is mandatory.
- Saul and Ducker demonstrated benefits by treating ICP above 15 mm Hg when compared to a group of patients treated for ICP above 25 mm Hg.[3]
- Marmarou et al. (1991) examined data from 428 patients in the Traumatic Coma Data Bank and calculated the ICP threshold most predictive of 6-month outcome using logistic regression.[6] The threshold that correlated best was 20 mm Hg, and this is the current level at which most centers begin treatment.
- Current opinion now regards cerebral perfusion pressure as a more important parameter, which should be monitored in concert with ICP.

Guidelines for ICP monitoring after trauma in adults include

- a GCS of 3–8 and
- an abnormal computed tomography (CT) scan

In the presence of GCS 3–8, and a normal CT scan, two or more of the following should prompt monitoring in any event:

- Age >40 years
- Unilateral/bilateral motor posturing
- Systolic BP <90 mmHg

Patients with GCS >8 may benefit from ICP monitoring if the CT scan demonstrates a significant mass lesion or treatment is required for associated injuries. Further, these are only guidelines, and clinical decisions should be individualized. For example, a patient with an abnormal head CT but a good clinical exam who needs prolonged anesthesia for other injuries may not meet criteria but might benefit from an ICP monitor because of the inability to follow the neurologic exam in the OR.

The role of ICP monitoring in adult brain trauma is clear; however, the role and clinical evidence for improved outcome is less clear in nontraumatic settings such as:

- Status epilepticus
- Fulminant hepatic failure
- Reye's syndrome
- Diffuse cerebritis
- Metabolic encephalopathies
- Cerebral infarction

In these conditions, the decision about whether to monitor ICP should be individualized and based on whether raised ICP is a problem, whether knowing ICP will change management, and whether there is a component of neurologic injury that is reversible if ICP is managed.

Methods of ICP Measurement

- Ventriculostomy
- Subdural catheter
- Epidural transducer
- Fiberoptic microtransducer

In modern clinical practice ventriculostomy coupled with a pressure transducer remains the gold standard for monitoring ICP because of accuracy and ease of calibration. CSF drainage for ICP control is an additional benefit. Disadvantages are that catheter placement can be difficult when the ventricles are small or shifted from the midline and the risk of infection rises in ventriculostomies after 5 days, although this risk can be lessened by tunneling the catheter under the skin. Current estimates have associated ventriculostomy with <2% hemorrhagic complications and <10% infective complications.[7]

One of the commonest methods of ICP measurement utilized in the modern NICU is the fiberoptic or "bolt" ICP monitor. The method is advantageous because of ease of placement, low morbidity, and the facility to add additional monitoring devices such as thermal probes or oxygen monitors (see later). One disadvantage is the lack of therapeutic CSF drainage.

Bolt placement is usually performed in the right frontal skull, although theoretically any location not overlying a dural sinus is acceptable.

- Monitor placement is conducted in the ICU or operating room under sterile conditions.
- A small (<1 cm) skin incision is made down to the skull bone.
- The periosteum is then stripped off the bone, and a twist drill burr hole is made using a commercial drill bit matched to the size of the bolt adapter. When the burr hole is complete, the bolt device is screwed into the skull, and then a dilator used to breach the dura and dilate a tract for the fiberoptic probe.
- The skin is then closed around the bolt, and the fiberoptic probe is zeroed at atmospheric pressure.
- The probe is then placed through a retaining cap ideally into the subarachnoid space, although parenchymal placement does not significantly affect observed values.
- Appropriate probe placement can be verified visually on the monitor screen by observing a good ICP waveform.
- The monitor can be connected directly to most bedside ICU monitors, and with continuous ABP monitoring, a continuous measure of CPP is possible.
- Fiberoptic transducers cannot be recalibrated externally; however, their accuracy in practice has proved excellent.[8]

Table 8.1. Comparison between different features of ventriculostomy and fiberoptic ICP monitoring

	Ventriculostomy	Fiberoptic bolt
Accuracy	Gold-standard, fluid couple	Subject to drift
Placement	Harder	Easier
Ease of use	Requires zeroing and height adjustment	No routine calibration steps needed
Risk of infection	Increases at >5 days	Low
Clinical utility	CSF drainage: treatment and measurement	Measurement only
Location	Lower risk of regional variation	Higher risk of regional variation
Management	Higher nursing burden	Lower nursing burden

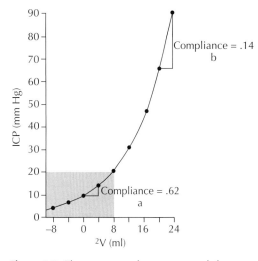

Figure 8.2. The pressure–volume curve and the pressure volume index describe the response of intracranial pressure to the addition of volume. The normal curve shows how compliance changes as greater volumes are added. The CSF system is in the phase of spatial compensation at point a (shaded area), as compared with spatial decompensation at point b.

Pressure–Volume Relationships

The relationship between intracranial volume and intracranial pressure is not linear. Pressure–volume relationships can be depicted by graphing the response of ICP to volume added into the neural axis (Fig. 8.2). In the normal adult this relationship describes a hyperbolic curve.

■ Along the flat portion of the curve, increases in volume affect ICP minimally because compensatory mechanisms can effectively maintain ICP in a normal range. This part of the curve is termed the "period of spatial compensation."

■ As volume is added the pressure changes per unit volume become increasingly large, and compliance lessens; this portion is called the "period of spatial decompensation." The reciprocal of the slope of this curve ($\Delta V/\Delta P$) represents the compliance of the system, which is maximal in the period of spatial compensation. The slope of the pressure–volume curve rises rapidly during spatial decompensation, and therefore compliance falls.

Clinically compliance can be measured by infusion or withdrawal of small volumes into the CSF space, with measures of the pressure response. Methods of continuous compliance measurement have been devised using multiple time-averaged small volume pulses. The Spiegelberg Compliance Monitor (Spiegelberg, Hamburg, Germany) is a commercially available device that measures compliance continuously when placed in the ventricle. Observing loss of compliance can herald increases in ICP and therefore allow earlier and more aggressive treatment of the brain at threat from ICP.

ICP Waveform Analysis

Whereas the ICP waveform can be evaluated by the characteristics of each individual wave and the momentary mean ICP, coupled with measures of compliance, there has been steady interest in evaluating continuous runs of ICP data for longer term trends and correlations using systems and waveform analysis techniques. Goals of this type of analysis include provision of a more sensitive assessment of the pathological state, and an early indicator of impending system change. These techniques have included spectral analysis, waveform correlation coefficients and system entropy.

These analytical techniques rely on the relationship between the ICP waveform and ABP waveform. The correlation coefficient between changes in BP and ICP is defined by Cosnyka et al. (1996) as the pressure reactivity index (PRx).[9]

■ PRx varies from low values (no association) to values approaching 1.0 (strong positive association).
■ With lower BP, lower blood vessel wall tension results in an increase in transmission of the BP waveform to the ICP.
■ Also with elevated ICP brain compliance is reduced, thereby increasing transmission of the BP waveform.
■ PRx has been implicated as a marker of autoregulatory reserve.

Approximate Entropy (ApEn) is a measure of system regularity/randomness devised for use in physiologic systems.[10] It measures the logarithmic likelihood that runs of patterns are similar over a given number of observations. Reductions in ApEn imply reduced randomness or increased order and have been associated with pathology in the cardiovascular, respiratory, and endocrine systems. Approximate Entropy analysis has been successfully applied under conditions of raised ICP for measuring changes in transmission of system randomness between the heart rate and the ICP waveform.[11]

MEASUREMENT OF CEREBRAL BLOOD FLOW

Matching CBF to cerebral tissue metabolic demand and avoiding ischemia is a critical feature of support in neurointensive care. Although it is currently difficult to measure metabolic demand, measurement of CBF is possible and should be considered in a wide group of patients. CBF can be measured

| • Directly | • Continuously |
| • Indirectly | • Discontinuously |

There is wide variability in the accuracy or interpretation of the different techniques, and extreme care should be taken in comparing data obtained with different methods. There are clearly ischemic thresholds of CBF that have been defined; however, these thresholds may vary under conditions of physiologic stress or pharmacologically induced hypometabolism (such as barbiturate coma).

Indirect Measures of CBF

Indirect methods of CBF measurement essentially include any marker of physiologic health of cerebral tissue. Specific examples including jugular venous oxygen saturation, tissue oxygen tension, and microdialysis are discussed later. However, the neurologic examination, EEG, and CPP are all potential markers of changes in CBF and should be viewed as such.

Direct Discontinuous Measures of CBF

The commonest discontinuous method of CBF measurement is based on assessment of the amount of measurable tracer that reaches the brain after peripheral injection.

■ Tracers can be divided into diffusible and nondiffusible depending on their ability to pass through the blood–brain barrier (BBB).
■ Tracers are required to cause a signal intensity change with a specified imaging modality.
■ CT, magnetic resonance imaging (MRI), and nuclear medicine contrast agents have been used in this technique.
■ The central volume principle is used to derive CBF from signal intensity change vs. time curves after injection using complex algorithms.[12]
■ Absolute CBF can only be measured in this way if a corresponding arterial concentration vs. time curve can be measured (arterial input function). Without this, semiquantitative or relative values of CBF only can be obtained.

Several imaging modalities have been clinically used to measure CBF.

XENON-ENHANCED CT

In this technique the diffusible contrast agent xenon is used. Baseline CT slices of the head are obtained. The patient then inhales a mixture of 28%

xenon and 72% oxygen for approximately 4 minutes. Sequential scanning of the same slices occurs during this inhalation period. Tissue attenuation vs. time data are then derived. The arterial concentration is proportional to the expired xenon concentration. Xenon-CT has been extensively studied, is relatively low cost, and is relatively easy to accomplish even in unstable patients. A relative disadvantage is a high sensitivity to motion artifact.

SPECT (SINGLE PHOTON EMISSION CT)

In SPECT scanning, the radioisotope technetium-99m (Tc-99m) is combined with a carrier molecule that is highly lipophilic such as hexamethyl-propyleneamine (HMPAO) or ethyl cysteinate dimer. Intravenously injected compound is taken up into brain tissue in an amount proportional to tissue blood flow. Tissue metabolism then ensures that Tc-99m remains in the tissue for several hours. Detection can then occur in a delayed fashion using a standard SPECT system, with scan times of approximately 5 minutes.

SPECT scanning has the advantages that it is easy to perform, takes only a few minutes of scan time, and most radiology departments already have appropriate hardware. However, there are limitations of this technique. Assembly of the compound takes a finite period of time and may even need to be ordered from an off-site location. The technique has a relatively coarse imaging matrix and therefore low resolution. While this reduces error from motion artifact, it also makes it difficult to determine precise anatomic location of areas of abnormality. Also, arterial data are difficult to acquire and therefore only relative CBF values can be acquired, and this may be misleading in states of global hypo- or hyperperfusion.

MR PERFUSION

"Dynamic Susceptibility Contrast Imaging," also called "first-pass" or "bolus tracking" MR perfusion imaging is based on very rapid acquisition of MR signal intensity data from the brain during the injection of a contrast agent. Ten to fifteen images are obtained as baseline before injection and then 20–40 images are obtained after injection at 1–2 seconds per image. The commonest contrast agent is a gadolinium chelate. Signal intensity–time curves are generated for each pixel in the image. CBF can then be calculated as described above by determination

of an arterial input function by focusing a region of interest over a major intracranial vessel.

Arterial spin labeling is another method of MR perfusion assessment. With this technique the intravascular tracer used is normal protons within the extracranial internal carotid artery that are saturated and spin-inverted electromagnetically using MRI. As these protons mix with normal protons in the brain there is a change in magnetization detectable on MR imaging.

There are several advantages to MR-based perfusion techniques, including the high level of anatomic accuracy and the ability to obtain multiple other sequences in conjunction such as MR angiography and diffusion weighted imaging. Relative disadvantages include possible errors in accuracy in the presence of a deficient BBB and a higher level of difficulty in unstable patients.

CT WITH IODINATED CONTRAST

A technique similar to MR perfusion has been described using iodinated CT contrast in combination with rapid repetitive CT scanning through slices of interest. One advantage of this technique is the relative ease of obtaining CT scans compared with MRI in a critically ill patient. A relative disadvantage is the potential nephrotoxic or allergic complications of an iodine contrast load. However, the dose of contrast required for this study is significantly less than for other studies such as abdomen/pelvis CTs or pulmonary angiography.

Continuous Measures of CBF

Continuous measures of CBF that have been clinically applied include:

- Transcranial Doppler
- Laser Doppler flow
- Thermal diffusion

Continuous measures of CBF have the advantage of detecting minute-by-minute variations in cerebral physiology; however, they universally tend to lose anatomic resolution in comparison with imaging techniques.

TRANSCRANIAL DOPPLER

Transcranial Doppler (TCD) actually measures CBF velocity in the major intracranial vessels. Briefly, ultrasound waves are transmitted through a bone

Table 8.2. Comparison between the features of direct and indirect measures of cerebral blood flow

	Time resolution	Anatomic resolution	Invasive	Accuracy
Direct				
Xe-CT	Approximately 5 minutes	++	None	++ / abs
Contrast CT	Approximately 5 minutes	+++	None	++ / abs
SPECT	Approximately 5 minutes	+	None	+ / rel
MRI	Approximately 2 minutes	++++	None	+++ / abs
LDF	Continuous	Local	None	++
Thermal	<1 minute	Local	Intracranial	++
Indirect				
TCD	Seconds	n/a	None	n/a
Sjvo$_2$	Continuous	n/a	Central IV	n/a
po$_2$	Continuous	n/a	Intracranial	n/a
Oximetry	Continuous	n/a	None	n/a
Microdialysis	>10 minutes	n/a	Intracranial	n/a

See text for the specifics of each method. Anatomic resolution and accuracy are not applicable to indirect methods, since they do not directly measure blood flow. For the accuracy column, / abs implies that absolute cerebral blood flow can be measured; / rel implies that only relative flow can be measured.

"window" such as the thin temporal bone, the orbit, or the foramen magnum. When these waves contact moving blood cells they are reflected back to a detector with an altered frequency. The TCD probe emits ultrasound waves in short pulses, and because ultrasound waves travel in tissue at a constant velocity, the depth of measurement can be varied by changing the time window for receiving reflected waves. The degree of frequency variation is affected by both direction and velocity of blood flow, following the Doppler principle. Most of the major intracranial vessels can be insonated, by varying both the angle of the probe through the chosen window and the depth of measurement.

- The most useful applications of this technology include monitoring patients for vasospasm after subarachnoid hemorrhage and confirmation of brain death.
- Changes in CBF can be inferred from changes in blood flow velocity and therefore TCD can be used as an indirect measure of CBF.
- Unfortunately, in up to 10% of the population suitable acoustic windows cannot be obtained.

- Also, accuracy of velocity measurement is dependent on probe angle, and therefore interobserver error can be high with this technique. Systems for rigidly mounting the probe to patients' heads have been devised.
- Also the constancy of relation between CBF and CBF velocity relies on a constant diameter of the artery, and a direct relation between blood flow in arteries of the circle of Willis and cortical blood flow. Under conditions of trauma or serious neurologic illness, both these assumptions may not be valid.

LASER DOPPLER FLOW

Laser Doppler measures of cerebral blood flow were first described by Williams et al. (1980).[13] A sensor affixed to a burr hole in the skull emits a monochromatic laser into brain parenchyma that is disrupted by the passage of red blood cells in a volume and concentration sensitive fashion. Blood flow can therefore be calculated by the extent of this disruption. Laser Doppler flow (LDF) does allow continuous monitoring; however, its sampling area is small (approximately 1 mm^3), it is highly dependent on the proximity of the probe to a blood vessel, only relative changes are measurable, and measurement has to take into account the patient's hematocrit. Recently combined probes that integrate an ICP monitor and a laser Doppler flow probe have been introduced (Neurosensor, Integra Lifesciences, Plainsboro, NJ).

THERMAL DIFFUSION

Thermal diffusion quantitatively measures the ability of cerebral tissue to dissipate heat, and directly relates this to CBF. It has a small sampling volume; however, readings are displayed in mL/100 g per minute. Two small thermistors coexist in a probe. The distal thermistor is heated by 2°. The greater the tissue blood flow, the greater is the ability to dissipate heat. Changes in the proximal thermistor are converted to a CBF reading. Commercial systems are available (SABER Series, Flowtronics Inc., Phoenix, AZ).

MEASURES OF CEREBRAL METABOLISM

Jugular Bulb Oximetry

The paired jugular veins carry deoxygenated blood away from the brain. Therefore measurement of jugular venous oxygen saturation ($SjvO_2$) is a broad measure of oxygen supply and consumption of cerebral tissue. Decreased supply (reduced CBF) or increased demand (increased tissue metabolism) both result in a reduction in $SjvO_2$.

- Central venous access through an internal jugular vein is required.
- A fiberoptic oximeter (Abbot Opticath, Abbot Laboratories, North Chicago, IL) is placed in a retrograde fashion into the jugular bulb.
- The normal range for $SjvO_2$ is 55–75%.
- Risks of placement include the risks of central venous access, carotid puncture, thrombosis, hematoma, and infection.

Studies have identified that episodes of jugular venous desaturation after traumatic brain injury are associated with a worse outcome. The use of $SjvO_2$ may allow for finer tuning of parameters such as cerebral perfusion pressure or lower limits of hyperventilation, where inappropriate selection of parameters may result in ischemia. However, one major disadvantage of $SjvO_2$ is that it is a global measure of CBF and may be quite insensitive to focal areas of ischemia.

Brain Oxygen Tension

Measurement of oxygen tension in brain tissue is possible at the bedside and this is a marker of mismatch between perfusion and metabolic demand and therefore indirectly CBF. Two commercially available systems allow measurement of tissue oxygen tension (pO_2): the LICOX catheter (LICOX, Integra Lifesciences, Plainsboro, NJ) and the Neurotrend catheter (Neurotrend, Codman, Raynham MA). Both rely on a special adaptation of a fiberoptic ICP monitoring bolt, using side-ports for additional probes.

- The LICOX system uses a polagraphic technique (a Clark electrode).
- The Neurotrend system uses an optical luminescence technique.
- It has been demonstrated that the 18 mL/100 g per minute ischemic threshold for cerebral tissue correlated with a tissue pO_2 of 22 mm Hg.[14]
- Normal brain tissue pO_2 has been recorded at approximately 40 mm Hg.

However, it is important to be aware of the limitations of this technique, namely, loss of anatomic information, lack of information about adequacy of tissue oxygenation, and no information about tissue oxygen usage. An increasing volume of data is being acquired about the role of primary mitochondrial dysfunction in neurocritical care, and if damaged mitochondria cannot utilize oxygen, then tissue pO_2 becomes redundant.

Transcranial Cerebral Oximetry

Pulse oximetry near-infrared spectroscopy (NIRS) has been used for many years to monitor systemic arterial oxygenation via finger, toe, or ear probes. A similar technique can be used noninvasively in the NICU to monitor regional cerebral oxygen saturation. NIRS relies on measuring the transmission and absorption of near-infrared light in the range of 700–1000 nm as it passes through tissue. Absorption is related to the concentration of tissue iron (hemoglobin) and copper (cytochrome aa3); however, oxygenated and deoxygenated hemoglobin have different absorption spectra.

Table 8.3. Relationship between measured tissue pO2, ICP, and jugular venous oxygen saturation and specific clinical problems in the injured brain, together with suggested clinical actions

	Clinical problem	Expected ICP	Expected SjvO2	Clinical action
Low tissue pO2 (<25 mm Hg)				
↑ Demand	↑ ICP	↑	= /↓	Treat ICP elevation
	Pain/agitation	↑	= /↓	Sedation/analgesia
	Seizures	↑	= /↓	EEG/antiepileptic
	Fever	↑	= /↓	Cool/Tylenol
↓ Delivery	↓ CPP	↑	↓	ICP Rx/pressors/volume
	Hypoxia	↑	↓	↑ FiO2, identify cause
	Anemia	=	= /↓	Transfuse
	Hyperventilation	= /↓	↓	Reduce hyperventilation
	Vasospasm	= /↑	↓	Treat vasospasm
High tissue pO2 (>50 mm Hg)				
↑ Delivery	Hyperemia	↑	↑	Hyperventilation
	Ventilator	=	= /↑	↓ FiO2
↓ Demand	Hypothermia	= /↓	↑	Elevate temperature
	Sedatives	= /↓	↑	Decrease sedation

■ Normal values have been reported ranging from 60% to 80%.

■ There are several commercially available systems such as the INVOS series (Somanetics Corp, Troy, MI) and the NIRO series (Hamamatsu Photonics, Japan).

Unlike regular pulse oximetry, information from the entire intracranial blood volume is reflected, including arteries, veins, and capillary beds. Also, the depth of light penetration in adults and the degree of scatter is very variable, and therefore there is a degree of unpredictability in the results, and studies so far have had conflicting results regarding the predictive value of changes in NIRS measures. There may also be significant contamination from extracranial blood flow.

Microdialysis

Microdialysis is a method by which metabolites in the extracellular space can be measured on a semicontinuous basis. As such it represents an elegant way to monitor tissue health through directly evaluating both substrates and products of metabolism. However, the technique is cumbersome and fraught with difficulties in analysis, which has made it not widely accepted for clinical use.

A semipermeable dialysis membrane is implanted in tissue and connected to an infusate of saline or artificial CSF. The membrane allows equilibration of the extracellular molecules with the dialysate, and therefore biochemical analysis of the dialysate in combination with the known flow rate through the system, allows determination of extracellular concentrations of biomolecules. Many markers have been analyzed, and the only limitations are the ability for the molecule to diffuse appropriately quickly through the membrane, and the existence of a technique to measure it. Some commonly evaluated markers have included glucose, lactate, pyruvate, and glutamate.

Again it is important to note that this technique is a focal measure of tissue biochemistry. Probe placement also exposes the tissue to a degree of local damage that can affect the obtained results. Absolute values are difficult to obtain and must be interpreted with caution. Also, only extracellular markers are measured, and these may or may not reflect intracellular biochemistry.

MULTIMODAL MONITORING IN THE ICU

It is apparent that there are many methods for measuring cerebral physiology in the ICU. The challenge ahead is to identify ways in which data from these multiple sources can be integrated and used to define treatment protocols that can ultimately improve patient outcome. This can be challenging as large volumes of data can be acquired, and there is still much to be learned about the pathophysiology of the injured brain. A simple algorithm relating changes in tissue oxygen, ICP, and jugular venous oxygen saturation is shown in Table 8.3. Extension and refinement of such algorithms will come as we begin to better understand the data yielded by the various monitoring techniques and the subtleties of the pathophysiologic processes that they are measuring.

REFERENCES

1. Miller JD. Volume and pressure in the craniospinal axis. *Clin Neurosurg.* 1975;**22**:76–105.
2. Lundberg N. Continuous recording and control of ventricular fluid pressure in neurosurgical practice. *Acta Psychiatr Neurol Scand.* 1960;**36** (Suppl 49):1–193.
3. Saul TG, Ducker TB. Effect of intracranial pressure monitoring and aggressive treatment on mortality in severe head injury. *J Neurosurg.* 1982 April;**56**(4): 498–503.
4. Miller JD, Becker DP, Ward JD, Sullivan HG, Adams WE, Rosner MJ. Significance of intracranial hypertension in severe head injury. *J Neurosurg.* 1977;**47**(4):503–16.
5. Rosner MJ, Rosner SD, Johnson AH. Cerebral perfusion pressure: management protocol and clinical results [see comments]. *J Neurosurg.* 1995 December; **83**(6):949–62.
6. Marmarou A, Anderson RL, Ward JD. Impact of ICP instability and hypotension on outcome in patients with severe head trauma. *J Neurosurg.* 1991;**75**:S59.
7. Clark WC, Muhlbauer MS, Lowrey R, Hartman M, Ray MW, Watridge CB. Complications of intracranial pressure monitoring in trauma patients. *Neurosurgery.* 1989; **25**(1):20–4.
8. Crutchfield JS, Narayan RK, Robertson CS, Michael LH. Evaluation of a fiberoptic intracranial pressure monitor [see comments]. *J Neurosurg.* 1990;**72**(3):482–7.
9. Czosnyka M, Kirkpatrick PJ, Pickard JD. Multimodal monitoring and assessment of cerebral haemodynamic reserve after severe head injury. *Cerebrovasc Brain Metab Rev.* 1996;**8**(4):273–95.
10. Pincus SM. Approximate entropy as a measure of system complexity. *Proc Natl Acad Sci USA.* 199;15; **88**(6):2297–301.
11. Beaumont A, Marmarou A. Approximate entropy: a regularity statistic for assessment of intracranial pressure. *Acta Neurochir Suppl.* 2002;**81**:193–5.
12. Ostergaard L. Principles of cerebral perfusion imaging by bolus tracking. *J Magn Reson Imaging.* 2005;**22**(6):710–7.
13. Williams PC, Stern MD, Bowen PD, et al. Mapping of cerebral cortical strokes in Rhesus monkeys by laser Doppler spectroscopy. *Med Res Eng.* 1980;**13**(2):3–5.
14. Doppenberg EM, Zauner A, Watson JC, Bullock R. Determination of the ischemic threshold for brain oxygen tension. *Acta Neurochir Suppl.* 1998;**71**:166–9.

9 Hemodynamic and Electrophysiological Monitoring

Rahul Nanchal, MD, Ahmed J. Khan, MD, and Todd Gienapp, MD

Hemodynamic monitoring simply defined is the measurement and analysis of biological signals emanating from the cardiovascular system. Therapies based on these signals are then titrated and physiologic response is measured. Ideally hemodynamic monitoring should involve a holistic approach. Oxygen delivery at both global and regional levels as well as tissue perfusion and cellular health should be assessed. Although easy to articulate, our ability to monitor in this fashion remains limited. Indeed it is sobering to reflect on the paucity of high-quality validation of the commonly used monitors. No randomized trials exist to prove that even monitoring of basic vital signs is beneficial. In fact none are likely to ever be conducted. That being said, in a field as heavily weighted on monitoring, technological advances have evolved over the past 30 years. New noninvasive techniques attempt to negate the necessity of indwelling vascular catheters. The pulmonary artery catheter remains a cornerstone of hemodynamic monitoring despite the persistent controversy about its efficacy. In this chapter, hemodynamic monitoring techniques and important physiologic concepts behind these methods are addressed.

PHYSIOLOGIC PRINCIPLES

The basic tenet of hemodynamic monitoring is to ensure adequate oxygenation at the cellular level. Physiologic signals obtained by various monitoring techniques are often manipulated to this end. Outside of experimental technologies it is not possible to monitor cellular hypoxia; hence global and sometimes regional variables are used.

Oxygen Delivery (D_{O_2}) and Oxygen Consumption ($\dot{V}_{O_2}$)

- D_{O_2} is determined by two factors: the cardiac output (CO) and the arterial content of oxygen (Ca_{O_2}).
- $D_{O_2} = CO \ (L/min) \times Ca_{O_2} \ (mL \ O_2/dL) \times 10$

Oxygen Content

Ca_{O_2} is the amount of oxygen carried in blood both in soluble and bound forms. The determinants are hemoglobin (Hgb), saturation of Hgb in arterial blood (Sa_{O_2}), and the oxygen dissolved in arterial blood. The oxygen carried in dissolved form is dependent on the solubility of oxygen in human plasma and the oxygen tension (Pa_{O_2}). Since the solubility coefficient is low, D_{O_2} depends mainly on Sa_{O_2} and little benefit is derived by increasing oxygen tension to more than 80 mm Hg secondary to the sigmoid nature of the oxyhemoglobin dissociation curve (Fig. 9.1).

- $Ca_{O_2} = [1.36 \times Hgb \ (grams/dL) \times Sa_{O_2}] + [0.003 \times Pa_{O_2}]$

Cardiac Output

Cardiac output (CO) is the product of heart rate (HR) and stroke volume (SV). Stroke volume in

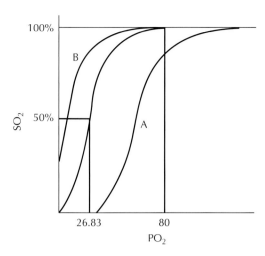

Figure 9.1. Oxyhemoglobin dissociation curve.

- Oxygen extraction ratio (OER) is calculated as $\dot{V}o_2/Do_2$
- Normal values of many of these parameters are given in Table 9.1.

DETERMINANTS OF CARDIAC FUNCTION

The foundations for determining cardiac performance were established more than a century ago by the Frank Starling relationship (Fig. 9.2). The curve generated is a description of the length–tension relationship which in the intact heart manifests as a ventricular function curve. Stroke volume is determined by a complex interaction of preload, afterload, and contractility. In truth these variables are intricately related; however, it is important to understand how each variable in theory can affect stroke volume.

turn depends on the determinants of cardiac performance namely preload, afterload, and cardiac contractility.

- CO (L/min) = HR (beats/min) × SV (L/beat)

Oxygen Consumption

Oxygen consumption ($\dot{V}o_2$) is the difference between oxygen delivered to the tissues and the oxygen returned to the right side of the heart. The determinants of mixed venous oxygen content (Cvo_2) are Hgb, oxygen saturation of Hgb in mixed venous blood (Svo_2), and arterial tension of oxygen in mixed venous blood (Pvo_2).

- Cvo_2 (mL/dL) = 1.36 × Hgb (grams/dL) Svo_2 + 0.003 × Pvo_2
- $\dot{V}o_2$ = CO × 1.36 × 10 × Hgb (in grams) × (Sao_2 – Svo_2)

Preload

This is the amount of end-diastolic stretch on myocardial muscle fibers. It is determined by the volume of blood filling the ventricle at end-diastole. In the absence of significant cardiac, pericardial, or pulmonary disease central venous pressure (CVP) and pulmonary artery occlusion pressure (PAOP) are reasonable surrogates of right ventricular and left ventricular end diastolic volumes, respectively.

Afterload

Afterload is defined as the sum of all forces against which the muscle fibers of both ventricles must

Table 9.1. Normal vlaues of oxygen delivery and consumption parameters

Parameters	Symbol	Normal range
Mixed venous oxygen saturation	Svo_2	70–75%
Oxygen saturation	Sao_2	96–100%
Mixed venous oxygen tension	Pvo_2	35–40 mm Hg
Mixed venous oxygen content	Cvo_2	13–16 mL o_2/dL
Oxygen delivery	Do_2	520–570 mL/min·m²
Oxygen uptake	$\dot{V}o_2$	110–160 mL/min·m²
Oxygen extraction ratio	o_2ER	20–30%

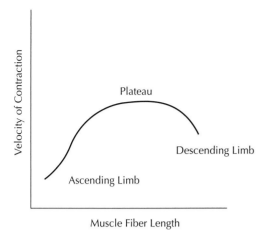

Figure 9.2. Frank-Starling curve.

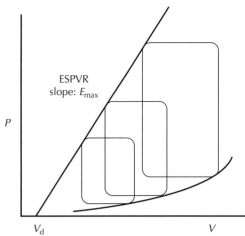

Figure 9.3. End-systolic pressure–volume relationship. (From Zhong *et al. BioMedical Engineering OnLine* 2005;**4**:10 doi:10.1186/1475–925X.)

shorten in order to eject blood into the arterial or pulmonary circulation. Multiple factors influence afterload such as vascular resistance, mass of blood in arteries, viscosity of blood, and compliance of arterial walls. As afterload increases stroke volume falls and myocardial oxygen consumption rises. Afterload is measured indirectly by obtaining pulmonary or systemic vascular resistances (PVR and SVR, respectively).

- SVR = MAP – CVP/CO × 80
- PVR= mPAP – PAOP/CO × 80
- MAP and mPAP are mean arterial pressure and mean pulmonary artery pressure, respectively.

Myocardial Contractility

Simply defined myocardial contractility is the ability of the heart to do work. Intuitively it means the inotropic state of the ventricle, however since mechanical behavior of the myocardium depends on loading conditions, ionotropic state is difficult to determine. End systolic volume to which a ventricle contracts is a linearly increasing function of end systolic pressure. Hence the end systolic pressure volume relationship (ESPVR) reasonable defines the contractile state of the ventricle (Fig. 9.3).

NONINVASIVE MONITORING

Electrocardiogram

The electrocardiogram (EKG) is probably the simplest of monitors and displays a wealth physiologic information and assists in monitoring arrhythmias, cardiac ischemia, electrolyte disturbances, etc.

Automated Blood Pressure Devices

These are used in every ICU to measure blood pressure cyclically over a set frequency. The methodology applied in auscultatory, oscillometric, or both. The oscillometric technique is most often used. Volume unloading technique and the arterial applanation tonometry technique are newer methods to measure blood pressure noninvasively but have not been extensively validated in clinical trials.

Esophageal Doppler

This device consists of an esophageal probe capable of continuous wave Doppler ultrasound. Thus real time flow in the aorta can be monitored continuously. By analyzing the Doppler flow signal and waveforms a variety of useful information such as stroke volume and the state of contractility can be derived.

Echocardiography

Both transthoracic and transesophageal echocardiography combined with Doppler imaging are powerful tools providing a plethora of sophisticated information on cardiovascular structure and function. The major limitation, however, is that it does not provide continuous data and is operator dependent.

INVASIVE MONITORING

Principles of Intravascular Pressure Measurement

Reliable pressure measurements and knowledge of artifacts that can lead to unreliable measurements is essential. The problem arises mainly with central venous pressure (CVP) and pulmonary artery occlusion pressure (PAOP) because range of normal clinical values is small and errors and become a large percentage of the true value.

Pressure Measurement

Pressure is measured in either millimeters of mercury (mm Hg) or centimeters of water (cm H_2O). Intravascular pressures are measured in mm Hg. Since mercury is about 13.6 times as dense as water, a change is transducer position of x cm will affect intravascular pressures by $x/1.36$ mm Hg.

Pressure was originally measured with columns of fluid but today it is measured with transducers. A transducer is essentially a Wheatstone's bridge consisting of a conducting membrane that is distorted by forces on its surface leading to change is resistance and hence current flowing through the membrane.

- Zeroing the transducer: The process of subtracting atmospheric pressure from measured pressure is called zeroing. This is achieved by opening the fluid-filled catheter system to atmosphere and adjusting the electronics so that starting pressure is atmospheric pressure and has a value of zero. This is important because otherwise measured pressures will vary with changes in atmospheric pressure and it would become necessary to keep a barometer in the unit to discern the reason for pressure changes

- Leveling: Pressure measurements in fluid-filled catheter systems are relative to an arbitrarily picked reference point. There is consensus that the midpoint of the right atrium be used as the reference. However, the reference point for arterial catheters in brain-injured patients while determining cerebral perfusion pressure (CPP) should ideally be at the level of the tragus. The measured pressure is determined by the height of the fluid column above the transducer. On initial zeroing the position of the stop cock that is opened to atmosphere is important for establishing a level or reference point, because on establishing an electronic zero the height of the fluid column above or below the transducer is canceled. After zeroing the catheter system the transducer system should remain fixed relative to the patient. If the bed is moved up or down x cm without the transducer the measured pressure decreased or increases by $x/1.36$ mm Hg, respectively. Leveling for measuring central venous pressures or ventricular pressures is an extremely important concept because small changes may lead to a wrong therapeutic decision.

- Transmural pressure: The heart and vascular structures within the thorax are surrounded by thoracic pressures. Similarly vascular structures in the abdomen are surrounded by intra-abdominal pressure. Thus the walls of the elastic structures within these cavities are stretched by the difference between the inside and outside pressure. This is called transmural pressure. The influence of pleural pressure, forced or active expiration, high levels of positive end-expiratory pressure (PEEP), and auto PEEP should be taken into account before interpretation of CVP, PAOP, or intra- abdominal pressure readings. Measurements of these pressure are always made at end-expiration while on or off positive pressure ventilation because pleural pressure in the absence of significant recruitment of expiratory muscles in closest to zero during this phase (Figs. 9.3 and 9.4).

DYNAMICS OF THE MONITORING SYSTEM (NATURAL FREQUENCY, DAMPING, AND THE FAST FLUSH TEST)

Arterial or venous pressure waves are complex waves created by summating individual sine waves of increasing frequency. The fundamental frequency is the first harmonic and occurs at the rate of the pulse. Subsequent harmonics are simply multiples of the fundamental frequency. A fluid-filled catheter system oscillates because of the pressure waves reflecting back and forth between the tip of the catheter and the transducer. The natural frequency of the catheter system is the frequency at which it oscillates maximally. If the natural frequency of the system is

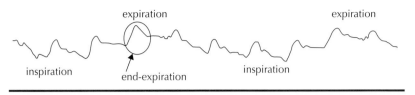

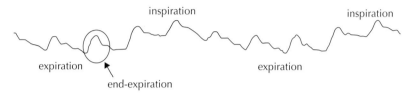

Figure 9.4. Measurement of vascular pressure during spontaneous and positive pressure breathing.

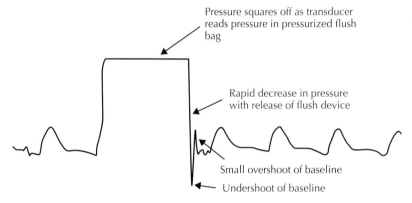

Figure 9.5. Square wave tracing of flush test.

close to any of the frequencies of the pressure waveform that is to be reproduced, the amplitude of the waveform form will be augmented (resonance). This will produce a distortion of the waveform with an artifactual increase in systolic pressure (ringing or pressure overshoot) and an artifactual decrease in diastolic blood pressure. To prevent this phenomenon the natural frequency of the catheter system should be at least six to ten times greater than the fundamental frequency of the pressure wave. Shorter and stiffer pressure monitoring tubing is associated with a higher natural frequency.

The damping coefficient determines how quickly an oscillating system comes to rest after having been set in motion. Some amount of damping is necessary so that characteristics of the waveform near

the natural frequency of the catheter system are not amplified. The natural frequency and damping coefficient of the system determine its dynamic characteristics. Overdamping diminishes and underdamping accentuates waveform transmission. Overdamping is usually caused by air bubbles in the system or kinking of the pressure tubing. Underdamping is caused by excessively long pressure tubing or numerous in line stopcocks.

- A fast flush or square wave test is often employed to test the damping of the system and optimize its dynamic response and performance.
- The maneuver involves opening and then rapidly closing the valve of the flush device. This produces a square wave tracing (Fig. 9.5).

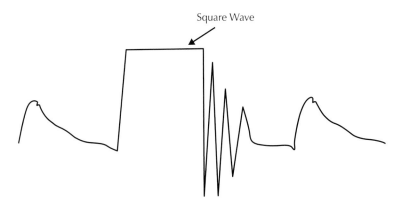

Figure 9.6. Underdamping of system.

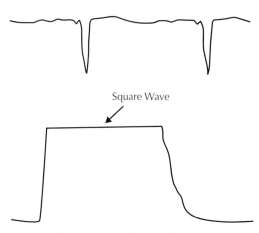

Figure 9.7. Overdamping of system.

- An optimally damped system displays one small undershoot and one small overshoot, followed by a return to normal waveform.
- Underdamped systems display multiple accentuated bounces while underdamped ones demonstrate an absence of bounce with a slurring of the square wave downstroke (Figs. 9.6 and 9.7).
- Inadequacy of the dynamic characteristics is corrected by removing air bubbles and blood clots, replacing kinked tubing, removing unnecessary stop cocks, and reducing the length of the tubing.

ARTERIAL PRESSURE MEASUREMENT

Indications for arterial cannulation include the need for reliable beat to beat measurement of blood pressure and frequent arterial blood sampling. Common sites of placement of an arterial cannula include radial, femoral, axillary, and dorsalis pedis arteries. The arterial waveform is generated by left ventricular

(LV) ejection and subsequent peripheral runoff. A slight pressure overshoot may be seen in the displayed waveform because monitoring systems in clinical practice are slightly underdamped. As the waveform moves more distally from the aorta harmonic resonance and pulse wave reflection cause distal pulse amplification causing the systolic pressure to be higher, diastolic pressure to be lower, and pulse pressure to be magnified peripherally. However, MAP remains close to that in the aortic arch and this is what should be taken into account clinically (Fig. 9.8).

Using the Arterial Waveform to Assess Fluid Responsiveness in Mechanically Ventilated Patients

The major therapeutic intervention in terms of hemodynamic optimization is fluid loading to normalize preload and maximize CO. However, fluid challenges fail to increase CO in about 50% of patients. The traditionally used static indices of preload (CVP and PAOP) remain poor predictors of fluid responsiveness. They fail to differentiate between patients who will or will not respond to a volume challenge.

During the inspiratory phase of a positive pressure breath venous return usually decreases secondary to an increase in upstream intrathoracic pressure and a waterfall effect on the venae cavae. Right ventricular (RV) stroke volume thus decreases. Conversely the LV stroke volume is augmented due to a decrease in afterload (decreased transmural aortic pressure) and an inspiratory squeezing of the blood in the pulmonary circulation enhancing pulmonary venous flow. The decrease in RV stroke volume leads to a decrease

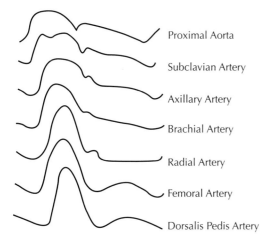

Figure 9.8. Waveforms at various sites of the body.

in LV stroke volume during the expiratory phase. These respiratory fluctuations in LV stroke volume are reflected in the arterial pressure waveform. Systolic arterial blood pressure thus varies cyclically during a positive pressure mechanical breath being maximal at end inspiration and minimal at end expiration.

■ Systolic pressure variation (SPV) is defined as the difference between the maximum inspiratory systolic and minimum expiratory systolic pressures. It is further characterized by dUP, which is the increase of pressure from baseline and dDOWN,

which is the decrease in pressure from baseline (Fig. 9.9).

■ Pulse pressure variation (PPV) is the difference between the maximal and minimal pulse pressures during the mechanical breath cycle. SPV, dDOWN, and PPV have all been found to be accurate predictors of volume responsiveness. PPV with a value of 13% best allows differentiation between responders and non responders with high specificity and sensitivity. Fluid responsiveness however does not automatically imply that volume is needed.

Keep in mind that these functional hemodynamic monitoring parameters are dependent on a passive mechanically ventilated patient with adequate tidal volume (at least 8 mL/kg). In addition, this is difficult to utilize in the face of cardiac arrhythmias especially atrial fibrillation where LV stroke volume changes beat to beat

PULMONARY ARTERY CATHETER

Since its introduction by Swan into clinical practice in 1970, the use of the pulmonary artery catheter (PAC) has remained shrouded in controversy. Some investigators called for a moratorium on its use following the study reported by Connors and associates that suggested an increased mortality, cost, and hospital stay associated with its

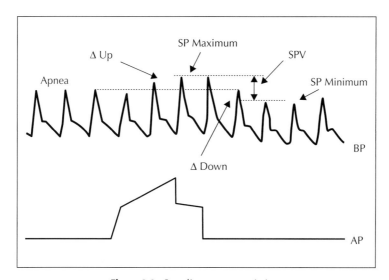

Figure 9.9. Systolic pressure variation.

Table 9.2. Hemodynamic parameters obtained from a PA catheter direct and indirect

Central venous pressure	CVP	1–6 mm Hg
Pulmonary capillary wedge pressure	PCWP	6–12 mm Hg
Cardiac index	CI	2.4–4 L/min·m²
Stroke volume index	SVI	40–70 mL/beat·m²
Left-ventricular stroke work index	LVSWI	40–60 g·m/m²
Right ventricular stroke work index	RVSWI	4–8 g·m/m²
Ejection fraction	RVEF	46–50%
End-diastolic volume	RVEDV	80–150 mL/m²
Systemic vascular resistance index	SVRI	1600–2400 dynes·s¹·cm⁵/m²
Pulmonary vascular resistance index	PVRI	200–400 dynes·s¹·cm⁵/m²

use. However, there was no mention about how hemodynamic data were obtained or used in this study. A more recent randomized controlled study in high-risk surgical patients conducted by Sandham and colleagues demonstrated no difference in mortality between the group that did or did not receive a PAC. The group that received a PAC had a higher incidence of pulmonary embolism. The most recent trial in acute lung injury (ALI) patients who were randomized to receive either a PAC or a central venous catheter, no benefit of the PAC could be demonstrated and routine use of the PAC in ALI was discouraged. Despite lack of absolute efficacy, the PAC in expert hands remains a valuable diagnostic tool. Nevertheless, nonexpert and indiscriminate use is ill advised. Adequate training should be provided to medical and nursing personnel about the appropriate use of the catheter.

The PAC provides a wealth of directly measured and derived physiologic data. Normal values are given in Table 9.2.

- Usually PAP and CVP are monitored continuously and PAOP, CO, and mixed venous oxygen saturation (Svo₂) are obtained intermittently.
- CO is calculated using the thermodilution technique.
- Some catheters have the ability to monitor Svo₂ and CO continuously.
- Volumetric PACs have the ability to measure RV end diastolic volumes but suffer the error of mathematical coupling through CO.

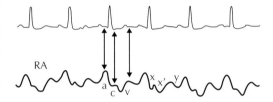

Figure 9.10. CVP waveform.

WAVEFORM ANALYSIS

Reading pressures right from the monitor is frequently erroneous and leads to misinterpretation. Since electrical activity of the heart governs all mechanical activity, waveforms should never be interpreted without the aid of a single-lead EKG tracing.

- CVP: This waveform is obtained from the right atrium and consists of 3 positive waves (a, c, and v) and two negative deflections (x and y) (Fig. 9.10). The a wave denotes atrial systole and occurs 80 milliseconds after the P wave on the EKG. The c wave denotes closure of the tricuspid valve, and the value of the CVP should ideally be read at the c wave. The v wave occurs due to passive filling of the atrium during ventricular systole and occurs after the T wave on the EKG. The x descent is due to atrial relaxation and the y descent denotes flow of blood from atrium to ventricle during tricuspid valve opening. If the c wave is not visible the value of the CVP is obtained by averaging the a wave. In abnormal

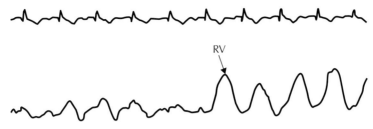

Figure 9.11. RV waveform.

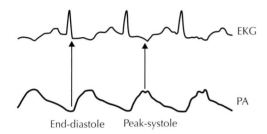

End-diastole   Peak-systole

Figure 9.12. PA waveform.

rhythms such as atrial fibrillation or paced rhythms where the *a* wave is not visible a line is drawn from the end of the QRS complex on the EKG down to the CVP tracing (Z point) and pressure is measured at this point.

■ Right ventricle: The RV waveform is characterized by a rapid upstroke to peak systole, a rapid downstroke, and a small terminal rise at end diastole (Fig. 9.11).

■ Pulmonary artery: As the PAC is advanced through the pulmonic valve into the pulmonary artery, the waveform changes. Peak systole of the PA and RV are similar. The characteristic change is a rise in diastolic pressure. The PA waveform consists of a rapid upstroke reflecting onset of RV ejection, a dicrotic notch denoting closure of the pulmonary valve, and a smooth progressive diastolic runoff (Fig. 9.12). Peak systole is found after the QRS complex but before the T wave. The PA and RV waveforms can be confused especially if the catheter tip has migrated back into the RV. Careful examination of the contour and diastolic pressure can usually discriminate between the two.

■ PAOP: The PAOP waveform, like the CVP, has three positive waves (*a, c,* and *v*) and two negative deflections (*v* and *y*). The *c* wave is usually not visible due to damping. The *a* wave occurs about

200 milliseconds after the P wave on the EKG (Fig. 9.13). This time delay is due to the longer distance the wave travels through the pulmonary circulation to the transducer. The *v* wave occurs after the T wave on the EKG and significantly later than the PAP waveform on the EKG tracing. Several entities such as mitral regurgitation can give rise to giant *v* waves. These giant waves can be mistaken for a PAP waveform. The key lies in timing with the EKG. Accurate timing can reliably distinguish between the two (Figs. 9.14 and 9.15). When reading the PAOP in the presence of a giant *v* wave, the *a* wave is averaged.

MEASUREMENT OF CARDIAC OUTPUT

Thermodilution Cardiac Output

Thermodilution CO is an indicator dilution technique which involves the injection of cold saline into the proximal port of the PAC. The resultant temperature drop is measured by a fast response thermistor near the catheter tip. A thermodilution curve is then generated and the area under the curve is inversely proportional to the CO. This method has been extensively validated, however the accuracy is reduced in the setting of tricuspid regurgitation, septal defects, poor technique and very low CO states.

Transpulmonary Cardiac Output

Transpulmonary CO involves injection of cold saline into the venous circulation through a central venous catheter. The resultant temperature change is measured by a thermistor equipped arterial catheter. CO is estimated using the Stewart Hamilton equation. The commercially available PiCCO system (Pulsion technologies) uses this technology.

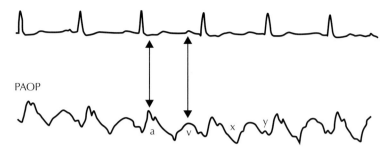

Figure 9.13. PAOP waveform.

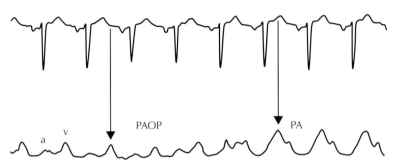

Figure 9.14. Large *v* wave in a pulmonary artery occlusion waveform.

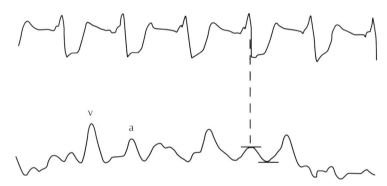

Figure 9.15. Timing measurement of vascular pressure waves with the EKG.

Pulse Contour Cardiac Output

Pulse contour CO assumes that the compliance and impedance variables of the arterial tree and aorta remain constant. The arterial waveform under these circumstances is dependent only on the LV stroke volume. Thus monitoring the contour of the arterial waveform can provide a beat-to-beat analysis of stroke volume. CO first needs to be measured via an alternative technique such as thermodilution and calibrated with the arterial pulse. Under conditions of rapidly changing arterial tone, this technique becomes unreliable.

Lithium Dilution Cardiac Output

Isotonic lithium chloride is used as an indicator and is injected as a small bolus either centrally or peripherally. A concentration–time curve is then generated using an ion-selective electrode attached to an arterial line. CO is then calculated via the lithium dose and the area under the concentration time curve.

Esophageal Doppler Cardiac Output

A Doppler probe placed in the esophagus monitors descending aortic blood flow. The velocity time

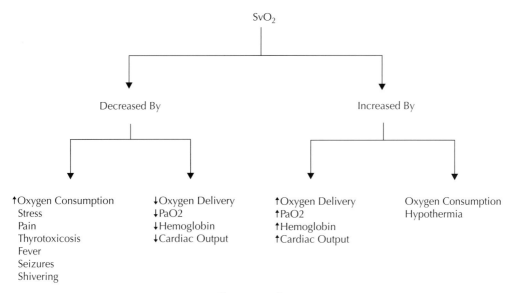

Figure 9.16. Sv_{O_2}

integral is then calculated based on Doppler shift of signals from the aorta. SV is then obtained by multiplying the cross-sectional area of the descending aorta with the velocity time integral. A correction factor is needed because not all the blood flow enters the descending aorta.

MONITORING TISSUE PERFUSION

Mixed Venous Oxygen Saturation (Sv_{O_2})

Shock represents an imbalance between Do_2 and $\dot{V}o_2$ wherein either supply is inadequate to meet demands or O_2 extraction or utilization is impaired.

- Sv_{O_2} is used as a surrogate maker for the adequacy of Do_2. It can be altered by changes in CO, Hgb, arterial oxygen saturation, or $\dot{V}o_2$ (Fig. 9.16).
- As Do_2 decreases, oxygen extraction increases to keep $\dot{V}o_2$ constant. Therefore blood returning to the right side of the heart has low oxygen content and a reduced Sv_{O_2}.

Thus a reduced Sv_{O_2} is indicative of global hypoxia and oxygen debt. This debt leads to anaerobic metabolism and lactate production, which has been associated with increased mortality. Though a low Sv_{O_2} is indicative of global hypoxia, it does not allow any inference about the cause. Rather it is an early sign of something being amiss and forces the physician to evaluate all aspects of either reduced Do_2 or increased Vo_2.

- Sv_{O_2} is usually measured intermittently by drawing blood from the pulmonary port of the PAC.
- Catheters using infrared oximetry based on reflection spectrophotometry have the ability to monitor Sv_{O_2} continuously.

Although a low value of Sv_{O_2} is suggestive of oxygen debt a high value does not necessarily indicate well being. Patients with severe sepsis or hepatic failure are frequently unable to utilize oxygen properly even if Do_2 is adequate (cytopathic hypoxia). In these cases Sv_{O_2} is often elevated while oxygen extraction is reduced. Monitoring Sv_{O_2} gives the clinician a global picture of tissue perfusion and does not provide information about the adequacy of regional Do_2 or oxygen extraction.

Monitoring superior vena cava oxygen saturation ($Sc\dot{V}o_2$) was used as a surrogate to Sv_{O_2} in a recent study of early goal directed therapy in patients with septic shock.

Gastric Tonometry

Tonometry is a method to equilibrate gas tension between two compartments. A nasogastric tube detects tissue carbon dioxide that diffuses into a saline/air-filled balloon. Air tonometry has a lesser equilibration time and is fully automated. The partial pressure of carbon dioxide (pco_2) is measured and the gastric intramucosal pH (pH_i) as well as the mucosal arterial difference in pco_2 is calculated. Both gastric mucosal acidosis as well as increased mucosal arterial pco_2 have been demonstrated to be markers of mesenteric dyoxia and markers of mortality and morbidity in critically ill patients. Optimization of pH_i and Pco_2 gap have been associated with improvements in morbidity and mortality

Sublingual Capnometry

This involves placing a CO_2 sensor under the tongue facing the sublingual mucosa. This technique may prove to be an early indicator of systemic perfusion failure in critically ill patients. In one study Marik and Bankov have demonstrated that sublingual pressure of CO_2 ($Pslco_2$) better differentiates between survivors and non survivors than lactate.

MONITORING THE MICROCIRCULATION

Although global hemodynamic monitoring is of value it may fail to detect subtle alterations in organ perfusion. The microcirculation plays a vital role in organ function supplying oxygen and nutrients. Microcirculatory oxygen delivery cannot be predicted by global measurements as hematocrit is lower in capillaries and is unevenly distributed at branch points. Microvascular alterations have been demonstrated in many pathological conditions such as ischemia, reperfusion injury, and sepsis. Orthogonal polarization spectral (OPS) and sidestream dark field (SDF) imaging techniques have recently been developed to visualize the microcirculation. They can be used in tissue protected by a thin epithelial layer with the sublingual mucosa being the most accessible. Studies have now demonstrated decreased density and impaired perfusion of small vessels and capillaries in severe sepsis compared to healthy controls. The impairment is more severe in non survivors and persistent alterations were associated with organ failure and death.

In subarachnoid hemorrhage, cortical vessel reactivity changed more in patients prone to developing vasospasm compared to patients who did not develop it.

Other techniques such as near infrared spectroscopy and laser Doppler flowmetry are currently under investigation.

Thus probing the microcirculation may be the next wave of hemodynamic monitoring with the

provision of a better understanding of pathophysiology of shock states and the development of therapies aimed at the microcirculation (e.g., activated protein C).

THE FUTURE OF HEMODYNAMIC MONITORING

The monitors of today present raw data without intelligent integration. It is clear that hemodynamic monitoring is only a piece of the puzzle. We must learn to think in terms of the entire organism. We should therefore design, test, and integrate closed loop systems that monitor at macroscopic, microscopic, and molecular levels. When derangements are detected effective therapies should be immediately and precisely titrated. As our knowledge of critical illness is refined, so will our ability to monitor and treat effectively.

REFERENCES

Barcroft J, Hill AV. The nature of oxyhaemoglobin with a note on its molecular weight. *J Physiol*. 1910;**39**(6):411–28.

Bernardin G, Tiger F, Fouché R, Mattéi M Continuous noninvasive measurement of aortic blood flow in critically ill patients with a new esophageal echo-Doppler system. *J Crit Care*. 1998;**13**(4):177–83.

Cholley BP, Singer M. Esophageal Doppler: noninvasive cardiac output monitor. *Echocardiography*. 2003;**20**(8):763–9.

Connors AF Jr, Speroff T, Dawson NV, et al. The effectiveness of right heart catheterization in the initial care of critically ill patients. SUPPORT Investigators. *JAMA*. 1996;**276**(11):889–97.

Gardner RM. Hemodynamic monitoring: from catheter to display. *Acute Care*. 1986;**12**(1):3–33.

Gibbs NC, Gardner RM. Dynamics of invasive pressure monitoring systems: clinical and laboratory evaluation. *Heart Lung*. 1988;**17**(1):43–51.

Gutierrez G, Palizas F, Doglio G, et al. Gastric intramucosal pH as a therapeutic index of tissue oxygenation in critically ill patients. *Lancet*. 1992;**339**(8787):195–9.

Jansen JR, Schreuder JJ, Mulier JP, Smith NT, Settels JJ, Wesseling KH. A comparison of cardiac output derived from the arterial pressurewave against thermodilution in cardiac surgery patients. *Br J Anaesth*. 2001;**87**(2):212–22.

John AD, Fleisher LA. Electrocardiography. the ECG. *Anesthesiol Clin*. 2006;**24**(4):697–715.

Kirton OC, Windsor J, Wedderburn R, Hudson-Civetta J, Shatz DV, Mataragas NR, Civetta JM. Failure of splanchnic resuscitation in the acutely injured trauma patient correlates with multiple organ system failure and length of stay in the ICU. *Chest*. 1998;**113**(4):1064–9.

Kumar A, Anel R, Bunnell E, et al. Pulmonary artery occlusion pressure and central venous pressure fail to predict ventricular filling volume, cardiac performance, or the response to volume infusion in normal subjects. *Crit Care Med*. 2004;**32**(3):691–9.

Kurita T, Morita K, Kato S, Kikura M, Horie M, Ikeda K Comparison of the accuracy of the lithium dilution technique with the thermodilution technique for measurement of cardiac output. *Br J Anaesth*. 1997;**79**(6):770–5.

Matthys K, Verdonck P. Development modeling of arterial applanation tonometry: a review. *Technol Health Care*. 2002;**10**(1):65–76.

Magder S. Clinical usefulness of respiratory variations in arterial pressure. *Am J Respir Crit Care Med*. 2004; **169**(2):151–5.

Marik PE, Bankov A. Sublingual capnometry versus traditional markers of tissue oxygenation in critically ill patients. *Crit Care Med*. 2003;**31**:818–22.

Michard F, Boussat S, Chemla D, et al. Relation between respiratory changes in arterial pulse pressure and fluid responsiveness in septic patients with acute circulatory failure. *Am J Respir Crit Care Med*. 2000;**162**(1):134–8.

Michard F, Teboul JL. Using heart-lung interactions to assess fluid responsiveness during mechanical ventilation. *Crit Care*. 2000;**4**(5):282–9.

Michard F, Teboul JL. Predicting fluid responsiveness in ICU patients: a critical analysis of the evidence. *Chest*. 2002;**121**(6):2000–8.

National Heart, Lung, and Blood Institute Acute Respiratory Distress Syndrome (ARDS) Clinical Trials Network, Wheeler AP, Bernard GR, Thompson BT, et al. Pulmonary-artery versus central venous catheter to guide treatment of acute lung injury. *N Engl J Med*. 2006;**354**(21):2213–24.

Pennings FA, Bouma GJ, Ince C. Direct observation of the human cerebral microcirculation during aneurysm surgery reveals increased arteriolar contractility. *Stroke*. 2004;**35**(6):1284–8.

Rivers E, Nguyen B, Havstad S; Early Goal-Directed Therapy Collaborative Group. Early goal-directed therapy in the treatment of severe sepsis and septic shock. *N Engl J Med*. 2001;**345**(19):1368–77.

Sagawa K, Suga H, Shoukas AA, Bakalar KM. End-systolic pressure/volume ratio: a new index of ventricular contractility. *Am J Cardiol*. 1977;**40**(5):748–53.

Sakka SG, Rühl CC, Pfeiffer UJ, Beale R, McLuckie A, Reinhart K, Meier-Hellmann1 A. Assessment of cardiac preload and extravascular lung water by single transpulmonary thermodilution. *Intens Care Med*. 2000;**26**(2):180–7.

Sakr Y, Dubois MJ, De Backer D, Creteur J, Vincent JL. Persistent microcirculatory alterations are associated with organ failure and death in patients with septic shock. *Crit Care Med*. 2004;**32**(9):1825–31.

Sandham JD, Hull RD, Brant RF. Canadian Critical Care Clinical Trials Group. A randomized, controlled trial of the use of pulmonary-artery catheters in high-risk surgical patients. *N Engl J Med*. 2003;**348**(1):5–14.

The Linacre Lecture on the Law of the Heart. London: Longmans, Green and Co, 1918.

Trzeciak S, Dellinger RP, Parrillo JE. Microcirculatory Alterations in Resuscitation and Shock Investigators. Early microcirculatory perfusion derangements in patients with severe sepsis and septic shock: relationship to hemodynamics, oxygen transport, and survival *Ann Emerg Med*. 2007;**49**(1):88–98.

10 Ischemic Stroke

May A. Kim, MD, Justin Wagner, MD, Clif Segil, MD, Reed Levine, MD,
and Gene Y. Sung, MD, MPH

Stroke is the third leading cause of death and the leading cause of disability in the United States. There are two major categories of strokes: ischemic and hemorrhagic. Approximately 80% of strokes are ischemic and 20% are hemorrhagic. Within these two major categories are subcategories of possible etiologies that fit under ischemic such as cardioembolism, large vessel thrombosis, and lacunar strokes. Hemorrhagic causes of stroke include hypertension, underlying aneurysmal or arteriovenous vascular malformations, ischemic stroke with hemorrhagic transformation, or metastatic primary tumors that bleed (i.e., melanoma, renal cell carcinoma, lung carcinoma, thyroid carcinoma). Neurocritical care units (NCCUs) have been gaining popularity among academic institutions in providing a higher level of care and expertise in the acute setting. In this chapter, we focus on the care of ischemic strokes in the NCCU.

EVALUATING THE STROKE PATIENT

- The treating physician must evaluate and establish airway patency.
  - If the airway appears to be unstable, the patient is in respiratory distress, or the patient's Glasgow coma scale (GCS) is <8, the patient needs endotracheal intubation, and mechanical ventilation should be instituted.
- Once airway is established, the systemic blood pressure should be evaluated.
  - Acute ischemic stroke patients very rarely present with hypotension; however, when present is usually associated with other medical problems such as sepsis, myocardial infarction, or dehydration.

- Before a decision is made to either lower blood pressure or provide an agent such as a vasopressor to elevate blood pressure in a suspected ischemic stroke patient, a swift history as well as neurologic examination need to be completed.

The most accepted way to evaluate a patient who comes into the emergency department with acute neurologic deficits consistent with stroke is the National Institutes of Health Stroke Scale (NIHSS).

- This scale evaluates different aspects of the neurologic exam including consciousness, language/speech, sensorimotor systems, visual fields, and neglect.
- The highest score possible is 42 and the higher the number indicates presumably either a large or more severe stroke. It is important to recognize and perform the NIHSS in the acute setting because it can help to determine patients eligible for aggressive medical management as well as provide a standardized and reproducible neurologic exam.

Once the NIHSS has been established, radiologic evaluation is important to determine the stroke type. Several imaging modalities are available for use in the acute ischemic stroke patient. These include head computed tomography (HCT), computed tomography angiography (CTA), magnetic resonance imaging (MRI), magnetic resonance angiography (MRA), and transcranial Doppler (TCD).

Head CT is the quickest scan to obtain to differentiate acute ischemic strokes from hemorrhagic strokes, subarachnoid hemorrhages, subdural hematomas, hydrocephalus, and cerebral edema.

The presence of hypodense areas involving >50% of the middle cerebral artery (MCA) territory within 5 hours of symptom onset or the entire MCA territory 24–48 hours after stroke onset is highly predictive of poor outcome and death in 80% of these patients. CTA of the head and neck is also a rapid scan in which includes a noncontrast HCT; contrast is then administered to assess the vasculature of the head and neck and whether a blockage is visible for possible intervention.

MRI is another imaging modality that has important diagnostic tools and has revolutionized the evaluation process of patients with acute ischemic stroke. Such modalities include the diffusion-weighted (DWI) and perfusion-weighted imaging (PWI). DWI measures the restricted diffusion of water molecules in the ischemic brain tissue, which can then be confirmed by the apparent diffusion coefficient (ADC). DWI is more sensitive than conventional MRI sequences to detect ischemic tissue, and can be positive within minutes after stroke onset. Abnormal areas appear hyperintense compared to normal brain tissue. The addition of PWI provides a better understanding of the hemodynamic characteristics of the ischemic brain.

Cerebral angiography is considered the "gold standard" radiologic method of choice to detect cerebral vessel occlusion and delineate the vascular anatomy. Advantages of this technique are the possibility of intra-arterial administration of medications (i.e., thrombolytic agents), and the performance of endovascular treatments (i.e., angioplasty or stent placement of stenosed arteries and clot retrieval).

Transcranial dopplers (TCDs) are useful in determining with a high degree of certainty vessel stenoses, vessel occlusion, and embolic signals originating in the heart or proximal cerebral vessels. It can also be useful for assessing colateral circulation and determining successful recanalization.

Patients with NIHSS ≥4 or any disabling deficit are potential candidates for thrombolytic therapy with intravenous (IV) tissue plasminogen activator (tPA), which is FDA approved if within 3 hours of symptom onset excluding all contraindications (Table 10.1). In the NINDS trial, patients with NIHSS values ≥18 seemed to have the worst clinical outcomes likely secondary to increased clot burdet in a proximal artery. In the NINDS trial, patients treated with IVtPa had improved clinical outcome at 3 months when compared with placebo and a symptomatic hemorrhage rate of ~6%.

Table 10.1. Indications/contraindications to IV tPA

Indications

1. Age >18 years old
2. Clinical diagnosis of ischemic stroke with a measurable neurologic deficit
3. Exact time of onset established to be <180 minutes before treatment

Contraindications

1. Evidence of intracranial hemorrhage on pretreatment HCT
2. Minor or rapidly improving symptoms
3. Presentation suggestive of SAH even with normal HCT
4. Seizure at onset of stroke (relative)
5. Platelet count <100,000
6. Received heparin within 48 hours and with elevated PTT
7. Known history of intracranial hemorrhage
8. Other stroke or serious head trauma within past 3 months
9. Major surgery within last 14 days
10. Sustained SBP >185 mm Hg
11. Sustained DBP >110 mm Hg
12. Aggressive treatment necessary to lower BP
13. Gastrointestinal or urinary tract hemorrhage within 21 days
14. Arterial puncture at noncompressible site within 7 days
15. Serum glucose <50 mg/dL or >400 mg/dL

From the Brain Attack Coalition: tPA Stroke Study Group Guidelines. http://www.stroke-site.org/guidelines/tpa_guidelines.html

Intra-arterial (IA) tPA may be administered within 6 hours of symptom onset if the patient angiographically demonstrates an arterial occlusion and no major early infarct signs on the baseline HCT scan or MRI for selected patients in centers with the appropriate neurologic and interventional expertise.

Mechanical thrombectomy with use of either the MERCI (Mechanical Embolus Removal in Cerebral Ischemia) device or the newer PENUMBRA device, which uses aspiration for by clot retrieval, may be performed up to 6–8 hours after symptom onset.

- Indications for mechanical thrombectomy are for patients in whom IV tPA has not resolved a visible clot, or in those whose neurologic exam has worsened or not improved with residual clot still visible on imaging.
- The devices themselves have been FDA approved for the *removal* of thrombus in the neurovasculature of patients who are experiencing the symptoms of ischemic stroke.
- The decision to try to remove a clot mechanically should be made on an individual patient basis depending on the NIHSS, underlying medical history, age, whether or not infarcted tissue is already seen on imaging modalities, and the risks versus benefits of recanalization.

INDICATIONS FOR ADMISSION TO THE NEUROCRITICAL CARE UNIT (NCCU)

Patients with acute ischemic stroke may be admitted to the NCCU for neurologic or medical reasons (Table 10.2).

- Patients treated with IV tPA are at risk for intracranial hemorrhage and require close monitoring for at least 24 hours, including frequent neurologic exams to assess if any worsening in clinical exam.
- The presence of intracranial hemorrhage after thrombolytics requires aggressive management of blood pressure to make sure there is no expansion of the hematoma (while maintaining proper cerebral perfusion), reverse any coagulopathies that may be present, and to watch for clinical signs of cerebral edema.
- The presence of a massive MCA infarct as determined by an NIHSS >18 and predictive HCT signs (>50% MCA territory) is an indication for close monitoring in the NCCU even if the patient appears to be stable in the emergency department. These patients may develop malignant cerebral edema and herniation, especially in the first 3–5 days of presentation, which carries a high mortality and has a high frequency of cardiac and pulmonary complications.
- Other neurologic conditions that warrant admission to the NCCU include crescendo transient ischemic attacks (TIAs) or limb-shaking TIAs (has a high incidence of ischemic stroke if untreated), progressive worsening of neurologic deficit (may

Table 10.2. Indications for admission to the NCCU after acute ischemic stroke

Neurologic

1. Post-thrombolysis
2. Massive cerebral infarction
3. Intracranial bleeding
4. Crescendo transient ischemic attacks
5. Progressive worsening of neurologic symptoms
6. Arterial dissection
7. Post-endovascular treatment
8. Cerebral vasospasm after subarachnoid hemorrhage

Non-neurologic

1. Respiratory failure
2. Mechanical ventilation for airway protection
3. Persistent hypotension
4. Intravenous drug management for hypertension
5. Aggressive pulmonary therapy
6. Cardiac infarction or arrhythmias
7. Severe systemic bleeding

From Sung GY. Emergency and Critical Care Management of Acute Ischemic Stroke. American Academy of Neurology, 2008.

benefit from the use of vasopressor agents to induce hypertension to increase cerebral perfusion), arterial dissection (requires hypervolemia and possibly hypertensive therapy), postendovascular therapy (high risk for embolization, and reocclusion), and cerebral vasospasm following subarachnoid hemorrhage wherein patients may require hypervolemic, hypertensive, and hyperdynamic therapy to help decrease the development of ischemic strokes.

Non–neurologic reasons for admission to the NCCU are those with respiratory failure, mechanical ventilation, vasopressor administration for hypotension, IV therapy for hypertension, cardiac abnormalities (i.e., infarction, ischemia, or arrhythmias), severe systemic bleeding after thrombolytic therapy, and need for aggressive pulmonary therapy.

ICU MANAGEMENT OF ACUTE ISCHEMIC STROKE

Blood Pressure Before and After IV/IA tPA

The management of arterial hypertension remains controversial. The goal of maintaining adequate cerebral perfusion must be balanced by minimizing the complications of hypertension. The blood pressure before administering IV tPA should be systolic blood pressures (SBP) <185 mm Hg or diastolic blood pressures (DBP) <110 mm Hg.

- Current guidelines recommend labetalol, nitropaste, or nicardipine infusions to help lower blood pressure to <185/110 mm Hg (Table 10.3).
- Goal blood pressure post IV/IA tPA or other acute reperfusion interventions should be SBP <180 and DBP <105 for at least the first 24 hours. The blood pressure is measured every 15 minutes for the first 2 hours and subsequently every 30 minutes for the next 6 hours, then hourly until 24 hours after treatment.
- During or after IV tPA, if SBP ranges from 180 to 230 mm Hg, or DBP ranges from 105 to 120 mm Hg then labetalol should be given. If SBP >230 mm Hg, or DBP 121–140 mm Hg, then labetalol or nicardipine may be used. If blood pressure remains uncontrolled with the use of the aforementioned agents, then one may consider the use of nitroprusside (Table 10.3). Nitrates and nitroprusside can lead to cerebral vasodilation and can increase intracranial pressures, so should be used with caution.

Excessively high blood pressure is associated with an increased risk of symptomatic hemorrhagic transformation. Failure to meet the blood pressure parameters may be one of the reasons why an increased risk of hemorrhagic complications occurs after administration tPA. The lower limit of blood pressure should be adequate to keep the cerebral perfusion pressure (CPP) >70 mm Hg.

No antiplatelets or antithrombotics should be given for 24 hours after receiving tPA. One should also avoid placing nasogastric tubes, indwelling bladder catheters, or intra-arterial pressure catheters for 24 hours as well. Many patients have a spontaneous decline in blood pressure within the first hours of stroke even without treatment, which may be the result of being in a less stressful environment (out of

emergency department, in quiet room), rest, bladder emptied, and pain is controlled.

There is a need for large, well-designed trials to clarify the management of arterial hypertension after acute stroke. There is controversy regarding the acute lowering of blood pressure in acute ischemic strokes as being beneficial in that lowering pressure reduces the formation of brain edema, lessens the risk of hemorrhagic transformation of infarction, prevents further vascular damage, and forestalls early recurrent strokes.

- However, Castillo et al. noted that the aggressive treatment of blood pressure (>20 mm Hg) may lead to worsening of the neurologic exam, higher rates of poor outcomes or death, and larger infarct volumes by reducing the perfusion pressures to infracted areas of the brain.
- A trial testing the utility of antihypertensive therapy in the setting of stroke (Controlling Hypertension and Hypotension Immediately Post-Stroke [CHHIPS]) study showed that stroke patients who were treated for hypertension had lower mortality after 3 months than patients who received a placebo.
  - ▷ Blood pressure reduction was not associated with deterioration in neurologic status at 72 hours.
  - ▷ Active treatment did not alter death or disability at 2 weeks.
  - ▷ The CHHIPS pilot data emphasizes the need for a full-scale trial to see if these encouraging preliminary results can be reproduced.
- Pending ongoing trials on whether acute lowering of blood pressure or keeping blood pressure high in the acute setting is better, the consensus is that emergency administration of antihypertensive agents should be withheld unless the DBP is >120 mm Hg or if the SBP is >220 mm Hg.
  - ▷ Lowering blood pressure should be done cautiously and a reasonable goal would be to lower it by 15–25% within the first day (post 24 hours tPA).
  - ▷ There is no data to support the administration of any specific antihypertensive agent, and the treating physician should select medications for lowering blood pressure in the acute stroke setting on a case-by-case basis based on any underlying medical conditions that would prohibit certain blood pressure medications (i.e., using beta-blockers in asthmatics).

Table 10.3 Blood pressure management before and after IV rtPA/acute intervention

Indication that patient is eligible for treatment with intravenous rtPA or other acute reperfusion intervention

Blood pressure level

Systolic >185 mm Hg or diastolic >110 mm Hg

Labetalol 10–20 mg IV over 1–2 minutes, may repeat × 1;

or

Nitropaste 1–2 inches;

or

Nicardipine infusion, 5 mg/h, titrate up by 2.5 mg/h at 5–15-minute intervals, miximum dose 15 mg/h; when desired blood pressure attained, reduce to 3 mg/h

If blood pressure does not decline and remains > 185/110 mm Hg, do not administer rtPA

Management of blood pressure during and after treatment with rtPA or other acute reperfusion intervention

Minitor blood pressure every 15 minutes during treatment and then for another 2 hours, then every 30 minutes for 6 hours, and then every hour for 16 hours

Blood pressure level

Systolic 180–230 mm Hg or diastolic 105 to 120 mm Hg

Labetalol 10 mg IV over 1–2 minutes, may repeat every 10–20 minutes, maximum dose of 300 mg;

or

Labetalol 10 mg IV followed by an infusion at 2–8 mg/min

Systolic > 230 Hg or diastolic 121–140 mm Hg

Labetalol 10 mg IV over 1–2 minutes, may repeat every 10–20 minutes, maximum dose of 300 mg;

or

Labetalol 10 mg IV followed by an infusion at 2–8 mg/min;

or

Nicardipine infusion, 5 mg/h, titrate up to desired effect by increasing 2.5 mg/h every 5 minutes to maximum of 15 mg/h

If blood pressure not controlled, consider sodium nitroprusside

Adapted from Adams HP Jr, Del Zoppo G, Alberts MJ, et al. Guidelines for the early management of patients with ischemic stroke: a scientific statement from the Stroke Council of the American Stroke Association. *Stroke.* 2007; **38**:1655–1711.

Glucose Control in the NCCU

Blood glucose should be checked in all suspected acute stroke patients when they are evaluated because hypoglycemia/hyperglycemia may mimic symptoms of ischemic stroke and may also lead to brain injury. Most patients who present to the emergency department with stroke symptoms usually have moderate elevations of glucose level in their serum even if they are not diabetic and it is usually from an acute stress response to the cerebrovascular event. The effect of high blood sugar in acute stroke patients is not completely understood but may be associated with increasing tissue acidosis from anaerobic glycolysis, lactic acidosis, and free radical production. It may also affect the blood–brain barrier and the development of brain edema.

- Baird et al. found that the effects of hyperglycemia (blood glucose level >200 mg/dL) during the first 24 hours after stroke independently predicted the expansion of the volume of ischemic stroke and poor neurologic outcomes.

■ Also reported was a 25% symptomatic hemorrhage rate in ischemic stroke patients who received tPA whose serum glucose was >200 mg/dL.

■ The desired level of blood glucose is in the range of 80–140 mg/dL.

While acute ischemic stroke patients are being monitored in the NCCU, serum glucose should be monitored every 4 hours and sliding scale of insulin or insulin drip begun if glucose >140. In patients who received tPA, admission glucose levels of 140 mg/dL was associated with poor outcomes; therefore, patients with blood glucose levels >140 should be treated with insulin.

■ The United Kingdom Glucose Insulin in Stroke Trial (GIST-UK) tested a solution of glucose/potassium/insulin to induce and maintain euglycemia after acute stroke to observe if it reduced death at 90 days.
  ▸ The study found no evidence to support acute management of raised blood glucose after stroke.
  ▸ However, some criticisms of this study were that the treatment, an IV infusion of glucose/potassium/insulin (GKI) had a significant impact on blood pressure lowering that could be potentially harmful as well as the fact that hypoglycemia was documented in 41% of patients.

■ Until more conclusive evidence is found, both hypoglycemia and hyperglycemia in acute stroke patients should continue to be avoided. A serum glucose level >140 mg/dL will trigger the administration of an insulin drip at our institution with close monitoring of serum glucose to avoid hypoglycemia .

Temperature Management in the NCCU

■ Fever in the setting of an acute ischemic stroke is associated with an increased risk of morbidity and mortality by increasing the metabolic demands of the brain, releasing neurotransmitters, and an increase in free radical production.

■ When a patient becomes febrile, the source of fever should be investigated by obtaining blood cultures, urine cultures, chest radiograph, and assessing line status (i.e., when lines were placed and whether that could be a nidus for infection).

■ Patients should be placed on acetaminophen 650 mg every 4–6 hours by mouth, per rectum, or by nasogastric tube when the temperature is >38°C.

■ If temperature is >38.5°C, a cooling blanket and ice packs may be used in addition to acetaminophen to lower the temperature to ≤37°C.

■ Several studies in the past used either aspirin or acetaminophen in achieving normothermia, or administered daily acetaminophen to febrile/afebrile patients in an attempt to improve neurologic outcomes.

■ To date, there are no data demonstrating that using medications to lower body temperature among febrile or afebrile patients improves neurologic prognosis after stroke. The goal in the NCCU is to maintain normothermia in the acute ischemic stroke patient.

Hypothermia has been shown to be neuroprotective in experimental and focal hypoxic brain injury models. It is thought that cooling the brain delays the depletion of energy stores, lessens intracellular acidosis, slows the influx of calcium into ischemic cells, suppresses the production of oxygen free radicals, and lessens the impact of excitatory amino acids. Hypothermia has been shown to reduce mortality and improve neurologic outcomes among patients with cardiac arrest (ventricular fibrillation). Hypothermia in the central nervous system may decrease intracranial pressure (ICP) by cerebral vasoconstriction and associated decrease in blood volume. It may act as an anticonvulsant as well. Results of studies using induced hypothermia in patients with malignant ischemic strokes in an attempt to improve neurologic outcome have been mixed.

Reith et al. (1996) prospectively enrolled 390 patients within 6 hours of stroke onset. They found that an association exists between body temperature and initial stroke severity, infarct size, mortality, and outcome. Mortality rates and neurologic outcome improved in the hypothermic group. For every 1°C increase in temperature, the risk of poor outcome doubled. Only randomized controlled trials of hypothermia can prove whether this relation is causal.

The COOL AID (Cooling for Acute Ischemic Brain Damage) trial tested whether endovascular cooling combined with meperidine, buspirone, and surface warming could achieve hypothermia rapidly in acute ischemic stroke patients. Induced moderate hypothermia was feasible using an endovascular cooling device in most patients with acute ischemic stroke. Further studies are still needed to determine if hypothermia improves neurologic outcome in acute ischemic stroke patients.

Currently, we do not routinely practice cooling patients with malignant ischemic infarcts unless there is difficulty controlling a patient's intracranial pressures. We discuss treatment options in malignant ischemic strokes in the latter part of this chapter.

There are several methods of cooling down the body as well as the brain. Cooling blankets are available but do not efficiently cool the body in a controlled manner, as is the case with other traditional methods such as ice water baths and fans. Newer methodologies utilize computer-regulated cooling units that circulate cool saline through an endovascular device or superconductive gel pads that circulate to effectively cool patients down to 33 or 34°C over a 24-hour period. The endovascular cooling devices have been used to effectively cool patients in a controlled fashion but require the placement of a large-bore catheter in the inferior vena cava via a femoral vein. The machine allows for the controlled rewarming of a patient no greater than 0.3°C/h up to 36.5–37°C to prevent the risk of cerebral edema.

- The use of paralytics and sedative agents are indicated to help prevent shivering during the cooling process and prevent the body from increasing its core temperature.
- The patient should be placed on deep venous thrombosis (DVT) prophylaxis 12 hours after the removal of the catheter and a lower extremity Doppler ultrasound may be obtained if a DVT is suspected because the use of an intravascular device predisposes one to DVTs (because of the large size of catheter).

Some of the side effects to therapeutic hypothermia are hypotension, cardiac arrhythmias, and infections. An intranasal cooling device in development that may effectively cool the brain and avoid some of the side effects delivers perfluorochemical spray via nasal tongs within minutes. The nasal cavity is cooled to 5°C, thus cooling the brain by conduction and by the cooled blood supply through this vascular region. Exciting devices are being developed and hopefully larger well designed trials will prove that hypothermia is safe and effective in the treatment of acute ischemic strokes.

Fluid Status Management and Nutrition in Acute Ischemic Strokes

The goal in the NCCU for acute ischemic stroke patients is to maintain euvolemia. Systemic dehydration may reduce cerebral edema but may worsen cerebral perfusion. Average maintenance fluid is 1 mL/kg per hour which is approximately 2000–2500 mL/day for adults. Normal saline is the intravenous fluid of choice in the NCCU. Hypotonic solutions can worsen cerebral edema and are avoided. Dextrose containing solutions are also avoided in that glucose is metabolized to lactic acid in the ischemic tissue by anaerobic metabolism and worsens cerebral injury. An ongoing trial (Albumin Therapy for Neuroprotection in Acute Ischemic Stroke [ALIAS]) is currently enrolling patients to determine if human serum albumin at 2 g/kg given over 2 hours to ischemic stroke victims within 5 hours of stroke onset, results in improved outcome at 3 months. The trial is expected to be completed in 2010. If this trial turns out to be positive then this would be the first neuroprotective agent that would improve outcome in acute ischemic stroke patients.

Nutrition is of utmost importance in the NCCU and the sooner it is initiated, the better the neurologic outcomes because metabolic activity is increased during times of stress. In patients who have acute ischemic strokes, a formal swallow evaluation should be done to assess whether or not the patient has difficulty swallowing and therefore may be an aspiration risk. Patients who have a decreased level of consciousness or fail their swallow study should have a nasogastric tube placed, nutrition consult, and nutritional preparations started. A good bowel regimen should also be implemented because delayed gastric emptying is common in the NCCU patients with head or spinal trauma. The use of narcotic agents for pain may also delay bowel movements, and laxatives should be started. Gastrointestinal prophylaxis should also be started in NCCU patients to protect the stomach lining from all the medications they receive by mouth or intravenously.

Deep Venous Thrombosis and Pulmonary Embolism prophylaxis

DVT and PE are frequent complications in stroke patients. Acute ischemic stroke patients with restricted movement because of weakness and who are bed-ridden should receive low dose heparin subcutaneously (SQ) or low molecular weight heparins SQ.

The PREVAIL (Prevention of Venous Thromboembolism After Acute Ischemic Stroke) was an open-label, randomized comparison of either enoxaparin 40 mg SQ once a day or unfractionated heparin (UFH) at 5000 units SQ every 12 hours in patients with ischemic stroke.

- The risk of both symptomatic intracranial bleeding and major extracranial bleeding was similar in both groups.
- A reduction seen of asymptomatic DVTs was seen in the enoxaparin group but the absolute increase in major extracranial bleeding was similar to the reduction in symptomatic DVT/PE.
- Low molecular weight heparins have been found to be equivalent to or better than UFH in preventing DVT.

In patients with an acute intracerebral hemorrhage or any contraindication to anticoagulants, intermittent pneumatic compression (IPC) devices or elastic stockings should be used initially. In stable patients with intracerebral hemorrhage, the use of low-dose SQ heparin can be started as soon as the second day post hemorrhage. This recommendation is based on one study and it puts more value on reducing the risks of thromboembolism and puts a lower value on minimizing the risk of cerebral rebleeding.

MANAGEMENT OF INTRACRANIAL BLEEDING AFTER THROMBOLYTIC THERAPY

The major risk of thrombolytic therapy is intracranial hemorrhage. Ongoing infusions of a thrombolytic should be stopped immediately if bleeding is suspected. A head CT without contrast is ordered immediately if intracranial hemorrhage is suspected. It is useful to distinguish between hemorrhagic transformation (petechial hemorrhage within an infarct) and parenchymal or symptomatic hemorrhage. It has been shown that if physicians do not adhere to recommended national guidelines for administration of thrombolytic therapy, the incidence of intracranial bleeding can increase.

- Blood should be immediately drawn to measure the patient's hematocrit, hemoglobin, PTT

(partial thromboplastin time), PT (prothrombin time), INR (international normalized ratio), platelet count, and fibrinogen.

- Blood should be typed and cross-matched if transfusions are needed (at least 4 units of packed red blood cells, 5–6 units of fresh frozen plasma, or 6–8 units of cryoprecipitate and 1 unit of donor platelets. These blood products should be available for emergent administration.
- Neurosurgery should also be consulted if evacuation is a consideration. Surgical evacuation of an ICH can be performed once the coagulopathy is corrected, size of hematoma is assessed, and location of hematoma is determined. Cerebellar hematomas that are >3 cm or large (>60 mL) lobar hematomas with mass effect should be evacuated emergently.

MANAGEMENT OF MALIGNANT HEMISPHERIC ISCHEMIC STROKES WITH CEREBRAL EDEMA AND/OR ELEVATED INTRACRANIAL PRESSURES

Cerebral edema in acute ischemic infarcts usually peaks in 48–72 hours and starts resolving by day 5. Treatment of cerebral edema is primarily medical and overlaps with that of elevated intracranial pressure (Table 10.4).

- First and foremost, one must assess the patient's ability to protect his or her airway if he or she starts to become less responsive.
  - Endotracheal intubation should be initiated if the patient appears to be in respiratory distress and if his or her Glasgow Coma Scale (GCS) is <8.
  - Short-acting medications should be used for intubation such as etomidate, thiopental, propofol, and lidocaine.
- Once controlled hyperventilation has been started, $PaCO_2$ of <25 should be avoided because of the possibility of cerebral ischemia. At the same time, MAP should be maintained with intravenous isotonic fluids and vasopressors if necessary to keep CPP >70 mm Hg, and the head of the bed elevated about 30 degrees.
- The use of an ICP monitoring device should be implemented especially when using osmotic agents to help decrease ICP.
  - Several devices are available for ICP monitoring: intraventricular catheters (IVCs), subarachnoid bolts, and fiberoptic transducers.

Table 10.4. Emergency management of elevated intracranial pressure (ICP)
*Elevation of the head of the bed at 30 degrees
*Osmotherapy
Mannitol 20% 0.25 g/kg to 0.5 g/kg every 4 hours
Hypertonic saline
*Barbiturates
Pentobarbital 10 mg/kg over 30 minutes
Thiopental 1.5 mg/kg to 3.5 mg/kg
*Paralysis
Vecuronium 0.1 mg/kg
Pancuronium 0.1 mg/kg
*Hyperventilation (temporary measure only)
Raise ventilation rate with a constant tidal volume
Goal partial pressure of carbon dioxide 30 to 35
*ICP monitor placement in patients with hydrocephalus or clinical deterioration secondary to elevated ICP
Goal ICP <20 mm Hg

Adapted from Broderick JP, Adams HP Jr, Barsan W, et al. Guidelines for the management of spontaneous intracerebral hemorrhage: a statement for healthcare professionals from a special writing group of the Stroke Council, American Heart Association. *Stroke.* 1999;30:905–15.
*External ventricular drain may be indicated in patients with or at risk for hydrocephalus.

- Osmotic agents such as mannitol are used to reduce the cerebral water content, decreasing serum viscosity, and thereby reducing ICP. It also decreases the viscosity of blood in the cerebral arterioles and induces vasoconstriction leading to reduction in ICP.
  - The initial dose is 0.5–2.0 g/kg and maintenance dose of 0.25 g/kg every 4–6 hours to keep serum osmolality between 310 and 320 mOsmol/L.
  - Serum sodium and osmolalities are usually checked every 6 hours when mannitol and/or hypertonic saline is used to help keep ICP <20 mm Hg.
- 3% hypertonic saline boluses may also be used to help lower ICP's as well. A bolus of 250 cc every 6 hours as needed to keep serum osmolality in the 310–320 mOsmol/L range can be given while trying to maintain euvolemia. An alternative to boluses would be to initiate a 3% hypertonic saline drip with a goal sodium of 145–155.
- Barbiturate coma can be instituted once all other medical maneuvers have failed but it is important to anticipate possible complications from this therapy: cardiac and blood pressure depression,

diminished interstitial peristalsis, sepsis, pneumonia, poikilothermia, and coagulopathies.

- Maintaining normothermia and euglycemia are also important in these patients.
- Decompressive hemicraniectomy by neurosurgery can also be considered on a case-by-case basis in those patients >50 years of age who were otherwise healthy with large territory infarcts that are unresponsive to maximal medical management.
  - For patients age 50 or younger with massive infarction involving >50% of MCA territory and associated with a decrease in consciousness who are therefore at high risk of developing malignant edema and who desire aggressive therapy, decompressive hemicraniectomy may be offered.

CONCLUSION

The close care that a neurocritical care unit provides for an acute ischemic stroke patient is important in the long-term prognosis and recovery from this devastating illness. The importance of blood pressure control before and after IV tPA, maintaining euglycemia, normothermia, euvolemia, and pre-venting cerebral edema/ increased ICPs to occur can all be monitored in the NCCU. Exciting new therapies such as induced hypothermia in acute ischemic stroke and whether or not blood pressure lowering in acute ischemic stroke is beneficial is in the near future. With time, many new options will be available for treating acute ischemic stroke patients in the NCCU which will take them out of the acute phase and on the road to rehabilitation.

REFERENCES

Adams HP Jr, Del Zoppo G, Alberts MJ, et al. Guidelines for the early management of patients with ischemic stroke: a sci-entific statement from the Stroke Council of the American Stroke Association. *Stroke*. 2007;**38**:1655–1711.

Albers, GW, Amarenco P, Easton JD, et al. Antithrombotic and thrombolytic therapy for ischemic stroke: the Eighth ACCP Conference on Antithrombotic and Thrombolytic Therapy. *Chest*. 2008; **133**(Suppl); 630–69.

Baird T, Parsons MW, Phanh T, et al. Persistent poststroke hyperglycemia is independently associated with infarct expansion and worse clinical outcome. *Stroke*. 2003; **34**:2208–14.

Castillo J, Leira R, García M, Serena J, Blanco M, Dávalos A. Blood pressure decrease during the acute phase of isch-emic stroke is associated with brain injury and poor stroke outcome. *Stroke*. 2004;**35**:520–6.

De Georgia MA, Krieger DW, Abou-Chebyl A, et al. Cooling for acute ischemic brain damage (COOL AID): a feasibility trial of endovascular cooling. *Neurology*. 2004;**63**:312–7.

Demchuck AM, Morgenstern LB, Krieger DW, et al. Serum glucose levels and diabetes predict tissue plasminogen activator-related intracerebral hemorrhage in acute ische-mic stroke. *Stroke*. 1999;**30**:34–39.

Gray CS, Hildreth AJ, Sandercock PA, et al. Glucose-potassium-insulin infusions in the management of post-stroke hyperglycemia: the UK Glucose Insulin in Stroke Trial (GIST-UK). *Lancet Neurol*. 2007;**6**:397–406.

Hypothermia After Cardiac Arrest Group. Mild therapeutic hypothermia to improve the neurologic outcome after car-diac arrest. *N Engl J Med*. 2002;**346**:549–56.

Katzan IL, Furlan AJ, Lloyd LE, et al. Use of tissue type plas-minogen activator for acute ischemic stroke. The Cleve-land area experience. *JAMA*. 2000;1151–8.

Lopez-Yunez AM, Bruno A, Zurru C, et al. Protocol violations in community based rt-PA use are associated with symp-tomatic intracerebral hemorrhage. *Stroke*. 1999;**30**:264.

Lyden P, Bott T, Tilley B, et al. Improved reliability of the NIH Stroke Scale using video training. *Stroke*. 1994;**25**:2220–26.

National Institute of Neurological Disorders, and Stroke rt-PA Stroke Study Groupf Tissue plasminogen activator for acute ischemic stroke. *N Engl J Med*. 1995;**333**:1581–7.

Quereshi AI, Bhardwaj MD, Uletowski JA. *Neurocritical care for the house officer. In ICU Care House Officer Series*. Edited by Helfaer M. Baltimore: Williams & Wilkins; 1998:65,92.

Reith J, Jorgenson HS, Pedersen PM, Nakayama H, Raaschou HO, Jeppesen LL, Olsen TS. Body temperature in acute stroke: relation to stroke severity, infarct size, mortality, and outcome. *Lancet* .1996;**347**(8999):422–5.

Sabin JA, Molina CA, Montaner J, Arenillas JF, Huertas R, Ribo M, Codina A, Quintana M. Effects of admission hypergly-cemia on stroke outcome in reperfused tissue plasmino-gen activator–treated patients. *Stroke*. 2003;**34**:1235.

Sherman DG, Albers GW, Bladin C, et al.; PREVAIL inves-tigators. The efficacy and safety of enoxaparin versus unfractionated heparin for the prevention of venous thromboembolism after acute ischaemic stroke (PREVAIL Study): an open-label randomised comparison. *Lancet*. 2007;**369**(9570):1347–55.

11 Intracerebral Hemorrhage

Natalia Rost, MD and Jonathan Rosand, MD, MSc

Intracerebral hemorrhage (ICH) is spontaneous nontraumatic bleeding into the brain parenchyma. Annually, approximately 65,000 people in the United States suffer an ICH, which accounts for 10–30% of all stroke cases across different ethnic groups.[1-3] ICH is the most fatal and least treatable form of stroke, causing, in addition, severe disability among survivors.[4,5] Patients with ICH uniformly require ICU management[6] and patients cared for in specialized neurologic intensive care units are less likely to die.[7,8] Although, as compared to ischemic stroke and subarachnoid hemorrhage, the pace of advances in management of ICH has been slow, recent results of clinical trials of recombinant factor VIIa (fVIIa) in acute ICH[9] have generated excitement.

Based on the underlying pathology of ruptured vessel that originates the bleeding, ICH is classified as primary or secondary. The majority of primary ICH result from a ruptured vessel as a consequence of chronic injury to the small cerebral vessels by sustained hypertension (hypertensive vasculopathy)[10-12] or abnormal protein deposition (cerebral amyloid angiopathy).[13-15] Secondary causes of ICH include underlying vascular malformations, ruptured saccular aneurysms, coagulation disorders, use of anticoagulants and thrombolytic agents, hemorrhage into a preexisting infarct, brain tumor, or infectious focus, and drug abuse (Table 11.1).[6,16,17]

EPIDEMIOLOGY AND RISK FACTORS

ICH is a common disorder that occurs in all populations. Estimates of overall incidence are 12–15 cases per 100 000 people per year,[4] slightly higher among men, young and middle-aged African-Americans,

and Asians.[2] Advanced age and hypertension are the most prevalent ICH risk factors accounting for up to 50% of cases.[1,16]

Hypertensive vasculopathy is usually the result of underlying arteriolosclerosis (thickening and damage to the arteriolar wall, also referred to as fibrohyalinosis or lipohyalinosis).[10]

- The most commonly affected arteries are the deep penetrators (medium-small arterioles, 100–600 μm in diameter) in the basal ganglia (putamen, caudate nucleus, or thalamus), pons, or cerebellum.[10,11,16] Their spontaneous rupture causes a typical pathologic and neuroimaging pattern of deep ICH (Fig. 11.1).
- Hypertensive vasculopathy can also affect more superficial vessels, leading to lobar hemorrhage.

Cerebral amyloid angiopathy (CAA) is the second most common cause of primary ICH, and may account for up to 35% of cases.[1,6] This angiopathy results from dynamic deposition of β-amyloid peptide within the walls of small-to-medium size vessels of the cerebral cortex, overlying leptomeninges, and cerebellum (Fig. 11.1).[18-20] Amyloid deposits contribute to vessel fragility and lead to spontaneous rupture, causing distinct pathological and neuroimaging pattern of lobar hemorrhages,[21] as well as microhemorrhages identified by MRI (Fig. 11.2).[21-23] CAA-associated ICH carries high risk of recurrence (10–20% per year).[21-23] In contrast, the risk of recurrent hypertensive ICH can be less than 2% per year, provided that hypertension is well controlled.[24,25] Among other risk factors for ICH, age, antithrombotic/anticoagulant use, excessive alcohol consumption, and hypocholesterolemia have been implicated.[1,6,16,17,26,27]

PATHOPHYSIOLOGY

ICH is a dynamic process that begins with cerebral vessel rupture. The precise mechanisms of early

Table 11.1. Etiology of secondary ICH

Aneurysm

Arteriovenous malformation

Anticoagulant and thrombolytic use

Cavernous angioma

Coagulation disorder

CNS vasculitis

Cocaine

Dural arteriovenous fistula

Dural sinus thrombosis

Hemorrhagic conversion of ischemic stroke

Intracranial neoplasm or infection

hematoma expansion are still poorly understood. Following initial vessel rupture, the accumulating volume of extravasated blood contributes to sudden rise in intracranial pressure (ICP), associated tissue distortion, and breakdown in blood–brain barrier leading, possibly, to secondary foci of hemorrhage at the periphery of the initial hematoma.[28] In addition, early tissue ischemia, poor venous outflow as well as propensity for local coagulopathy due to the role of plasmin and fibrin degradation products along with continued bleeding from the primary ruptured vessel have been suggested as the possible contributors to expansion of the initial clot.[28-31]

Early hematoma growth is a common and deleterious event associated with high neurologic morbidity and poor clinical outcome[32,33] (Fig. 11.3).

■ Based on computed tomography (CT) data, more than one-third of ICH patients whose initial CT scan is obtained within 3 hours of symptom onset, develop a clinically significant increase in hematoma volume (>33%).[33,34]

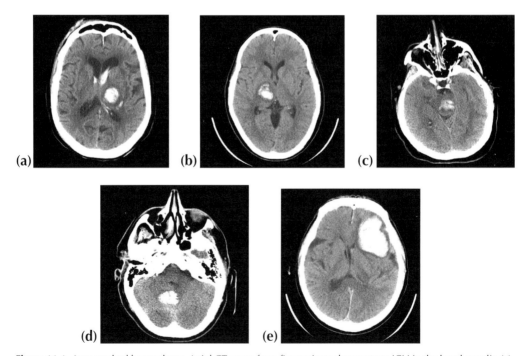

(a) (b) (c)

(d) (e)

Figure 11.1. Intracerebral hemorrhage. Axial CT scans from five patients demonstrate ICH in the basal ganglia (**a**), thalamus (**b**), pons (**c**), cerebellum (**d**), and the lobar brain regions (**e**).

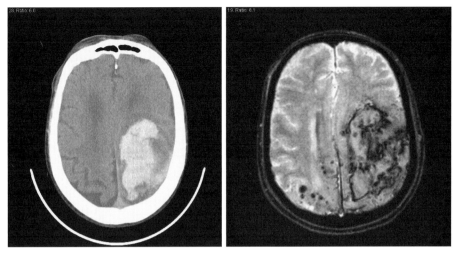

Figure 11.2. MRI characteristics of cerebral amyloid angiopathy. This patient's head CT revealed a left fronto-parietal lobar hemorrhage (*left panel*). Follow-up gradient-echo (*susceptibility*) sequenced MRI revealed numerous punctate microhemorrhages (*right panel*), suggesting underlying cerebral amyloid angiopathy. (Adapted from Goldstein JN, Greenberg SM, Rosand J. Emergency management of intracerebral hemorrhage. *Continuum* 2006;**12**(1):13–29.)

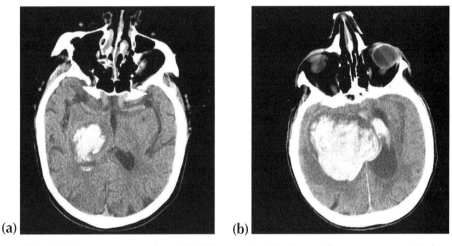

Figure 11.3. Early hematoma expansion. Initial CT scan taken 50 minutes after symptom onset **(a)** showing right-sided cerebral hematoma, which is significantly increased on repeat head CT at 160 minutes **(b)**, including intraventricular extension.

■ Hematoma expansion is also detected in those who present beyond 3 hours, although with reduced frequency.[35]

The primary mechanism of injury due to ICH appears to be mass effect from the hematoma itself.[32,33] As measured by poor functional outcome, the neurologic damage is proportional to the volume of hematoma, i.e., the amount of blood that extravasates from the ruptured vessel intraparenchymally.[32-34] When ICH occurs in patients receiving anticoagulation, hematoma expansion has been observed in half of patients, regardless of time of presentation.[35] This expansion appears to be an important contributor to the high mortality of warfarin-related ICH.[29,35]

The significance of perihematomal hypodensity often observed on CT remains poorly understood.[36,37] This hypodensity, often referred to as edema, appears as early as 1 hour after the bleeding event and can persist up to 2 weeks or more.[37,38] It may result from the extrusion of plasma that results from clot formation[39] and/or the inflammatory response to cerebral clot formation, when thrombin-rich plasma permeates brain parenchyma and triggers inflammatory cascade with activation and expression of cytotoxins, inflammatory mediators, induction of matrix metalloproteases,[40,41] leukocyte recruitment,[40] and disruption of the blood–brain barrier.[42,43]

PROGNOSIS

ICH is one of the deadliest acute neurologic disorders, with 1-year mortality rates approaching 50%.[6,44] The majority of patients who survive have some degree of residual neurologic disability, with only 20% regaining independence within 6 months.[44,45]

Hematoma volume, Glasgow Coma Score (GCS) on presentation, intraventricular extension, use of warfarin, advanced age, and infratentorial location of the hemorrhage appear to predict 30-day and 1-year mortality (Table 11.2).[35,46,47] However, because withdrawal of aggressive measures is commonly sought by family members and physicians in the setting of ICH, clinical care withdrawn from patients within the first 24 hours becomes the single most important predictor of survival after ICH.[7] This last point requires careful consideration because physicians' judgment of poor prognosis remains imprecise, raising the possibility that bias introduced by "self-fulfilling prophecies" probably affects most studies of ICH outcome.[48] However, the key question for most patients and their family members is not the likelihood of death, but the likelihood of log-term disability should the patient survive. More recently published data addressed both the issues of functional outcome (rather than mortality) and care withdrawal bias in patients with ICH.[50] This approach to ICH outcome and prognosis is both clinically relevant and practical in research considerations.

DIAGNOSIS

ICH should be considered in any patient with acute and rapidly developing focal neurologic deficits, particularly when there are signs or symptoms of rising ICP (headache, decreased levels of arousal, nausea and vomiting).[1,6,51] Emergent evaluation with head CT should be initiated immediately.

Noncontrast head CT scan is a highly sensitive and specific neuroimaging tool in diagnosis of ICH.[52-54]

Table 11.2. The ICH score

Component of ICH score	Points
GCS score	2
3–4	2
5–12	1
13–15	0
ICH volume, cm³	
>30	1
<30	0
IVH	
Yes	1
No	0
Infratentorial origin of ICH	
Yes	1
No	0
Age, years	
>80	1
<80	0
Total ICH score 0–6:	
Score	30 day mortality
0	0%
1	13%
2	26%
3	72%
4	97%
5	100%

GCS score, Glasgow Coma Scale score on initial presentation; ICH volume: Hematoma volume on initial CT; IVH, presence of any intraventricular hemorrhage; ICH score: No patient, in this study or others, has received a score of 6. This likely reflects the fact that infratentorial hematomas have a limited space in which to expand to >60 mL of blood.

Adapted from Hemphill JC 3rd, Bonovich DC, Besmertis L, et al. The ICH score: a simple, reliable grading scale for intracerebral hemorrhage. Stroke. 2001;**32**:891–7.

- Hematoma location, size, intraventricular extension, presence of hydrocephalus, and/or mass effect can be quickly and reliably assessed on CT alone.
- ICH volume can be estimated by using the *ABC*/2 method,[55] where *A* is the greatest hemorrhage diameter by CT, *B* is the diameter 90 degrees to

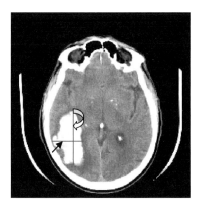

Figure 11.4. Using *ABC/2* method for ICH volume measurement. On axial head CT, multiply *A* = larest hematoma diameter (*curved left arrow*), *B* = largest diameter perpendicular to *A* (*thin arrow*), and *C* = number of slices containing ICH (each is usually 0.5 cm, and divide total by 2). Volume is expressed in milliliters.

A, and *C* is the approximate number of CT slices with hemorrhage multiplied by slice thickness in cm (Fig. 11.4).

If underlying aneurysm or AVM is suspected, CT angiography (CTA) or catheter angiography will provide diagnostic information.[54,56,57] As a general rule, angiography should be especially considered in those patients <55 years old without chronic hypertension or whose neuroimaging characteristics of the hematoma include atypical topographical and morphometric features.[58] For example, Sylvian

fissure hemorrhage may frequently obscure MCA aneurysm as an underlying etiology (Fig. 11.5).

MRI can be as sensitive as CT in detecting blood products without loss of specificity;[59] however, its role in ICH is currently limited to the nonacute setting since it seldom offers information unavailable from CT that can assist with acute decision making.

- MRI is most frequently used as an adjunct tool to elucidate an underlying etiology (e.g., evidence of microhemorrhages consistent with CAA; presence of arteriovenous malformation or venous cavernoma; or potentially, causal hemorrhagic neoplasm).[54,60]
- MRI may frequently be delayed to allow for better visualization of brain parenchyma, as the blood products continue to be reabsorbed for up to 8–12 weeks after the acute ICH.

MANAGEMENT

Current management of ICH focuses on urgent support of vital function, prevention of hematoma expansion, reduction of mass effect, minimizing of secondary neurologic injury, and prevention of nosocomial complications.[61] This approach is usually taken in several integrated steps, as outlined below:

- Urgent clinical and radiographic evaluation, leading to a diagnosis of ICH
- Airway and circulation support

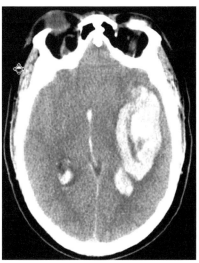
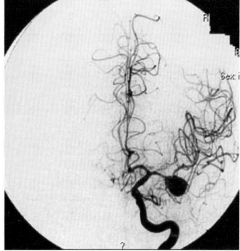

Figure 11.5. Left Sylvian fissure hemorrhage (*left panel*) obscuring left middle cerebral artery aneurysm diagnosed by angiography (*right panel*).

Table 11.3. Sample Rapid Sequence Intubation (RSI) for patients at risk for elevated intracranial pressure

Time	Step
Zero minus 10 minutes	Preparation
Zero minus 5 minutes	Preoxygenation (100% O_2 for 5 minutes)
Zero minus 3 minutes	Pretreatment
	Vecuronium 0.01 mg/kg*
	Lidocaine 1.5 mg/kg
	Fentanyl 3 µg/kg (slowly)
Zero	Paralysis with induction
	Etomidate 0.3 mg/kg**
	Succinylcholine 1.5mg/kg*
Zero plus 45 seconds	Placement
	Sellick's maneuver
	Laryngoscopy with intubation
	End-tidal CO_2 confirmation
Zero plus 2 minutes	Postintubation management
	Ventilation

*May substitute rocuronium 1.0 mg/kg or vecuronium 0.15 mg/kg for succinylcholine. If so, omit vecuronium during pretreatment.
**May substitute thiopental 3.0 mg/kg for etomidate in patients who are hemodynamically stable or hypertensive.
Reprinted with permission from Walls RM. Airway. In: Marx JA, ed. *Rosen's Emergency Medicine: Concepts and Clinical Practice*. 5th edition. St. Lois: C.V. Mosby, 2002: 2–21. Copyright Elsevier (2002).

■ Reversing coagulopathy and consideration of acute hemostatic therapy, should it become available
■ Controlling blood pressure
■ Preventing hyperglycemia, hypotension, and pyrexia
■ Management of elevated ICP
■ Seizure prophylaxis
■ Neurosurgical evaluation

1. **Assess vital function.**

Any patient arriving to the hospital with suspected cerebral hemorrhage constitutes an emergency.

■ Initial management includes a swift clinical evaluation, including assessment of the patient's ability to protect his or her airway.
■ Early intubation is essential for patients with impaired arousal, which raises risk of aspiration, hypoxemia, and hypercarbia.[62]

▶ For this purpose, ultra-short-acting neuromuscular blockade or sedative-hypnotics agents are preferred to allow for rapid return of motor control and assessment of neurologic deficits (Table 11.3).[63]
■ Since the act of endotracheal intubation may cause transient ICP elevation and, as such, contribute to worsening of mass effect or development of cerebral ischemia due to reduction in cerebral blood flow (CBF) special care should be taken to choose medications that will minimize this effect (Table 11.4).[64]
▶ Etomidate is known to have the least impact on blood pressure and should be used for induction.
▶ Although thiopental has cerebroprotective and anticonvulsant properties, its use should be limited in patients with ICH due to its tendency to cause hypotension because of its venodilatory and myocardial depressor effects.

Table 11.4. Sedating agents for the mechanically ventilated patient

Agent	Class	Dose	Frequency of dosing
Propofol	Alkylphenol	5–80 µg/kg per minute	Continuous infusion
Fentanyl	Opioid	2–3 µg/kg	q0.5–1h
Morphine	Opioid	0.01–0.15 mg/kg	q1–2h
Hydromorphone	Opioid	10–30 µg/kg	q1–2h
Midazolam	Benzodiazepine	0.02–0.1 mg/kg	q0.5–2h
Diazepam	Benzodiazepine	0.03–0.1 mg/kg	q0.5–6h
Lorazepam	Benzodiazepine	0.02–0.06 mg/kg	q2–6h

Adapted from Goldstein JN, Greenberg SM, Rosand J. Emergency management of intracerebral hemorrhage. *Continuum.* 2006;**12**(1):13–29.

Table 11.5. Glasgow Coma Scale

Best motor response	Best verbal response	Best eye-opening response
Obeys commands (6)	Oriented (5)	Spontaneously open (4)
Localizes to pain (5)	Confused (4)	Opens to speech (3)
Withdraws to pain (4)	Inappropriate words (3)	Opens to pain (2)
Flexion to pain (3)	Incomprehensible (2)	None (1)
Extension to pain (2)	None (1)	
None (1)		

Points are in parentheses.
Adapted from Teasdale G, Jennet B. Assessment of coma and impaired consciousness: a practical scale. *Lancet.* 1974;**2**:81–4.

▷ If paralysis is used with induction, pretreatment with a defasciculating dose of a competitive neuromuscular blocker (e.g., pancuronium or vecuronium) should be administered before succinylcholine dose.

2. **Measure GCS, FUNC score**[49] **and ICH score** (Tables 11.2 and 11.5).

3. **Establish acute comorbidities** (acute myocardial injury; hypertensive emergency; arrhythmia; blood dyscrasia, etc.) based on initial clinical exam and vital signs monitoring.

4. **STAT laboratory investigation**: Prothrombin time/international normalized ratio (PT/INR), partial thromboplastin time (PTT), complete blood count (CBC) with platelets, D-dimer, fibrinogen, electrolytes, blood urea nitrogen/creatinine (BUN/Cr), glucose, liver function tests, type and screen to blood bank, toxicology screen for young patients or those with history of substance abuse. Each of these laboratory values may have an impact on diagnosis or management of ICH.

5. **Arrange for STAT head CT scan.** Topographic and morphologic properties of the hematoma (volume, location, mass effect, midline shift, associated abnormalities within the brain suggestive of secondary ICH) will alert the viewer to the etiology of the ICH and its further management.[51-54] The *ABC*/2 method can rapidly and reliably estimate ICH volume (Fig. 11.4).[55]

6. **Neurosurgical evaluation**. Cerebellar ICH is a neurosurgical emergency.[65] In addition, patients with lobar ICH who demonstrate progressive clinical deterioration may be considered for hematoma evacuation, although randomized trials have not demonstrated benefit in this setting.[66]

External ventricular drains (EVD) are frequently used in patients intraventricular hemorrhage as

Table 11.6. Differential diagnosis of ICH

Spontaneous (primary) ICH	• No suspicion for underlying lesion • No further radiologic studies maybe necessary. • Likely etiology: HTN vs. CAA
ICH secondary to aneurysmal rupture	• Considered when the hematoma is situated in the region of the MCA bifurcation or extends down to a vessel of the circle of Willis • CTA or other vascular imaging should be performed. • If an aneurysm is confirmed, contact neurosurgery immediately and follow SAH guidelines for BP and airway control.
ICH secondary to underlying tumor, AVM, cavernous malformation, or venous sinus thrombosis	• Additional brain imaging is necessary to exclude an underlying lesion. • Both contrast CT or contrast MRI may be useful initially and several weeks later once hemorrhage products have begun to be reabsorbed. • Management of each condition will depend on underlying etiology.
Hemorrhagic conversion of ischemic infarction	• Additional brain imaging with MRI (and DWI if available) may be needed to confirm the underlying ischemic etiology in regions that were not subject to hemorrhagic transformation. • Regions of subtle petechial hemorrhage that are not visible on unenhanced CT but easily seen on MR gradient echo susceptibility sequences have an unclear significance with respect to initiation of antithrombotic therapy. • If acute ischemic stroke is suspected (onset <12 hours), contact acute stroke team immediately.

Adapted from the MGH Acute Stroke Service Guidelines for Emergency Department Management of Brain Hemorrhage (http://www.stopstroke.org).

well as in those with suspected elevated intracranial pressure (ICP), deteriorating levels of consciousness, CT evidence of mass effect or hydrocephalus, and in patients in whom neurologic examination cannot be followed. Patients with intraventricular blood may benefit from direct application of thrombolytic agents through indwelling ventricular catheters.[67]

7. **Consider the differential diagnosis** based on the preliminary evaluation (Table 11.6). Based on the ICH etiology, specific management guidelines will apply.

8. **Correct coagulopathy**. There are multiple sources of coagulopathy which may contribute to hemorrhage and hematoma expansion, including blood dyscrasias (thrombocytopenia, prolonged PT/PTT associated with liver failure and poor nutritional status) as well as anticoagulation with warfarin, heparin, or heparinoids; or use of direct thrombin inhibitors. Antiplatelet agents increase the risk of ICH slightly[68] but their effect on outcome appears to be limited.[35] Management of these conditions is addressed separately.

a. Anticoagulation with **warfarin** increases risk of ICH and worsens the severity of disease, approximately doubling its mortality.[31] This mortality appears to be related to hematoma expansion due to prolonged bleeding, which is commonly observed in patients with anticoagulation-related ICH.[29,31,69] Therefore, early reversal of coagulopathy, although of unproven benefit, is critical.[70] Reversal of anticoagulation is usually achieved by concomitant

---

Table 11.7. Sample guidelines for emergent reversal of coagulopathy in ICH

Patients on warfarin:

1. Administer fresh frozen plasma (FFP) 10 mL/kg over 90 minutes.

   a. Each unit of FFP contains 200 mL.

   b. Prothrombin complex concentrate 50 units/kg can be substituted.

2. Administer vitamin K 10 mg IV over 10 minutes.

3. Repeat INR at 4 hours.

   a. If INR is >1.3, administer a second dose of FFP (10 mL/kg over 90 minutes).

   b. Otherwise, check INR every 6 hours for 24 hours.

4. Repeat INR at 8 hours.

   a. If INR is still >1.3, evaluate for disseminated intravascular coagulation (DIC).

   b. Otherwise, check INR every 6 hours for 24 hours.

Patients on heparin:

Administer protamine 10–50 mg IVP over 1–3 minutes.

Patients with platelet disorders:

1. Thrombocytopenia (platelet count <100,000/µL):

   a. Consider platelet transfusion depending upon severity

2. Von Willebrand syndromes:

   a. Administer 0.3 µg/kg DDAVP IV over 30 minutes.

   b. Consider VWF factor concentrate.

3. Recent antiplatelet agent use such as ASA or clopidogrel:

   a. Consider 1 dose (6 unit equivalent) of platelets.

Current guidelines for our institution can be found at http://www.stopstroke.org.

Adapted from Goldstein JN, Greenberg SM, Rosand J. Emergency management of intracerebral hemorrhage. *Continuum*. 2006;**12**(1):13–29.

---

administration of clotting factor replacement therapy and vitamin K, since clotting factors have a limited half-life (Table 11.7).

- Most authors recommend fresh frozen plasma (FFP) or a concentrate of specific clotting factors (prothrombin-complex concentrates, or PCC) as a means of early repletion of vitamin K–dependent clotting factors.[71,72]

  ▶ Administration of FFP at 10 mL/kg is very rarely associated with a risk of volume overload and congestive heart failure. Depending on the clinical condition of the patient, however, judicious administration of diuretics may be indicated.[73]

- If FFP is administered without concomitant vitamin K, the effect will dissipate in 6–8 hours. FFP should therefore never be used without concomitant vitamin K for ICH.

  ▶ Intravenous vitamin K is the preferred route of administration, due to its accelerated absorption, and oral vitamin K should always be administered when the intravenous route is unavailable.[72] When administered at the rate not exceeding 1 mg/min, it is associated with a very small risk of severe allergic reaction.[71–73]

- Reversal of anticoagulation by any means (vitamin K FFP or PCC) is associated with a risk of thrombosis depending on the patient's underlying indication for anticoagulation. Regardless of the choice of agent and protocol used, frequent reevaluation of the INR is critical to guide continued correction of coagulopathy.[72,73]

Follow-up therapy should include a STAT PT/INR every 4 hours during the first 24 hours of hospitalization, then every 6 hours up to 36 hours of hospitalization, and then as needed.

- If the INR is more than 1.4 at 4 hours, a second dose of vitamin K 10 mg IV can be given, as well as second dose of FFP (10 ml/kg over 90 minutes).
- If the INR remains above 1.4 at 8 hours, the possibility of disseminated intravascular coagulation should be considered.[74]

b. Anticoagulation with standard (unfractionated) **heparin** may similarly increase risk of continued bleeding and hematoma expansion and it is prudent to initiate its immediate reversal with protamine sulfate, a specific antidote, which is administered at a dose of 1.0–1.5 mg per 100 units/h of heparin, if administered within 30 minutes of cessation of heparin infusion; or 0.5 mg of protamine sulfate for every 100 units/h of heparin, if administered between 30–45 minutes of cessation of heparin infusion. There is a risk of anaphylactic reaction to protamine, especially in diabetic patients who have been exposed to insulin. Of note, FFP is equally effective for temporary reversal of heparin effects but its use is nonspecific and inefficient due to heparin's short half-life.[71–73]

- The plasma half-life of heparin averages 1–2 hours in healthy adults. However, the half-life of the drug increases with increasing doses.
- After IV administration of heparin sodium 100, 200, or 400 units/kg, the plasma half-life of the drug averages 56, 96, and 152 minutes, respectively.
- The plasma half-life of the drug is decreased in patients with liver impairment but may be prolonged in cirrhotic patients.
- In anephric patients or patients with severe renal impairment, the half-life of heparin may be slightly prolonged.
- Thus, to follow up initial treatment, STAT PTT every 1 hour for the next 4 hours, and then every 4 hours through 12 hours of hospitalization, and then at least every 24 hours for 3 days of hospitalization is required.[74]

9. **Other anticoagulation agents**: c. Strategies for reversal of **low molecular weight heparin** (LMWH), should include protamine sulfate, although it only negates about 60% of the anti-factor Xa activity of LMWH. Protamine, however, has negligible effects on danaparoid (a mixture of anticoagulant glycosaminoglycans used to treat heparin-induced thrombocytopenia) and fondaparinux (a synthetic antithrombin-binding pentasaccharide with exclusive antifactor Xa activity). For patients who have received enoxaparin, use 1 mg of protamine for each milligram of enoxaparin; if PTT prolonged 2–4 hours after the first dose, consider additional dose of 0.5 mg for each milligram of enoxaparin. With dalteparin or tinzaparin: 1 mg of protamine for each 100 anti-Xa IU of dalteparin or tinzaparin; if the PTT prolonged 2–4 hours after first dose, consider additional dose of 0.5 mg for each 100 anti-Xa IU of dalteparin or tinzaparin.[71–74]

d. There are no specific reversal agents for the **direct thrombin inhibitors** (argatroban, lepirudin, bivalirudin, ximelagatran) at this time. Antifibrinolytic agents, such as ε-aminocaproic acid (Amicar) can be considered.[75]

(e) **Platelet disorders** are managed based on the underlying etiology. Our practice is to reserve platelet transfusion for patients who are taking acetylsalicylic acid (ASA) in addition to warfarin.[74] There are no data to suggest whether platelet repletion is required, if patients are using other agents with antiplatelet action (ADP inhibitors such as clopidogrel and ticlopidine; PDE III inhibitors such as cilostazol; IIb/IIIa inhibitors such as abciximab, ebtifibatide, and tirofiban; and adenosine reuptake inhibitors such as dipyridamole).

(f) Among **noniatrogenic platelet disorders**, thrombocytopenia (platelet count <100,000/μL) is treated with repeated platelet transfusion until the platelet count exceeds 100,000/μL.[74]

- Patients with von Willebrand syndrome should be given 0.3 μg/kg DDAVP, as an intravenous infusion over 30 minutes. Transfusion of von Willebrand factor concentrate should then be administered, in consultation with transfusion medicine or hematology specialist. DDAVP is also known to benefit patients with uremic platelet dysfunction,[76] congenital platelet function disorders, and recent ingestion of antiplatelet agent combination (e.g., ASA and clopidogrel).
- Mechanism of action of DDAVP is thought to be of general endothelial stimulant for factor VIII, prostaglandin I_2, and plasminogen-activated release.

Table 11.8. American Heart Association/American Stroke Association recommendations for blood pressure management in spontaneous ICH

a. If SBP is >200 mm Hg or MAP is >150 mm Hg, then consider aggressive reduction of blood pressure with continuous intravenous infusion, with frequent blood pressure monitoring every 5 minutes.

b. If SBP is >180 mm Hg or MAP is >130 and there is evidence of or suspicion of elevated ICP, then consider monitoring ICP and reducing blood pressure using intermittent or continuous intravenous medication to keep cerebral perfusion pressure >60–80 mm Hg.

c. If SBP is >180 mm Hg or MAP is >130 and there is not evidence of or suspicion of elevated ICP, then consider a modest reduction of blood pressure (e.g., MAP of 110 mm Hg or target blood pressure of 160/90 mm Hg) using intermittent or continuous intravenous medication to control blood pressure, and clinically reexamine patient every 15 minutes. .

Adapted from Broderick JP, Connoly S, Feldman E, et al. Guidelines for the management of spontaneous intracerebral hemorrhage in adults: 2007 update. A Guideline from the American Heart Association/American Stroke Association Stroke Council, High Blood Pressure Research Council, and the Quality of Care and Outcomes in Research Interdisciplinary Working Group. *Stroke.* 2007;**38**:2001–23.

Table 11.9. Blood pressure management in ICH (suggested IV medications)

Labetalol	Up to 100 mg/h by intermittent bolus doses of 5–20 mg or continuous drip (2–8 mg/min, maximum 300 mg/day)
Esmolol	250 μg/kg as a load; then continuous infusion of 25–300 μg/kg per minute
Nitroprusside	0.1–10 μg/kg per minute (continuous infusion only)
Nicardipine	5 mg/h increased by 2.5 mg/h q15min to max 15 mg/h (continuous infusion)
Hydralazine	5–20 mg q30min as an IV load, or 1.5–5.0 μg/kg per minute continuously
Enalapril	1.25–5 mg IV bolus q6h (first test dose should be 0.625 mg to avoid the risk of precipitous blood pressure lowering)

Adapted from Broderick JP, Connoly S, Feldman E, et al. Guidelines for the management of spontaneous intracerebral hemorrhage in adults: 2007 update. A Guideline from the American Heart Association/American Stroke Association Stroke Council, High Blood Pressure Research Council, and the Quality of Care and Outcomes in Research Interdisciplinary Working Group. *Stroke.* 2007;**38**:2001–2023.

This direct and local effect on vessel walls may produce an increase in platelet adhesion, and thus, decreasing the bleeding time in patients with platelet dysfunction.

10. **Management of hypertension.** Controversy surrounds the initial treatment of hypertension in patients with acute ICH, due in part to conflicting data suggesting both decrease and increase in mortality associated with such treatment.[77–79] Acute ICH patients commonly have elevated blood pressure (BP).[80] BP elevation has, in some studies, been shown to be associated with increased risk of neurologic deterioration and poor outcome,[80,81] leading to long-standing recommendations for BP reduction in acute ICH. High BP has also been observed in the patients with hematoma expansion; however, there is no conclusive evidence of whether this raised BP is a cause or consequence of this expansion.[77]

While lowering of blood pressure in acute ICH is hypothetically aimed at minimizing risk of hematoma expansion, this BP reduction may also reduce cerebral blood flow (CBF) and, consequently, contribute to ischemia in already compromised cerebral parenchyma.[78,79,82] A standard approach to BP management in patients with severely elevated pressures has been proposed and is currently summarized in the American Heart Association/American Stroke Association guidelines (Table 11.8).[82]

An ideal antihypertensive agent in acute ICH would minimize cerebral vasodilatation in order to prevent increase in cerebral blood volume (CBV), ICP increase, and CBF decrease (Table 11.9).[74] Among widely available medications, labetalol carries the least of cerebrovascular side effects and is the most commonly used in the emergency setting. It can be administered in repeated bolus doses or continuous intravenous infusion. Other agents such as nicardipine or esmolol can also be used; however, hydralazine and sodium nitroprusside should be avoided, at first, due to their propensity to cause cerebral vasodilation and increased ICP. In all cases of ICH, systolic BP should be maintained above 90 mm Hg to avoid decrease in CBF and additional cerebral ischemia of perihematomal zone. Alternatively, mean arterial pressure (MAP) or cerebral perfusion pressure (CPP) may be selected as a target variable to follow in monitoring of the effective antihypertensive therapy.

11. **Management of hypotension**. Low systemic blood pressure may carry equal, and possibly worse, neurologic risks in patients with ICH. Etiology of hypotension must be established and treated aggressively to prevent impairment of CBF and worsening of cerebral ischemia. Volume repletion with isotonic crystalloid boluses or colloids is the first approach, and requires monitoring of central venous pressure (CVP) for effectiveness. If hypotension persists after correction of volume deficit, continuous infusion of vasopressors should be considered, particularly for low systolic blood pressure such as that <90 mm Hg (Table 11.10).[74] If CVP is normal or elevated in the setting of hypotension, then further evaluation of cardiac function using a pulmonary artery catheter or noninvasive measures is indicated.

12. **Glycemic control**. Hyperglycemia may worsen outcome in ICH.[83] Patients should therefore be monitored and treated several times daily for any elevation in blood sugar.[84] In monitored settings, continuous insulin infusions are ideal for maintaining normoglycemia (Table 11.11).

13. **Pyrexia control**. Sustained fever after ICH is likely to be associated with poor outcome.[17] Potential sources of infection have to be investigated thoroughly at fever onset.[85] Several sources recommend antipyretics (such as acetaminophen 650 mg every 6 hours) for sustained fever in excess of 38°C (101.4°F) or external cooling procedures;[4,74] however, evidence to support efficacy of these interventions in patients with ICH is lacking.

Table 11.10. Management of hypotension in ICH

Some suggested medications:	
Phenylephrine	2–10 µg/kg per minute
Dopamine	2–20 µg/kg per minute
Norepinephrine	0.05–0.2 µg/kg per minute

Adapted from the MGH Acute Stroke Service Guidelines for Emergency Department Management of Brain Hemorrhage (http://www.stopstroke.org).

Table 11.11. Insulin titration in critical care setting (the Portland Protocol)

Blood glucose	Action
<75 mg/dL	Stop insulin. Give 25 mL of dextrose 50% water (D50w) and recheck BG every 30 minutes. When BG reaches >150 mg/dL, restart at 50% of previous rate.
75–100 mg/dL	Stop insulin. Recheck BG every 30 minutes. When levels reach >150 mg/dL, restart at 50% of previous rate unless the dose is <0.25 U/h.
101–125 mg/dL	If <10% lower than last BG, decrease rate by 0.5 U/h. If >10% lower than last BG, decrease rate by 50%. If neither occurs, continue current rate.
126–175 mg/dL	Same rate
176–225 mg/dL	If lower than last BG, continue the same rate. If higher than last BG, increase rate by 0.5 U/h.
>225 mg/dL	If >10% lower than last BG, continue same rate. If <10% lower than last BG or if higher than last BG, increase rate by 1 U/h.

Adapted from: www.starrwood.com/research/insulin.html (the Albert Starr Academic Center for Cardiac Surgery. The Portland Protocol for Continuous Intravenous Insulin Infusion in Post Operative Diabetic Cardiac Surgery Patients. March 2001).

Table 11.12. Emergency management of elevated ICP

1. Elevation of the head of the bed at 30 degrees
2. Osmotherapy
   a. Mannitol 20% 0.25–0.5 g/kg every 4 hours
   b. Hypertonic saline
3. Barbiturates
   a. Pentobarbital 10 mg/kg over 30 minutes
   b. Thiopental 1.5–3.5 mg/kg
4. Paralysis
   a. Vecuronium 0.1 mg/kg
   b. Pancuronium 0.1 mg/kg
5. Hyperventilation (temporary measure only)
   a. Raise ventilation rate with a constant tidal volume
   b. Goal pco_2 30–35
6. ICP monitor placement in patients with hydrocephalus or clinical deterioration secondary to elevated ICP
   a. Goal ICP <20 mm Hg
7. External ventricular drain may be indicated in patients with or at risk for hydrocephalus

Adapted from Goldstein JN, Greenberg SM, Rosand J. Emergency management of intracerebral hemorrhage. *Continuum.* 2006;**12**(1):13–29.

14. **Management of elevated ICP**. Increased intracranial pressure (ICP) is common in patients with ICH.[86,87] Elevated ICP is usually recognized by progressively worsening level of arousal, or development of worsening or new neurologic deficit accompanied by evidence of mass effect ("midline shift," edema, hydrocephalus, or herniation) on neuroimaging.

Emergent management of elevated ICP in a rapidly deteriorating patient includes:

1. Proper head positioning (elevated to 30 degrees)
2. Rapid infusion of 20% mannitol at 1.0–1.5 g/kg
3. Hyperventilation (increase in ventilation rate with constant tidal volume) of the patient to a pco_2 of 30–35 mm Hg[86,87]

These are temporary measures designed to lower ICP quickly and effectively, until a definitive treatment can be instituted. In this case, a neurosurgical intervention such as EVD, or craniotomy may prove life-saving [4,17,61] (Table 11.12).

For patients in whom the neurologic exam cannot be followed, and elevated ICP is suspected, early invasive ICP monitoring offers additional diagnostic

and therapeutic advantage.[88] Early neurosurgical consultation is essential to prevent cerebral herniation, the most detrimental of ICH complications.

Goal ICP is less than 20 mm Hg, while CPP is optimal when maintained above 70 mm Hg. Options for continued medical therapy in patients who are not deemed to be surgical candidates or in whom CSF drainage with EVD is insufficient include:

a. Osmotherapy (20% mannitol 0.25–0.5 g/kg every 4 hours or hypertonic saline (NaCl), 30 mL of 23% or continuous infusion of 3% NaCl)
b. Use of barbiturates (pentobarbital 10 mg/kg over 30 minutes or thiopental 1.5 mg/kg to 3.5 mg/kg
c. Pharmacologic paralysis with vercuronium or pancuronium (both 0.1 mg/kg)[74,89]

15. **Seizure prophylaxis**. Patients with ICH have an estimated 30-day risk of clinically evident seizure activity of 8%, with lobar ICH being an independent predictor of early seizure onset.[90] Up to 2% of ICH patients will develop convulsive status epilepticus after their index event, and up to 28% of continuously monitored stuporous or comatose ICH patients will develop some sort of epileptiform activity during the first 72 hours after admission.[90–92]

Table 11.13. Anticonvulsant agents commonly used for seizure prophylaxis

Agent	Initial dose	Protein binding (%)	Metabolism	Goal serum levels
Phenytoin	20 mg/kg IV	90	Hepatic	15–20 µg/mL
Fosphenytoin	20 mg PE/kg IV	90	Hepatic	15–20 µg/mL
Phenobarbital	20 mg/kg IV	20–60	Hepatic	10–30 µg/mL
Valproate	15–20 mg/kg IV	90	Hepatic	50–100 µg/mL
Levetiracetam	500–1000 mg PO	<10	Renal	None

Adapted from Goldstein JN, Greenberg SM, Rosand J. Emergency management of intracerebral hemorrhage. *Continuum.* 2006;**12**(1):13–29.

Seizure activity is associated with neurologic deterioration, progressive mass effect, and worse clinical outcomes in these patients;[90] however, the benefit of primary prophylactic use of anticonvulsive therapies has not been demonstrated.

- The American Stroke Association guidelines recommend seizure prophylaxis in selected ICH patients (large supratentorial hematoma; evidence of subarachnoid or subdural hemorrhage; evidence of traumatic brain injury; decreased levels of consciousness) for 1 month, and then discontinuation, if seizure-free.[4]
- Multiple antiepileptics are available for use in the intensive care setting (Table 11.13), with phenytoin and fosphenytoin being most commonly used and easy to dose according to serum levels.

16. **Role of neurosurgery.** Cerebellar surgery is life-saving and deficit sparing, with surgical evacuation of cerebellar hemorrhage >3 cm in diameter considered standard.[65] The recently reported STICH (Surgical Trial in Intracerebral Hemorrhage) trial showed that emergent surgical evacuation of hematoma within 72 hours did not improve outcome as compared to a standard conservative management;[66] however, neurosurgical intervention is worth considering in selected patients. In particular, young patients with large lobar hematomas, who deteriorate rapidly due to mass effect, are likely to benefit from craniotomy with hematoma evacuation and duraplasty to follow. Treatment of intraventricular hemorrhage with local instillation of thrombolytics via indwelling intraventricular catheters is a plausible experimental approach.[67] Clinical trials will be needed to evaluate the benefit of newer neurosurgical interventions.

CONCLUSION

From its onset, ICH is a dynamic illness that requires frequent and thorough reassessment. Once the diagnosis of ICH is made, urgent intervention to reduce hematoma volume or prevent its expansion can be life-saving. These patients uniformly require early intensive care provided through the collaborative effort of emergency personnel, neurologic, neurosurgical, and intensive care unit staff. The development of specialized neurocritical care and recent advances in understanding and management of ICH have resulted in improvement in outcome for patients with this devastating disease. Future improvements in the management of ICH may include early hemostatic therapy with fVIIa as well as the application of refined neurosurgical interventions.

REFERENCES

1. Kase CS, Mohr JP, Caplan LR. *Intracerebral hemorrhage. In* Barnett H, Mohr J (eds), *Stroke: Pathophysiology, diagnosis, and management.* Philadelphia: Churchill Livingstone, 1998, pp 649–700.
2. Flaherty ML, Woo D, Haverbuch M, et al. Racial variations in location and risk of intracerebral hemorrhage. *Stroke.* 2005;**36**:934–7.
3. Albers GW, Amarenco P, Easton JD, et al. Antithrombotic and thrombolytic therapy for ischemic stroke: the Seventh ACCP Conference on Antithrombotic and Thrombolytic Therapy. *Chest.* 2004;**126**:483S–512S.
4. Broderick JP, Adams HP, Barsan W, et al. Guidelines for the management of spontaneous intracerebral

hemorrhage: a statement for healthcare professionals from a special writing group of the Stroke Council, American Heart Association. *Stroke.* 1999;**30**:905–15.

5. Flaherty ML, Haverbusch M, Sekar P, et al. Long-term mortality after intracerebral hemorrhage. *Neurology.* 2006;**66**(8):1182–6.

6. Qureshi AI, Tuhrim S, Broderick JP, et al. Spontaneous intracerebral hemorrhage. *N Engl J Med.* 2001;344: 1450–60.

7. Diringer MN, Edwards DF. Admission to a neurologic/ neurosurgical intensive care unit is associated with reduced mortality rate after intracerebral hemorrhage. *Crit Care Med.* 2001;**29**:635–40.

8. Mirski MA, Chang CW, Cowan R. Impact of a neuroscience intensive care unit on neurosurgical patient outcomes and cost of care: evidence-based support for an intensivist-directed specialty ICU model of care. *J Neurosurg Anesthesiol.* 2001;**13**: 83–92.

9. Mayer SA, Brun NC, Begtrup K, et al. Recombinant activated factor VII for acute intracerebral hemorrhage. *N Engl J Med.* 2005;**352**:777–85.

10. Fisher CM. Pathological observations in hypertensive intracerebral hemorrhage. *J Neuropathol Exp Neurol.* 1971; **30**:536–50.

11. Brott T, Thalinger K, Hertzberg V. Hypertension as a risk factor for spontaneous intracerebral hemorrhage. *Stroke.* 1986;**17**:1078–83.

12. Thrift AG, McNeil JJ, Forbes A, et al. Three important subgroups of hypertensive persons at greater risk of intracerebral hemorrhage. *Hypertension.* 1998;**31**: 1223–9.

13. Greenberg SM, Vonsattel JP, Stakes JW, et al. The clinical spectrum of cerebral amyloid angiopathy: presentations without lobar hemorrhage. *Neurology.* 1993;**43**(10): 2073–9.

14. Greenberg SM, Rebeck GW, Vonsattel JP, et al. Apolipoprotein E epsilon 4 and cerebral hemorrhage associated with amyloid angiopathy. *Ann Neurol.* 1995; **38**(2):254–9.

15. Greenberg SM. Amyloid angiopathy. *Neurology.* 1997;**48**(1):291.

16. Woo D, Broderick JP. Spontaneous intracerebral hemorrhage: epidemiology and clinical presentation. *Neurosurg Clin N Am.* 2002;**13**:265–79.

17. Mayer SA, Rincon F. Treatment of intracerebral haemorrhage. *Lancet Neurol.* 2005;**4**(10):662–72.

18. Greenberg SM, Vonsattel JP. Diagnosis of cerebral amyloid angiopathy. Sensitivity and specificity of cortical biopsy. *Stroke.* 1997;**28**(7):1418–22.

19. Greenberg SM, Vonsattel JP, Segal AZ, et al. Association of apolipoprotein E epsilon2 and vasculopathy in cerebral amyloid angiopathy. *Neurology.* 1998;**50**(4):961–5.

20. Alonso NC, Hyman BT, Rebeck GW, et al. Progression of cerebral amyloid angiopathy: accumulation of amyloid-beta40 in affected vessels. *J Neuropathol Exp Neurol.* 1998;**57**(4):353–9.

21. O'Donnell HC, Rosand J, Knudsen KA, et al. Apolipoprotein E genotype and the risk of recurrent lobar intracerebral hemorrhage. *N Engl J Med.* 2000;**342**:240–5.

22. Greenberg SM, Finkelstein SP, Shaeffer PW. Petechial hemorrhages accompanying lobar hemorrhage: detection by gradient-echo MRI. *Neurology.* 1996;**46**(6): 1751–4.

23. Greenberg SM, Eng JA, Ning M, et al. Hemorrhage burden predicts recurrent intracerebral hemorrhage after lobar hemorrhage. *Stroke.* 2004;**35**:1415–20.

24. Hypertension Detection, and Follow-Up Program Cooperative Group. Five-year findings of the hypertension detection and follow-up program III: reduction in stroke incidence, *JAMA.* 1982;**247**:633–8.

25. Arakawa S, Saku Y, Ibayashi S, et al. Blood pressure control and recurrence of hypertensive brain hemorrhage. *Stroke.* 1998;**29**:1806–9.

26. Thrift AG, Donnan GA, McNeil JJ. Heavy drinking, but not moderate or intermediate drinking, increases the risk of intracerebral hemorrhage. *Epidemiology.* 1999;**10**:307–12.

27. Segal AZ, Chiu RI, Eggleston-Sexton PM, et al. Low cholesterol as a risk factor for primary intracerebral hemorrhage: a case-control study. *Neuroepidemiology.* 1999; **18**:185–93.

28. Mayer SA. Ultra-early hemostatic therapy for intracerebral hemorrhage. *Stroke.* 2003;**34**:224–9.

29. Rosand J, Eckman MH, Knudsen KA, et al. The effect of warfarin and intensity of anticoagulation on outcome of intracerebral hemorrhage. *Arch Intern Med.* 2004;**164**:880–4.

30. Mayer SA, Lignelli A, Fink ME, et al. Perilesional blood flow and edema formation in acute intracerebral hemorrhage: a SPECT study. *Stroke.* 1998;**29**:1791–8.

31. Rosand J, Eskey C, Chang Y, et al. Dynamic single-section CT demonstrates reduced cerebral blood flow in acute intracerebral hemorrhage. *Cerebrovasc Dis.* 2002;**14**:214–20.

32. Broderick JP, Brott TG, Duldner JE, et al. Volume of intracerebral hemorrhage: a powerful and easy-to-use predictor of 30-day mortality. *Stroke.* 1993;**24**:987–93.

33. Davis SM, Broderick J, Hennerici M, et al. Hematoma growth is determinant of mortality and poor outcome after intracerebral hemorrhage. *Neurology.* 2006;**66**:1175–81.

34. Brott T, Broderick J, Kothari R, et al. Early hemorrhage growth in patients with intracerebral hemorrhage. *Stroke.* 1997;**28**:1–5.

35. Flibotte JJ, Hagan N, O'Donnell J, et al. Warfarin, hematoma expansion, and outcome of intracerebral hemorrhage. *Neurology.* 2004;**63**:1059–64.

36. Xi G, Wagner KR, Keep RF, et al. Role of blood clot formation on early edema development after experimental intracerebral hemorrhage. *Stroke.* 1998;**29**:2506–8.

37. Gebel JM, Jauch EC, Brott TG, et al. Relative edema volume is a predictor of outcome in patients with hyperacute spontaneous intracerebral hemorrhage. *Stroke.* 2002;**33**:2636–41.

38. Mayer SA, Sacco RL, Shi T, et al. Neurologic deterioration in noncomatose patients with supratentorial intracerebral hemorrhage. *Neurology.* 1994; **44**: 1379–84.

39. Levine JM, Snider R, Finkelstein D, et al. Early edema in warfarin-related intracerebral hemorrhage. *Neurocrit Care*. 2007;**7**(1):58–63.

40. Zazulia AR, Diringer MN, Derdeyn CP, et al. Progression of mass effect after intracerebral hemorrhage. *Stroke*. 1999;**30**:1167–73.

41. Power C, Henry S, Del Bigio MR, et al. Intracerebral hemorrhage induces macrophage activation and matrix metalloproteinases. *Ann Neurol*. 2003;**53**:731–42.

42. Abilleira S, Montaner J, Molina CA, et al. Matrix metalloproteinase-9 concentration after spontaneous intracerebral hemorrhage. *J Neurosurg*. 2003;**99**:65–70.

43. Schellinger PD, Fiebach JB, Hoffmann K, et al. Stroke MRI in intracerebral hemorrhage: is there a perihemorrhagic penumbra? *Stroke*. 2003;**34**:1674–9.

44. Vermeer SE, Algra A, Franke CA, et al. Long-term prognosis after recovery from primary intracerebral hemorrhage. *Neurology*. 2002;**59**:205–9.

45. Counsell C, Boonyakarnkul S, Dennis M, et al. Primary intracerebral hemorrhage in the Oxfordshire community stroke project. 2. Prognosis. *Cerebrovasc Dis*. 1995;**5**:26–34.

46. Fujii Y, Takeuchi S, Sasaki O, et al. Multivariate analysis of predictors of hematoma enlargement in spontaneous intracerebral hemorrhage. *Stroke*. 1998;**29**: 1160–6.

47. Hemphill JC, Bonovich DC, Besmertis L, et al. The ICH score: a simple, reliable grading scale for intracerebral hemorrhage. *Stroke*. 2001;**32**:891–7.

48. Becker KJ, Baxter AB, Cohen WA, et al. Withdrawal of support in intracerebral hemorrhage may lead to self-fulfilling prophecies. *Neurology*. 2001;**56**: 766–72.

49. Hemphill JC, Newman J, Zhao S, et al. Hospital usage of early do-not-resuscitate orders and outcome after intracerebral hemorrhage. *Stroke*. 2004; **35**: 1130–4.

50. Rost NS, Smith EE, Chang Y, et al. Prediction of Functional outcome in patients with primary intracerebral hemorrhage: the FUNC score. *Stroke*. 2008; **39**(8): 2304–9.

51. Caplan, LR. Intracerebral hemorrhage. In Caplan LR (ed), *Caplan's Stroke: A Clinical Approach*, 3rd ed. Boston: Butterworth-Heinemann, 2000, pp 383–418.

52. Weisberg LA. Computerized tomography in intracerebral hemorrhage. *Arch Neurol*. 1979; **46**:422–6.

53. Broderick JP, Brott T, Tomsick T, et al. Ultra-early evaluation of intracerebral hemorrhage. *J Neurosurg*. 1990;**72**: 195–9.

54. Smith EE, Rosand J, Greenberg SM. Hemorrhagic stroke. *Neuroimaging Clin N Am*. 2005;**15**:259–72.

55. Kothari RU, Brott T, Broderick JP, et al. The ABCs of measuring intracerebral hemorrhage volumes. *Stroke*. 1996;**27**:1304–5.

56. Murai Y, Takagi R, Ikeda Y, et al. Three-dimensional computerized tomography angiography in patients with hyperacute intracerebral hemorrhage. *J Neurosurg*. 1999;**91**:424–31.

57. Zhu X, Chan MS, Poon WS. Spontaneous intracranial hemorrhage: which patients need diagnostic cerebral

58. Laissy JP, Normand JP, Monroe M, et al. Spontaneous intracerebral hematoma from vascular causes. *Neuroradiology*. 1991;**33**:291–5.

59. Kidwell CS, Chalela JA, Saver JL, et al. Comparison of MRI and CT for detection of acute intracerebral hemorrhage. *JAMA*. 2004;**292**:1823–30.

60. Atlas SW, Thulborn KR. Intracranial hemorrhage. In *Atlas SW (ed), Magnetic Resonance Imaging of the Brain and Spine*, 3rd ed. Philadelphia: Lippincot Williams & Wilkins, 2002, pp 773–832.

61. The European Stroke Initiative Writing Committee (EUSI). Recommendation for the Management of Intracranial Hemorrhage – Part I: Spontaneous Intracerebral Hemorrhage. *Cerebrovasc Dis*. 2006;**22**: 294–316.

62. Gujjar AR, Deibert E, Manno EM, et al. Mechanical ventilation for ischemic stroke and intracerebral hemorrhage: indications, timing, and outcome. *Neurology*. 1998;**51**:447–51.

63. Walls RM. Airway. In Marx JA, Harkberger RS, Walls RM (eds), *Rosen's Emergency Medicine: Concepts and Clinical Practice*. 5th ed. St. Louis: C.V. Mosby, 2002, pp 2–21.

64. Roppolo LP, Walters K. Airway management in neurological emergencies. *Neurocrit Care*. 2004;**1**:405–14.

65. Ott KH, Kase CS, Ojemann RG, et al. Cerebellar hemorrhage: diagnosis and treatment, a review of 56 cases. *Arch Neurol*. 1974;**31**:160–7.

66. Mendelow AD, Gregson BA, Fernandes HM, et al. Early surgery versus initial conservative treatment in patients with spontaneous supratentorial intracerebral haematomas in the International Surgical Trial in Intracerebral Haemorrhage (STICH): a randomised trial. *Lancet*. 2005;**365**:387–97.

67. Naff NJ, Hanley DF, Keyl PM, et al. Intraventricular thrombolysis speeds blood clot resolution: results of a pilot, prospective, randomized, double-blind, controlled trial. *Neurosurgery*. 2004;**54**:577–83.

68. He J, Whelton PK, Vu B, et al. Aspirin and risk of hemorrhagic stroke: a meta-analysis of randomized controlled trials. *JAMA*. 1998;**280**(22):1930–5.

69. Steiner T, Diringer M, Rosand J. Intracerebral hemorrhage associated with oral anticoagulant therapy: current practices and open questions. *Stroke*. 2006;**37**:256–62.

70. Goldstein JN, Thomas Sh, Frontiero V, et al. Timing of fresh frozen plasma administration and rapid correction of coagulopathy in warfarin-related intracerebral hemorrhage. *Stroke*. 2006;**37**:1–5.

71. Fredricksson K, Norrving B, Stromblad LG. Emergency reversal of anticoagulation after intracerebral hemorrhage. *Stroke*. 1992;**23**:972–7.

72. Ansell J, Hirsh J, Dalen J, et al. Managing oral anticoagulation therapy. *Chest*. 2001;**119**:225–385.

73. Hanley JP. Warfarin reversal. *J Clin Pathol*. 2004; **57**: 1152–9.

74. http://www.massgeneral.org/stopstroke/home.htm

angiography? A prospective study of 206 cases and review of the literature. *Stroke*. 1997;**28**:1406–9.

75. Piriyawat PML, Yawn DH, Hall CE, et al. Treatment of acute intracerebral hemorrhage with epsilon aminocaproic acid: a pilot study. *Neurocrit Care.* 2004;**1**:47–52.

76. Mannucci PM, Remuzzi G, Pusineri F, et al. Deamino-8-D-arginine vasopressin shortens the bleeding time in uremia. *N Engl J Med.* 1983;**308**:8–12.

77. Ohwaki K, Yano E, Nagashima H, et al. Blood pressure management in acute intracerebral hemorrhage: relationship between elevated blood pressure and hematoma enlargement. *Stroke.* 2004;**35**:1364–7.

78. Jauch EC, Lindsell CJ, Adeoye O, et al. Lack of evidence for an association between hemodynamic variables and hematoma growth in spontaneous intracerebral hemorrhage. *Stroke.* 2006;**37**(8):2061–5.

79. Qureshi AI, Mohammed YM, Yahia IM, et al. A prospective multicenter study to evaluate feasibility and safety of aggressive antihypertensive treatment in patients with acute intracerebral hemorrhage. *J Intens Care Med.* 2005;**20**:34–42.

80. Fogelholm R, Avikainen S, Murros K. Prognostic value and determinants of first-day mean arterial pressure in spontaneous supratentorial intracerebral hemorrhage. *Stroke.* 1997;**28**:1396–1400.

81. Willmot M, Leonardi-Bee J and Bath Pmw. High blood pressure in acute stroke and subsequent outcome: a systematic review. *Hypertension.* 2004;**43**:18–24.

82. Broderick JP, Connoly S, Feldman E, et al. Guidelines for the management of spontaneous intracerebral hemorrhage in adults: 2007 update. A Guideline from the American Heart Association/American Stroke Association Stroke Council, High Blood Pressure Research Council, and the Quality of Care and Outcomes in Research Interdisciplinary Working Group *Stroke.* 2007;**38**:2001–23.

83. Passero S, Ciacci G, Ulivelli M. The influence of diabetes and hyperglycemia on clinical course after intracerebral hemorrhage. *Neurology.* 2003;**61**:1351–6.

84. van den Berghe G, Wouters P, Weekers F, et al. Intensive insulin therapy in the critically ill patients. *N Engl J Med.* 2001;**345**:1359–67.

85. Commichau C, Scarmeas N, Mayer SA. Risk factors for fever in the neurologic intensive care unit. *Neurology.* 2003;**60**:837–841.

86. The Brain Trauma Foundation, The American Association of Neurological Surgeons, The Joint Section on Neurotrauma and Critical Care, Guidelines for the management of traumatic brain injury. *J Neurotrauma.* 2000;**17**:457–549.

87. McKinley BA, Parmley CL, Tonneson AS. Standardized management of intracranial pressure: a preliminary clinical trial. *J Trauma.* 1999;**46**:271–9.

88. Adams RE, Diringer MN. Response to external ventricular drainage in spontaneous intracerebral hemorrhage with hydrocephalus. *Neurology.* 1998; **50**:519–523.

89. Goldstein JN, Greenberg SM, Rosand J. Emergency management of intracerebral hemorrhage. *Continuum.* 2006;**12**(1):13–29.

90. Passero S, Rocchi R, Rossi S, et al. Seizures after spontaneous supratentorial intracerebral hemorrhage. *Epilepsia.* 2002;**43**:1175–80.

91. Vespa PM, O'Phelan K, Shah M, et al. Acute seizures after intracerebral hemorrhage: a factor in progressive midline shift and outcome. *Neurology.* 2003; **60**:1441–6.

92. Claassen J, Mayer SA, Kowalski RG, et al. Detection of electrographic seizures with continuous EEG monitoring in critically ill patients. *Neurology.* 2004;**62**: 1743–8.

12 Cerebral Venous Thrombosis

Magdy Selim, MD, PhD

Thrombosis of the cerebral veins and sinuses (CVT) is often challenging to diagnose owing to the broad spectrum and variability of clinical symptoms and signs on initial presentation. Delayed diagnosis of CVT can have devastating consequences, while early diagnosis can facilitate timely initiation of effective treatment to improve the prognosis. This chapter highlights the pathogenesis and risk factors for CVT, clinical and radiologic diagnosis, and treatment strategies and options.

CVT AS A DISTINCT CEREBROVASCULAR DISEASE

The estimated incidence of CVT is three to four cases per one million people per year, much less common than its arterial counterpart. In contrast to arterial occlusions:

- Patients with CVT tend to be younger (mean age is mid-30s to 40s). However, CVT can also develop in elderly patients with debilitating diseases and neonates and infants suffering from dehydration.
- Women are more likely than men to develop CVT, especially at a young age. This is attributed to puerperium, pregnancy, and use of oral contraceptives.
- Patients with CVT have lower frequencies of traditional risk factors, such as hypertension, diabetes, and cardiac disease.
- The clinical course and evolution of CVT is often slow and indolent, and progression of symptoms is the rule.

CAUSES AND PATHOPHYSIOLOGY OF CVT

Table 12.1 lists the conditions that can cause or predispose to CVT. The presence of any of these conditions should alert physicians and raise suspicion to the possibility of CVT. These conditions predispose to CVT by inducing:

- Hypercoagulability
- Low-flow state within the affected sinus or vein
- Extrinsic compression or invasion of a venous sinus
- Intravascular volume depletion

CLINICAL PRESENTATION OF CVT

Onset: Abrupt onset is uncommon, and is mostly seen in infectious and obstetrical cases. A slow, progressive course is seen in most patients.

Symptoms and signs: Symptoms are often subtle early on, and are variable. Some cases may be completely asymptomatic at onset. Table 12.2 summarizes the most common symptoms and signs of CVT. The clinical findings may relate to occlusion of the venous structures and subsequent venous congestion and secondary increase in intracranial pressure (ICP), or specific involvement of certain structures. CVT should be suspected and evaluated in ALL patients with "benign" intracranial hypertension or pseudo-tumor cerebri

Table 12.1. Causes of CVT

Infective (septic) causes

- Intracranial infections, such as meningitis, encephalitis, dural and epidural empyemas, and abscesses
- Paracranial infections, such as dental, paranasal sinuses, mastoids, and face or scalp infections
- Systemic infections, such as endocarditis, septicemia, viral, fungal, or parasitic infections

Noninfective causes

- Head trauma
- Dural arteriovenous malformation
- Compression or injury of internal jugular vein
- Neoplasms, such as systemic adenocarcinomas, leukemia, and lymphoma, or intracranial tumors that about on venous sinuses including meningiomas
- Pregnancy and puerperium
- Inflammatory gastrointestinal diseases, such as ulcerative colitis and Crohn's disease
- Inflammatory tissue diseases, such as sarcoidosis, Wegener's granulomatosis, Behçet's disease, systemic lupus erythematosus, and giant cell arteritis
- Postsurgery and -spinal procedures, such as epidural anesthesia and lumbar puncture
- Hematologic disorders predisposing to hypercoagulability, such as polycythemia, paroxysmal nocturnal hemoglobinuria (PNH), thrombocythemia, and sickle cell disease
- Nephrotic syndrome
- Volume depletion from dehydration, malnutrition, cachexia, or blood loss, particularly in the neonates and elderly
- Congenital heart disease and cardiac insufficiency
- Medications, such as oral contraceptives, hormonal therapy, steroids, and L-asparaginase
- Coagulation disorders, acquired or inherited
- "Idiopathic"

DIAGNOSIS OF CVT

The first step in diagnosing CVT is to suspect it! The following "red flags" should raise suspicion for CVT:

- Personal or family history of recurrent deep vein thromboses, pulmonary embolism, unexplained miscarriages, or known condition predisposing to hypercoagulability
- Symptoms and signs of increased ICP (headache, vomiting, papilledema, altered level of alertness) in the absence of an obvious intracranial mass lesion or infection
- Presence of dural AV fistula (approximately 40% of patients with dural AVF also have CVT)
- Young age and absence of traditional risk factors for stroke

- Pregnant and puerperal women
- Development of symptoms after procedural manipulations of the internal jugular vein
- Unexplained intracerebral hemorrhage: The majority of venous infarcts are hemorrhagic. There are no pathognomonic features to hemorrhagic venous infarcts, and it is not uncommon to label them as "intraparenchymal hemorrhages" on initial evaluation. However, (1) multiplicity; (2) nonarterial territory; (3) subcortical localization; (4) ill-defined appearance; (5) surrounding edema out of proportion to the suspected age and size of hemorrhage and lack of radiologic evidence of underlying neoplasm; and (6) bilateral involvement of the thalami or basal ganglia should raise suspicion for possible CVT.

Table 12.2. Symptoms and signs of CVT
Symptom/sign comments
Headache: Usually the earliest, and may be the only, symptom. It is the most frequent symptom, being present in up to 91% of patients. It has no typical characteristics, and may be mistaken for chronic headache, thunderclap headache, and even migraine with visual symptoms. It is caused by distension of the occluded sinus and elevated ICP.
Seizures can be focal or generalized, and are usually secondary to a cortical venous infarct. Seizures occur in 10–63% of patients with CVT.
Altered alertness is uncommon at presentation, but almost 44% of patients will have an alteration in level of alertness (drowsiness – confusion – coma) at some time during the course of the disease. It may be attributed to increased ICP, postictal state, or bilateral involvement of the thalami in patients with deep vein thrombosis.
Signs of elevated ICP: These include headache, sixth nerve palsy, transient visual obscuration, and vomiting. Papilledema can be seen in 7–80% of patients with CVT. Up to 38% of patients diagnosed with pseudotumor cerebri show angiographic evidence of lateral sinus thrombosis.
Focal signs: These vary considerably depending on the sinus(es) affected and location of the associated venous infarction. Hemiparesis is the most common finding. Other less common findings include aphasia, neglect, hemianopia, and ataxia.
Sinus-specific presentation
Cavernous sinus thrombosis: Characteristic presentation, often with a variable combination of chemosis, ptosis, proptosis, headache or retro-orbital pain, diplopia due to involvement of CN III or VI, and signs of involvement of CN V1 and V2. Cavernous sinus is the most frequent dural sinus to become infected, usually after facial, sphenoid air sinus, or dental infections.
Lateral sinus thrombosis: The presentation of septic cases is quite characteristic.
There is often evidence of acute or chronic ear infections (fever "picket fence" – earache – draining ears with pus or drum perforation – neck pain and tenderness along the anterior border of the ipsilateral sternocleidomastoid). Diplopia and retro-orbital eye pain from involvement of CN V and VI may be present. Signs of increased ICP are more commonly seen than focal signs and symptoms.
Deep vein of Galen thrombosis: Classical presentation is that of acute coma or stupor, stiffness of the limbs, and decerebrate posturing or extensor spasms, due to bilateral involvement of the thalami and basal ganglia. Other features may include abulia or akinetic mutism.
Cerebellar venous thrombosis: The presentation is similar to a posterior fossa tumor, with incoordination, central nerve palsies, and signs of elevated ICP.
Rolandic cortical vein thrombosis: The presentation is characterized by hemiparesis (leg > arm), and sparing of face and speech. Hypertonia is often present in the leg and a cramp in the hand. Focal cortical sensory deficits may be elicited in the hand.

Although rarely used in clinical practice today, the Toby-Ayer test may help to suggest the diagnosis of CVT, particularly of the lateral sinus. The test is performed by monitoring the cerebrospinal fluid (CSF) pressure during a lumbar puncture. Pressure is applied to the neck to compress the internal jugular veins; this reduces venous outflow from the cranium and raises the intracranial pressure. A spinal puncture will displace CSF into the spinal sac and cause the measured CSF pressure to rise rapidly. This is not seen if a spinal block to the flow of CSF is present. No increase in CSF pressure during external compression of the internal jugular vein on the affected side, and an exaggerated response on the patent side, is suggestive of CVT.

Brain imaging is essential to confirm the diagnosis of CVT suspected on clinical grounds. Imaging should include the brain parenchyma and the sinuses and veins. The administration of contrast is always required to increases the ability of computerized axial tomography (CT) in diagnosing CVT. The administration of contrast is also advocated to increase the reliability of magnetic resonance imaging (MRI) in confirming the diagnosis.

- Plain CT shows nonspecific, subtle abnormalities in most patients later proven to have CVT. It primarily helps to rule out other pathologies.
  - ▸ Contrast administration, together with CVT, significantly improves the reliability of CT in diagnosing CVT.
  - ▸ The most common CT sign of CVT is the "empty delta sign" seen on postcontrast images as a bright triangle (representing the dilated collaterals) surrounding a central hypointense core (representing the clot) in the superior sagittal, lateral, and straight sinuses.
- Multimodal MRI is more sensitive than CT, and is currently the imaging modality of choice for diagnosing CVT. The main sign of CVT on MRI is the lack of expected flow signal void on T1- and T2-weighted images.
- Direct imaging of the sinuses and veins, by CT or MR venograms (CTV or MRV), is almost always required to provide the definitive diagnosis of CVT.
- The commonly used time-of-flight MRV can suffer from in-plane flow signal loss leading to false-positive diagnoses of CVT. Other pitfalls are the absence or hypoplasia of the anterior portion of the superior sagittal or transverse sinuses (normal variants that can simulate thrombosis on MRV). The use of gadolinium-enhanced MRV or CTV may aid is visualizing sinuses or smaller veins with low flow to avoid false-positive diagnosis of sinus occlusion.
- The use of conventional angiogram to diagnose CVT, once the gold standard, should be reserved for patients in whom CTV or MRV are inconclusive, especially those with suspected isolated cortical vein thrombosis.

ETIOLOGICAL DIAGNOSIS

The underlying cause of CVT is usually apparent in most cases, on careful review of the patient's history and comorbid conditions. In cases in which no immediate obvious cause is apparent, extensive workup is often required because the underlying cause may require specific treatment. The initial step in evaluation should include:

Routine blood laboratories

- Complete blood cell count and smear:
  - ▸ Anemia may indicate malignancy or paroxysmal nocturnal hemoglobinuria (PNH).
  - ▸ High hematocrit may indicate dehydration or polycythemia.
  - ▸ High platelet count may indicate thrombocythemia.
  - ▸ Leukocytosis may indicate an underlying infection.
  - ▸ Macrocytosis may highlight an underlying vitamin B_{12} or folate deficiency and associated hyperhomocysteinemia.
- Erythrocyte sedimentation rate (ESR): Elevated ESR may be indicative of an underlying inflammatory illness.
- Electrolytes
- Renal function
- Coagulation parameters: Abnormalities in coagulation parameters may point to an underlying coagulopathy; for example, prolonged partial thromboplastin time (PTT) may uncover antiphospholipid antibody syndrome.
- Antinuclear antibody
- Serum protein electrophoresis: The presence of monoclonal gammopathy may uncover underlying myeloproliferative disorder.
- Stool guaiac: A positive test may uncover undetected colon cancer.
- D-dimer: Elevated d-dimer may be suggestive of venous thromboembolism, but this is neither sensitive nor specific.

Workup for Acquired and Hereditary Thrombophilias

Acquired and congenital abnormalities of coagulation are the most common causes of CVT, and should be an integral part of evaluations for all patients with confirmed diagnosis of CVT. Fewer than 10% of cases of venous thromboembolism, of undetermined cause upon initial evaluation, are attributed to an inherited coagulation disorder.

- The most common causes of acquired thrombophilias are:
  - ▸ Malignancy and myeloproliferative disorders
  - ▸ Antiphospholipid antibody syndrome

- ▶ Recent surgery
- ▶ Pregnancy
- ▶ Medications, such as female hormonal replacement and chemotherapy
- ▶ Sickle cell disease
- Factor V Leiden mutation is the most common inherited thrombophilia, followed by prothrombin gene mutation, then deficiencies of protein C and S, and antithrombin III.
- It is recommended that coagulation workup proceeds in consecutive tiers to avoid unnecessary costs.
- **First tier**: Factor V Leiden/activated protein-C resistance, G20210A-prothrombin gene mutation, antithrombin III deficiency, protein C and S deficiency, fibrinogen, serum homocysteine, and lupus anticoagulant and anticardiolipin antibodies.
- **Second tier**: This includes evaluation for plasminogen, plasminogen-activator and – activator inhibitor levels, deficiency of plasma glutathione peroxidase, factor VIII levels, and Russell viper venom. These tests should be performed if the first tier tests are unrevealing, yet suspicion remains high for a congenital thrombophilia as in the case of a strong family history, recurrent thromboembolic events, or presentation at a very young age.
  - ▶ The timing of coagulation studies is important. Ideally, these tests should be performed before anticoagulation is started because heparin can reduce antithrombin III activity; warfarin reduces both protein C and S levels; and either treatment can influence lupus anticoagulant assays.
  - ▶ The level of some of these coagulation factors may fluctuate after acute thrombosis. Therefore, it is recommended that the coagulation work-up be repeated a few months after cessation of anticoagulation therapy in patients in whom the initial evaluation fails to detect thrombophilia.

Ancillary Tests

These may include electroencephalogram (EEG), serological bacteriological tests, malignancy workup, or lumbar puncture.

- The main value of EEG is to rule out seizures in patients with altered alertness and to demonstrate superimposed epileptic discharges requiring initiation of antiepileptic therapy.
- Cultures and bacteriologic studies may be required in infective cases to determine the offending pathogen and appropriate antibiotics. *Staphylococcus aureus* accounts for up to 70% of cases of septic sinus thrombosis.
- Search for occult malignancy may be required in older patients in whom the above workup is unrevealing.
- Cerebrospinal fluid (CSF) examination is often of little diagnostic value in patients with CVT. It is often abnormal with elevated protein, leukocytosis, and some red blood cells. It is helpful to exclude meningeal infections or carcinomatous meningitis as a cause for CVT. Also, the presence of the above abnormalities in patients with "benign" intracranial hypertension should alert the physician to the possibility of CVT. The main utility of lumbar puncture in patients with CVT is therapeutic to remove CSF to reduce elevated ICP.

DIFFERENTIAL DIAGNOSIS OF CVT

The differential diagnosis of CVT includes:

1. Arterial stroke
2. Intracerebral hemorrhage
3. Brain tumor
4. CNS infections
5. Migraine
6. Pseudotumor cerebri

The differential diagnosis for cavernous sinus thrombosis includes:

1. Orbital cellulites
2. Carotid-cavernous fistula
3. Dural AV fistula
4. Tolosa–Hunt syndrome

MANAGEMENT OF CVT

The management of CVT is directed toward measures to: (1) control elevated ICP, seizures, and other complications; (2) treat the underlying cause; and (3) use anticoagulation or thrombolytic therapy to maintain patency of the venous sinuses and prevent progressive occlusion of venous drainage from the brain.

The priority of treatment during the acute phase is to stabilize the patient's condition and to prevent or reverse elevated ICP, brain edema, and herniation. These are best managed in the intensive care setting and include:

1. ABC (Airway – Breathing – Circulation) management: Gentle intravenous hydration is often required to prevent dehydration and to maintain euvolemia.
2. Management of ICP: This should proceed in a stepwise fashion, as follows:
   a. Head of bed positioned ≥30 degrees
   b. Aggressive treatment of fever
   c. Osmotherapy with mannitol and/or hypertonic saline
   d. Consideration of barbiturate coma, in refractory cases
   e. Hematoma evacuation, intraventricular catheter with external drain placement, or decompressive craniotomy.
   f. Repeated lumbar puncture for CSF removal, treatment with acetazolamide, and placement of a lumboperitoneal shunt may be required in patients with persistent elevation of ICP.
3. The use of prophylactic antiseizure medications during the acute phase is debatable. Life-long treatment with antiepileptics is not required since seizures rarely recur beyond the acute phase.

Antithrombotics play an important role in the management of CVT during the acute phase.

■ Most experts recommend the use of intravenous heparin, with a target PTT value of 80–100 seconds, as the first-line therapy during the acute phase to prevent the progression of venous thrombosis and pulmonary embolism. Acute heparinization does not seem to worsen the condition of patients with hemorrhagic infarcts, and may be associated with a reduction in the risk of death and dependency.
■ Selective, endovascular, catheter-guided, local thrombolysis with or without mechanical clot aspiration should be reserved for patients who

deteriorate despite adequate heparinization, or those presenting with rapid onset of coma.
■ Oral anticoagulation with warfarin is recommended following the acute phase for 3–6 months, and for life when a prothrombotic condition is detected.

Prevention of recurrent venous thromboembolism requires appropriate treatment of the underlying cause, if detected, for example, antibiotics in infective cases, bloodletting in polycythemia, and discontinuation of prothrombotic medications such as oral contraceptives and L-asparaginase.

PROGNOSIS FOR CVT

The disease is treatable; 57–86% of patients achieve complete functional recovery with treatment. The mortality ranges from 5% to 18%, and the recurrence rate is 12–14%.

The factors associated with poor prognosis include:

1. Extremes of age (infancy and advanced age)
2. Abrupt onset with coma and focal deficits
3. Extensive thrombosis of the deep venous system

CONCLUSION

Cerebral venous thrombosis is a potentially fatal disease and is often difficult to diagnose with certainty based on clinical grounds alone. Imaging of the brain and venous sinuses is required to confirm the diagnosis. Early clinical suspicion can lead to rapid diagnosis and treatment, which are essential to minimize morbidity and improve survival.

REFERENCES

Ayanzen RH, Bird CR, Keller PJ, McCully FJ, Theobald MR, Heiserman JE. Cerebral MR venography: normal anatomy and potential diagnostic pitfalls. *AJNR.* 2000;**21**:74–8.

Biousse V, Bousser MG. Cerebral venous thrombosis. *Neurologist.* 1999;**5**:326–49.

Bousser MG. Cerebral venous thrombosis. *Stroke.* 1999;**30**: 481–3.

Bousser MG, Ferro JM. Cerebral venous thrombosis: an update. *Lancet Neurol.* 2007;**6**(2):162–70.

Einhaupl K, Bousser MG, de Bruijn SF, Ferro JM, Martinelli I, Masuhr F, Stam J. EFNS guideline on the treatment of cerebral venous and sinus thrombosis. *Eur J Neurol.* 2006;**13**(6):553–9.

Provenzale JM, Joseph GJ, Barboriak DP. Dural sinus thrombosis: findings on CT and MR Imaging and diagnostic pitfalls. *AJR.* 1998;**170**:777–83.

Stam J. Thrombosis of the cerebral veins and sinuses. *N Engl J Med.* 2005;**352**:1791–8.

Stam J, De Bruijn SF, DeVeber G. Anticoagulation for cerebral sinus thrombosis. *Cochrane Database Syst Rev.* 2002;(4):CD002005.

13 Subarachnoid Hemorrhage

Matthew Miller, MD and Grant Sinson, MD

EPIDEMIOLOGY

Subarachnoid hemorrhage (SAH) includes the subset of intracranial hemorrhage that lies in the space between the thin arachnoid layer and pia mater. In the United States, the vast majority of SAH is caused by traumatic injury. Estimated prevalence of traumatic brain injury (TBI) worldwide is between 150 and 250 per 100,000 population per year. From 12% to 53% (a realistic figure is probably 40%) of traumatic brain injury patients have subarachnoid hemorrhage on initial computerized tomography (CT) scanning. Based on these data, approximately 240,000 persons in the United States suffer traumatic SAH per year.

The presence of traumatic SAH has a significant impact on patient outcome. In fact, the development of vasospasm – which has been demonstrated in various studies by angiography and transcranial Doppler – occurs in approximately 5–40% of head injuries with SAH. In one study, 10 (7.7%) of 130 head-injured patients who displayed SAH on initial CT scanning developed delayed ischemic neurologic deficits (DINDs), reportedly all attributable to vasospasm. In addition, severely head-injured patients (defined as Glasgow Coma Scale [GCS] score of 8 or less on admission, or deterioration to that level within 48 hours of admission) with SAH on CT scanning have a statistically significant increase in risk of death, with an odds ratio of 2.39.

In contrast to traumatic SAH, spontaneous SAH occurs less frequently, and its etiology is more diverse:

- Ruptured intracranial aneurysm (75–80%)
- "Angiogram negative SAH" (7–10%)
- Cerebral arteriovenous malformations (AVMs; 4–5%)
- Vasculitis
- Carotid or vertebral artery dissection
- Ruptured arterial infundibulum (rare)
- Coagulation disorders (rarely cause SAH, more likely to cause intraparenchymal hemorrhage or subdural hemorrhage [SDH])
- Cerebral venous thrombosis
- Spinal AVM
- Cocaine use
- Sickle cell disease
- Pituitary apoplexy
- Tumor

The highest reported incidences of aneurysmal SAH (aSAH) come from Japan and Finland and occur at a rate of 16 per 100,000 per year. In the United States, the incidence is approximately 6 per 100,000, or a total of 18,000 events per year.

Incidence of aSAH peaks in the 55–60-year-old age group. Aneurysmal SAH is often neurologically devastating and carries a poor prognosis, as evidenced by the following statistics:

- 10–12% of patients die before reaching the hospital and 45–50% of patients die within the first 30 days.
- Of the surviving patients, 30% have moderate to severe disability and 66% of patients who undergo successful aneurysm clipping do not return to the same quality of life as before the SAH.

RISK FACTORS

Numerous factors have been identified that increase the risk of aSAH. These include:

- Increasing age
- Smoking: Relative risk is 3.0 for men, 4.7 for women
- African American
- Moderate to excessive alcohol intake
- Hypertension
- Cocaine use
- Autosomal dominant polycystic kidney disease (ADPKD)
- Fibromuscular dysplasia (FMD)
- Arteriovenous malformations
- Moyamoya disease
- Connective tissue disease: Ehlers-Danlos type IV, Marfan's syndrome, pseudoxanthoma elasticum
- Multiple family members with intracranial aneurysms
- Coarctation of the aorta
- Osler–Weber–Rendu syndrome
- Atherosclerosis
- Bacterial endocarditis

If both risk factors of smoking and hypertension are present in the same patient, the rate of spontaneous SAH is increased 15-fold.

CLINICAL PRESENTATION

The clinical presentation of aneurysmal SAH is usually quite distinctive. The classic description of a patient with SAH is one who describes his or her headache as the "worst headache of my life". This often manifests as a sudden, severe, and unremitting headache, accompanied by nausea and vomiting. Photophobia, neck stiffness, and back pain can occur as a result of meningeal irritation. Meningismus may be present consisting of nuchal rigidity or positive Brudzinski or Kernig signs. Impairment of consciousness may occur, as well as focal neurologic deficits.

- An oculomotor nerve palsy often accompanies a posterior communicating artery aneurysm.
- An abducens nerve palsy may accompany a posterior cerebral artery aneurysm.

Hemiplegia or hemiparesis may result from cerebral infarction. Approximately 4.5–8% of patients will either present with seizure, or develop seizures as a result of aSAH. Obtundation or coma may be present as the neurologic grade worsens.

In 33–70% of cases, a history of severe headache occurs 2–3 weeks before presentation. Known as "warning headache" or "sentinel leak", this theoretically represents a small hemorrhage from the offending aneurysm that quickly stops or clots weeks before the catastrophic event. In the primary care setting, studies have shown that 25% of patients who complain of an acute, severe, paroxysmal headache will have an aSAH.

DIAGNOSIS

In cases of unusually severe headache, CT scanning should be performed. This modality has a 97.5% sensitivity rate for identifying SAH. Patients with a negative head CT but a high index of suspicion should be considered for lumbar puncture. In those with SAH, the red blood cell (RBC) count is usually >100,000 cells/mm^3 in the third tube of the cerebrospinal fluid (CSF) collection, and xanthochromia is present.

- It is commonly quoted that the presence of xanthochromia is a sensitive indicator for SAH; however, it has been shown that simple visual inspection of CSF for xanthochromia is not sensitive or specific.
- More sensitive and specific is the measurement of excess bilirubin content in the CSF sample. When red blood cells are released into the subarachnoid space, hemolysis with release of oxyhemoglobin occurs. Oxyhemoglobin is then enzymatically converted to bilirubin, which can be quantitated using spectrophotometry.
- CSF bilirubin concentration peaks at 24–48 hours and can persist for 2–4 weeks. Apperloo et al. demonstrated a method of spectrophotometric analysis of CSF that achieved 100% sensitivity and 100% specificity for aSAH.

In a patient diagnosed with SAH, it is essential to determine the etiology so that proper treatment can be instituted. In cases of aSAH, noncontrasted CT studies characteristically show hemorrhage patterns suggesting the location of aneurysmal rupture. Often, there is extensive hemorrhage into the lateral sylvian fissures or anterior interhemispheric fissure.

Ruptured posterior circulation aneurysms show hemorrhage in the fourth ventricle in up to 85% of cases and to a lesser extent the third ventricle. Occasionally, the only finding with a ruptured posterior circulation aneurysm is intraventricular blood. Therefore, in patients with a negative angiogram, occult aneurysm should be suspected if there is extensive extravasation of blood into the anterior interhemispheric fissure, the lateral sylvian fissure, or the ventricles. The following are modalities currently used in clinical practice for imaging of intracerebral aneurysms.

■ CT angiography (CTA) is especially well suited for imaging aneurysms. An intravenous dose of iodinated contrast is given as a timed bolus to produce images of the intracranial vessels. Current high-resolution helical CT scanners are able to rapidly obtain images, allowing high-definition 3-dimensional images that aid in diagnosis (Fig. 13.1). CTA is 95% sensitive and 83% specific for aneurysms 2.2 mm and larger.
   ▸ This modality is especially advantageous to the neurosurgeon because of its ability to show bony anatomical relationships and 3-dimensional structure of the aneurysm.
   ▸ Its drawbacks are that intravenous contrast must be given, and thus the test is contraindicated in patients with renal failure or iodinated contrast dye allergy.
■ Magnetic resonance angiography (MRA) produces images of the intracranial vasculature by detecting a specific range of blood flow velocity, allowing isolation of intracranial arteries (Fig. 13.2).
   ▸ MRA is 86% sensitive and 84% specific in detecting aneurysms >3 mm in diameter.
   ▸ MRA takes longer to perform, produces degraded image quality with patient motion, and does not show bony detail.
   ▸ Its advantage is that it does not require intravenous contrast agents.
■ Conventional cerebral angiography is the "gold-standard" for imaging of intracranial aneurysms (Fig. 13.3). Angiography provides exceptional resolution, can detect small aneurysms and infundibuli, and demonstrates dynamic flow of cerebral vasculature and of the aneurysm itself.
   ▸ Cerebral angiography is negative in 10–15% of patients with spontaneous SAH. Reasons for negative angiography include vasospasm,

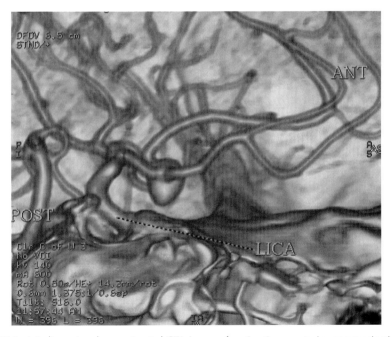

Figure 13.1. A 3-dimensional reconstructed CTA image of an 8 × 6 mm anterior communicating artery aneurysm is shown (note the right internal carotid artery has been subtracted from the image to improve visualization of the aneurysm). Surrounding bony detail is well demonstrated. (See also figure in color plate section.)

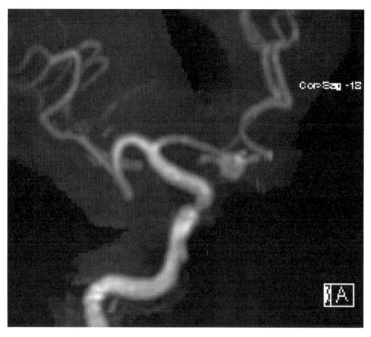

Figure 13.2. A 3-dimensional time-of-flight (TOF) MRA image of a 7 × 7 mm anterior communicating artery aneurysm. No surrounding bony anatomy is shown in MRA images.

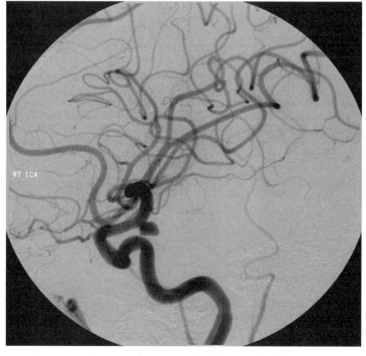

Figure 13.3. Conventional angiographic image of a right supraclinoid ICA aneurysm is shown.

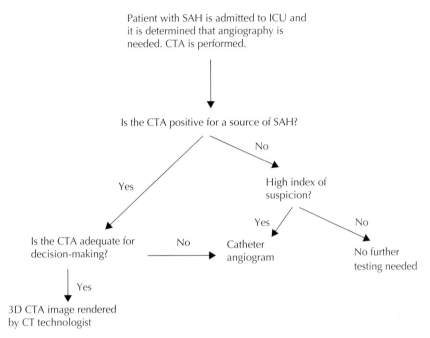

Figure 13.4. Flow diagram for choosing an imaging modality in cases of spontaneous SAH.

thrombosis of the aneurysm, poor-quality study, or nonaneurysmal subarachnoid hemorrhage (see section entitled "Angiogram-Negative Subarachnoid Hemorrhage").

▸ Repeat angiography should be done in 1–2 weeks on a case-by-case basis if the initial study is negative. Repeat angiography detects an aneurysm in an additional 16% of cases, but in cases of pretruncal nonaneurysmal subarachnoid hemorrhage (PNSAH), repeat angiography is not indicated.

An example algorithm for decision making in diagnostic imaging for patients with spontaneous SAH is shown in Figure 13.4.

PROGNOSTIC INDICATORS

At least 37 different SAH grading scales have been proposed in the past, aiming to stratify patients into risk categories based on presenting signs and symptoms. The scale most commonly used in clinical practice is the Hunt and Hess grading scale, proposed in 1968 (Table 13.1).

The correlation of Hunt and Hess grade to the development of DIND is shown in Table 13.2.

In 1981, a committee was formed by the World Federation of Neurological Surgeons (WFNS) to create a universal subarachnoid hemorrhage grading scale (Table 13.3). The WFNS grading system attempts to reduce interobserver variability by basing its grading on GCS score and presence of aphasia, hemiparesis, or hemiplegia.

Initial WFNS predicts GOS score, with significant differences among patients in Grade 1 versus grade 2 and 3 versus grade 4 and 5. Correlation of WFNS score and GOS score of 294 consecutive patients at 1 month after discharge is shown in Table 13.4.

Fisher grade is explained in detail in the section entitled "Vasospasm". Its correlation to poor GOS score at 1 month is shown in Table 13.5.

Age at the time of aneurysm rupture is a significant indicator of morbidity and mortality. Incidence of vasospasm and rebleeding is identical to the younger age group, but outcome is unfavorable (GOS score 1–3)≥ in 60.4% of patients age 70 years or older versus 34.5 % in patients younger than 70.

Volume of SAH is a statistically significant predictor of 30-day mortality. In the series reported by Broderick, 3 (10%) of 29 patients with ≤15 cm^3 of subarachnoid hemorrhage died within 30 days,

Table 13.1. Modified Hunt and Hess SAH Grading Scale

Grade	Signs and symptoms	Percent risk of death as originally reported by Hunt and Hess
0	Unruptured aneurysm	
1a	No acute meningeal signs, fixed neuro deficit	
1	Asymptomatic or mild HA or mild nuchal rigidity	11
2	Cranial nerve palsy, moderate to severe HA, nuchal rigidity	26
3	Drowsiness, confusion, or mild focal neurologic deficit	37
4	Stupor, moderate or severe hemiparesis, early decerebrate	71
5	Deep coma, decerebrate, moribund appearance	100

Table 13.2. Hunt and Hess severity correlation to DIND

Hunt and Hess grade	% of patients who develop DIND
1	22
2	33
3	52
4	53
5	74

Table 13.4. WFNS grade correlation to 1 month GOS score

WFNS Grade	Percentage of patients with poor outcome at 1 month after discharge (GOS 1–3)
1	20
2	53
3	70
4	85
5	93

Table 13.3. World Federation of Neurological Surgeons (WFNS) SAH Grading Scale

Grade	GCS score	Presence of aphasia, hemiparesis, or hemiplegia
0 – intact aneurysm	–	–
1	15	–
2	13–14	–
3	13–14	+
4	7–12	+/–
5	3–6	+/–

From Drake CG. Progress in cerebrovascular disease: management of cerebral aneurysm. Stroke 1981;**12**:273–83 and Teasdale GM, Drake CG, Hunt W, et al. A universal subarachnoid hemorrhage scale: report of a committee of the world federation of neurosurgical societies. *J Neurol Neurosurg Psychiatry*. 1988;**51**:1457.

Table 13.5. Fisher Grade correlation to 1 month GOS score

Fisher Grade	Percentage of patients with poor outcome at 1 month after discharge (GOS 1–3)
1	20
2	22
3	66
4	52

whereas 7 (86%) of 8 patients with ≥50 cm³ died within 30 days.

PATHOPHYSIOLOGY/ETIOLOGY

The exact pathophysiology of congenital (also known as berry or saccular) intracranial aneurysms is debatable. The consensus view holds that a congenital defect of the internal elastic lamina and tunica media of an intracranial vessel can become distended with time, and turbulent blood flow can cause a saccular outpouching at the area of defect. Pathologic specimens show an absence of internal elastic lamina and tunica media at the site of aneurysm formation.

Maximal wall stress and turbulent flow is greatest at a curve in the wall of the parent artery or at a bifurcation site of the parent artery. If a congenital defect of the internal elastic lamina is present, it is possible that an aneurysm will form, pointing in the direction of blood flow. Predisposing cerebral blood vessels to aneurysm formation is the fact that they lie in the subarachnoid space with no supportive connective tissue. As aneurysms enlarge, the risk of rupture increases according to LaPlace's law, which states that wall stress increases as the radius of a sphere increases.

From 15% to 33.5% of patients had multiple aneurysms (16% of patients had 2 aneurysms, 3–4% had 3 aneurysms, and 1–2% had 4 aneurysms) in the International Subarachnoid Aneurysm Trial (ISAT). To determine which aneurysm bled, consider the following:

1. Distribution of blood on CT
2. Area of vasospasm on angiography
3. Irregularities in the shape of the aneurysm
4. Larger aneurysms are more likely to rupture.

Common locations for saccular aneurysms:

- 85–95% in the carotid system/anterior circulation:
  ▶ Anterior communicating artery (ACoA) 30%
  ▶ Posterior communicating artery (P-Comm) 25%
  ▶ Middle cerebral artery (MCA) 20%
  ▶ Internal carotid artery (ICA) 15%
- 5–15% in the posterior circulation
  ▶ 10% basilar artery including basilar bifurcation, BA-SCA, BA-VA junction, AICA
  ▶ 5% vertebral artery – VA-PICA junction
  ▶ 1% PCA

Congenital aneurysms are the most common cause of spontaneous SAH; however, numerous other causes for aneurysms and SAH exist, including:

- Traumatic aneurysm – pseudoaneurysm at site of vessel wall injury
- Giant aneurysm – aneurysm >2.5 cm diameter
- Vein of Galen aneurysm/malformation – typically presents as heart failure in an infant in the first few weeks of life
- Mycotic aneurysm – infectious cause of aneurysm (usually bacterial) and commonly occur at distal MCA sites and the vertebrobasilar system.
- AVM – intranidal aneurysms or arterialized venous channels are usually the source of hemorrhage.
- Dural AV-fistula – risk of hemorrhage is highest when blood flow is retrograde to cortical vessels.
- Perimesencephalic/pretruncal nonaneurysmal SAH

From 75% to 85% of spontaneous SAHs are due to ruptured aneurysms; however, in 7–10% of cases, no aneurysm is found. These cases are classified as "angiogram negative SAH". This classification contains a very heterogeneous group of diseases and is discussed in detail at the end of the chapter. The most common among these is pretruncal nonaneurysmal SAH (PNSAH), which is responsible for 50–75% of all "angiogram negative SAH". The natural history of PNSAH is relatively benign compared to aSAH and its treatment is therefore less aggressive.

MANAGEMENT AND TREATMENT OF SAH AND ITS COMPLICATIONS

Rebleeding

Other than the initial hemorrhage, rebleeding is the highest cause of mortality in patients with an initial aSAH. According to the cross-sectional study by Broderick et al., 22% of aSAH mortalities occur as a result of rebleeding. An estimated 3000 deaths occur in North America per year due to rebleeding. In untreated ruptured cerebral aneurysms, the risk of rebleeding varies according to the time from initial hemorrhage:

- The risk is 4% in the first 24 hours and 1.5% per day for the following 13 days.
- The total risk of rebleeding is 15–20% in the first 14 days and 50% at 6 months.

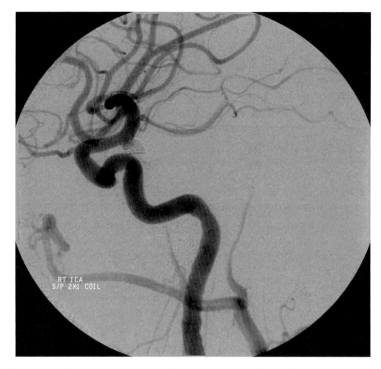

Figure 13.5. The same aneurysm as Figure 13.3, after coil embolization with GDCs.

■ In the long term, rebleeding occurs at 3% per year and its associated mortality is 2% per year.

Higher Hunt and Hess grade at admission is associated with increased risk of rebleeding. Evidence for and against increased risk of rebleeding exists for preoperative ventriculostomy or lumbar drain placement.

Treatment for prevention of rebleeding is aneurysm obliteration. Options for treatment include open aneurysm clipping and, more recently available, endovascular coil embolization procedures (Fig. 13.5) with Guglielmi detachable coils (GDCs). There is considerable ongoing debate regarding which treatment modality yields better results for short-term complications, long-term outcome, and durability of aneurysm obliteration.

The randomized, controlled, multicenter ISAT has provided evidence that coil embolization yields improved survival and functional status at 1 year after treatment in patients with ruptured cerebral aneurysms.

■ 23.5% of patients treated by endovascular means versus 30.9% of patients treated with open surgery were either dead or functionally dependent (as defined by a score of 3–6 on the modified Rankin scale) at 1 year after treatment with a relative risk reduction of 23.9% for the endovascular group.

■ Patients with poor neurologic grade (WFNS 4 and 5) as well as patients with posterior circulation and MCA aneurysms were underrepresented in this study; therefore, the benefit of endovascular treatment is not known for these patients.

The durability of endovascular procedures is not as well studied as that of surgical clipping owing to its recent emergence; however, at 7-year follow-up, there is no statistical difference in rebleeding rate in the endovascular group compared to the surgical group. Continued evaluation of the two treatment modalities is needed but it is certain that each case should be evaluated on an individual basis. Each aneurysm should be evaluated by a neurosurgeon and neurointerventional specialist to determine the proper course of treatment with consideration of the clinical circumstances relative to the patient.

Hydrocephalus

Hydrocephalus after aSAH may be separated into communicating and obstructive hydrocephalus. Communicating hydrocephalus occurs when blood in the subarachnoid space interferes with reabsorption at the arachnoid granulations and pial surface. CSF production exceeds CSF reabsorption and increased ventricular volume results.

Obstructive hydrocephalus occurs when the Sylvian aqueduct or the fourth ventricle at the foramina of Luschka and/or Magendie is occluded by blood products. CSF is not drained from the ventricles into the subarachnoid space and CSF production exceeds ventricular outflow. Posterior circulation aneurysms are more likely to occlude the fourth ventricle; therefore, obstructive hydrocephalus is more common in these patients.

■ Clinical deterioration with enlarging ventricles by CT scan can be classified as hydrocephalus only when other causes are ruled out, such as vasospasm, infarction, hyponatremia, sepsis, hypoxia, cerebral edema, and seizure.
■ Of the 20% of patients with aSAH who develop enlarged ventricles by CT, only 30–60% of those patients demonstrate neurologic deterioration.
■ In addition, 50% of patients with altered level of consciousness due to hydrocephalus will improve spontaneously. Therefore, if neurologic condition permits, external ventricular drain (EVD) placement may be avoided.

Concern that ventriculostomy or lumbar drainage increases the risk of rebleeding exists because CSF drainage theoretically increases transmural pressure on the aneurysm wall. Some authors state that ICP should be maintained from 20 to 25 cm if CSF drainage is performed. However, other studies show there is no increased rate of rebleeding with preoperative ventriculostomy placement.

Chronic hydrocephalus may occur after aSAH. Increased likelihood of chronic hydrocephalus occurs when there is presence of intraventricular blood during the initial SAH. A preliminary study has shown that intraventricular hemorrhage can be safely reduced in volume after intraventricular tissue plasminogen activator (tPA) administration. Currently there are no data to show that intraventricular tPA reduces the incidence of chronic hydrocephalus.

Vasospasm

Vasospasm is a major cause of morbidity and mortality in patients who survive the initial hemorrhage. Of all patients with spontaneous SAH, 6% die and another 7% have major neurologic deficits as a result of vasospasm. Delayed ischemic neurologic deficit (DIND) occurs when vasospasm is severe enough to cause significant reductions of cerebral blood flow (CBF) to a focal area of the brain. Clinically, the patient develops a neurologic deficit that matches the vascular distribution of vasospasm. If severe, the areas of reduced CBF may cause infarction of brain tissue, causing permanent deficit.

The amount and distribution of blood on the initial CT scan predicts which patients will develop clinically apparent neurologic deficits and a scale was first described by Fisher in 1980 (Table 13.6). Fisher Grades 1, 2, and 4 have a very low incidence of clinically apparent vasospasm (0 of 18 cases) whereas Fisher Grade 3 frequently (23 of 24 cases) heralds severe, symptomatic vasospasm.

In a study by Howington, cocaine use within 24 hours of presentation with aSAH raised the risk of vasospasm significantly, from 27.8% (20/72) in nonusers to 77.8% (28/36) in cocaine users. The vasoactive properties of cocaine likely influence the propensity for developing clinically relevant vasospasm. Poor GOS score (1–3) was seen in 91.7% (33/36) of cocaine users versus 27.8% (20/72) in the noncocaine user group.

The Hijdra scale grades the amount of cisternal blood and intraventricular blood separately and has an improved correlation with delayed cerebral ischemia (DCI) and outcome (GOS at 3 months) over the Fisher grading system. Total score is calculated by evaluating 10 cisterns and fissures (frontal interhemispheric, bilateral lateral sylvian fissures, bilateral basal sylvian fissures, bilateral ambient cisterns, quadrigeminal cistern, right and left halves of the suprasellar cistern) for the presence or absence of blood (Fig. 13.6). Also, each ventricle is graded for blood. Total Hijdra score has been correlated to DCI and GOS (Table 13.7).

Vasospasm generally occurs on days 4–20 after initial hemorrhage and virtually never occurs before day 3. To diagnose vasospasm, one must first rule out other potential causes of neurologic deterioration in the patient with aSAH, which include hydrocephalus, cerebral edema, seizure,

Table 13.6. Fisher's original series of patients and the frequency of occurrence of vasospasm in relation to Fisher Grade

Grade	Subarachnoid blood distribution	Number of cases	No angiographic vasospasm	Slight-moderate angiographic vasospasm	Severe angiographic vasospasm	Clinical sign of vasospasm (DIND)
1	None	11	7	2	2	0
2	Thin distribution with vertical layers <1mm	7	4	3	0	0
3	Thick – localized clots or vertical layers >1mm thick	24	0	1	23	23
4	Diffuse or no SAH, but with Intracerebral or intraventricular hemorrhage	5	3	2	0	0

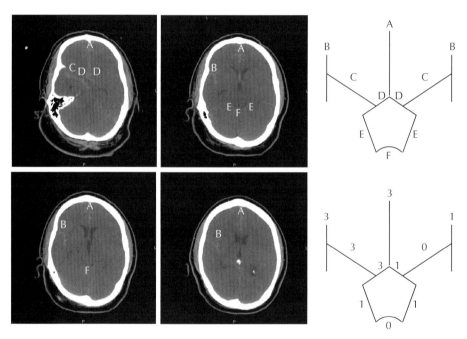

Figure 13.6. Hijdra Grade is calculated by evaluating a total of 10 cisterns and fissures for the presence of blood (0 = no blood; 1 = small amount of blood; 2 = moderately filled with blood; 3 = completely filled with blood; total score 0–30.) **(A)** Frontal interhemispheric; **(B)** bilateral lateral sylvian fissures; **(C)** bilateral basal sylvian fissures; **(D)** right and left halves of the suprasellar cistern; **(E)** bilateral ambient cisterns; **(F)** quadrigeminal cistern. Separately, each ventricle is graded for blood. 0 = no blood; 1 = small sediment in posterior part of ventricle; 2 = partially filled with blood; 3 = totally filled with blood; total score 0–12. The total score for the CT scan shown in the figure is: anterior interhemispheric fissure (3) + right lateral sylvian fissure (3) + right basal sylvian fissure (3) + left lateral sylvian fissure (1) + left basal sylvian fissure (0) + right suprasellar cistern (3) + left suprasellar cistern (1) + right ambient cistern (1) + left ambient cistern (1) + quadrigeminal cistern (0) + left occipital horn sediment (1) = 17.

Table 13.7. Correlation of total Hijdra scale score to DCI and 3-month GOS score (24)

Total Hijdra score	Percentage with DCI	Percentage poor GOS (1–3) at 3 months
0–14	8	10
15–28	24	28
29–42	30	56

From Hijdra A, Brouwers PJ, Vermeulen M, van Gijn J. Grading the amount of blood on computed tomograms after subarachnoid hemorrhage. *Stroke*. 1990; **21**:1156–61.

Table 13.8. Lindegaard ratio

Mean MCA velocity (cm/s)	MCA:ICA ratio	Interpretation
<120	<3	Normal
120–200	3–6	Mild vasospasm
>200	>6	Severe vasospasm

hyponatremia, hypoxia, and sepsis. Vasospasm can be demonstrated radiographically with transcranial Doppler, cerebral angiography, or CT angiography. Transcranial Doppler velocities must be considered in the context of the Lindegaard ratio, which compares the blood flow velocities of the MCA to those in the ICA (Table 13.8).

VASOSPASM TREATMENT

Clinically apparent vasospasm typically results in a neurologic deficit that correlates to a specific vascular distribution. Therapies that elevate the systolic blood pressure (SBP) may reduce these symptoms by increasing CBF in the vascular distribution of vasospasm either via collateral circulation or via the narrowed vessels that are constricted. Because rebleeding may be caused by elevated SBPs, aggressive blood pressure elevation should be induced only after the ruptured aneurysm has been secured. At that time, vasospasm can be treated with hyperdynamic or "triple H" therapy, which includes hypertension, hypervolemia, and hemodilution

Table 13.9. Parameters for "triple H" therapy

"Triple H" treatment parameters
SBP 200
Hematocrit .30–35
CVP 10–12
PCWP 14–16
Arterial line
P-A catheter
Stool softeners

(Table 13.9). Before securing the aneurysm, normotension should be maintained (SBP 100–140).

There is currently a lack of Class I evidence, however, to support the use of hypervolemic therapy and hemodilution. Hemodilution fails to consistently show prevention of cerebral infarction.

- Numerous potential complications occur as a result of hyperdynamic therapy including pulmonary edema, myocardial ischemia, hyponatremia, renal failure, indwelling catheter-related complications, cerebral hemorrhage, and cerebral edema.
- Patients should be managed on an individual basis by monitoring central venous pressure (CVP), mean arterial pressure (MAP), pulmonary-capillary wedge pressure (PCWP), and renal function, thereby ensuring adequate perfusion of all end-organs.
- SBP elevation may be induced while monitoring the patient vigilantly for complications of treatment.
- In cases in which vasospasm is the cause of neurologic deterioration, a proper response may be to aggressively increase the blood volume and SBP.

Administration of a hypertonic saline bolus (2 mL/kg of 23.4% saline) has been shown to improve CBF, CPP, and to decrease ICP significantly at 90 and 180 minutes after administration. This may play a role in improving outcomes in patients with aSAH who experience decreases in regional cerebral blood flow (rCBF) due to vasospasm. This treatment is limited by hyperchloremia, hyperosmolality, and hypernatremia.

The use of selective calcium channel blockers, such as nimodipine, is a treatment option for patients at risk for symptomatic vasospasm. It is thought that the action of selective calcium channel blockers decreases the incidence of DIND by preventing cerebral arterial smooth muscle contraction. Nimodipine has been shown, by meta-analysis, to improve outcomes by measure of GOS; however, its use has failed to show any significant difference with respect to overall mortality in patients treated with the drug. Most studies included in the meta-analysis treated patients for 21 days of total nimodipine therapy; therefore, this is the recommended time for nimodipine treatment. The dosage and frequency of nimodipine are often limited by its tendency to reduce blood pressure and the drug should be held until SBP goals are met.

Sympatholytics such as metoprolol or clonidine are theoretically advantageous by blocking the vasospasmogenic adrenergic response of the intracranial vasculature. No Class I evidence exists to support the use of these drugs.

When hyperdynamic therapies and pharmacologic therapies fail to reverse neurologic deficit attributable to vasospasm, endovascular and surgical treatments are then considered.

- There is some evidence that early angioplasty achieves substantial clinical improvement. Rosenwasser reports that there is a 70% sustained clinical improvement if intra-arterial balloon angioplasty is performed within 2 hours of symptom onset; and 40% sustained clinical improvement when performed 2 hours after symptom onset (53).
- Intra-arterial papaverine injections, which relaxes cerebral vasculature smooth muscle directly when injected, has variable reported benefits. Clinical improvement ranges from 33% to 80%, and is more likely to derive transient improvement of vasospasm versus balloon angioplasty, often requiring multiple treatments.
- Investigational intra-arterial pharmacologic therapies exist. Intra-arterial verapamil and intra-arterial nicardipine both have longer-lasting clinical improvement when compared to papaverine.

Some surgical or invasive interventions are aimed at removing blood products after aSAH. Direct contact with intracerebral vessels is likely a major contributor to vasospasm development; thus removal of blood products may be beneficial. Treatment options include:

- CSF drainage to remove intraventricular blood products
- Lumbar drainage to enhance blood product removal by increasing CSF circulation

- Irrigation of basilar cisterns at time of aneurysm clipping to remove blood products
- Fenestration of the lamina terminalis (theoretically enhances CSF circulation to remove blood products from the intraventricular space)

Hyponatremia

Hyponatremia occurs frequently in the setting of SAH, likely secondary to elevated brain natriuretic peptide (BNP) and atrial natriuretic peptide (ANP). These peptides cause cerebral salt wasting (CSW), which is characterized by hyponatremia in the setting of hypovolemia. Urine osmolality can be normal or inappropriately high and urine sodium is invariably high. Serum electrolytes may be identical to patients with the syndrome of inappropriate antidiuretic hormone (SIADH).

- In CSW patients, treatment should include fluid and sodium replacement, which is contrary to treatment of patients with SIADH.
- Volume status must be assessed clinically, by PCWP, or by CVP before instituting treatment.
- Specific treatments include normal saline or 2–3% saline fluid replacement and (optional) oral or nasogastric (NG) salt tablet administration.
- If the hyponatremia is acute and symptomatic (seizure or altered level of consciousness), it should be treated promptly without consideration of the rapidity of serum sodium correction.
- In patients with hyponatremia of chronic or unknown duration, correction should be slow because of the possibility of central pontine myelinolysis (CPM). An initial correction of 10%, followed by correction of 10 mEq/L every 24 hours is recommended.

SIADH is a potential cause of hyponatremia in the setting of aSAH. ADH elevation in aSAH is transient; therefore, CSW is more likely in this patient population. Typically in SIADH, patients will be euvolemic or hypervolemic. The urine osmolality will be high despite serum hyponatremia and low serum osmolality. Treatment of SIADH in the setting of aSAH is not straightforward.

- In patients without aSAH, vasospasm is not a concern and total fluid may be restricted to <1 L per day.

In patients with aSAH intravascular volume must be sufficient to maintain cerebral perfusion. Therefore, sodium replacement by IV, PO, or NG is preferred over fluid restriction.

The presence of hyponatremia is a poor prognostic indicator for patient outcome and incidence of vasospasm. Patients with hyponatremia have three times the incidence of DCI after SAH than normonatremic patients.

Seizure

Although once reported to be as high as 20–30%, more recent data suggests the risk of seizure after aSAH is lower, at approximately 4.5–8%. Likely secondary to these initial figures, two thirds of all aSAH patients throughout the world between 1991 and 1997 received antiepileptic drug (AED) treatment. AED treatment may not be necessary in most of these patients.

Seizures have been studied in relation to timing of aneurysm surgery. In patients undergoing aneurysm clipping, 1.5% of seizures occur in the immediate postoperative period (first 14 days) whereas 3.0% occur in long-term follow-up (11 months – 5 years, average 2.4 years). This argues against prophylactic use of AEDs in the acute setting for patients with aSAH. In addition, Baker et al. (1995) showed that there is likely no benefit in preventing the development of long-term epilepsy by starting AEDs before seizures begin. Moreover, after adjustment for study center, WFNS grade, age, and SBP, use of AEDs are associated with a poorer GOS score at 3 months (OR = 1.56), and higher rates of symptomatic vasospasm (OR 1.87), cerebral infarction (1.33), and T >38°C on day 8 (1.36). Therefore, the use of AEDs in patients with aSAH is still in question, and likely should not be used in every patient who presents with aSAH.

- While AEDs may prevent an initial seizure, incidence in the first 14 days is quite low.
- In addition, early AED use is unlikely to prevent the development of epilepsy.
- More studies are necessary, but if AEDs are chosen, they should be used for the short-term only.

Deep Venous Thrombosis

Sequential compression devices (SCDs) should be used routinely in patients before definitive aneurysm treatment, unless a contraindication exists such as preexisting deep venous thrombosis (DVT). After aneurysm treatment, either subcutaneous heparin (5000 U SQ tid) or low molecular weight heparin (Lovenox 40 mg SQ daily) is more effective at preventing DVT than SCDs alone.

Outcome

In 1988, the World Federation of Neurological Surgeons Committee on a Universal Subarachnoid Hemorrhage Grading Scale adopted the WFNS neurologic grading scale as shown above in Table 13.3. The same committee adopted the Glasgow Outcome Scale to be used for classification of outcome in patients with SAH (Table 13.10). (Note: In some clinical studies, the numerical order is reversed.)

Outcome is fairly poor for aSAH as a whole. Sixty-six percent of patients who undergo successful aneurysm clipping do not return to the same quality of life as before SAH. 20% of survivors have moderate to severe disability, and the overall mortality of aSAH is 45–50%.

Rosengart has recently reported independent variables that are prognostic for poorer Glasgow outcome scale (GOS 1–3) score 3 months after aSAH (odds ratio in a multivariate logistic regression analysis shown in parentheses):

- Increasing age (1.5)
- Poorer WFNS grade on admission (1.74)
- Ruptured posterior circulation aneurysm (1.09)
- Anticonvulsant use (1.37)

Table 13.10. Glasgow Outcome scale designed for use in patients who suffer SAH

GOS Grade	Neurologic status
1	Dead
2	Vegetative
3	Severely disabled; conscious but totally dependent on others
4	Moderately disabled; patient has neurologic impairment but is independent
5	Good recovery; resumption of normal activities

- Elevated body temperature: >38°C on hospital day 8 (1.81)
- Previous history of hypertension (1.41), myocardial infarction (1.58), or previous SAH (1.51)
- Symptomatic vasospasm (1.75)
- Cerebral infarction (5.38)

Lagares showed that initial loss of consciousness at the time of hemorrhage imparted a relative risk of 4 for having a poor GOS score (1–3) at 1 month (34).

Angiogram-Negative Subarachnoid Hemorrhage

Angiogram-negative SAH defines a subset of diseases that present with SAH without a congenital aneurysm as the cause. Some of the causes are reviewed in the following subsections.

TRAUMA

Blood is confined to the ambient cistern, usually unilateral and located at the tentorial margin. There is a history of trauma with a negative angiogram. Hemorrhage is typically due to grazing of a vein against the tentorial edge. Angiography is seldom done in the circumstance of traumatic SAH. However, if it is unclear whether the traumatic event occurred prior to the loss of consciousness, a CTA should be performed to rule out aneurysmal SAH, which may have circumstantially caused the traumatic brain injury.

If the subarachnoid hemorrhage pattern appears similar in distribution to that of an aneurysm (such as blood contained in the chiasmatic, anterior interhemispheric, or sylvian cisterns), then a CTA should be performed to ensure than an aneurysm does not go undiagnosed in the setting of trauma.

VERTEBRAL ARTERY DISSECTION

Hypertension coexists in one third of patients diagnosed with vertebral artery dissection. Dissection should be suspected in patients with recent history of neck trauma or unusual neck movements (such as chiropractic manipulation).

- Lower cranial nerve palsies, Horner's syndrome, or lateral medullary syndrome can occur.
- Diagnosis requires identification of luminal narrowing (string sign), intimal flap, or double lumen.
- Rebleeding occurs in 30% of patients and is fatal in half of these.

INSUFFICIENT ANGIOGRAPHIC EXAMINATION

Ruptured posterior circulation aneurysms show hemorrhage in the fourth ventricle in up to 85% of cases and to a lesser extent the third ventricle. Occasionally, the only finding in a patient with a ruptured posterior circulation aneurysm is intraventricular blood. Imaging of the posterior circulation is technically difficult despite four-vessel angiography; adequate visualization of both vertebral arteries, including bilateral posterior–inferior cerebellar arteries (PICA), is crucial.

When anterior communicating artery (ACommA) aneurysms are very small (<3 mm) they may be difficult to identify by CTA or conventional angiography. In a series of 130 patients, one 2-mm ACommA aneurysm was not seen on initial review of CTA, but was seen on initial angiography. Three-dimensional reconstruction aided in post hoc recognition of the aneurysm on CTA. Di Lorenzo reported two cases of spontaneous SAH with negative angiography for aneurysm. Both patients were found to have ACommA aneurysms at operation. Three-dimensional digital-subtraction angiography may have helped to improve recognition of the aneurysm in these cases.

OCCULT ANEURYSM

Occult aneurysms may occur because of vasospasm, thrombosis of the aneurysm, or a poor-quality study and should be suspected in patients with extensive extravasation of blood into the anterior interhemispheric fissure, the lateral sylvian fissure, or the ventricles. Repeat angiography is diagnostic in 16% of cases.

DURAL AVM

Tentorial-based dural AVMs may hemorrhage into the basal cisterns, mimicking aSAH. Angiography of the external carotid arteries is critical as feeding vessels may arise exclusively from this artery.

SPINAL AVM

10% of spinal AVMs present with SAH. High cervical AVMs may mimic an intracranial source of SAH with hemorrhage into the basal cisterns and ventricles. History of severe arm, shoulder, or lower neck pain is suggestive of the diagnosis. MRI may be used for screening if this etiology is suspected.

MYCOTIC ANEURYSM

Endocarditis may cause aneurysms of the distal MCA. However, 10% are located on the proximal MCA. Hemorrhage of the proximally located aneurysms may appear similar to a ruptured saccular aneurysm. Mycotic aneurysms of the MCA are typically treated with long courses of IV antibiotics, and may be clipped or treated by endovascular means on a delayed basis.

Mycotic aneurysms caused by aspergillosis are usually located on the proximal vertebrobasilar or internal carotid artery. The rupture of these aneurysms causes hemorrhage into the basilar cisterns and is frequently fatal.

PITUITARY APOPLEXY

Patients present with headache, nausea, vomiting, meningismus, and decreased visual acuity or diplopia. Endocrine derangements may occur, corticosteroid deficiency being the most life-threatening. CT demonstrates hemorrhage in the pituitary fossa. A pituitary adenoma is also usually demonstrable via MRI.

PERIMESENCEPHALIC SAH/PRETRUNCAL NONANEURYSMAL SAH

This entity is termed pretruncal nonaneurysmal subarachnoid hemorrhage (PNSAH) because the anatomic localization of blood is centered at the prepontine cistern, anterior to the brainstem (truncus cerebri). Hemorrhage is restricted to the perimesencephalic cisterns which include the interpeduncular, crural, ambient, and quadrigeminal cisterns, and should not extend significantly into the lateral sylvian fissures or the anterior interhemispheric fissure. An estimated 50–75% of aneurysm-negative SAH cases are attributed to PNSAH. The etiology is unknown, but may involve rupture of a small perimesencephalic vein or capillary. PNSAH has a good prognosis, with no incidence of rebleeding in 37 patients followed for a mean of 45 months. Another study showed no rebleeding in 169 patients with 8–51-month follow-up. Vasospasm occurred in 1–5% of patients, and is attributed to cerebral angiography in the vast majority of these patients.

DIAGNOSIS

- Compared to aSAH, patients tend to be predominantly male, less hypertensive, and younger.
- Angiography is negative.
- There should be no occurrence of sentinel headache or loss of consciousness.
- Photophobia, severe headache, and meningismus may be present.
- Strenuous activity precedes the event in 33% of cases.
- Headache onset is more gradual than aSAH (minutes rather than seconds)
- Subarachnoid blood should be localized to the prepontine, interpeduncular, and carotid cisterns. Blood in the chiasmatic, interhemispheric, or sylvian cisterns is not compatible with pretruncal nonaneurysmal subarachnoid hemorrhage. There should be no significant intraventricular hemorrhage.
- There are no focal neurologic deficits.
- 20% of patients will have acute ventriculomegaly on initial CT scan, but will most likely not manifest symptoms.
- Rebleeding does not occur.

TREATMENT

- Because of the low risk of rebleeding or cerebral infarction, aggressive hyperdynamic treatment is not indicated.
- Treatment should follow clinical symptoms.
- Institute cardiac monitoring.
- Monitor electrolytes closely.
- Patients should be advised to use a stool softener.
- Calcium channel blockers and anticonvulsants are not indicated.
- Antihypertensives are not indicated.
- Do not force bedrest or restrict activity.
- Repeat angiography is not necessary if the patient fits all of the diagnostic criteria for PNSAH.
- Patients may return to their normal daily activities.
- Patients should be informed of the benign nature of their disease.

Future Directions

VASOSPASM

Vasospasm contributes significantly to morbidity and mortality in aSAH; therefore, it is the focus of ongoing research directed toward novel therapies. Numerous parenteral investigatory treatments exist:

- Nitric oxide
- Endothelin antagonists

- Inflammatory antagonists
- Serine protease inhibitors
- Statins
- Antioxidants
- IV magnesium

Cervical sympathetic block with locoregional anesthesia at the superior cervical ganglion has been shown in small clinical trials to be efficacious at improving rCBF in the territory of vasospasm.

HYDROCEPHALUS

Intraventricular tPA administration after aSAH with intraventricular hemorrhage (IVH) reduces the incidence of shunt dependence, decreases hospital length of stay, and improves Glasgow outcome scale scores. Intraventricular tPA seems to be safe in patients with secured aneurysms and is effective at reducing the amount of intraventricular blood clot.

ENDOVASCULAR TREATMENT

Endovascular treatment of aneurysms continues to advance with newer technologies and resultant ability to coil aneurysms previously untreatable. Initially, endovascular techniques allowed coil embolization of aneurysms with a dome-to-neck ratio of 2 or greater. However, with balloon-assisted and now stent-assisted coil embolization, aneurysms with wide necks may be treated with endovascular techniques. Incidence of thromboembolic events is increased to roughly 10% with both balloon-assisted and stent-assisted techniques.

- Hydrocoil – platinum coil coated with a polymer that swells 3- to 9-fold on contact with blood to improve coil packing density
- Matrix coil (polyglycolic acid/lactide) – accelerated aneurysm fibrosis and neointimal formation without parent artery stenosis
- Neuroform stent – Nitinol stent with limited radial force on deployment.
- Growth-factor eluting stents: vascular endothelial growth factor, transforming growth factor β, fibroblast growth factor
- Gene therapy delivery via stent

REFERENCES

Allen GS, Ahn HS, Preziosi TJ, et al. Cerebral arterial spasm—a controlled trial of nimodipine in patients with subarachnoid hemorrhage. *N Engl J Med.* 1983;**308**:619–24.

Apperloo JJ, van der Graaf F, Dellemijn PL, Vader HL. An improved laboratory protocol to assess subarachnoid haemorrhage in patients with negative cranial CT scan. *Clin Chem Lab Med.* 2006;**44**:938–48.

Atlas SW. MR angiography in neurologic disease. *Radiology.* 1994;**193**:1–16.

Auer LM, Mokry M. Disturbed cerebrospinal fluid circulation after subarachnoid hemorrhage and acute aneurysm surgery. *Neurosurgery.* 1990;**26**:804–8; discussion 808–9.

Baker CJ, Prestigiacomo CJ, Solomon RA. Short-term perioperative anticonvulsant prophylaxis for the surgical treatment of low-risk patients with intracranial aneurysms. *Neurosurgery.* 1995;**37**:863–70; discussion 870–1.

Barker FG 2nd, Ogilvy CS. Efficacy of prophylactic nimodipine for delayed ischemic deficit after subarachnoid hemorrhage: a metaanalysis. *J Neurosurg.* 1996;**84**:405–14.

Bidzinski J, Marchel A, Sherif A. Risk of epilepsy after aneurysm operations. *Acta Neurochir (Wien).* 1992;**119**:49–52.

Biller J, Toffol GJ, Kassell NF, Adams HP Jr, Beck DW, Boarini DJ. Spontaneous subarachnoid hemorrhage in young adults. *Neurosurgery.* 1987;**21**:664–7.

Bonita R. Cigarette smoking, hypertension and the risk of subarachnoid hemorrhage: a population-based case-control study. *Stroke.* 1986;**17**:831–5.

Broderick JP, Brott TG, Duldner JE, Tomsick T, Leach A. Initial and recurrent bleeding are the major causes of death following subarachnoid hemorrhage. *Stroke.* 1994;**25**:1342–7.

Broderick JP, Brott T, Tomsick T, Miller R, Huster G. Intracerebral hemorrhage more than twice as common as subarachnoid hemorrhage. *J Neurosurg.* 1993;**78**:188–91.

Di Lorenzo N, Guidetti G. Anterior communicating aneurysm missed at angiography: report of two cases treated surgically. *Neurosurgery.* 1988;**23**:494–9.

Doberstein CE, Hovda DA, Becker DP. Clinical considerations in the reduction of secondary brain injury. *Ann Emerg Med.* 1993;**22**:993–7.

Dorsch NW, Young N, Kingston RJ, Compton JS. Early experience with spiral CT in the diagnosis of intracranial aneurysms. *Neurosurgery.* 1995;**36**:230–6; discussion 236–8.

Drake CG. Progress in cerebrovascular disease: management of cerebral aneurysm. *Stroke.* 1981;**12**:273–83.

Eisenberg HM, Gary HE Jr, Aldrich EF, et al. Initial CT findings in 753 patients with severe head injury. A report from the NIH traumatic coma data bank. *J Neurosurg.* 1990;**73**:688–98.

Ekelund A, Reinstrup P, Ryding E, et al. Effects of iso- and hypervolemic hemodilution on regional cerebral blood flow and oxygen delivery for patients with vasospasm after aneurysmal subarachnoid hemorrhage. *Acta Neurochir (Wien).* 2002;**144**:703–12; discussion 712–3.

El Khaldi M, Pernter P, Ferro F, et al. Detection of cerebral aneurysms in nontraumatic subarachnoid haemorrhage: role of multislice CT angiography in 130 consecutive patients. *Radiol Med (Torino).* 2007;**112**:123–37.

Fang H. A comparison of blood vessels of the brain and peripheral blood vessels. In Wright IS, Millikan CH (eds), *Cerebral Vascular Diseases*. New York: Grune & Stratton, 1958, pp 17–22.

Fisher CM, Kistler JP, Davis JM. Relation of cerebral vasospasm to subarachnoid hemorrhage visualized by computerized tomographic scanning. *Neurosurgery*. 1980;**6**:1–9.

Greene KA, Marciano FF, Johnson BA, Jacobowitz R, Spetzler RF, Harrington TR. Impact of traumatic subarachnoid hemorrhage on outcome in nonpenetrating head injury. part I: A proposed computerized tomography grading scale. *J Neurosurg*. 1995;**83**:445–52.

Harrigan MR. Cerebral salt wasting syndrome: a review. *Neurosurgery*. 1996;**38**:152–60.

Hasan D, Vermeulen M, Wijdicks EF, Hijdra A, van Gijn J. Management problems in acute hydrocephalus after subarachnoid hemorrhage. *Stroke*. 1989;**20**:747–53.

Hijdra A, Brouwers PJ, Vermeulen M, van Gijn J. Grading the amount of blood on computed tomograms after subarachnoid hemorrhage. *Stroke*. 1990;**21**:1156–61.

Hop JW, Rinkel GJ, Algra A, van Gijn J. Case-fatality rates and functional outcome after subarachnoid hemorrhage: a systematic review. *Stroke*. 1997;**28**:660–4.

Howington JU, Kutz SC, Wilding GE, Awasthi D: Cocaine use as a predictor of outcome in aneurysmal subarachnoid hemorrhage. *J Neurosurg*. 2003;**99**:271–5.

Hsiang JN, Liang EY, Lam JM, Zhu XL, Poon WS. The role of computed tomographic angiography in the diagnosis of intracranial aneurysms and emergent aneurysm clipping. *Neurosurgery*. 1996;**38**:481–7; discussion 487.

Hunt WE, Hess RM. Surgical risk as related to time of intervention in the repair of intracranial aneurysms. *J Neurosurg*. 1968;**28**:14–20.

Kassell NF, Drake CG. Review of the management of saccular aneurysms. *Neurol Clin*. 1983;**1**:73–86.

Koebbe CJ, Veznedaroglu E, Jabbour P, Rosenwasser RH. Endovascular management of intracranial aneurysms: current experience and future advances. *Neurosurgery*. 2006;**59**:S93–102; discussion S3–13.

Komotar RJ, Zacharia BE, Valhora R, Mocco J, Connolly ES Jr. Advances in vasospasm treatment and prevention. *J Neurol Sci*. 2007, Oct 15; **261**(1–2):134–42.

Kroll M, Juhler M, Lindholm J. Hyponatraemia in acute brain disease. *J Intern Med*. 1992;**232**:291–7.

Kusske JA, Turner PT, Ojemann GA, Harris AB. Ventriculostomy for the treatment of acute hydrocephalus following subarachnoid hemorrhage. *J Neurosurg*. 1973; **38**:591–5.

Lagares A, Gomez PA, Lobato RD, Alen JF, Alday R, Campollo J. Prognostic factors on hospital admission after spontaneous subarachnoid haemorrhage. *Acta Neurochir (Wien)*. 2001;**143**:665–72.

Leon-Carrion J, Dominguez-Morales Mdel R, Barroso y Martin JM, Murillo-Cabezas F. Epidemiology of traumatic brain injury and subarachnoid hemorrhage. *Pituitary*. 2005;**8**:197–202.

Linn FH, Wijdicks EF, van der Graaf Y, Weerdesteyn-van Vliet FA, Bartelds AI, van Gijn J. Prospective study of sentinel headache in aneurysmal subarachnoid haemorrhage. *Lancet*. 1994;**344**:590–3.

Lynch JR, Wang H, McGirt MJ, et al. Simvastatin reduces vasospasm after aneurysmal subarachnoid hemorrhage: results of a pilot randomized clinical trial. *Stroke*. 2005;**36**:2024–6.

McGirt MJ, Lynch JR, Parra A, et al. Simvastatin increases endothelial nitric oxide synthase and ameliorates cerebral vasospasm resulting from subarachnoid hemorrhage. *Stroke*. 2002;**33**:2950–6.

McIver JI, Friedman JA, Wijdicks EF, et al. Preoperative ventriculostomy and rebleeding after aneurysmal subarachnoid hemorrhage. *J Neurosurg*. 2002;**97**:1042–4.

Milhorat TH. Acute hydrocephalus after aneurysmal subarachnoid hemorrhage. *Neurosurgery*. 1987;**20**:15–20.

Molyneux A, Kerr R, Stratton I, et al. International subarachnoid aneurysm trial (ISAT) of neurosurgical clipping versus endovascular coiling in 2143 patients with ruptured intracranial aneurysms: a randomised trial. *Lancet*. 2002;**360**:1267–74.

Molyneux AJ, Kerr RS, Yu LM, et al. International subarachnoid aneurysm trial (ISAT) of neurosurgical clipping versus endovascular coiling in 2143 patients with ruptured intracranial aneurysms: a randomised comparison of effects on survival, dependency, seizures, rebleeding, subgroups, and aneurysm occlusion. *Lancet*. 2005;**366**:809–17.

Okawara SH. Warning signs prior to rupture of an intracranial aneurysm. *J Neurosurg*. 1973;**38**:575–80.

Osborn AG. Intracranial aneurysms. In *Handbook of Neuroradiology*, St. Louis Mosby-Yearbook, 1991, pp 79–84.

Petzold A, Keir G, Sharpe LT. Spectrophotometry for xanthochromia. *N Engl J Med*. 2004;**351**:1695–6.

Rhoton AL. Anatomy of saccular aneurysms. *Surg Neurol*. 1981;**14**: 59–66.

Rinkel GJ, Feigin VL, Algra A, van Gijn J. Circulatory volume expansion therapy for aneurysmal subarachnoid haemorrhage. *Cochrane Database Syst Rev*. 2004;(4): CD000483.

Rinkel GJ, van Gijn J, Wijdicks EF. Subarachnoid hemorrhage without detectable aneurysm. A review of the causes. *Stroke*. 1993;**24**:1403–9.

Rinkel GJ, Wijdicks EF, Vermeulen M, Hageman LM, Tans JT, van Gijn J. Outcome in perimesencephalic (nonaneurysmal) subarachnoid hemorrhage: a follow-up study in 37 patients. *Neurology* 1990;**40**:1130–2.

Ronkainen A, Hernesniemi J, Puranen M, et al. Familial intracranial aneurysms. *Lancet* 1997;**349**:380–4.

Rosengart AJ, Huo JD, Tolentino J, et al. Outcome in patients with subarachnoid hemorrhage treated with antiepileptic drugs. *J Neurosurg.*.2007;**107**:253–60.

Rosengart AJ, Schultheiss KE, Tolentino J, Macdonald RL. Prognostic factors for outcome in patients with aneurysmal subarachnoid hemorrhage. *Stroke*. 2007;**38**:2315–21.

Rosenwasser RH, Armonda RA, Thomas JE, Benitez RP, Gannon PM, Harrop J. Therapeutic modalities for the management of cerebral vasospasm: timing of endovascular options. *Neurosurgery*. 1999;**44**:975–9; discussion 979–80.

Ross JS, Masaryk TJ, Modic MT, Ruggieri PM, Haacke EM, Selman WR. Intracranial aneurysms: Evaluation by MR angiography. *AJR Am J Roentgenol*. 1990;**155**: 159–65.

Schievink WI, Wijdicks EF. Pretruncal subarachnoid hemorrhage: an anatomically correct description of the perimesencephalic subarachnoid hemorrhage. *Stroke*. 1997;**28**:2572.

Schwartz TH, Solomon RA. Perimesencephalic nonaneurysmal subarachnoid hemorrhage: review of the literature. *Neurosurgery*. 1996;**39**:433–40; discussion 440.

Taneda M, Kataoka K, Akai F, Asai T, Sakata I. Traumatic subarachnoid hemorrhage as a predictable indicator of delayed ischemic symptoms. *J Neurosurg*. 1956;**84**:762–8.

Teasdale GM, Drake CG, Hunt W, et al. A universal subarachnoid hemorrhage scale: report of a committee of the world federation of neurosurgical societies. *J Neurol Neurosurg Psychiatry*. 1988;**51**:1457.

Treggiari MM, Romand JA, Martin JB, Reverdin A, Rufenacht DA, de Tribolet N. Cervical sympathetic block to reverse delayed ischemic neurological deficits after aneurysmal subarachnoid hemorrhage. *Stroke*. 2003;**34**:961–7.

Tseng MY, Al-Rawi PG, Czosnyka M, et al. Enhancement of cerebral blood flow using systemic hypertonic saline therapy improves outcome in patients with poor-grade spontaneous subarachnoid hemorrhage. *J Neurosurg*. 2007;**107**:274–82.

van Calenbergh F, Plets C, Goffin J, Velghe L: Nonaneurysmal subarachnoid hemorrhage: Prevalence of perimesencephalic hemorrhage in a consecutive series. *Surg Neurol*. 1993;**39**:320–3.

van Gijn J, Hijdra A, Wijdicks EF, Vermeulen M, van Crevel H. Acute hydrocephalus after aneurysmal subarachnoid hemorrhage. *J Neurosurg*. 1985;**63**:355–62.

van Gijn J, van Dongen KJ, Vermeulen M, Hijdra A. Perimesencephalic hemorrhage: a nonaneurysmal and benign form of subarachnoid hemorrhage. *Neurology*. 1985;**35**:493–97.

van Norden AG, van Dijk GW, van Huizen MD, Algra A, Rinkel GJ. Interobserver agreement and predictive value for outcome of two rating scales for the amount of extravasated blood after aneurysmal subarachnoid haemorrhage. *J Neurol*. 2006;**253**:1217–20.

Varelas PN, Rickert KL, Cusick J, et al. Intraventricular hemorrhage after aneurysmal subarachnoid hemorrhage: pilot study of treatment with intraventricular tissue plasminogen activator. *Neurosurgery*. 2005;**56**:205–13; discussion 205–13.

Weir B, Grace M, Hansen J, Rothberg C. Time course of vasospasm in man. *J Neurosurg*. 1978;**48**:173–8.

Wijdicks EF, Ropper AH, Hunnicutt EJ, Richardson GS, Nathanson JA. Atrial natriuretic factor and salt wasting after aneurysmal subarachnoid hemorrhage. *Stroke*. 1991;**22**:1519–24.

Wijdicks EF, Schievink WI, Burnett JC Jr. Natriuretic peptide system and endothelin in aneurysmal subarachnoid hemorrhage. *J Neurosurg*. 1997;**87**:275–80.

Wijdicks EF, Schievink WI, Miller GM. Pretruncal nonaneurysmal subarachnoid hemorrhage. *Mayo Clin Proc*. 1998;**73**:745–52.

Wijdicks EF, Vermeulen M, Hijdra A, van Gijn J. Hyponatremia and cerebral infarction in patients with ruptured intracranial aneurysms: is fluid restriction harmful? *Ann Neurol*. 1985;**17**:137–40.

Wilkinson IM. The vertebral artery. extracranial and intracranial structure. *Arch Neurol*. 1972;**27**:392–6.

Wirth FP. Surgical treatment of incidental intracranial aneurysms. *Clin Neurosurg*. 1986;**33**:125–35.

Wise BL. Syndrome of inappropriate antidiuretic hormone secretion after spontaneous subarachnoid hemorrhage: a reversible cause of clinical deterioration. *Neurosurgery*. 1978;**3**:412–4.

Yamashita K, Kashiwagi S, Kato S, Takasago T, Ito H. Cerebral aneurysms in the elderly in yamaguchi, japan. analysis of the Yamaguchi data bank of cerebral aneurysm from 1985 to 1995. *Stroke*. 1997;**28**:1926–31.

Yoon DY, Choi CS, Kim KH, Cho BM. Multidetector-row CT angiography of cerebral vasospasm after aneurysmal subarachnoid hemorrhage: comparison of volume-rendered images and digital subtraction angiography. *AJNR Am J Neuroradiol*. 2006;**27**:370–7.

Youmans JR, ed. *Neurological Surgery*, 3rd ed. Philadelphia: WB Saunders, 1990.

14 Status Epilepticus

Marek A. Mirski, MD, PhD, and Panayiotis N. Varelas, MD, PhD

Traditionally, status epilepticus (SE) has been arbitrarily defined as either a single generalized seizure lasting greater than 30 minutes, or a group of repetitive seizures between which the patient had not fully recovered. Recently, exactly when a prolonged seizure or set of recurrent seizures is deemed to have become SE has further evolved. In light of data now demonstrating the time-dependent risk of early neuronal injury, and the necessity to treat this disorder prior to irreversible cerebral insult, shorter seizure epochs have been emphasized.[1] Since typical seizures last no longer than 1–2 minutes, and injury can be documented histologically by 30 minutes, it is reasonable to consider as SE any seizure events greater than 5–10 minutes in length.[2] This epoch has been now adopted by both the American Academy of Neurology and the American Epilepsy Society.

THE PHENOTYPE OF STATUS EPILEPTICUS

There are three main subtypes of SE:

- The most common is generalized convulsive SE (GCSE).
- Focal Motor SE (FMSE), or epilepsy partialis continuans, is relatively uncommon and typically manifests as continuous motor twitching of a single limb or side of face.
- It is not clear whether FMSE may result in substantive injury to the cerebral cortex.
- Reasonable attempts at control are advocated, but high-risk therapies such as induced pharmacologic coma are rarely considered appropriate.
- Nonconvulsive SE (NCSE) incorporates a variety of continuous non-motor electrical paroxysms,

often described as complex-partial SE, subtle SE, non tonic-clonic SE, or subclinical SE.

- A diminishment of the neurologic exam secondary to the seizure is the common theme in this under recognized seizure subtype, but may range between awake/ambulatory to coma.
- The label of NCSE has been given even to conditions where a seizure state is questionable, as in the case of severe anoxic/ischemic encephalopathy with bilateral periodic lateralizing epileptiform discharges (PLEDS).
- Although GCSE must be treated aggressively, it remains unclear whether permanent morbidity has been attributed to NCSE.[3-5] In the purest form, NCSE is typically benign with no permanent neurologic sequelae. On the other spectral end, some advocate treating PLEDS although such paroxysms in the setting of anoxia typically portend a poor neurologic outcome.

EPIDEMIOLOGY

Approximately 150,000 patients in the United States are diagnosed with SE each year. Although it remains the most severe seizure diagnosis, SE is in fact, an uncommon admission diagnosis (0.2%), certainly much less than the incidence of seizures overall that may occur as a complication of other medical illness (3.3%). The mortality from SE approximates 20–25.[6] The above data fail to include NCSE, despite the fact that this non-motor seizure group is becoming increasingly appreciated, particularly in the hospital setting. Recent data suggests that up to 5–10 of comatose patients in an ICU that have been examined by EEG were in NCSE.[5] Other investigators have evidence to suggest that the incidence of nonconvulsive seizures may be as high as 34% of neurologic ICU patients, and it is only for a lack of monitoring that these seizures are not detected.[6]

ANATOMIC CORRELATE

Seizures present phenotypically in a number of forms and all occur as a consequence of local excitatory aberrations of the cerebral cortex.

- As simple focal motor or sensory paroxysms in a limb or face, SE in such cases constitutes focal SE.
- To the other end of the range are the primary and secondarily generalized seizures, where consciousness is affected and convulsions may occur throughout the face and extremities. The patient invariably falls, as axial rigidity is not maintained.
- In primary GTCS, a focus cannot be identified and the seizure appears to be global from the outset, whereas a focal cortical nidus is often noted in seizures that "secondarily" generalize. The "primary" generalized seizures (example: absence) probably utilize brain stem/subcortical structures in the mediation and propagation of the paroxysmal activity.
- Complex-partial seizures are focal seizures anatomically, but the sensorium and cognitive function are affected as a consequence of the affected cortex. Occurring in the temporal lobe and particularly in the region of the hippocampus, a noninteractive condition presents where memory is disturbed and automatisms such as lip smacking, blinking, or repetitive hand movements are commonplace.
- Regardless of seizure type, the continuous form (SE) represents a unique seizure event. Not self-terminating, the cortical chemical milieu has undergone alterations during the early seizure stages that undermine the brain's ability to promote neuronal inhibition within the seizure network that will stop the paroxysmal activity.[8,9] The so-called "inhibitory surround" normally present to thwart aberrant excitation breaks down. Positive reinforcement also occurs, so that prolonged seizures become increasingly more difficult to self-terminate.[8]

ETIOLOGY

The vast majority of the cortical synapses are believed to be inhibitory (γ-aminobutyric acidergic [GABAergic]). Uncontrolled activation of cortical neurons usually comes from disinhibition, although over-excitation can occur from some triggers. This disinhibition, and lowering of the seizure threshold, may be a consequence of a large number of conditions (Table 14.1). The specific triggers of SE may be due to primary pathology in the patient, or from iatrogenic causes. Although primary neurologic pathology such as ischemic stroke, intracerebral hemorrhage, central nervous system (CNS) infections, and brain tumors disturb normal cortical integrity and therefore raise the risk for seizures, some of the most common causes in a hospital setting are due to sepsis, drug toxicity, renal failure, electrolyte disorders, and cardiovascular disease.[6]

Seizures from neurologic injury are common, and occur most often as a result of stroke (ischemic or hemorrhagic) or trauma (contusions, subdural hemorrhages).

- Although the risk of seizures from ischemic stroke is not high – approximately 3% per year, the large numbers of stroke patients (500,000–700,000/year) ensures that the incidence of new cases nationwide remains appreciable.[10,11]
- Prophylaxis is generally not recommended, as the risk of SE appears lower than the hazard of drug toxicity.
- A similar risk for seizures and SE follows traumatic brain injury. Seizures may manifest either early in the course (<1 week) or develop during the late recovery period or after discharge.
- Although a recent population-based study observed a 2.1% incidence of seizures following full recovery from head injury,[12] the incidence of early seizures appears to be higher.
- Two reports noted early seizures occurring in 4.1% of patients with moderate closed head injury and 3.6% when the injury was severe.[13,14] Almost half of the seizures occurred during the first 24 hours. Such a risk of seizures includes presentation as SE.
- Head injury comprises approximately 5% of all cases of SE admitted to a hospital.[15]
- Once a seizure occurs, especially if it is of late onset (>1 week), the risk of recurrence is high,

Table 14.1. Common etiologies of seizures and status epilepticus

▶ **Neurologic Pathology**

Neurovascular
  Stroke
  Arteriovenous malformations
  Hemorrhage
Tumor
  Primary
  Metastatic
Central nervous system infection
  Abscess
  Meningitis
  Encephalitis
Inflammatory disease
  Vasculitis
  Acute disseminated encephalomyelitis
Traumatic brain injury
  Contusion
  Hemorrhage
Primary epilepsy
Primary central nervous system metabolic disturbance (inherited)

▶ **Complications of Critical Illness**

Hypoxia/ischemia
Drug/substance toxicity
  Antibiotics
  Antidepressants
  Antipsychotics
  Bronchodilators
  Local anesthetics
  Immunosuppressives
  Cocaine
  Amphetamines
Drug/substance withdrawal
  Barbiturates
  Benzodiazepines
  Opioids
  Alcohol
Infection fever (febrile seizures)
Metabolic abnormalities

Hypophosphatemia
Hyponatremia
Hypoglycemia
Renal/hepatic dysfunction
Hypophosphatemia
Surgical injury (craniotomy)

approaching 90%. Late onset seizures are also a greater predictor of significant long-term morbidity and poor outcome than those occurring early in the postinjury phase.

Regarding medical causes for SE, drug toxicity and withdrawal (especially alcohol), are significant drug conditions inducing SE.

■ Up to 15% of hospital-based seizures are linked to medication toxicity, and up to 45% if one includes the iatrogenic complications of acute withdrawal of medications (primarily opiates and benzodiazepines) prescribed in the hospital setting.[16]
■ Seizures from drug toxicity and withdrawal represent a disproportionate number of SE cases.
■ 50% may be attributed to anticonvulsant noncompliance, alcohol, or other medications.
■ The withdrawal syndrome imposes rebound excitation, which has been documented as an up-regulation of the glutamatergic system.
■ Drug-induced seizures are usually generalized tonic–clonic convulsions and occur either as single or multiple episodes within the first 48 hours.

Aside from withdrawal from alcohol, opiates, and benzodiazepines, drug-induced SE ranks low as a precipitant. Several classes of drugs do, however, pose an SE risk, and such occurrences are typically observed in the hospital setting.

■ The penicillins, and related antibiotics structurally containing the β-lactam, have been long associated with convulsant mechanisms by antagonizing the $GABA_A$ Cl^- channel.
■ The use of penicillins – especially penicillin G – has been shown to pose a risk for inducing convulsions (0.5%), and SE is often precipitated thereafter.
■ Renal insufficiency is an important predisposing factor for β-lactam drug toxicity, by concentrating plasma and CNS levels of the drugs.[17]

- The carbapenem complex imipenem/cilastatin has been shown in rats to induce convulsive behavior at lower serum concentrations than even penicillin G, and has been reported to carry the highest risk for seizures of 1.8–6.0%.[18] Carbapenems such as meropenem and biapenem have lower convulsant risks compared to imipenem owing to their weaker affinity for the $GABA_A$ receptor.

Occasionally, medication toxicity or withdrawal from the psychotropic agents such as the antidepressants or antipsychotics may induce seizures (0–4% risk) and SE (much lower overall risk). The antidepressant category is particularly large, with many agents and mechanisms of action.

- All of the serotonin selective reuptake inhibitors carry a low risk potential, as do trazodone, doxepin, and the monoamine oxidase inhibitors (MAO).
- Drugs with medium risk include the tricyclics and buproprion, while at the other end, maprotiline and amoxapine are considered high risk.[19]
- Of the antipsychotics, perhaps the phenothiazines, in particular chlorpromazine, carry the greatest risk (3–5%), mostly because of its frequent use rather than any selective proconvulsant action.

In the nonpsychotropic category of medications, theophylline (risk 8–14% in theophylline toxic patients) is particularly notable for provoking the onset of drug resistant SE because its excitatory mechanism is not via antagonism of GABA inhibition, which usually is effectively treated with benzodiazepines.

Both benzodiazepines and barbiturates have been advocated but with little clinical support of efficacy. General anesthesia and hemodialysis have also been advocated. Despite these measures, the mortality may be as high as 50%.

Local anesthetics constitute another class of agents that may precipitate SE. These drugs induce seizures via antagonism at the Na^+ channel.

- Lidocaine is most often the cause owing to its ubiquitous use as an antiarrhythmic and in a variety of forms for providing local anesthesia (spray, topical, subcutaneous, intravenous, epidural, intrathecal).
- The risk of seizures from local anesthetics is well correlated with serum concentration, and is close to linearly dose-dependent.

- At therapeutic levels for the treatment of arrhythmias and as an anesthetic supplement (1–5 mg/L), the incidence of seizures is very low, whereas at concentrations of 8–12 mg/L, seizures become relatively common.
- Although convulsions are usually a result of high-dose intravenous injection or directly into the CNS as in spinal anesthesia, seizures have been reported after intratracheal instillation for bronchoscopy or even after topical application.

Aside from direct cerebral pathology or drug related seizures, metabolic abnormalities constitute another common factor in SE, including hyponatremia, hypocalcemia, hypophosphatemia, uremia, and hypoglycemia.

- Hypo-osmolarity, rather than hyponatremia itself, leads to increased nervous system excitability by strengthening both excitatory synaptic communication in neocortex and field effects among the entire cortical population.
- The risk of seizures and SE in patients with renal failure correlates with the degree of uremic encephalopathy. The treatment of renal failure may also lower seizure threshold as a result of a dialysis disequilibrium syndrome caused by cerebral edema.
- Hypoglycemia induces neocortical hyperexcitability, either through an osmotic effect or by increasing or decreasing glutamate and GABA concentrations respectively.

If a patient is admitted to the hospital with a diagnosis of SE, then the likely causes are from anticonvulsant noncompliance, alcohol withdrawal, infection, or other drug toxicity.[2]

- In the ICU, between 5 and 10 percent of cases of SE are due to infections, either primary within the CNS – abscess, encephalitis, meningitis, or systemic – sepsis, vasculitis.[20]
- The most common causes of "refractory SE" are probably anoxic-ischemic encephalopathy or viral encephalitis, and most of the latter cases the etiology is rarely assigned to a specific virus, despite gene amplification techniques.
- Less common etiologies of "refractory SE" include carcinomatosis, paraneoplastic syndromes, and genetic disorders.[21]

MORBIDITY

The need to diagnose and effectively treat SE is imperative. Status epilepticus is a neurologic emergency for two reasons: there is a serious risk of systemic complications leading to poor clinical outcome as well as the very real potential for direct neuronal injury as a consequence of unremitting seizure activity (Table 14.2).

- Convulsive SE, particularly those expressed as paroxysms with severe motor contractions, may lead to acidosis, hyperthermia, rhabdomyolysis and trauma with consequent higher morbidity and mortality. Aspiration may be a concomitant risk as there may be loss of protective airway reflexes.
- Clinical studies have convincingly concluded that the duration of seizures of more than one hour is an independent predictor of poor outcome (odds ratio of almost 10).[22] Prolonged seizures increase the risk of cerebral damage due to excitotoxicity, intracellular Ca^{2+} accumulation and apoptosis, epileptogenic synaptic reorganization and sprouting, and the depletion of energy stores with inhibition of protein and DNA synthesis.[23]

The brain is not a homogeneous organ with respect to susceptibility to the effects of SE. Certain regions of brain are more vulnerable than others,

and these regions typically have high density of excitatory amino acid receptors.[24]

- Such areas include the hippocampal complex, pyramidal cells of the cerebellum, amygdala, thalamus, and middle cortical lamina.
- Injury to these areas may lead to permanent dysfunction in memory, balance, affect, and a general diminution in cognition.

MONITORING

The scalp EEG is the definitive diagnostic and monitoring tool for the management of SE. Not only does it serve to confirm ongoing electrical seizure activity, which must be ruled out even in the absence of any other paroxysmal clinical manifestations, but the EEG is critical for monitoring of the therapeutic response. There are distinctive EEG features of the various subtypes of SE[25,26] (Table 14.3). In particular it is important to recognize NCSE which may not present with any other implicating stigmata. In light of NCSE having a variable electrical appearance, specific criteria for its EEG diagnosis have been proposed[26] (Table 14.4).

There continues to be ongoing controversy regarding some EEG waveforms as to their consideration of

---

Table 14.2. Associated complications of generalized convulsant status epilepticus

▶ **Systemic**

Acidosis

Hyperthermia

Rhabdomyolysis

Renal failure

Arrhythmias

Trauma

Impaired V/Q (ventilation-perfusion ratio) matching

Pneumonia/aspiration

▶ **Neurologic**

Direct excitotoxic injury

Epileptogenic foci

Synaptic reorganization

Impaired protein synthesis

Table 14.3. Typical electroencephalogram presentation of generalized convulsant status epilepticus and nonconvulsant status epilepticus

▶ **Classic Generalized Convulsant Status Epilepticus**

Generalized spike or sharp wave pattern that – begins from a normal background rhythm. Status epilepticus is characterized by an unremitting spike activity or, more commonly, a crescendo-decrescendo pattern of major motor ictal periods interspersed with lower voltage paroxysmal activity. No abrupt termination or "postictal depression" is observed as following simple seizures.

▶ **Nonconvulsant Status Epilepticus**

EEG is variable with a number of EEG patterns being recognized. Generally, seizures such as complex-partial status resemble their non–status epilepticus counterparts.

EEG = electroencephalogram.

Table 14.4. Electroencephalogram criteria for nonconvulsive seizures

Nonconvulsive seizure type	Electroencephalogram criteria
Primary	1. Repetitive generalized or focal spikes, sharp waves, spike-and-wave, or sharp-and-slow complexes at greater than 3/s
	2. As above but less than 3/s, but also meeting criteria 4 (below)
	3. Sequential rhythmic waves along with secondary criteria 1, 2, 3 +/– 4
Secondary	1. Incrementing onset: increase in voltage and/or increase/decrease in frequency
	2. Decremental offset: decrease in voltage or frequency
	3. Postdischarge slowing or voltage attenuation
	4. Significant improvement in clinical state or electroencephalogram with anticonvulsant therapy

Adapted from Brenner RP.[26] Is it status? *Epilepsia*. 2002;**43**:S103–13.

representing a seizure state. Perhaps the most difficult to qualify are the periodic lateralizing epileptic discharges (PLEDS if unilateral, BIPLEDS if bilateral/independent, and PEDS if focal or bilateral/uniform) and triphasic waves (TW). Many epileptologists regard PLEDS in this context as being an interictal event, while others disagree and consider them as continuation of the seizure. The presence of PLEDS at a minimum suggests severe underlying neuronal injury, with BIPLEDS even worse (mortality of 61% in the latter group compared to 29% in the former).

- It is imperative that patients suspecting of having SE be closely monitored by EEG.
- It is not only useful to make the diagnosis (especially in NCSE), but also necessary to evaluate for residual, nonclinical epileptiform activity during therapy.
- Often, the motor component of SE subsides yet leaving continued paroxysmal epileptiform EEG activity. Some clinical reports suggest residual electrographic seizures in almost 50% of patients with GCSE, and a 10–20% incidence of NCSE in those patients treated for GCSE with cessation of motor seizure activity.

TREATMENT FOR STATUS EPILEPTICUS

The adage "seizures beget seizures" pertains well to SE: the longer SE continues, the more difficult it becomes to terminate. The local, cortical inhibitory circuits that are normally present and assist in limiting seizure duration become ineffective during SE. Seizures themselves augment this disinhibition, possibly due to early neuronal injury. As a consequence, the longer duration of SE, the more difficult it is to terminate.

- At the onset of suspicion of SE, provisions for airway protection and supplemental oxygen and ventilation, hemodynamic monitoring, and dependable intravenous access are mandatory. Often patients lose their ability to protect their airway, due to the effect of prolonged seizures or to the medications given to treat SE.
- Close hemodynamic monitoring is also mandatory to ensure appropriate visceral and cerebral perfusion pressure in the face of cardiodepressant drugs.

The mainstay for pharmacologically treating SE includes potentially a variety of drug classes: the benzodiazepines, phenytoin, valproic acid, levetiracetam, barbiturates, propofol, and the inhalational anesthetics [2,27-31] (Lowenstein, 1999)(Table 14.5). Prompt termination of electrical seizure activity is the goal, and if necessary, induction of electrocerebral flat, or near flat (i.e., "burst-suppression") EEG record.

1. First-line therapy for GCSE is the benzodiazepines.[28] Although the drug lorazepam as most efficacious, the three commonly used benzodiazepines

Table 14.5.	Initial drug therapy for status epilepticus first-line agents	
Benzodiazepines	Elimination time(time = 1/2 hours)	Recommended dosage range
Lorazepam	15	0.05–0.1 mg/kg
Midazolam	2–4	0.05–0.2 mg/kg
Diazepam	20	0.1–0.4 mg/kg
Second-line Agents		
Second-line Intravenous Anticonvulsant	Dosage	Target serum level
Phenytoin (PHT)	15–20 mg/kg	15–20 µg/mL
Fosphenytoin (fPHT)	15–20 mg/kg PE	15–20 µg /mL
Valproate (VPA)	15–20 mg/kg	50–100 µg/mL
Levetiracetam	1000–1500 mg q12h	? 10–30 µg/mL
PE = phenytoin equivalents.		

– lorazepam, midazolam, and diazepam – all are potentially effective in appropriate doses.

■ Benzodiazepines are effective in about 65% of the time in stopping GCSE.
■ The benzodiazepines are valued for their rapid penetration into the brain, and they are potent GABA$_A$ agonists, which results in inhibition of signal transmission.
■ Diazepam is very lipid soluble and rapidly redistributes away from serum into tissue. Effectively, a bolus dose will last only 5–10 minutes. However, terminal drug elimination drug takes many hours and is the longest of the three agents.[32] In addition, the hepatic intermediate yields a compound that possesses GABA-agonist activity of 15–20% of diazepam, and its plasma half-life is approximately 96 hours. Thus, such kinetics and metabolism result in only brief seizure control yet a prolonged sedative effect if large dosages are required.
■ Midazolam, as diazepam, is highly lipophilic, but is cleared by the liver more rapidly, resulting in faster clearance.
■ Lorazepam has greater water solubility than either of the other two drugs, prolonging its serum half-life, and is clinically effective for 4–6 hours. For immediate therapy of SE, and to provide for longer prophylaxis against recurrence, lorazepam remains the drug of choice.

■ Diazepam or midazolam still offer a niche where rapid termination of seizure activity is accomplished, followed by transition to a nonsedating anticonvulsant (such as phenytoin, valproic acid, or levetiracetam) in an effort to recover the neurologic exam. At times, continuous infusion of a short-acting benzodiazepine like midazolam may be considered.[29]

2. Benzodiazepines are almost never used as the sole agent to treat SE. Even if effective, tachyphylaxis to this class of drug precludes their use in monotherapy as a chronic anticonvulsant. In approximately 25–50% of the time in treating SE, the benzodiazepines themselves are insufficient to terminate the seizures. Thus, additional medications are in order in either case. The second-line agents commonly used are phenytoin, fosphenytoin, and valproic acid, primarily due to both their proven efficacy as well as availability in an intravenous formulation (Table 14.5).

■ Fosphenytoin is a phosphate ester prodrug of phenytoin. Once administered, fosphenytoin is metabolized to phenytoin within a few minutes. Advantages to its use include both the ability to administer the drug IV and IM as well as fewer local adverse effects, especially a greatly reduced risk of severe phlebitis that can occur with intravenous phenytoin. Although fosphenytoin may be infused up to three times faster than phenytoin, the enzymatic conversion required to release free phenytoin results in similar kinetics as an equivalent dose of phenytoin.

■ Most recently we have seen the introduction of levetiracetam as an IV formulation. Although little data exists as to its efficacy in acute seizure management, especially SE, this drug may prove useful in critical care and emergency departments as an adjunctive therapy following benzodiazepines. Once seizures are controlled, monotherapy for seizures is advocated to lessen the complications of drug interactions, which is of considerable concern in the ICU.

3. In cases of SE precipitated by medications, the benzodiazepines and barbiturates should be considered first-line options because of their action primarily as GABA agonists (Table 14.6).

■ Phenytoin is not particularly effective against most drug-induced convulsions, especially those triggered by β-lactam antibiotics.
■ Hemodialysis may be a consideration if seizures are resistant, particularly if renal failure complicates drug elimination.

As noted previously, convulsions and SE from theophylline toxicity carry a high risk of morbidity and mortality. Hemoperfusion, dialysis, and activated charcoal all have their advocates for acute therapy, and some experts believe aggressive measures be initiated if theophylline serum levels reach 100 mg/mL. Isoniazid is another drug that requires nonconventional therapeutics. Owing to its action as an antagonist to pyridoxal phosphate, treatment includes intravenous pyridoxine.

4. Oral anticonvulsants, such as gabapentin, lamotrigine, topiramate and vigabatrin, have little data in support of efficacy against SE, are difficult to administer in acute situations, but may offer some adjunctive benefit in the control of recurrent or resistant seizures (Table 14.7). The newer classes of agents vary with respect to their mechanism of clearance and elimination.

5. When seizures continue despite treatment with benzodiazepines and high therapeutic doses of the second-line intravenous anticonvulsant agents, a state of "refractory SE" is said to exist. 85% of SE cases are effectively treated with benzodiazepines and intravenous phenytoin, valproate or phenobarbital;

Table 14.6. Therapies for specific drug-induced status epilepticus

Drug precipitating status epilepticus	Treatment options
Antibiotics: penicillins, β-lactams, fluoroquinolones	Benzodiazepines, hemodialysis
Theophylline	?Midazolam, hemodialysis
Isoniazid	Intravenous pyridoxine

Adapted from Varelas PN, Mirski MA.[33] Seizures in the adult intensive care unit, *J Neurosurg Anesthesiol.* 2001;**13**:163–75.

Table 14.7. Indications for oral anticonvulsant drugs as adjuvant agents in refractory status epilepticus

Drug	Primary generalized	Partial
Lamotrigine	Yes	Yes
Gabapentin		Yes
Felbamate*	Yes	Yes
Topiramate		Yes
Tiagabine		Yes
Vigabatrin†	Yes	Yes

* Restricted use due to aplastic anemia.
† Not available in the United States.
Adapted from Varelas PN, Mirski MA. Seizures in the adult intensive care unit. *J Neurosurg Anesthesiol.* 2001;**13**:163–75.

only 15% remain resistant and require additional pharmacologic strategies.[34] EEG suppression is usually required to permit normal brain circuitry to reestablish, especially the return of cortical inhibitory networks. For this reason, a drug-induced period of EEG suppression is introduced, historically with the short-acting barbiturates (hence the term "barbiturate coma"). Continuous EEG monitoring is considered a standard of patient care in this setting, as is invasive hemodynamic management and respiratory care.

■ Regarding specific agents to provide for initial management continuing on to EEG suppression, a number of therapies have proven successful (Table 14.8). The barbiturates remain popular,

---

Table 14.8. Common algorithm for management of status epilepticus

▶ **Medical and Pharmacologic Treatment for Status Epilepticus**

Preserve airway and oxygenation by intubation. Order EEG to be available during therapy.

Measure finger-stick blood glucose and administer IV glucose if <40–60 mg/100 dL.

Immediate benzodiazepines: IV lorazepam 5–10 mg, diazepam 20–40 mg, or midazolam 5–20 mg over 5 minutes.

Phenytoin loading dose 20 mg/kg at 50 mg/min or fosphenytoin 20 mg/kg PE (phenytoin equivalents) at 150 mg/min. Goal serum level 15 mg/dL to 20 mg/dL.

Continuous EEG if available.

If seizures continue, phenytoin or fosphenytoin (additional 5–10 mg/kg or 5–10 mg/kg PE). Goal serum level 20–25 mg/dL.

▶ **Refractory Status Epilepticus: Several Options**

Rapid pharmacologic burst suppression/coma with hemodynamic support: propofol 2 mg/kg and 150 µg/kg per minute to 200 µg/kg per minute infusion or thiopental 4 mg/kg and 0.3 mg/kg per minute to 0.4 mg/kg per minute.

Midazolam 0.2 mg/kg followed by 0.1–0.2 mg/kg per hour may be used as an alternative to propofol or thiopental.

Valproate 60–70 mg/kg may be tried.

Pentobarbital 5–10 mg/kg followed by 1–10 mg/kg per hour is a common recipe for long-term burst-suppression requirement.

▶ **Weaning from Electroencephalogram Seizure Suppression**

Using continuous EEG, maintain in status epilepticus suppressed state (true burst-suppression may be, but not required) for 12–48 hours before attempting to withdraw from pharmacologic coma.

Ensure adequate anticonvulsant levels of selected agents for chronic seizure control. Aim for high levels of the fewest number of anticonvulsant agents. The most common agents are phenytoin and valproate.

Wean infusion, and follow EEG as background rhythm begins or increases. If breakthrough seizures recur, rebolus using 30–70% as necessary of original bolus amount required of infusion drug.

Readjust anticonvulsant serum level or add additional agents before another wean attempt.

It is not uncommon for more than one adjustment to be made before a successful wean.

EEG = electroencephalogram; IV = intravenous.

Adapted from Varelas PN, Mirski MA. Seizures in the adult intensive care unit. *J Neurosurg Anesthesiol.* 2001;**13**:163–75.

---

referring specifically to pentobarbital, thiopental, or phenobarbital.

■ Thiopental has the shortest plasma half-life with initial dosing, owing to its lipophilic nature and rapid redistribution kinetics. However, should treatment for SE require several days of EEG suppression, the long drug clearance of thiopental becomes problematic.

■ Pentobarbital is commonly selected over thiopental, owing to its greater water solubility and matched plasma kinetics and elimination as compared to thiopental. Thus, if the EEG suppression period is planned for a few hours, then thiopental is a good choice. For duration of several days of therapy, a commonly selected period of EEG suppression, neurointensivists commonly select pentobarbital.

■ Plasma levels are targeted to approximately 10–20 µg/mL, with the ultimate guide being the EEG record.

■ Typically a "burst-suppression" record is targeted, with the suppression periods ranging from 5 to 30 seconds. This burst-suppression time is continued for 24–48 hours as an initial attempt, during which time anticonvulsant drugs are maintained at high levels, and supplemental agents in combination may be considered.

- When the patient is weaned off the barbiturate, the EEG record is examined for recurrence of SE. If resurgence is noted, return to burst-suppression is accompanied by an increase in dosage of the mainstay anticonvulsant drug or change in type or number of these agents.

- Pentobarbital, like thiopental, is not truly considered to be an anticonvulsant. By accepted definition, an anticonvulsant is a drug that helps to treat or prevent seizures in dosages or serum levels that do not substantively disturb level of consciousness or cognition. Pentobarbital has no efficacy against seizures other than to suppress the EEG of cortical transmission. Thus, mainstay anticonvulsants such as phenytoin, valproate, etc. are mandatory in any planned regimen of "barb coma". An exception is when phenobarbital is the barbiturate, which is the only drug of this class that is indeed an anticonvulsant. However, because of its very long plasma half-life of up to 144 hours, phenobarbital "burst-suppression" is undertaken only when a projected coma state and ICU stay of >1–2 weeks are projected and acceptable. In such cases, high dose phenobarbital has a track record of some success.[31,35,36]

- Also used with varying degrees of success in refractory cases of SE have been the volatile anesthetic gases or other IV anesthetic induction agents such as propofol. Recently, ketamine and trials of electroconvulsive therapy have been tried with some anecdotal promise.[37,38]

- Particularly popular during the past 10 years has been the use of propofol as an initial agent for "burst-suppression." Like the short-acting anesthetic barbiturates (thiopental, pentobarbital) propofol's antiseizure mechanism appears due, in part, to GABA neurotransmission. Its popularity is owed to it very short half-life, because of its enormous plasma volume of distribution (up to 600 L, highly lipophilic) and very rapid clearance.

- The use of this drug may promote faster emergence and extubation than use of high-dose barbiturates once SE has been terminated. Propofol may thus be considered over the barbiturates in appropriate circumstances[39]

- A cautionary note need be made with reference to the numerous ICU reports of systemic acidosis and hepatic and other organ failure linked to high-dose propofol (anesthetic ranges of 100 μg/kg per minute to 300 μg/kg per minute) when used in uninterrupted fashion for several days to weeks. Thus, when it is desirable to attempt a brief EEG suppression period of a few hours before returning to an active EEG state, then propofol may be an excellent short-acting selection. For longer periods, use of more traditional barbiturates is probably wise.

- A period of EEG suppression of at least 8–12 hours is typically maintained during the first attempt before weaning of the barbiturates or anesthetic agents. All such therapies have profound effects on systemic vascular resistance. Thus, almost without exception, cardiovascular support with pressors or ionotropes is required to maintain hemodynamic parameters within the normal range. The neurologic exam is virtually without any positive findings when patients are in deep drug-induced coma. The patients may appear neurologically "brain dead," albeit a sluggish pupillary light reflex is occasionally preserved. Patient neurologic monitoring by evoked potentials often continues to demonstrate preservation of peripheral and central signals even with a flat cortical EEG.

ANTICONVULSANT TOXICITY

Anticonvulsant medications commonly introduce idiosyncratic and dose-dependent drug-induced side effect that may be harmful, especially in a critical care setting. Anticonvulsants are typically heavily protein bound, and the free serum drug is the active moiety. In low albumin states, free drug concentrations may be significantly increased even in the face of normal total serum drug concentrations, and monitoring of free drug is warranted in such patients.

- In cases of potential drug fever, an elevated eosinophil count can be helpful in distinguishing an infection from a drug effect. Commonly, however, a trial with another anticonvulsant is often necessary.

- Carbamazepine toxicity may present in biphasic fashion: acutely and subacutely as a consequence

Table 14.9. Alteration in drug plasma levels with combination anticonvulsant use

Added drug	% Bound	Phenytoin	Phenobarbital	Carbamazepine	Valproate	Benzodiazepines
Effect on plasma levels of primary agents						
Phenytoin	90		~	↓	↓	
Phenobarbital	45	↑, then ↓		~	↓	↓
Carbamazepine	75	~	~	↓	↓	↓
Valproate	90	↓ *	↑	~ or ↑ **		↑
Benzodiazepines		↓	~		~	

*↑ Free DPH level.
**Epoxide.
% Bound = percentage serum protein bound; ↓ = decrease; ↑ = increase; ~ = variable.
Adapted from Varelas PN, Mirski MA. Seizures in the adult intensive care unit. *J Neurosurg Anesthesiol.* 2001;**13**:163–75.

of increasing levels of the toxic intermediate 10, 11-epoxide metabolite.[40]

- Additional common acute, dose-dependent toxicities include transient leukopenia and thrombocytopenia (carbamazepine/valproate), megaloblastic anemia (phenytoin), and syndrome of inappropriate antidiuretic hormone (SIADH) (carbamazepine).

Idiosyncratic reactions of anticonvulsants may contribute to patient morbidity. Hypersensitivity is common with anticonvulsants, especially phenytoin and carbamazepine, with clinical features of fever, rash and eosinophilia.[40] Other drug effects that may occur (all are uncommon) include hepatic failure, pancreatitis (particularly valproic acid), agranulocytosis, aplastic anemia, Stevens-Johnson syndrome, and a lupus-like syndrome.[40]

- Severe hepatic dysfunction may rarely occur with valproic acid therapy secondary to a toxic metabolic intermediate.[41]
- This potentially fatal action is best correlated in children younger than 2 years of age receiving aspirin and polypharmacy for seizure control.

Renal dysfunction may greatly perturb the clearance of anticonvulsants, especially to phenytoin and valproate when the glomerular filtration rate falls below 10 mL/min. Phenobarbital and carbamazepine are not greatly affected.[40] During dialysis, phenytoin levels are not dramatically affected as with phenobarbital.

The interaction between anticonvulsants and other pharmaceuticals can pose a serious problem in the ICU where SE is managed.[42] Prominent effects of the former compounds are their action on hepatic metabolism and protein binding, leading to altered kinetics of other agents.

- Phenytoin, carbamazepine, and phenobarbital are all potent stimulators of hepatic enzyme systems, and can affect concentration of other medications, including concomitantly administered anticonvulsant drugs (Table 14.9).
- Phenytoin may reduce the plasma concentration of carbamazepine and valproic acid, whereas interaction with phenobarbital is variable.
- Valproic acid inhibits the metabolism of phenobarbital and carbamazepine (including the epoxide metabolite), which may result in increased serum levels.
- Carbamazepine increases the hepatic metabolism of diazepam and valproic acid.
- Phenytoin also decreases in the effectiveness of warfarin and theophylline (Table 14.10). Similarly, phenobarbital results in decreased levels of warfarin, theophylline, and cimetidine.[42]

Table 14.10. Effects of anticonvulsant drugs on commonly used medications

Effect on plasma levels or clinical effectiveness of primary agents					
Added drug	Warfarin	Theophylline	Steroids	Haloperidol	Lithium
Phenytoin	↓	↓	↓		
Phenobarbital	↓	↓	↓	↓	
Carbamazepine	↓	↓	↓	↓	↑

↓ = decrease, ↑ = increase.
Adapted from Varelas PN, Mirski MA. Seizures in the adult intensive care unit. *J Neurosurg Anesthesiol.* 2001;**13**:163–75.

Table 14.11. Other common drug effects on anticonvulsants

Added drug	Phenytoin	Carbamazepine
Salicylates	↑	
Erythromycin		↑
Chloramphenicol	↑	
Trimethoprim	↑	
Isoniazid	↑	↑
Propoxyphene	↑	↑
Amiodarone	↑	
Diltiazem, verapamil		↑
Cimetidine	↑	↑
Ethanol	↓	
Rifampicin	↓	
Digoxin	↓	
Cyclosporine	↓	
Warfarin	↓	
Theophylline	↓	
Glucocorticosteroids	↓	

↓ = decrease, ↑ = increase in plasma levels.
Adapted from Varelas PN, Mirski MA. Seizures in the adult intensive care unit. *J Neurosurg Anesthesiol.* 2001;**13**:163–75.

Whereas anticonvulsant drugs may alter the kinetics of other drugs, so too can different medications interfere with the absorption, distribution, and elimination of these anti-seizure agents (Table 14.11).[40] For example, amiodarone, isoniazid, and chlorpromazine all decrease the hepatic metabolism of many drugs. Phenytoin, due to its popularity as an ICU medication, is commonly affected. Conversely, drugs that may decrease phenytoin levels include digoxin, cyclosporine, corticosteroids, warfarin, and theophylline. Aluminum hydroxide, magnesium hydroxide, and calcium antacids decrease the absorption of enterally administered phenytoin.

CONCLUSION

Status epilepticus represents a true neurologic emergency. Particularly challenging is the diagnostic component of SE management, when NCSE is considered, or when EEG is not immediately available and only subtle clinical evidence is present. The ability to recognize and treat SE is critical, however, as there exists clear evidence for potential grave neurologic injury when seizures persist. However, the treatment of seizures itself may impose new patient toxicity, and requires appropriate toxicity/benefit evaluation, as well as proper drug selection.

SUGGESTED READINGS

1. Lowenstein DH, Bleck T, Macdonald RL. It's time to revise the definition of status epilepticus. *Epilepsia.* 1999;**40**: 120–2.

2. Lowenstein DH, Aminoff MJ, Simon RP. Barbiturate anesthesia in the treatment of status epilepticus: clinical experience with 14 patients. *Neurology.* 1988;**38**: 395–400.

3. DeLorenzo RJ, Waterhouse EJ, Towne AR, et al. Persistent nonconvulsive status epilepticus after the control of convulsive status epilepticus. *Epilepsia.* 1998;**39**:833–40.

4. Kaplan PW. Assessing the outcomes in patients with nonconvulsive status epilepticus: nonconvulsive status epilepticus is underdiagnosed, potentially overtreated, and confounded by morbidity. *J Clin Neurophysiol.* 1999;**16**:341–52.

5. Towne AR, Waterhouse EJ, Boggs JG, et al. Prevalence of nonconvulsive status epilepticus in comatose patients. *Neurology.* 2000;**54**:340–5.

6. Bleck TP, Smith MC, Pierre-Louis SJC, et al. Neurologic complications of critical medical illness. *Critical Care Med.* 1993; **21**:98–103.

7. Jordan KG. Continuous EEG and evoked potential monitoring in the neuroscience intensive care unit. *J Clin Neurophysiol.* 1993;**10**:445–75.

8. Fountain NB, Lothman EW. Pathophysiology of status epilepticus. *J Clin Neurophysiol.* 1995;**12**:326–42.

9. Coulter DA, DeLorenzo RJ. Basic mechanisms of status epilepticus. *Adv Neurol.* 1999;**79**:725–33.

10. Arboix A, Garcia-Eroles L, Massons JB, Oliveres M, Comes E. Predictive factors of early seizures after acute cerebrovascular disease. *Stroke.* 1997; **28**:1590–4.

11. Rumbach L, Sablot D, Berger E, Tatu L, Vuillier F, Moulin T. Status epilepticus in stroke: report on a hospital-based stroke cohort. *Neurology.* 2000;**54**:350–4.

12. Annegers JF, Hauser A, Coan SP, Rocca WA. A population-based study of seizures after traumatic brain injuries. *N Engl J Med.* 1998;**338**:20–4.

13. Lee ST, Lui TN, Wong CW, Yeh YS, Tzaan WC. Early seizures after moderate closed head injury. *Acta-Neurochir-Wien.* 1995;**137**:151–4.

14. Lee ST, Lui TN, Wong CW, et al. Early seizures after severe closed head injury. *Can J Neurol Sci.* 1997;**24**:40–3.

15. Lowenstein DH. Status epilepticus: an overview of the clinical problem. *Epilepsia.* 1999;**40** (S1):S3–8.

16. Alldredge BK, Simon RP. Drugs that can precipitate seizures. In Resor SR Jr, ed. *The Medical Treatment of Epilepsy.* New York: Marcel Dekker, 1992, pp 497–523.

17. Wallace KL Antibiotic-induced convulsions. *Crit Care Clin.* 1997;**13**:741–61.

18. Norby SR. Neurotoxicity of carbapenem antimicrobials. *Drug Safety.* 1996;**15**:87–90.

19. Rosenstein DL, Nelson JC, Jacobs SC. Seizures associated with antidepressants: a review. *J Clin Psychiatry.* 1993;**54**:289–97.

20. Wijdicks EFM, Sharbrough FW. New-onset seizures in critically ill patients. *Neurology.* 1993;**43**:1042–4.

21. Bleck TP. Refractory status epilepticus. *Curr Opin Crit Care..* 2005;**11**:117–20.

22. Towne AR, Pellock JM, Ko D, DeLorenzo RJ. Determinants of mortality in status epilepticus. *Epilepsia.* 1994;**35**:27–34.

23. Sloviter RS. Status epilepticus-induced neuronal injury and network reorganization. *Epilepsia.* 1999;**40**:S34–9; discussion S40–1.

24. Wasterlain CG, Fujikawa DG, Penix L, Sankar R. Pathophysiological mechanisms of brain damage from status epilepticus. *Epilepsia* 1993;**34** (S1):S37–53.

25. Niedermeyer E, Lopes da Silva F, eds. *Electroencephalography. Basic Principles, Clinical Applications, and Related Fields,* 3rd ed. Baltimore: Williams & Wilkins, 1993.

26. Brenner RP. Is it status? *Epilepsia.* 2002;**43**(S3): S103–13.

27. Lowenstein DH. Treatment options for status epilepticus. *Curr Opin Pharmacol.* 2005;**5**(3):334–9.

28. Treiman DM, Meyers PD, Walton NY, et al. A comparison of four treatments for generalized convulsive status epilepticus. Veterans Affairs Status Epilepticus Cooperative Study Group. *N Engl J Med.* 1998;**339**: 792–8.

29. Kumar A, Bleck TP. Intravenous midazolam for the treatment of refractory status epilepticus. *Crit Care Med.* 1992;**20**:483–8.

30. Mackenzie SJ, Kapadia F, Grant IS. Propofol infusion for control of status epilepticus. *Anaesthesia.* 1990;**45**:1043–5.

31. Mirski MA, Williams, MA, Hanley DF. Prolonged pentobarbital and phenobarbital coma for refractory generalized status epilepticus. *Crit Care Med.* 1995;**23**: 400–4.

32. Mirski MA, Muffelman B, Ulatowski JA, Hanley DF. Sedation for the critically ill neurologic patient. *Crit Care Med.* 1995;**23**:2038–53.

33. Varelas P, Mirski MA. Seizures in the ICU, *J Neurosurg Anesthesiol.* 2001;**13**:163–75.

34. Bleck TP. Management approaches to prolonged status epilepticus. *Epilepsia.* 1999 **40**(S1):S59–63.

35. Crawford TO, Mitchell WG, Fishman LS, et. al. Very high dose phenobarbital for refractory status epilepticus in children. *Neurology.* 1988;**38**:1035–40.

36. Mirski MA. Rapid treatment of status epilepticus with low dose pentobarbital. *Crit Care Rep.* 1989;**1**: 150–6.

37. Ubogu EE, Sagar SM, Lerner AJ, Maddux BN, Suarez JI, Werz MA. Ketamine for refractory status epilepticus: a case of possible ketamine-induced neurotoxicity. *Epilepsy Behav.* 2003;**4**:70–5.

38. Carrasco Gonzalez MD, Palomar M, Rovira R. Electroconvulsive therapy for status epilepticus. *Ann Intern Med.* 1997;**127**:247-8.

39. Stecker MM, Kramer TH, Raps EC, O'Meeghan R, Dulaney E, Skaar DJ. Treatment of refractory status epilepticus with propofol: clinical and pharmacokinetic findings. *Epilepsia.* 1998;**39**:18-26.

40. Dreifuss FE. Toxic effects of drugs used in the ICU. Anticonvulsant agents. *Crit Care Clin.* 1991;**7**:521-32.

41. Gram L, Bentsen KD. Hepatic toxicity of antiepileptic drugs. *Rev Acta Neurol Scand.* 1983;**S97**:81-90.

42. Leppik IE, Wolff DL. Antiepileptic medication interactions. *Neurol Clin.* 1993;**11**:905-21.

15 Nerve and Muscle Disorders

Edward M. Manno, MD

Neuromuscular diseases and respiratory failure are common processes encountered in both neurologic and medical intensive care units. Problems can be encountered anywhere along the peripheral nervous system. Neurogenic respiratory failure can be localized to diseases of the motor neuron, peripheral nerve, neuromuscular junction, or muscle.

This chapter provides a broad overview of the clinical presentation of neuromuscular respiratory failure and reviews diagnostic criteria and treatment for specific neuromuscular diseases.

NEUROMUSCULAR RESPIRATORY FAILURE: CLINICAL FEATURES

Patients with neuromuscular respiratory weakness need to be closely followed with pulmonary function tests. These should include at least vital capacities, negative inspiratory forces, and expiratory flow volumes. Part of the need for close monitoring is due to the often unreliability of the clinical exam.

- The clinical signs and symptoms of patients with neuromuscular failure may differ and can present with varying signs and symptoms of respiratory, bulbar, or appendicular weakness.
- Patients may complain of dyspnea or a vague sense of uneasiness. Brow sweating is common.
- In many circumstances a patient with neuromuscular failure will develop the typical signs and symptoms of respiratory difficulties (tachypnea, tachycardia, accessory muscle use, decreased cough, etc.).

A patient with a rapidly ascending paralysis, an acute dysautonomia, or neuromuscular junction inhibition may not be able to manifest the signs and symptoms typically encountered in a patient with impending respiratory arrest secondary to primarily pulmonary processes. **Thus a decision on the timing of endotracheal intubation should be based on the decline of pulmonary function tests and not necessarily on the clinical presentation of the patient.** In the above circumstances patients may appear well until the need for urgent intubation.

- Respiratory insufficiency and vital capacities follow a typical progressive pattern.
- Normal tidal volumes are approximately 65–70 mL/kg. An initial decrease in tidal volumes may not be clinically apparent.
- An intrinsic cough is lost at vital capacities below 30 mL/kg. Decreasing tidal volumes at this point will lead to progressive atelectasis. Arterial blood gases at this stage of respiratory failure will reveal only a subtle drop in the partial pressure of oxygen.
- Pulmonary shunting occurs at vital capacities below 15 mL/kg with a notable decrease in oxygenation.
- Hypercapnia is a late sign of neuromuscular respiratory insufficiency developing as vital capacities drop below 10 mL/kg.

Decreasing vital capacities, however, may be less specific than other pulmonary function tests for neuromuscular respiratory insufficiency. Difficulties with patient compliance and variable effort may complicate the interpretation of vital capacities.

- The flow volume loops of patients with neuromuscular respiratory failure appear similar to patients with chronic obstructive pulmonary disease.

- A prolonged tail at the end of exhalation may contribute significantly to the volume of the vital capacity. If the respiratory technician is unaware of these technicalities, the actual vital capacity may be underestimated.

Neck flexor strength appears to correlate best with overall neuromuscular respiratory strength. It is difficult to quantify respiratory strength on the clinical exam; however, a rough estimate of a vital capacity can be elicited by having the patient take a deep breath and count to the highest number they can during exhalation.

- A count of 30 approximates a vital capacity of 2 L.
- Some coaching may need to occur to assure proper technique.

Negative inspiratory forces are probably the best measure of respiratory strength. They are less likely to be misinterpreted, easier to perform, and more reproducible.

- The negative inspiratory force requires that a patient is able to make a tight seal with his lips around the testing device.
- Patients with facial weakness due to a Miller–Fisher variant of Guillain–Barré or myasthenia gravis may not be able to perform this test properly.

The timing of endotracheal intubation is important and should be performed electively based on declining respiratory parameters. Wijdicks has advocated the 20–30–40 rule suggesting that patients with a vital capacity less than 20 mL/kg, a negative inspiratory force < 30 cm H_2O, or a negative expiratory force of < 40 cm H_2O should be intubated. The rate of decompensation should also be considered in the decision for endotracheal intubation.

SPECIFIC NEUROMUSCULAR DISEASES ENCOUNTERED IN THE INTENSIVE CARE UNIT

Amyotrophic Lateral Sclerosis

Amyotrophic lateral sclerosis (ALS) is a progressive degenerative disease of unknown etiology that leads to loss of motor neurons in the cortex, brain stem, and spinal cord. Clinically both upper and lower motor neurons are affected.

- A progressive muscle weakness with fasciculation, atrophy, spasticity is the typical presentation.
- Distinct criteria have been developed for the diagnosis.
- Electromyography reveals diffuse fasciculations and motor involvement.
- The disease needs to be differentiated from cervical spondylosis, thyroid disease, vitamin deficiencies, benign fasciculations, enzyme deficiencies, and multifocal motor neuropathy with conduction block, polymyositis, and other motor neuron diseases.

The diagnosis is usually well established before admission to an intensive care unit however on rare occasions respiratory insufficiency is the presenting symptomatology. A variant form of ALS can present with predominantly bulbar symptoms leading to progressive difficulties with swallowing. Aspiration pneumonia under these circumstances may be the initial presentation to an intensive care unit.

The mean survival after diagnosis is approximately 4 years. There is no known cure and only one drug has shown mild slowing of the disease.

- Riluzole is best used early in the course of the disease.
- It is however expensive and has many side effect. Liver function tests need to be monitored every 3 months for the first year and every 6 months after that.

If a patient elects to continue mechanical ventilation after the diagnosis is secured, plans for tracheostomy and home ventilation can be made.

Guillain–Barré Syndrome

Guillain–Barré syndrome (GBS) remains the most common disease etiology of acute paralysis. The syndrome commonly used as a synonym for acute inflammatory demyelinating polyneuropathy (AIDP) encompasses various forms of acute sensory and motor axonal clinical variants. An autoimmune humoral mediated attack of a wide range of myelin glycolipids is the most common mechanism for the disease. The disease affects the peripheral nervous system, so the longest peripheral nerves of the body are the most likely to be affected. Clinically, this results in an ascending distal to proximal weakness; however, limb and cranial nerve weakness can vary significantly.

- GBS can be preceded by a respiratory or gastrointestinal illness however up to 30% of patients will report no prior illnesses.
- Distal paraesthesias are common before the development of weakness.
- Weakness can progress rapidly over hours, requiring emergent intubation or progress slowly over days and weeks.
- The process of demyelination rarely persists beyond 3 weeks of symptom onset.
- A particular severe axonal form of the disease is found after infection with *Campylobacter jejuni*.

The clinical diagnosis is supported by the finding of elevated cerebrospinal fluid (CSF) protein and usually less than 10 white cells per mm³. Historically, the lack of CSF cellularity helped differentiate GBS from poliomyelitis. Today the lack of cellularity is helpful to differentiate GBS from West Nile myelitis. Nerve conduction studies are consistent with demyelination with prolonged F waves and slowed conduction velocities.

An acute dysautonomia, most frequently seen in the more aggressive presentation of the disease, can occur and can be life threatening.

- The most common form of dysautonomia is a mild to moderate sustained hypertension that usually responds to modest treatment with antihypertensives.
- Care must be taken to avoid overtreatment of the hypertension, which can subsequently lead to hypotension as the autonomic nervous system recovers. Large fluctuations in blood pressure can occur and need to be judiciously treated.
- A variety of cardiac arrhythmias can be encountered including ventricular tachycardia and fibrillation. The most ominous arrhythmia is bradycardia and asystole. A small percentage of patients will require pacemaker placement.

Treatment is largely supportive. Fluid resuscitation, however, is often helpful because dysautonomia is worsened in patients that are volume depleted. Endotracheal intubation should occur electively based on declining respiratory function tests. Noninvasive forms of ventilation have not been helpful in preventing endotracheal intubation.

- Patients may need to remain intubated for several weeks depending on the extent of peripheral nerve involvement.

- A pulmonary function score obtained 12 days after intubation can be helpful in predicting which patient will need long-term mechanical ventilation.
  - This is obtained by summating the scores of the patients' vital capacity and negative and expiratory pressures.
  - This score is obtained at the time of intubation and is compared to a score obtained at 12 days after intubation. If the score is improved it is likely that the patient will be extubated within 2 weeks.
  - If the score is worse long term mechanical ventilation will likely be needed. Elective tracheostomy could then be planned.

Both plasma exchange and intravenous immunoglobulin treatments (IVIG) have been shown to be equally effective treatments for GBS. The clinical endpoints in the studies evaluating patients with GBS were the time when mechanical ventilation was no longer required and the day of ambulation. Both occurred earlier with IVIG and plasma exchange. Anecdotally, clinical improvement may occur faster with plasma exchange.

- Plasma exchange of 2–4 L is a standardized treatment. Five treatments provided every other day is the usual regimen, although some advocate more aggressive plasma exchanges early in the treatment. Treatment is more effective if started within 2 weeks of the onset of symptoms.
- IVIG is given in doses of 0.4 g/kg daily for 5 days.

There are advantages to each of the treatment strategies. Practically, IVIG is more commonly available and is easier to administer. Plasma exchange usually requires the placement of a central venous catheter. Care must be used in patients with congestive heart failure to avoid fluid overload. Potential side effects include:

- Aseptic meningitis
- Pseudohyponatremia
- Renal failure
- Thromboembolic complications.
- In rare cases an anaphylactic reaction can occur in patients who are IgA deficient.
  - Close hemodynamic monitoring, however, is essential particularly in the early treatments as hypotension is common during treatment.

■ Plasma exchange is avoided in patients with severe dysautonomia.

There is no evidence to suggest that combining plasma exchange and IVIG improves long term outcome beyond treatment with plasma exchange or IVIG alone. Similarly, additional courses of IVIG or plasma exchange have not been shown to be more effective than single courses. Despite the lack of evidence combined and additional treatments are often employed in patients who do not show any anticipated improvements.

Corticosteroids are not helpful in the treatment of GBS. However, a careful history must be obtained to differentiate GBS from the more chronic form of the disease. Chronic inflammatory demyelinating polyneuropathy (CIDP) is responsive to treatment with corticosteroids. Clues in the history suggesting CIDP include subtle paraesthesias or weakness that may have preceded the current illness by a few weeks or months.

Clinical improvement or a decrease in the progression of the disease is usually seen after a week of treatment. The long-term prognosis and the rate of recovery depend on the extent and degree of demyelination and axonal damage. Demyelination, even if severe, will usually recover completely if the underlying axonal structure remains intact. Incomplete recovery can be expected if there is severe axonal damage or transection of the peripheral nerves.

Table 15.1. ICU management of Guillain–Barré syndrome

1. Admit to ICU for progressive appendicular weakness or respiratory weakness for observation.
2. Check EKG, CXR, and baseline laboratory values.
3. Follow vital capacities and negative and positive expiratory forces every 3–8 hours.
4. Place an arterial line and follow arterial blood gases.
   a. If dysautonomia is present:
      i. liberalize intravenous fluids as tolerated
      ii. Aggressive electrolyte replacement for hypokalemia, hypocalcemia, or hypomagnesemia
      iii. Vasopressor support or intravenous antihypertensive medication for blood pressure control as needed.
      iv. Anti cardiac dysrhythmia medications as needed
      v. Consider placement of a temporary pacemaker if bradycardia is problematic.
5. Intubate electively for decreasing pulmonary function tests or the development of hypercapnia.
6. Start IVIG or place central access and start plasma exchange.
   a. Plasma exchange protocols can be initiated every other day for five treatments or every day for 3 days followed by every other day for two additional treatments.
7. Initiate intensive care unit orders
   a. Place nasogastric tube and initiate enteral feeding
      i. Consider metoclopramide 10 mg intravenous or per nasogastric tube every 6 hours if gastrointestinal residuals are high.
      ii. Initiate bowel regimen to ensure regular bowel movements.
      iii. Observe for any abdominal distention.
   b. Start measures for gastrointestinal and deep venous thrombosis prophylaxis.
   c. Initiate chest physiotherapy and physical therapy regimen.
   d. Assess for pain regularly.
   e. Psychological support. Encourage regularly, consider notifying Guillain–Barré support groups.
8. Attempt weaning regimen when appendicular strength or respiratory muscle strength appears to be improving.
9. Check pulmonary function tests 12 days after intubation. Consider elective tracheostomy for long term ventilatory support if pulmonary function tests are worse than on the day of intubation.

General supportive measures for the long-term intensive care unit patient should be initiated. These include:

- Deep venous thrombus prophylaxis
- Gastrointestinal prophylaxis
- Early initiation of enteral nutrition: An adynamic ileus may make enteral nutrition difficult. This will occasionally respond to metoclopramide 10–20 mg given intravenously every 6–8 hours.
- Pain is occasionally problematic and may be unresponsive to narcotics.
  - ▸ Non steroidal anti-inflammatory medications are often helpful.
  - ▸ In recalcitrant cases isolated doses of methyl-prednisolone (60 mg) can be tried.
  - ▸ Psychological support is important.

Weaning and extubation criteria are not as well established as intubation criteria. In general intermittent mandatory ventilator rates and/or pressure support is gradually decreased until a patient can breathe on their own with minimal support. This usually occurs when a patient can generate 12–15 mL/kg tidal volumes. A t-piece trial that is tolerated for 30 minutes is generally indicative of extubation success.

Myasthenia Gravis

Myasthenia gravis (MG) is an autoimmune disease of unknown etiology. In this disease antibodies are formed against the postsynaptic acetylcholine receptor at the neuromuscular junction. It can be diagnosed at all ages but has a bimodal distribution in young women and older men. A genetic predisposition for HLA, A1, DRW3, and B12 genotypes is reported. Thymomas occur in 10% of patients with MG.

- The diagnosis is determined by the clinical presentation along with laboratory and electrophysiologic support.
- Many patients will display improvement in muscle strength when tested with Edrophonium. The testing, however, is often unreliable and needs to be performed by a skilled observer.
- Eighty five percent of patients with MG will have detectable antibodies to the acetylcholine receptor. About half of the seronegative patients with

MG will have detectable specific muscle tyrosine and kinase antibodies.
- A decremental pattern on EMG provides localization for neuromuscular junction failure.
- The most sensitive diagnostic test for MG is the single fiber EMG, which displays an increase in jitter. Jitter is the variability in time between normal synaptic transmissions which will increase with progressive neuromuscular failure.

The hallmark presentation of MG is evidence for multiple areas of muscle fatigue. The most active muscles are usually affected earliest in the clinical course. Diplopia, ptosis, and dysphagia are thus the most common presenting signs and symptoms with appendicular weakness occurring later in the clinical course of the disease. The Myasthenia Gravis Foundation of America has developed a grading scale of 1–5 for worsening disease. Patients requiring mechanical ventilation are listed as grade 5.

The most common reason for a patient with MG to be admitted to an ICU is for respiratory monitoring during a myasthenic crisis. The reasons for MG exacerbation are many and include preceding respiratory illnesses, surgery, or during the initiation of steroid therapy. Many authors advocate prophylactic plasma exchange in patients with MG before any major surgery. In about one third of patients no definable reasons can be found.

There are a number of pharmacologic agents that should be avoided in patients with disease of the neuromuscular junction. A list can usually be obtained through the hospital pharmacist.

- In general aminoglycosides and quinidine should be avoided.
- Other drugs with relative contraindications include the calcium channel blockers, lithium, and chlorpromazine.
- The cephalosporins and penicillins decrease calcium entry into the presynaptic junction and thus limit acetylcholine release into the synaptic junction.

Close respiratory monitoring with vital capacities and negative inspiratory pressures is crucial. Unlike in GBS, some patients with MG exacerbation can avoid endotracheal intubation with the use of bilevel positive airway pressure (BiPAP) if treatment is initiated early.

- Endotracheal intubation should occur electively based upon declining muscle strength and pulmonary function tests.
- Pharmacologic paralysis should be avoided during intubation since recovery can be prolonged.
- Life-threatening hyperkalemia can develop if succinylcholine is used for pharmacologic paralysis.

The differentiation between myasthenic crisis and cholinergic crisis in the ICU is often moot since the initial treatments will be the same. The initial treatment will be to stop the pyridostigmine. In patients in whom bronchial secretions or diarrhea is problematic, atropine or glycopyrrolate can be used.

Myasthenic crisis is treated with either plasma exchange or IVIG in regimens and dosages similar to those outlined for GBS.

- Some retrospective studies suggest that plasma exchange may be superior to IVIG in acute myasthenic crisis; however, larger trials have showed similar benefits.
- There is limited evidence that sequential treatment with plasma exchange and IVIG may provide some additional benefit.
- A newer form of plasma exchange using a resin that selectively absorbs acetylcholine receptor antibodies has shown promise but is not widely available.
- If no improvement is seen after 5 days of treatment prednisone at 60 mg/day is started.
  - About 5–10% of patients may transiently worsen after the initiation of treatment.
  - If the patient is not intubated close monitoring of respiratory function will be needed during the first few days after initiation of treatment.
- Long-term immunosuppression is reserved for recalcitrant cases and includes the use of cyclosporin or mycophenolate mofetil.

The ICU treatment of MG has been one of the Neuro ICU success stories with mortality dropping from about 30% to 5% over the last few decades (Table 15.2). Early intubation preventing aspiration and aggressive treatments are most likely responsible for this decline. Dysautonomia can occur with MG and along with sepsis and medical complications account for most of the mortality.

Botulism

Botulism is caused by a toxin produced by the anaerobic bacterium *Clostridium botulinum*. It is most commonly encountered as wound botulism in the United States in intravenous drug abusers. Botulism is also found in improperly sterilized foods (usually canned).

- The diagnosis is usually based on a history of an ingested food or purulent wound. This is followed by nausea and vomiting.
- Weakness and anticholinergic symptoms start 6–24 hours later. Anticholinergic symptoms include dry mouth, urinary retention, pupillary dilation, and a dysautonomia that is followed by the development of bulbar weakness and a descending paralysis.
- Respiratory failure can develop rapidly.

The toxin is believed to interfere presynaptically with the release of acetylcholine into the neuromuscular junction, although the exact mechanism of how this occurs is unknown. The EMG evolves over time. Findings may not be present early but include decreased compound muscle action potentials (CMAP) in at least two muscles, a 20% facilitation of CMAP with stimulation that is prolonged for at least 2 minutes, and no postactivation exhaustion. The single-fiber EMG shows increase jitter.

Treatment is primarily supportive. Diaminopyridine, which facilitates the release acetylcholine, is helpful but will not affect the underlying process. An antitoxin is available from the Centers for Disease Control and Prevention (CDC) but must be given within 24 hours of the onset of symptoms.

CRITICAL ILLNESS POLYNEUROPATHY

Critical Illness polyneuropathy (CIP) is a distal axonopathy that develops in patients with systemic inflammatory response syndrome (SIRS) or after sepsis. It was originally described in patients in the medical ICU who were unable to be weaned from mechanical ventilation despite resolution of their primary pulmonary process.

- Clinically, patients present with a flaccid areflexic limbs but with intact cranial nerves.
  - There is marked distal atrophy and wasting of the musculature.

Table 15.2. ICU management for an acute myasthenic crisis

1. Admit to ICU for observation of respiratory function.
2. Assess airway if dysphagia is a prominent symptom.
3. If secretions are problematic or a cholinergic crisis is considered than discontinue the pyridostigmine.
4. Check EKG, CXR, and baseline laboratory values.
5. Follow vital capacities, and negative and positive expiratory forces every 3–8 hours.
6. Place an arterial line and follow arterial blood gases.
   a. If dysautonomia is present:
      i. Liberalize intravenous fluids as tolerated
      ii. Aggressive electrolyte replacement for hypokalemia, hypocalcemia, or hypomagnesemia.
      iii. Vasopressor support or intravenous antihypertensive medication for blood pressure control as needed
      iv. Anticardiac dysrhythmia medications as needed
7. Intubate electively for decreasing pulmonary function tests or the development of hypercapnia.
   a. Avoid pharmacologic paralysis if possible.
   b. Consider a trial of BiPAP if respiratory decline has been slow and treatment has been initiated.
8. Place central access and start plasma exchange.
   a. Plasma exchange protocols can be initiated every other day for five treatments or every day for 3 days followed by every other day for two additional treatments.
   b. If no improvement, initiate a 5-day course of IVIG.
   c. Start prednisone 60 mg every day.
   d. Consider long-term immunosuppressive medications.
9. Initiate ICU orders.
   a. Place nasogastric tube and initiate enteral feeding and bowel regimen.
   b. Start measures for gastrointestinal and deep venous thrombosis prophylaxis.
   c. Initiate chest physiotherapy and physical therapy regimen.
   d. Treat infections as needed. Check with pharmacy to use antibiotics least likely to affect the neuromuscular junction.
10. Attempt weaning regimen when appendicular strength or respiratory muscle strength appears to be improving.
   a. Restart pyridostigmine 60 mg every 4–6 hours.
   b. Start glycopyrrolate 1 mg every 8 hours if diarrhea or increases secretions are problematic.

▸ Sensation is grossly preserved, as patients will grimace in response to painful stimulation.
▸ Respiratory muscle strength is compromised. The phrenic nerves can be directly involved.
■ Nerve conduction studies reveal preserved motor nerve conduction velocities with decreased nerve and muscle amplitudes. Sensory nerve action potentials are variably involved but are generally less affected than the motor action potentials. Sensory nerve conduction velocities are unaffected. The EMG reveals variable fibrillation potentials and sharp waves with a poor recruitment pattern.
■ The CSF is normal and nerve biopsy reveals distal greater than proximal axonal degeneration without evidence for inflammation.

The extent of the axonopathy is related to the severity and the length of time a patient is septic. CIP has been correlated with hyperglycemia, hypoalbuminemia, and increased ICU length of stay. Differentiation of this axonopathy from the

Table 15.3. Characterization of neuromuscular conditions associated with critical illness

Condition	Incidence	Clinical features	Electrophysiologic findings	Serum creatine kinase	Muscle biopsy	Prognosis
Critical illness polyneuropathy (CIP)	Common after Sepsis	Flaccid areflexia, intact sensory exam	Decreased amplitudes of NCS. Normal conduction velocities.	Usually normal	Denervation atrophy	Variable
CIM – Myosin loss	Common after neuromuscular blockade and steroid use	Flaccid quadriplegia	Abnormal muscle fibrillations	Mildly elevated	Loss of myosin filaments	Good
CIM- Rhabdomyolysis	Rare	Severe diffuse muscle weakness	Normal NCS and EMG	Markedly elevated	Diffuse muscle necrosis	Variable
CIM – Disuse atrophy	Common	Diffuse muscle wasting	Normal NCS and EMG	Normal	Normal or type II atrophy	Good
Combine CIP and CIM	Common	Flaccid limbs and muscle wasting	Combined CIP and CIM findings	Variable	Denervation atrophy	Variable

Adapted from Reference

CIP = critical illness polyneuropathy; CIM = critical illness myopathy; EMG = electromyography; NCS = nerve conduction studies.

axonal form of GBS is made clinically. CIP develops only after sepsis while the axonal form of GBS predates admission to an ICU.

The etiology of CIP is speculative. The leading theory is that sepsis leads to impairment of the nerve microcirculation. Cytokines released during sepsis can lead to endoneural edema which is worsened by hypoalbuminemia and hyperglycemia. This edema increases the distance oxygen must diffuse to provide energy for the peripheral nerve. Bioenergetic studies in muscle during sepsis support this concept. The peripheral nerve requires energy for axonal transport of nutrients. Decreased energy reserves would result in a dying back axonopathy.

There is no specific treatment for CIP other than aggressive treatment of the underlying sepsis.

▹ IVIG has been tried in a small series of patients.
▹ Intensive insulin treatment decreased the risk of CIP in a series of brain-injured patients.
▹ Activated protein C and CIP has not been studied.
▹ The prognosis of CIP depends upon the extent of the axonopathy. More severe case will take longer to regenerate and may be incomplete.

Critical Illness Myopathy

Critical illness myopathy (CIM) is a term used to describe a series of myopathies encountered in the critically ill patient. It is commonly seen in patients with pharmacologic paralysis and in transplant patients.

■ The major feature is flaccid weakness of all of the extremities including the neck flexors, facial muscles, and diaphragm.
■ Ophthalmoplegia is less common.
■ Myalgias are rare and the creatinine kinase enzyme is variably elevated.
■ Sensory and motor nerve potentials are normal but muscle fibrillations and sharp waves are present.
■ CMAPs are decreased.
■ Direct muscle stimulation is often helpful in differentiating CIP from CIM.
  ▹ In CIP direct muscle stimulation will show normal muscle potentials.
  ▹ In CIM muscle potentials will be decreased.

Two forms of myopathy can occur after pharmacologic paralysis and corticosteroid use.

■ An acute quadriplegic myopathy has been described in patients with status asthmaticus that receive corticosteroids and paralysis. Muscle biopsy reveals complete loss of myosin between the actin filaments.
■ An acute rhabdomyolysis can also occur. Muscle necrosis can be severe leading to life threatening hyperkalemia, hypocalcemia, and acute renal failure.

CIP and CIM can occur separately or coincidentally. Disuse atrophy with muscle wasting is common with CIP and represents a coincident myopathy related to denervation. Muscle biopsy can be helpful in differentiating the type of myopathy.

Weaning from mechanical ventilation will not be useful if the source of muscle weakness is denervated muscle or severe rhabdomyolysis. Alternatively, reinnervated but deconditioned muscle can respond to a weaning protocol. Prognosis in CIM is dependent on the underlying pathology. Disuse atrophy and myosin loss will recover. Severe denervation and rhabdomyolysis has a more uncertain prognosis.

REFERENCES

Bolton CF. Neuromuscular complications of sepsis. *Intens Care Med.* 1993;**19**:S58–63.

Bolton CF. Neuromuscular manifestations of critical illness. *Muscle Nerve.* 2005;**32**(2):140–63.

Clawson LL, Lechtzin N. Amyotrophic lateral sclerosis. In Johnson RT, Griffin JW, McArthur JC (eds), *Current Therapy in Neurologic Disease*, 6th ed. St. Louis: C. V. Mosby, 2002, pp 314–21.

Gajdos P, Chevret S, Toyka K. Plasma exchange for myasthenia gravis *Cochrane Database Syst Rev.* 2002;(4):CD002275.

Gajdos P, Chevret S, Toyka K. Intravenous immunoglobulin for myasthenia gravis. *Cochrane Database Syst Rev.* 2006;(2):CD002277.

Gajdos P, Tranchant C, Clair B, et al. Myasthenia Gravis Clinical Study Group. Treatment of myasthenia gravis exacerbation with intravenous immunoglobulin: a randomized double-blind clinical trial. *Arch Neurol.* 2005;**62**(11):1689–93.

Henderson RD, Lawn ND, Fletcher DD, McClelland RL, Wijdicks EF. The morbidity of Guillain-Barre syndrome admitted to the intensive care unit. *Neurology.* 2003;**60**(1):17–21.

Hughes RA, Raphael JC, Swan AV, van Doorn PA. Intravenous immunoglobulin for Guillain-Barré syndrome. *Cochrane Database Syst Rev.* 2006;(1):CD002063.

Hughes RA, Wijdicks EF, Barohn R, et al. Quality Standards Subcommittee of the American Academy of Neurology. Practice parameter: immunotherapy for Guillain-Barré syndrome: report of the Quality Standards Subcommittee of the American Academy of Neurology. *Neurology.* 2003;**61**(6):736–40.

Newsome-Davis J. Diseases of the neuromuscular junction. In Asbury AK, McKhann GM, McDonald WI. (eds), *Diseases of the Nervous System. Clinical Neurobiology.* Philadelphia: WB Saunders, 1992, pp 197–212.

Oomes PG, Jacobs BC, Hazenberg MP, Banffer JR, van der Meche FG. Anti-GM1 IgG antibodies and Campylobacter bacteria in Guillain-Barré syndrome: evidence of molecular mimicry. *Ann Neurol.* 1995;**38**(2):170–5.

Rabinstein A, Wijdicks EF. BiPAP in acute respiratory failure due to myasthenic crisis may prevent intubation. *Neurology.* 2002;**59**(10):1647–9.

Raphael JC, Chevret S, Hughes RA, Annane D. Plasma exchange for Guillain-Barré syndrome *Cochrane Database Syst Rev.* 2002;(2):CD001798.

Ropper AH. Critical Care of Guillain-Barre syndrome. In *Neurological and Neurosurgical Critical Care.* 3rd ed. New York: Raven Press, 1993, pp 363–82.

Sharshar T, Chevret S, Bourdain F, Raphael JC. French Cooperative Group on Plasma Exchange in Guillain-Barré syndrome. Early predictors of mechanical ventilation in Guillain-Barré syndrome. *Crit Care Med.* 2003;**31**(1):278–83.

Van den Berghe G, Schoonheydt K, Becx P, Bruyninckx F, Wouters PJ. Insulin therapy protects the central and peripheral nervous system of intensive care patients. *Neurology.* 2005;**64**:1348–53.

Wijdicks EFM. Guillain-Barré syndrome. In *The Clinical Practice of Critical Care Neurology*, 2nd ed. Oxford University Press, 2003, pp 403–21.

Wijdicks EF, Borel CO. Respiratory management in acute neurologic illness. *Neurology.* 1998;**50**(1):11–20.

Wijdicks EF, Roy TK. BiPAP in early arre syndrome may fail. *Can J Neurol Sci.* 2006;**33**(1):105–6.

Wolfe GI, Barohn RJ, Foster BM, et al. Myasthenia Gravis-IVIG Study Group. Randomized, controlled trial of intravenous immunoglobulin in myasthenia gravis. *Muscle Nerve.* 2002;**26**(4):549–52.

Zochodne DW, Bolton CF, Wells GA, et al. Critical illness polyneuropathy A complication of sepsis and multiple organ failure *Brain.* 1987;**110**:819–41.

16 Head Trauma

Fernanda Tagliaferri, MD, Christian Compagnone, MD, and
Thomas A. Gennarelli, MD

EPIDEMIOLOGY

Traumatic brain injury (TBI) is a major cause of morbidity, mortality, and healthcare expense in the United States and Europe. Each year approximately 1 million head-injured patients are treated and released from United States emergency departments (EDs). The incidence rate of hospitalized plus fatal TBI in the United States (103 per 100,000 population) is considerably lower than in Europe (235 per 100,000 population). The mortality rate remains similar for the United States and Europe (15–20 per 100,000 population/year).

- In the United States, transportation-related crashes (involving motor vehicles, bicycles, pedestrians, and recreational vehicles) accounted for 49% of all TBIs; falls accounted for an additional 26% and firearm use (including suicide attempts) accounted for 10% of all TBIs.
- In Europe, transportation-related crashes are still the main cause of injury. However, falls represents approximately 40% of injuries and violence/assaults fewer than 5%.

CLASSIFICATION OF TBI

The Glasgow Coma Scale (GCS; Table 16.2) is widely used to evaluate the severity of brain injuries. This scale corresponds to the definition of coma as no eye opening (E < 2), no verbal utterances (V < 3), and not following commands (M < 6). However, the assessment of the components of the GCS is limited by widespread use of sedation and intubation before hospital arrival.

- TBI is stratified according to the GCS score as mild (scores 14–15), moderate (9–13), or severe (3–8).
- Increased severity of injury on admission is associated with an increased rate of death or vegetative state and a decreased rate of good recovery.

However, mild TBI does not necessarily guarantee a good recovery, and an initial severe TBI will not definitely evolve to severe disability. Thornhill et al. reported an increased dependency in 28% of mild injury survivors, 30% moderate injury survivors, and 45% severe injury survivors, whereas Whitnall et al. clearly demonstrated that 11% of severely disabled patients at 1 year after injury evolved to good recovery in 5–7 years, and 23% of them evolved to moderate disability.

An important difference exists between penetrating and blunt head injuries. Penetrating head injuries may result from gunshot wounds, stab wounds, and other forms of trauma. In penetrating head injuries the skull and dura mater are compromised. Blunt head injuries result from mechanical forces (direct tissue deformation, linear/rotary stress, and compression) transmitted to intracranial structures that may produce traumatic brain injuries, hemorrhage, or cranial nerve lesions. According to Kraus et al., patients with penetrating brain injuries are 6.58 times more likely to die than those with blunt head injuries. Overall, of all patients with head injury admitted to hospital approximately 14% will not survive.

PRIMARY INJURIES

Primary injury is the neurologic damage that occurs at the moment of impact. It is the immediate consequence of head contact or the effect of induced head motions.

Diffuse Axonal Injury

A typical lesion associated with rapid rotational head motion is diffuse axonal injury (DAI). It depends on inertial forces that are commonly produced by motor vehicle crashes. These inertial forces are a result of rapid head rotational motions, which deform the white matter and lead to DAI, often referred to as "shearing" brain injury. Coma is the most common immediate impairment that has been associated with the severity of DAI. Gennarelli et al. demonstrated that DAI can be a sole cause of posttraumatic coma.

■ The "gold standard" for the diagnosis of DAI is the microscopic examination of the tissue that typically reveals a multitude of swollen and disconnected axons.

■ Computed tomography (CT) scan is limited in the detection of DAI; however, indirect signs could lead to the diagnosis of DAI. In the acute phase CT may show multiple petechial foci of hemorrhage commonly found in the central third of the brain, especially in the hemispheric subcortical lobar white matter, corpus callosum, basal ganglia, brain stem, and cerebellum.

■ Because of the poor sensitivity of CT in detection of DAI, magnetic resonance imaging (MRI) may be helpful as soon as feasible to evaluate better the extent of the injury.

Focal Parenchymal Injuries

CONTUSIONS

Focal lesions result in damage of capillaries or other tissue components (glial cells, nerve cells, etc.). Contusions can develop in the zone of the impact (coup contusions), evolve in the opposite side of the impact (contre-coup contusions), or can be present in deep structures (intermediate coup contusions). Contusions are also associated with fractures or may be due to the impact of the tentorium with bone structure of the foramen magnum in the herniation contusions.

■ On CT scan, contusions generally appear as a hemorrhagic core surrounded by an edematous low-density area.

■ A wide range of cerebral blood flow (CBF) was found in and around the majority of contusions.

■ The low pericontusional values suggest that much of this tissue is viable but vulnerable to secondary injury and ischemia. Some authors compare the low-density pericontusional area with the penumbra zone in stroke.

POSTTRAUMATIC INTRACEREBRAL HEMATOMA

Intracerebral hematoma (ICH) is a hematoma >2 cm in contact with the cortex. The incident in autopsy reports is approximately 15%. The cause is the rupture of blood vessels (single or multiple) at the moment of trauma.

EXTRACEREBRAL HEMATOMAS

EPIDURAL/EXTRADURAL HEMATOMA. Epidural/extradural hematoma (EDH) is the presence of blood between the inner surface of the skull and the dura mater, as a consequence of rupture of arteries and meningeal vessels. It is frequently associated with temporal fractures. On CT scans, EDH appears as a biconvex lenticular shape. In 20% of patients, there is a lucid interval (normal neurologic examination) before the clinical worsening.

SUBDURAL HEMATOMA. Acute subdural hematoma (SDH) is the presence of blood in the subdural space. It is usually due to the rupture of the bridging veins or cortical arteries. It could also be associated with brain surface contusions and bleeding in the subdural space.

TRAUMATIC SUBARACHNOID HEMORRHAGE. Traumatic subarachnoid hemorrhage (tSAH) represents bleeding into the subarachnoid space after craniocerebral trauma, as consequence of rupture of cortical arteries, veins and capillaries from brain surface contusions. The Traumatic Coma Data Bank and the European Brain Injury Consortium report an incidence of tSAH of 40%.

SECONDARY INJURIES. All neurologic damage does not occur immediately at the moment of impact (primary injury) but evolves afterwards (delayed injury). Low oxygen delivery in hypotension, hypoxia, edema, intracranial hypertension, or changes in CBF or cascades that involve delayed cellular damage account for development of secondary injuries. It is important to prevent the secondary injuries because these will increase the odds of unfavorable outcome.

HYPOTENSION AND HYPOXIA

In 1993, a study based on the Traumatic Coma Data Bank revealed the influence of secondary brain insults on outcome. The occurrence of at least one episode of hypotension (SBP < 90 mm Hg) from the time of injury through resuscitation was associated with a doubling of mortality and a marked increase in morbidity. More than 10 years later, the IMPACT study demonstrated that hypoxia and hypotension are still relatively common on admission, with an observed overall prevalence of 20% and 18%, respectively. In this study, hypotension increased the odds of death by 2.62 times (95% CI 1.99, 3.47) while hypoxia increased the odds of death by 2.02 (95% CI 1.61, 2.55). Each was an independent predictor of an adverse outcome in a multivariate analysis.

HYPERTHERMIA

Hyperthermia in the neurointensive care setting is very common. Hyperthermia can occur from central dysregulation of body temperature due to hypothalamic injury or from extracranial infection or inflammatory process. Kilpatrick et al. reported that more than 50% of TBI patients had at least one febrile episode ($T > 38.5^0$C) during the stay in the ICU. Hyperthermia after TBI is known to increase morbidity and mortality.

HYPERGLYCEMIA

Severely head-injured patients frequently develop hyperglycemia usually due to stress or brain-induced catecholamine release and the elevated serum glucose level may aggravate ischemic insults and worsen the neurologic outcome. Early hyperglycemia (>170 mg/dL) was associated with poor outcomes for patients with severe traumatic brain injury. Therefore, a tight control of serum glucose without reduction of nutritional support may improve the prognosis for these critically ill patients.

HYPONATREMIA

In acute hypotonic hyponatremia, water enters the brain and causes cerebral edema. Owing to the rigidity of the cranium, this cellular swelling can lead to serious complications, including seizures, coma, brainstem herniation, respiratory arrest, and even death.

SEIZURES

Posttraumatic seizures (PTS) are classified as immediate, early, or late when seizures occur within 24 hours, 7 days, or longer than 7 days after injury, respectively. The overall incidence of PTS in all levels of TBI severity is 5–7%. However, the incidence of PTS in severe blunt TBI is 11% and up to 35–50% in penetrating TBI. According to Vespa et al., seizures occur in 22% of the moderate to severe brain-injured patients. In the article, more than half of the seizures were nonconvulsive and were diagnosed on the basis of EEG studies alone. This is important to keep in mind when inexplicable increases in intracranial pressure (ICP) occur or when an inexplicable low GCS is present. In the acute period, seizures may precipitate adverse event in the injured brain because of elevations in the intracranial pressure, blood pressure changes, and changes in the oxygen delivery.

Patients with significantly elevated risk for posttraumatic seizures are those with:

- Evacuation of a subdural or epidural hematoma
- Surgery for an intracerebral hematoma
- GCS <8
- Depressed skull fracture that was not surgically elevated
- Dural penetration by injury
- At least one nonreactive pupil
- Cortical contusion and parietal lesions on CT scan

Early seizures increase the risk for late seizures. For those reasons, prophylactic use of anticonvulsant medication is indicated for the first 7 days after injury.

Monitoring

Neuromonitoring is extensively discussed in Chapter 8 (intracranial pressure and cerebral blood

Table 16.1. Indications for ICP monitoring

Indications for ICP monitoring in severely head injured patients
• Abnormal CT scan
– Presence of Haematoma or Contusions
– Edema or Swelling
– Compression of basal cisterns
• Normal CT scan and two or more risk factors.
– Age greater than 40 years
– Abnormal motor movements
– Arterial Hypotension (systolic lower than 90 mm Hg)

flow monitoring) and Chapter 9 (hemodynamic monitoring). In this chapter we briefly review the indications for ICP monitoring.

Unfortunately, clinical examinations have low sensitivity and low specificity for diagnosis of high ICP. CT scans in the acute phase have a high positive but a low negative predictive value. Patients with a GCS ≤8 and normal CT scan have a 10–15% incidence of high ICP. In the presence of risk factors (age >40 years, abnormal motor movements, or arterial hypotension) this incidence rate increases up to 60%. The indications for ICP monitoring in severely head injured patients are shown in Table 16.1. At this time, there are no guidelines for the treatment or monitoring of moderate head injured patients. In these cases, the monitoring of ICP should be evaluated individually according to the clinical and radiological findings.

In the last few years, different types of monitoring have been developed in addition to the ICP. CBF can be measured by means of xenon CT, CT perfusion, positron emission tomography (PET), or MRI and indirectly by transcranial Doppler. Metabolic rate ($pTio_2$, microdialysis, and PET) and electric activity (EEG, visual evoked potential [VEP], brain stem auditory evoked potential [BAEP], etc.) can also be monitored. A multimodal monitoring (association of diverse techniques of monitoring) had been advised to increase sensibility and specificity in detecting complications such as ischemia. However, there is no evidence that multimodal monitoring improves outcome.

Physical Examination

Adequate airway, oxygenation, ventilation, and circulation should be ensured. The neurologic examination should immediately assess the level of consciousness, focal deficits, and signs of herniation. The Glasgow Coma Scale (GCS) evaluates the response to stimuli in patients with craniocerebral injuries. The parameters are eye opening, motor response, and verbal response (Table 16.2). Asymmetric motor responses (spontaneous or stimulus induced) have localizing value.

Herniation occurs when mass lesions or edema causes shifts in brain tissue. Failure to recognize herniation sings will cause irreversible brain damage and death. These signs depend on the type of herniation. Clinical evaluation should focus on headache, nausea, vomiting, transient visual obscurations, alterations in consciousness, focal deficits, and respiratory irregularity or apnea.

If the patient already has an altered level of consciousness and is intubated, herniation should be suspected if the patient develops hypertension, bradycardia, anisocoria (asymmetric pupils), focal deficits, or posturing of the extremities. Serial examinations with pupil size and light reactivity (Table 16.3) must be performed and documented to identify neurologic deterioration early.

Hemotympanum, postauricular hematoma (Battle's sign), periorbital hematoma (raccoon eyes), and cerebrospinal fluid (CSF) otorrhea/rhinorrhea are indicative of basilar skull fracture. If those signs are present DO NOT place a nasogastric/nasotracheal tube.

The neurologic examination should also include a careful search for penetrating wounds. Foreign objects should NOT be moved. Active bleeding from scalp wounds can result in significant blood loss. Initial therapy involves application of direct pressure and inspection of the wound to exclude bone involvement. Neurosurgical consultation is indicated for patients with GCS <8 to evaluate an ICP catheter placement or whenever a contusion, intracranial hematoma, cervical fracture, skull fractures, penetrating injuries, or focal neurologic deficits are present.

When possible, the trauma and past medical history should be assessed. The trauma history should focus on the time of injury, mechanism of trauma, loss of consciousness, occurrence of a lucid interval

Table 16.2. Glasgow Coma Scale

Eye opening		Motor response		Verbal response	
Spontaneous	4	Obeys	6	Oriented	5
To speech	3	Localized	5*	Confused	4
To pain	2	Withdraws	4	Inappropriate	3
None	1*	Abnormal flexion	3	Incomprehensible	2*
–	–	Extensor response	2	None	1
–	–	None	1	–	–

* Needed to defined "coma."

Table 16.3. Pupil examination

Pupil size	Uni/bilateral	Light reactive	Probable cause
Large	Bilateral	None	Brain death*
Large (>1 mm of difference in pupil diameter)	Unilateral	Poor	Uncal herniation Eye contusion Focal seizures Anticholinergic droplets
Large	Bilateral	Present	Pain Seizures Drugs (atropine, norepinephrine, dopamine)
Midposition	Bilateral	None	Transtentorial herniation.
Small	Bilateral	Present (difficult to evaluate)	Narcotic agents Metabolic encephalopathy Thalamic or pontine lesions
Small (<1 mm)	Bilateral	Present (difficult to evaluate)	Acute pontine lesions

* When no ocular injury is present.

(which suggests expanding hematoma), amnesia (which is related to the severity of the blow), possible hypoxia or hypotension, seizures and prehospital/ED treatment. The past medical history should focus on allergies, comorbid factors, medications, and last oral intake.

Treatment

MEDICAL TREATMENT
By the time a patient is admitted to the ICU, several things should already have been accomplished (Table 16.4). If the patient arrives to the ICU without a complete initial resuscitation, the ABCDE must be started as soon as possible.

The indications for ICU admission are summarized in Table 16.4. These indications should be considered as a guideline and not as exclusive criteria. On arrival in ICU, the severity assessment should be repeated and the monitoring systems required and the ICU treatment plan should be determined (Table 16.4).

MECHANICAL VENTILATION:
Endotracheal intubation is mandatory for every patient with a GCS ≤8 and others with respiratory insufficiency based on extracranial injury, comorbid diseases, or age. If the GCS is >8, endotracheal intubation should be evaluated individually. The importance of an adequate oxygenation in a TBI patient has been stressed previously in this chapter.

Table 16.4. ICU admission

Before ICU admission	Indications for ICU admission	Upon arrival in ICU

• ABCDE*
 • Initial severity assessment
   – GCS
   – Pupils
   – CT
 • Initial blood laboratory studies
   – Cross-match
   – blood chemistries,
   – hematologic analysis
   – coagulation profile
   – blood gas
   – toxicologic analysis
   – Urinalysis
   – β-human chorionic gonadotropin level if the patient is a woman of childbearing age
 • Initial diagnosis
 • Initial treatment plan
   – Medical
   – Emergency surgery
	• Head Injury Severity
	   – GCS≤8
	   – GCS>8 + risk of evolving lesions
	   – Secondary injuries
	     • Hypoxia
	     • Hypotension
	     • Seizures, etc
	 • Extracranial injury severity
	   – Life threatening
	   – Potentially life threatening
	 • Co-morbid factors
	   – Age: Children and elderly
	   – Illnesses requiring monitoring
	     • Hypertension
	     • Diabetes
	     • Chronic respiratory failure
	     • Chronic Cardiac failure
	     • Neurologic problems, etc
	   – Chronic drug treatment
	     • Anticoagulant Agent
	     • Platelet-inhibitors Agents (ASA)
		• Repeat severity assessment
		 • Determine monitoring systems required
		   – Hemodynamic
		   – ICP
		   – CBF
		   – SjO_2
		   – EEG
		   – $PtiO_2$
		   – Microdialysis
		   – Further imagines
		 • Determine treatment plan
		   – Mechanical ventilation
		   – Fluid types and volumes
		   – Vasopressors
		   – ICP and CPP goals
		   – Check blood laboratory values
		   – Body T** goals
		   – ATB prophylaxis**
		   – FAST HUG***
		     • **F**eeding
		     • **A**nalgesia
		     • **S**edation
		     • **T**hromboembolic prophylaxis^
		     • **H**ead-of-bed elevation†
		     • Stress **U**lcer Prevention‡
		     • **G**lucose control

* Initial resuscitation (airway, breathing, circulation, disability, exposure).
** According to the injuries.
*** Vincent JL. Give your patient a fast hug (at least) once a day. *Crit Care Med.* 2005; **33**(6): 1225–9.
^ Pneumatic compression stockings.
† Check spinal cord lesions.
‡ If needed.

- The Pao_2 should be maintained above 60 mm Hg and the O_2 saturation above 90%.
- At the same time, the $Paco_2$ should be maintained at 35–40 mm Hg because reduction of $Paco_2$ causes arterial vasoconstriction and reduction of CBF.
  - Flow may already be reduced in the first 24 hours after injury, and its further reduction by hypocarbia may produce brain ischemia.
  - After 24 hours, this occurs rarely because flow usually is restored to almost normal.
  - Therefore, the use of prophylactic hyperventilation should be avoided because it can compromise cerebral perfusion.

FLUIDS TYPES

The American college of Surgeons suggests the rapid infusion of 2 liters of Ringer's lactate as initial resuscitative crystalloid bolus in every polytrauma patient. Crystalloids primary fill the interstitial space; therefore edema is an expected outcome of resuscitation. In head injury patients, dilutional hypo-osmolarity may worsen brain edema and may cause pulmonary edema as well. Colloid fluids are more efficient than crystalloids in expanding plasma volume. However, whether to use colloids or crystalloids is a controversy that has existed for decades. There is no evidence from randomized controlled trials that resuscitation with colloids reduces the risk of death, compared to resuscitation with crystalloids in trauma patients. Colloids are not associated with an improvement in survival and are more expensive than crystalloids. In any case, in the first day after brain injury, autoregulation of CBF to blood pressure changes is commonly abnormal, so overhydration is to be avoided because too much fluid volume can cause hypertension and consequent increased CBF, cerebral blood volume, and ICP.

INTRACRANIAL PRESSURE AND CEREBRAL PERFUSION PRESSURE

According to the guidelines ICP treatment should be initiated at an upper threshold of 20–25 mm Hg and the cerebral perfusion pressure (CPP) (MAP – ICP) should be maintained at a minimum of 60 mm Hg (Fig. 16.1). In children and decompressed patients, ICP treatment should be started at an upper threshold of 15 mm Hg. High values of ICP were associated with poor outcome.

It is important to understand why ICP is high before starting the treatment. Often this is associated with neurologic worsening defined by the occurrence of one or more of the following objective criteria:

- A spontaneous decrease in the GCS motor score of ≥2 points (compared with the previous examination)
- A new loss of pupillary reactivity
- Interval development of pupillary asymmetry of ≥2 mm
- Deterioration in neurologic status sufficient to warrant immediate medical or surgical intervention

An unknown expanding mass lesion can cause high ICP refractory to medical treatment. Poor

positioning, agitation, hyperthermia, hypoventilation, or noxious stimuli can cause an ICP increase that can be easily corrected.

Early posttraumatic seizures can be prevented with anticonvulsants. Phenytoin and carbamazepine are recommended in high-risk patients as a treatment option in the first week after trauma.

- The recommended *phenytoin* loading dose is 10–20 mg/kg via IV infusion.
- The rate of IV administration should not exceed 50 mg/min because of cardiac depression.
- A typical initial maintenance dose is 4–6 mg/kg per day IV, divided into 2 or more doses.
- Continuous monitoring of the electrocardiogram, blood pressure, and respiratory function is essential during loading dose administration.
- Therapeutic serum concentrations are 10–20 μg/ mL.

Ventricular drainage of CSF, when available, is the first step in the treatment of high ICP.

If the ICP remains high, ventilation may be adjusted to a mild hyperventilation for a short period of time. If mild hypocapnia is ineffective in controlling ICP, mannitol can be used. Effective doses of mannitol 20% range from 0.25 g/kg to 1 g/ kg body weight IV × 1.

- Mannitol will cause hyperosmolarity, dehydration, and fluid imbalance.
- A Foley catheter and a central venous pressure monitoring are essential in these patients, and fluid replacement, osmolarity, and electrolyte controls are mandatory.
- If osmolarity exceeds 320 mOsmol, there is a risk of acute tubular necrosis and acute renal failure.

Mannitol is known to cause "opening" in the blood–brain barrier, meaning that mannitol molecules can pass into the brain, causing a reversed osmotic gradient leading to fluid flow into the brain and brain swelling. A Cochrane review reported that mannitol therapy for raised ICP may have a detrimental effect on mortality when compared to hypertonic saline (HS). HS has been demonstrated to reduce ICP in TBI patients with high ICP when is used from 3% to 23.4%.

- A central venous line and a tight serum sodium control are required.

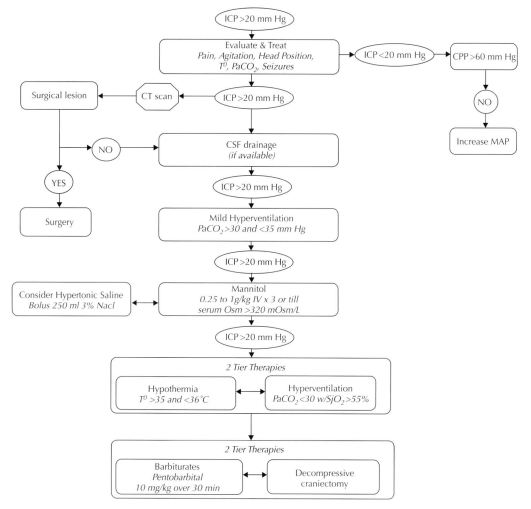

Figure 16.1. Algorithms for high ICP treatment. (Adapted from Brain Trauma Foundation guidelines.)

- Serum sodium should not be increased more or decreased less than 10 mEq/L over 24 hours for the risk of producing central pontine myelinolysis

    When there is an acute neurologic deterioration or if ICP is refractory to sedation, paralysis, CSF drainage, and mannitol or HS, second tier therapies might be necessary. There is no consensus about which one should be the first in the algorithm. We suggest starting with hyperventilation or hypothermia, considering them less risky than barbiturate therapy and decompressive craniectomy.

- Severe hyperventilation therapy ($Paco_2 \leq 30$ mm Hg) should be monitored with jugular venous

oxygen saturation ($Sjo_2 < 55\%$) to identify risk of ischemia. CBF monitoring may complete the diagnosis of ischemia.

- Hypothermia.
- High-dose barbiturate therapy might be considered in hemodynamically stable patients with refractory high ICP.
    ▸ The Guidelines recommends the Eisenberg pentobarbital protocol.
        ▹ The loading dose of *pentobarbital* is 10 mg/kg over 30 minutes or 5 mg/kg per hour for 3 hours, and the maintenance dose is 1 mg/kg per hour.
    ▸ In some countries where pentobarbital is not available, thiopental could be used.

▷ The loading dose of *thiopental* is 10–20 mg/kg IV slow bolus followed by 3–5 mg/kg per hour IV via continuous infusion.

▷ A lower loading dose of 5–11 mg/kg IV slow bolus followed by 4–6 mg/kg per hour IV via continuous infusion may also be effective.

▶ Barbiturate therapy requires *extreme* attention to the MAP because of unpredictable cardiac effects that produce hypotension. Therefore, pressure support may be required to keep MAP and CPP normal. ICP, mean arterial pressure, cerebral perfusion pressure, and EEG burst suppression should be monitored.

▶ Some authors consider propofol as an alternative to barbiturates for high ICP. The loading dose of propofol is 1–2 mg/kg IV followed by 2–10 mg/kg per hour IV as a continuous infusion. Continuous MAP, EEG and serum triglycerides must be monitored. Surgical decompressive craniectomy is discussed later.

SURGICAL TREATMENT

In the 2006 Guidelines, an international panel of experts, analyzed the current evidence for surgical treatment of TBI. As expected, they were unable to define treatment standards because all reported papers were at the level of simple options. The cause, at least in part, would be that the randomization of patients with large hematomas in a non-surgical arm is not compatible with the best clinical practice or current ethical standards. In the following text, we summarize agreements and uncertainties regarding surgical indications in traumatic brain injury.

GENERAL INDICATIONS FOR MASS EVACUATION

The decision to perform surgery is related to many factors. Clinical status (especially neuroworsening) and CT parameters (lesion volume >30 mL, midline shift >5 mm, cisternal compression and lesion location) are the most important factors to decide the surgery. As a guideline, a hematoma volume >25 cm³ should be considered for surgical evacuation. However, in a clinical context it is only another variable to consider. As any lesion may eventually evolve, surgical indication is a dynamic process. Neither a good clinical status on admission nor a small hematoma on the first CT scan can exclude subsequent surgical indications.

EXTRADURAL HEMATOMA

The small acute extradural hematoma (EDH; <30 cm³, with <15 mm thickness), with <5 mm midline shift, in patients without neurologic deficits, can be managed conservatively. However, according to Sullivan et al., 23% of EDH initially managed conservatively evolves within 8 hours after injury. As a consequence, all the patients treated conservatively, must be followed with at least a second CT obtained within 6 hours from injury.

SUBDURAL HEMATOMA

Small subdural hematoma (SDH; <10 mm) with a midline shift <5 mm may be managed conservatively. In these cases, the patients must be controlled clinically, and comatose patients should be monitored with an ICP device.

INTRACEREBRAL HEMATOMAS AND CONTUSIONS

Intracerebral hematomas (ICH) and contusions constitute the lesions more frequently evacuated at some distance from injury. Surgical treatments are based on clinical deterioration, CT evolution and/or ICP increases. The risk factors for enlargement of ICH are coagulation disorders, older age, SAH, and GCS at admission. Particular attention must be paid to frontal or temporal contusions which may enlarge dramatically in the first 48 hours. For this reason, a second CT scan is always necessary.

DECOMPRESSIVE CRANIECTOMY

When general treatment and first tier maneuvers fail to control ICP, second tier measures such as decompressive craniectomy (DC) should be considered. DC generates an increase in cranial volume by removing bone and opening the dura.

■ It is important to perform a large decompression. Large craniectomies (12 × 15 cm) were associated to better outcome and lower incidence of delayed intracranial hematoma, incisional hernia and CSF fistula than small craniectomies.

■ Several studies were published about the use of DC for high ICP treatment with wide differences in terms of inclusion criteria, timing and techniques.

■ A recent Cochrane review identified a single randomized trial affecting death and disability. This study includes 27 pediatric patients enrolled in a 7-year period. There is only reduced evidence (case report and small series) that DC affects the outcome in adult cohort.

■ There are some clinical trials on going (Rescue and Decra). Meanwhile, the use of DC should be based on the patient's characteristics and on the intensive care physician and neurosurgeon experience.

REFERENCES

American College of Surgeons CoT. *Advanced Trauma Life Support Manual*. Chicago; 1997.

Brain Trauma Foundation. The American Association of Neurological Surgeons. The Joint Section on Neurotrauma and Critical Care. Initial management. *J Neurotrauma*. 2000;**17**(6–7):463–9.

Bullock R, Chesnut RM, Clifton G, et al. Guidelines for the management of severe head injury. Brain Trauma Foundation. *Eur J Emerg Med*. 1996;**3**(2):109–27.

Bullock MR, Chesnut R, Ghajar J, et al. Surgical management of traumatic parenchymal lesions. *Neurosurgery*. 2006;**58**(3 Suppl):S25–46; discussion Si–iv.

Chesnut RM, Marshall SB, Piek J, Blunt BA, Klauber MR, Marshall LF. Early and late systemic hypotension as a frequent and fundamental source of cerebral ischemia following severe brain injury in the Traumatic Coma Data Bank. *Acta Neurochir Suppl (Wien)*. 1993;**59**:121–5.

Compagnone C, Murray GD, Teasdale GM, et al. The management of patients with intradural post-traumatic mass lesions: a multicenter survey of current approaches to surgical management in 729 patients coordinated by the European Brain Injury Consortium. *Neurosurgery*. 2005;**57**(6):1183–92; discussion 1183–92.

Diringer MN, Zazulia AR. Hyponatremia in neurologic patients: consequences and approaches to treatment. *Neurologist*. 2006;**12**(3):117–26.

Geffroy A, Bronchard R, Merckx P, Seince PF, Faillot T, Albaladejo P, Marty J. Severe traumatic head injury in adults: which patients are at risk of early hyperthermia? *Intens Care Med*. 2004;**30**(5):785–90.

Gennarelli TA, Champion HR, Copes WS, Sacco WJ. Comparison of mortality, morbidity, and severity of 59,713 head injured patients with 114,447 patients with extracranial injuries. *J Trauma*. 1994;**37**(6):962–8.

Gennarelli TA, Thibault LE, Adams JH, Graham DI, Thompson CJ, Marcincin RP. Diffuse axonal injury and traumatic coma in the primate. *Ann Neurol*. 1982;**12**(6):564–74.

Guerrero JL, Thurman DJ, Sniezek JE. Emergency department visits associated with traumatic brain injury: United States, 1995–1996. *Brain Inj*. 2000;**14**(2):181–6.

Jeremitsky E, Omert LA, Dunham CM, Wilberger J, Rodriguez A. The impact of hyperglycemia on patients with severe brain injury. *J Trauma*. 2005;**58**(1):47–50.

Jiang JY, Gao GY, Li WP, Yu MK, Zhu C. Early indicators of prognosis in 846 cases of severe traumatic brain injury. *J Neurotrauma*. 2002;**19**(7):869–74.

Jiang JY, Xu W, Li WP, et al. Efficacy of standard trauma craniectomy for refractory intracranial hypertension with severe traumatic brain injury: a multicenter, prospective, randomized controlled study. *J Neurotrauma*. 2005;**22**(6):623–8.

Kilpatrick MM, Lowry DW, Firlik AD, Yonas H, Marion DW. Hyperthermia in the neurosurgical intensive care unit. *Neurosurgery*. 2000;**47**(4):850–5; discussion 855–6.

Kraus JF, Peek-Asa C, McArthur D. The independent effect of gender on outcomes following traumatic brain injury: a preliminary investigation. *Neurosurg Focus*. 2000; **8**(1):e5.

Lam AM, Winn HR, Cullen BF, Sundling N. Hyperglycemia and neurological outcome in patients with head injury. *J Neurosurg*. 1991;**75**(4):545–51.

Langlois J, Rutland-Brown W, Thomas K. *Traumatic Brain Injury in the United States: Emergency Department Visit, Hospitalizations, and Deaths*. Atlanta, Georgia: Centers for Disease Control and Prevention, National Center for Injury Prevention and Control; 2004.

Martin RJ. Central pontine and extrapontine myelinolysis: the osmotic demyelination syndromes. *J Neurol Neurosurg Psychiatry*. 2004;**75**(Suppl 3):iii22–8.

McHugh GS, Engel DC, Butcher I, et al. Prognostic value of secondary insults in traumatic brain injury: results from the IMPACT study. *J Neurotrauma*. 2007; **24**(2):287–93.

Morris GF, Juul N, Marshall SB, Benedict B, Marshall LF. Neurological deterioration as a potential alternative endpoint in human clinical trials of experimental pharmacological agents for treatment of severe traumatic brain injuries. Executive Committee of the International Selfotel Trial. *Neurosurgery*. 1998;**43**(6):1369–72; discussion 1364–72.

Roberts I, Alderson P, Bunn F, Chinnock P, Ker K, Schierhout G. Colloids versus crystalloids for fluid resuscitation in critically ill patients. *Cochrane Database Syst Rev*. 2004;(4):CD000567.

Sahuquillo J, Arikan F. Decompressive craniectomy for the treatment of refractory high intracranial pressure in traumatic brain injury. *Cochrane Database Syst Rev*. 2006;(1):CD003983.

Statham PF, Johnston RA, Macpherson P. Delayed deterioration in patients with traumatic frontal contusions. *J Neurol Neurosurg Psychiatry*. 1989;**52**(3):351–4.

Stocchetti N, Pagan F, Calappi E, et al. Inaccurate early assessment of neurological severity in head injury. *J Neurotrauma*. 2004;**21**(9):1131–40.

Sullivan TP, Jarvik JG, Cohen WA. Follow-up of conservatively managed epidural hematomas: implications for timing of repeat CT. *AJNR Am J Neuroradiol*. 1999; **20**(1):107–13.

Tagliaferri F, Compagnone C, Korsic M, Servadei F, Kraus J. A systematic review of brain injury epidemiology in Europe. *Acta Neurochir (Wien)*. 2006;**148**(3):255–68; discussion 268.

Taylor A, Butt W, Rosenfeld J, et al. A randomized trial of very early decompressive craniectomy in children with traumatic brain injury and sustained intracranial hypertension. *Childs Nerv Syst.* 2001;**17**(3):154–62.

Teasdale G, Jennett B. Assessment of coma and impaired consciousness. A practical scale. *Lancet.* 1974;**2**(7872):81–4.

Teasell R, Bayona N, Lippert C, Villamere J, Hellings C. Post-traumatic seizure disorder following acquired brain injury. *Brain Inj.* 2007;**21**(2):201–14.

Temkin NR. Risk factors for posttraumatic seizures in adults. *Epilepsia.* 2003;44 Suppl **10**:18–20.

Temkin NR, Dikmen SS, Winn HR. Management of head injury. Posttraumatic seizures. *Neurosurg Clin N Am.* 1991;**2**(2):425–35.

Thornhill S, Teasdale GM, Murray GD, McEwen J, Roy CW, Penny KI. Disability in young people and adults one year after head injury: prospective cohort study. *BMJ.* 2000; **320**(7250):1631–5.

Thurman DJ, Alverson C, Dunn KA, Guerrero J, Sniezek JE. Traumatic brain injury in the United States: a public health perspective. *J Head Trauma Rehabil.* 1999;**14**(6):602–15.

Vespa PM, Nuwer MR, Nenov V, et al. Increased incidence and impact of nonconvulsive and convulsive seizures after traumatic brain injury as detected by continuous electroencephalographic monitoring. *J Neurosurg.* 1999;**91**(5):750–60.

Vincent JL. Give your patient a fast hug (at least) once a day. *Crit Care Med.* 2005;**33**(6):1225–9.

Wakai A, Roberts I, Schierhout G. Mannitol for acute traumatic brain injury. *Cochrane Database Syst Rev.* 2005;(4): CD001049.

Whitnall L, McMillan TM, Murray GD, Teasdale GM. Disability in young people and adults after head injury: 5–7 year follow up of a prospective cohort study. *J Neurol Neurosurg Psychiatry.* 2006;**77**(5):640–5.

17 Encephalopathy

Angelos Katramados, MD and Panayiotis N. Varelas, MD, PhD

Encephalopathy is a common complication of systemic illness or direct brain injury. It can manifest as a spectrum that begins with subtle cognitive changes, progresses as a full-blown syndrome of brain dysfunction, and eventually leads to coma or brain death (the latter two are described in separate chapters). In this chapter, we focus on the detection, etiologic diagnosis, and management of noncomatose, critically ill, encephalopathic patients. Their condition has been traditionally known with several interchangeable names such as acute confusional state, acute organic brain syndrome, and acute cerebral insufficiency, but is most commonly referred to as delirium.

Delirium contributes significantly to lengthened hospital stay, increased morbidity and mortality, increased overall medical costs, and worse long-term neurocognitive outcomes. Despite the awareness of its existence since the earliest historical medical documents, timely detection, workup, and appropriate management continue to present challenges for the treating physicians. Delirious patients in the Intensive Care Unit (ICU) form a particularly understudied population with unique characteristics.

- Delirium has been described as an acute alteration of consciousness and higher cognitive functions.
- It typically develops over a short period of time and has a fluctuating course.
- It is a well-defined syndrome that may be precipitated by several diverse pathological processes.
- The current edition of the *Diagnostic and Statistic Manual* (DSM-IV TR) lists criteria for the diagnosis of delirium due to a general medical condition (Table 17.1).[1]

The incidence of delirium has been estimated as between 5% and 40% for hospitalized patients in general and between 11% and 80% for critically ill patients. Other studies have reported a lower incidence of about 30%, after the exclusion of patients maintained in purposeful drug-induced sedation.

Among hospitalized, critically ill patients, delirium typically develops in those who have predisposing risk factors such as:

- Older age (older than 70 years)
- Male gender
- Poor functional status
- Malnutrition
- Substance abuse
- Premorbid medical conditions or cognitive impairment
- Polypharmacy
- Physical restraints
- Visual or hearing impairment
- Prior history of delirium

These factors have been found to correlate with the possibility and extent of functional recovery after the resolution of the acute insult.

ETIOLOGY

Several diverse pathological processes, which can precipitate delirium in vulnerable patients, are listed in Table 17.2. Those are broadly classified in diagnostic categories. Even though there are multiple and additive etiologies in most delirious patients, it is frequently possible to distinguish a primary disease process that can be the focus of treatment strategies.

Table 17.1. DSM-IV-TR diagnostic criteria for delirium due to a general medical condition

A. Disturbance of consciousness (i.e., reduced clarity of awareness of the environment) with reduced ability to focus, to sustain, or to shift attention.

B. A change in cognition (such as memory deficit, disorientation, or language disturbance) or the development of a perceptual disturbance that is not better accounted for by a preexisting, established, or evolving dementia.

C. The disturbance develops over a short period of time (usually hours to days) and tends to fluctuate during the course of the day.

D. There is evidence from the history, physical examination, or laboratory findings that the disturbance is caused by the direct physiologic consequences of a general medical condition.

From American Psychiatric Association. Task Force on DSM-IV. *Diagnostic and Statistical Manual of Mental Disorders*: DSM-IV-TR, 4th ed. Washington, DC: American Psychiatric Association; 2000.

Table 17.2. Etiology of delirium

Vascular	Ischemic stroke, transient ischemic attack, subarachnoid hemorrhage, intracerebral hemorrhage, epidural hematoma, subdural hematoma, cerebral venous thrombosis, myocardial infarction, pulmonary embolism, extreme hypertension/hypotension.
Infectious	Meningitis, encephalitis, cerebral abscess, neurosyphilis, Lyme disease, systemic sepsis, HIV infection and complications, pneumonia, urinary tract infection,
Inflammatory	CNS lupus erythematosus, Giant cell arteritis, neurosarcoidosis.
Neoplastic	Systemic cancer, paraneoplastic syndromes, CNS tumors, carcinomatous meningitis.
Legal and illegal drugs	Anticholinergics, narcotics, benzodiazepines, barbiturates, anesthetics, digitalis, corticosteroids, antiparkinsonian, antiepileptics, immunosuppressants (tacrolimus), recreational drugs (abuse or withdrawal), over-the-counter medications, herbal preparations
Recent surgery	Cardiac, orthopedic, CNS surgery, other invasive procedures
Trauma	Traumatic brain injury, multiple organ trauma, air or fat embolism.
Metabolic	Liver failure, uremia, hypoglycemia, hyperglycemia, electrolyte abnormalities, hypercarbia, hypoxia
Endocrine	Thyroid, parathyroid, pituitary, adrenal gland dysfunction, uncontrolled diabetes, pancreatitis.
Epileptic	Postictal conditions, status epilepticus (convulsive or nonconvulsive)
Nutritional	Thiamine, B_{12}, folic acid deficiencies,
Hereditary	Mitochondrial disorders (MELAS)
Miscellaneous	Anemia, dehydration, volume overload, burns, chronic obstructive pulmonary disease (COPD), migraine, sensory deprivation, sleep deprivation, posterior reversible encephalopathy syndrome, Reye syndrome

Particularly in the ICU population, most underlying processes are the ones responsible for the initial hospitalization and ICU admission. However, ICU delirium is often the result of environmental factors or iatrogenic interventions. The use of psychoactive medications (especially opiate narcotics and benzodiazepines) is common in critically ill patients and strongly correlates with the development of delirium. Other important factors are the sleep disruption in an ICU environment, bladder catheterization, physical restraints, sensory deprivation, and frequent invasive vascular access procedures.

CLINICAL FEATURES OF DELIRIUM

Delirium syndromes share many common clinical features, regardless of the underlying etiology. As described in the DSM-IV criteria:

- An alteration in the level of consciousness should be present. This is not as severe as in coma, where there is a profound impairment of arousal. It may range from paradoxical agitation (hyperactive delirium) to sedation and stupor (hypoactive delirium).
- Attention impairment is one of the hallmarks of delirium. This can manifest as difficulty maintaining attention (distractibility) or shifting the focus of attention (perseveration). This is typically tested by asking the patient to perform serial subtractions, multistep commands or assessing digit span.
- Fluctuation of symptomatology is also a prominent characteristic of delirium. Symptoms frequently worsen at night, often in association with a sleep–wake reversal. At times, patients may intermittently seem cognitively intact, something that may contribute to the delayed detection of the condition.
- Hallucinations, disorientation, and perceptual distortions often dominate the clinical picture, particularly in the hyperactive type. Visual hallucinations and illusions are most common and may result in attempts to dislodge endotracheal tubes or IV lines, thus compromising patient safety.
- Disorders of thought processes and memory are frequent and may need to be differentiated from an underlying dementia. Patients with delirium are more likely to have disorganized thinking, even to the point of incoherent speech, as well as immediate and recent memory impairment.

STANDARDIZED DETECTION

Delirium is frequently diagnosed in a delayed fashion, particularly in the ICU setting. Often, other lifesaving procedures take precedence in the patient's management and preclude serial assessments of the mental status. Many critically ill patients are nonverbal or even mechanically ventilated, and the evaluation of their higher cognitive functions is, thus, extremely difficult. Moreover, pharmacologic sedation is often an integral part of treatment in the neurocritical setting and further confounds the clinical presentation.

Several standardized delirium detection scales have been devised to assist in the early detection and management of delirium. They are, ideally, performed in a short amount of time, can be applied repeatedly, and can be delivered by nursing care providers. Only two of them have been specifically developed to assess critically ill patients:

1. The Confusion Assessment Method for the Intensive Care Unit (CAM-ICU),[2] which is an adaptation of the original Confusion Assessment Scale for mechanically ventilated patients and
2. The Intensive Care Delirium Screening Checklist (ICDSC)[3]

The implementation of these screening tools depends on local institutional criteria. Both scales are easy to use, have high accuracy and inter-rater reliability and assist communication between members of the healthcare team. The effect of early detection and management in achieving improved long-term outcomes remains to be proven.

DIAGNOSTIC EVALUATION

No single cognitive manifestation of delirium is specific to a particular etiology. "Hepatic encephalopathy," "septic encephalopathy," and "uremic encephalopathy" can all present with the same mental status impairments. Uncertain associations have been proposed between motoric subtypes (hypoactive, hyperactive or mixed delirium) and pathophysiology. Anticholinergic drug intoxication has been correlated with hypoactive delirium, while alcohol withdrawal or thyroid hyperactivity with hyperactive delirium.

However, additional historical, clinical, laboratory and imaging data are almost always required for differential diagnosis.

1. History: This can be of invaluable help, particularly in cases of drug intoxication, withdrawal,

trauma, or anoxia. Most of the time, historical information needs to be obtained and/or confirmed with family members, previous healthcare providers, or bystanders.

▸ The medication list should always be reviewed. Information about over-the-counter or herbal medications is not readily provided and should be specifically sought.

▸ Knowledge of the past medical history may reveal chronic conditions that frequently result in metabolic encephalopathies, if uncontrolled.

▸ Recent surgical procedures can easily precipitate delirium, although other causes still need to be evaluated.

▸ The presence of dementia is particularly relevant, because it can predispose to delirium and can be associated with increased risk of infections or seizures.

▸ Review of the history of present illness may reveal prior systemic symptoms suggestive of a metabolic encephalopathy, or focal neurologic symptoms associated with a structural central nervous system (CNS) lesion.

2. Clinical examination: A thorough general and neurologic clinical examination is very important. Alterations of vital signs are very frequent in infections or drug intoxications. A detailed examination of organ systems (gastrointestinal, genitourinary, pulmonary, cardiac, skin) can reveal an otherwise occult source of infection.

▸ Nuchal rigidity is a sensitive indicator of meningeal irritation.

▸ Cranial nerve dysfunction and lateralized neurologic signs are highly suggestive of a focal structural process (particularly a lesion in the right hemisphere or the territory of the posterior circulation).

▸ Fluent aphasia, psychosis, or mood disorders can mimic delirium.

▸ The patient should be carefully observed for the present of subtle convulsive activity in previously undetected complex partial status epilepticus.

3. Laboratory investigations: Laboratory tests that can be considered are included in Table 17.3.

▸ Laboratory evidence of infection should be aggressively pursued, particularly in elderly, debilitated patients who may not demonstrate clinical signs of inflammation.

Table 17.3. Laboratory investigations

Complete blood count with differential, ESR and CRP
Serum electrolytes, BUN, glucose
Thyroid hormone evaluation
Liver function tests, amylase, lipase, ammonia
Troponin levels
HIV ELISA
Arterial blood gases
Cerebrospinal fluid evaluation including cytology.
Body fluid cultures (blood, urine, stool, sputum, CSF)
Culture of indwelling catheters.
Serum and urine toxicology

ESR = erythrocyte sedimentation rate; CRP = C-reactive protein; BUN = blood urea nitrogen; ELISA = enzyme-linked immunosorbent assay.

▸ Serum and urine toxicology may reveal the presence of many drugs of abuse, as well as toxic levels of tricyclic antidepressants, antiepileptics, anticholinergics, digoxin, and other medications.

▸ Hypoxia and hypoglycemia are life-threatening conditions and their immediate identification and treatment are important for a good outcome.

▸ Cerebrospinal fluid evaluation should be performed with even the lowest suspicion of primary CNS involvement from infection and inflammation, or if the etiology is uncertain. There are very few contraindications to the procedure and they can be safely excluded by appropriate clinical examination and neuroimaging.

4. Other studies: An electrocardiogram (EKG) and a chest radiograph are inexpensive tests, which should always be performed in the evaluation of delirium.

5. Electroencephalogram (EEG): Several EEG characteristics are associated with etiologies of delirium, although most of them are not entirely specific.

▸ Ongoing electrographic seizures are diagnostic of nonconvulsive status epilepticus and are necessary in the correct detection and treatment of this condition. Otherwise, focal epileptiform discharges are associated with a higher risk of localization-related epilepsy but do not necessarily indicate the cause of the current event.

▸ Increased beta activity is associated with use of sedating medications, particularly benzodiazepines.

▸ Lateralized slowing and asymmetry could be the result of a hemispheric lesion.

▸ Triphasic waves are observed in metabolic encephalopathies, particularly of hepatic or uremic etiology.

▸ Finally, EEG is very useful in assessing the severity of encephalopathy and the response to medical interventions.

6. Neuroimaging: Computed tomography (CT) imaging of the brain is readily available in most settings and can exclude many structural abnormalities responsible for delirium. Recent advances of CT imaging with CT angiography can provide detailed images of the intracranial circulation in a noninvasive manner. Magnetic resonance imaging (MRI) can provide significantly more information than CT, but many critically ill patients cannot tolerate the study. Diffusion-weighted MRI can reveal areas of acute ischemia, while diffuse gadolinium enhancement is highly sensitive for blood–brain barrier disruption, even without a focal lesion. Neuroimaging has become an irreplaceable component of the diagnostic workup of delirium.

MANAGEMENT

The management of delirium in the ICU setting is particularly challenging. Many of the medically necessary procedures can precipitate delirium. The need for analgesia and sedation should be balanced against the risk of delirium, which is a side effect of all psychoactive medications. Optimally, management involves several different steps that can be implemented simultaneously through the coordinated efforts of the entire healthcare team.

1. Primary prevention of delirium. The patient, if awake, should be frequently oriented to time and place. Dim lighting at night can help

maintain normal sleep patterns. Eyeglasses and hearing aids should be asked for and brought by family members. Sensory stimuli should be kept at a comfortable level, avoiding overstimulation or sensory deprivation. If continuous iatrogenic sedation is required, daily awakening trials should be attempted to facilitate timely ventilator weaning, mobilization, and clinical monitoring. Clinical protocols can help prevent infection spread and fluid volume depletion. The presence of family members or a sitter should be encouraged and physical restraints should be avoided, when possible.

2. Identification of patients at high risk for developing delirium. Patients with multiple risk factors are particularly susceptible to developing delirium and have worse cognitive and overall clinical outcomes. Flexible clinical protocols that target these patients should be in place, providing a better yield for the resources of each institution.

3. Early detection of syndrome, even when only prodromal symptoms are evident. It is possible, but not clearly proven yet, that early detection in the ICU setting allows for better long-term outcomes. The presence of fragments of the delirium syndrome may alert physicians to the possibility of a subclinical process that will soon complicate clinical management.

4. Identification and treatment of underlying etiologies. Early treatment of infections, volume status maintenance, and reversal of other treatable causes are paramount to the treatment of delirium. Particular attention should be directed to life-threatening conditions such as hypoxia or hypoglycemia. IV thiamine should be administered before dextrose in suspected hypoglycemia.

5. Environmental modifications, nonpharmacologic management. The same principles for primary prevention should continue to be applied after delirium has been identified. Physical restraints are often necessary in this setting, but the continued need for them should be assessed frequently.

6. Symptomatic pharmacologic management. Pharmacologic management for delirium should be initiated with low doses of medications, and titrated according to clinical response. Patients should be monitored

Table 17.4. Common medications used to treat delirium

Drug	Dose	Comments
Haloperidol	Younger patients 2–5 mg IV q2h Older patients 0.5–1 mg IV q2h	Extrapyramidal side effects QTc prolongation
Risperidone	Younger patients 0.75–3 mg PO/day Older patients 0.25–0.5 mg PO q12h	Can induce delirium QTc prolongation
Olanzapine	Younger patients 3–7.5 mg PO/day Older patients 2.5–5 mg PO at night	Not to be used with age >70 years Increases glucose levels Less QTc prolongation
Quetiapine	Younger patients 25–100 mg PO/day Older patients 12.5 mg PO at night	QTc prolongation, but can be used following haloperidol-induced prolonged QTc.
Lorazepam	0.5–2 mg IV/PO q8h	Monitor sedation level and respiratory rate.

QTc = QT interval corrected for heart rate.

serially for improvement of symptoms or clinical toxicity. Table 17.4 shows the most common medication used. Available classes include:

a. First-generation (typical) antipsychotics: These remain the first line of pharmacologic treatment for delirium.
  ▷ High-potency antipsychotics (haloperidol, droperidol) are preferable to the low-potency ones (phenothiazines) because they cause less sedation.[4] Specifically, a titrating regimen of IV haloperidol has been recommended for the treatment of delirium in critically ill patients.[5]
  ▷ A baseline EKG should be obtained for any patient who is treated for delirium with antipsychotics. QT prolongation (>450 ms or >25% of baseline) could lead to torsades de pointes even with low doses.
  ▷ Oral administration of medications is often impossible. The IV route is usually preferred, but IM administration may be necessary in case of severe agitation or lack of IV access. The IM or PO routes, however, may increase the risk for extrapyramidal side effects compared to IV administration (due to hepatic "first pass").
b. Second-generation (atypical) antipsychotics: Increasing clinical and research data

support the use of atypical antipsychotics in delirium. Increased efficacy over typical antipsychotics in the treatment of delirium has not been clearly demonstrated.
  ▷ There are concerns of increased mortality in patients with concurrent dementia (which frequently predisposes to or coexists with delirium).
  ▷ The lack of IV formulations limits their use in critically ill patients who need acute symptomatic control. Risperidone is available in a liquid form and can be administered through nasogastric tubes. Clozapine should not be used because of its anticholinergic effects, a contraindication in delirium, which is considered a state of increased dopamine and decreased acetylcholine levels.
c. Benzodiazepines: These have a role in the treatment of delirium associated with withdrawal of alcohol, benzodiazepines or b-hydroxybutyric acid (GHA), intoxication of sympathomimetic substances (cocaine, phencyclidine), neuroleptic malignant syndrome, as well as seizure-related delirium.
  ▷ Benzodiazepines are not recommended in the routine management of delirious patients and they may, in fact, precipitate paradoxical agitation in vulnerable patients.

▷ Combination therapy with antipsychotics has been proposed, but, particularly in the elderly, a simplified regimen should be used.

▷ The risk of respiratory depression is significant in the critical care setting.

▷ If benzodiazepines are used, shorter-acting agents (midazolam, lorazepam) without active metabolites are preferable to longer-acting ones (chlordiazepoxide).

7. Mechanical ventilation: Extreme agitation can be associated with cardiovascular instability and hypoxia in the critical care setting. If such symptoms are not effectively controlled with medications, mechanical ventilation with sedation and, even, muscle paralysis becomes an option, until underlying etiologies are identified and reversed. Propofol infusion up to 75 μg/kg per minute has been recommended because of its immediate onset and fast elimination.

CONCLUSIONS

Encephalopathy is an index of acute CNS dysfunction, in susceptible patients. It is usually precipitated by multiple underlying etiologies, which are not immediately apparent and should be actively investigated. If untreated, neurologic damage may progress to coma or brain death. Early detection and treatment has the potential of improving long-term outcomes. Effective management is multimodal and requires coordination of the entire healthcare team. Standardized evaluation and treatment protocols have been recommended, but treatment should be individualized to the particular needs of the critically ill patient.

REFERENCES

1. American Psychiatric Association. Task Force on DSM-IV. *Diagnostic and Statistical Manual of Mental Disorders*: DSM-IV-TR, 4th ed. Washington, DC: American Psychiatric Association; 2000.
2. Ely EW, Inouye SK, Bernard GR, et al. Delirium in mechanically ventilated patients: validity and reliability of the confusion assessment method for the intensive care unit (CAM-ICU). *JAMA.* 2001;**286**(21):2703–10.
3. Bergeron N, Dubois MJ, Dumont M, Dial S, Skrobik Y. Intensive Care Delirium Screening Checklist: evaluation of a new screening tool. *Intens Care Med.* 2001;**V27**(5):859–64.
4. American Psychiatric Association. Practice guideline for the treatment of patients with delirium. *Am J Psychiatry.* 1999;**156**(5 Suppl):1–20.
5. Jacobi J, Fraser GL, Coursin DB, et al. Clinical practice guidelines for the sustained use of sedatives and analgesics in the critically ill adult. *Crit Care Med.* 2002; **30**(1):119–41.

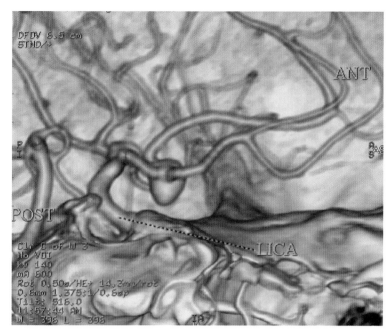

Figure 13.1. A 3-dimensional reconstructed CTA image of an 8 × 6 mm anterior communicating artery aneurysm is shown (note the right internal carotid artery has been subtracted from the image to improve visualization of the aneurysm). Surrounding bony detail is well demonstrated.

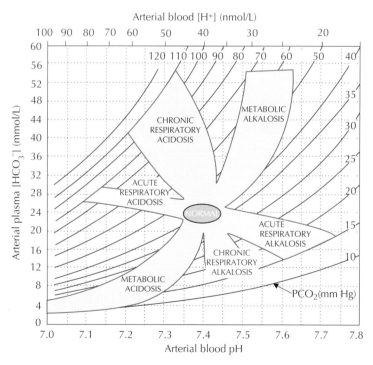

Figure 28.1. Acid–base nomogram (map). From *Brenner and Rector's The Kidney*, 8th ed.

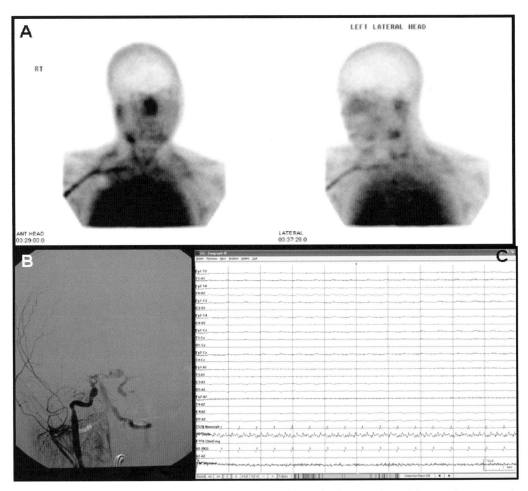

Figure 18.1. Confirmatory tests consistent with the diagnosis of brain death. **(A)** Radionuclide scan shows no perfusion of the brain, despite circulation in the neck and thorax. **(B)** Cerebral angiogram showing an AP view of a right carotid artery injection of contrast dye. The extracranial vessels are visualized with the injection, but there is no intracerebral perfusion beyond the circle of Willis. Contrast travels up the right carotid artery to the circle of Willis, then crosses to the left carotid and basilar arteries. (Courtesy of Phillipe Gailloud.) **(C)** EEG tracing shows electrocerebral silence. (Courtesy of Adam Hartman.)

18 Coma and Brain Death

Jennifer L. Berkeley, MD, PhD and Romergryko G. Geocadin, MD

Coma and impaired consciousness are common presentations in neurocritical care. This chapter reviews the definitions of different levels of awareness and discusses the diagnosis and management of comatose patients.

DEFINITIONS

- **Coma** is a state of unresponsiveness to external or internal stimuli in which a patient lies with eyes closed unaware of the environment. Although this definition seems quite straightforward, coma actually lies on a continuum of disorders of consciousness.
- **Consciousness**, defined as a state of awareness of both the self and the environment, is composed of two key elements: arousal and content.[1]

  - **Arousal** is mediated by the ascending reticular activating system that localizes to the rostral pons, midbrain, thalamus, and hypothalamus, and is characterized by wakefulness or alertness.
  - **Content**, on the other hand, requires the higher-level structures of the cerebral cortex and its connections to subcortical white matter, and is composed of affective and cognitive functions such as attention, memory, motivation, and executive function.

RATING IMPAIRED CONSCIOUSNESS

 Disruptions to either the reticular activating system or bilateral cortices can therefore result in impaired consciousness, and the extent of the damage determines where on the spectrum of consciousness a patient may lie. Several scales have been created to rate the severity of impaired consciousness.

- The most widely used is the Glasgow Coma Scale (GCS), which was originally designed for use in trauma; it assigns a number from 3 to 15, where 15 is normal with no impaired consciousness and 3 is comatose or worse.[2] The GCS, however, does not take into account several aspects of the neurologic exam, such as brain stem reflexes, and the verbal score is limited by intubation or aphasias.
- More recently a new scoring system, the FOUR (Full Outline of UnResponsiveness) score, has been adopted.[3]
- Table 18.1 compares the two scales.

SPECTRUM OF ALTERED CONSCIOUSNESS

Terms such as stuporous, obtunded, and lethargic are widely used to describe the spectrum of disorders of consciousness. These terms, however, are subjective with substantial inter-rater variability and therefore should not be used as basis for diagnosis or therapy. An exact description of a patient's response to a specific stimulus such as "follows simple commands" or "withdraws right arm with nail bed pressure" should be used instead. A change in the quality of the patient's response may suggest a clinical change that could require further investigation or interventions. Below are definitions of some of the more commonly used terms.

Table 18.1. Comparison of FOUR Score and GCS

FOUR Score (Full Outline of Unresponsiveness)	GCS (Glasgow Coma Scale)
Eye response	**Eye response**
4 = eyelids open or opened, tracking, or blinking to command	4 = eyes open spontaneously
3 = eyelids open but not tracking	3 = eye opening to verbal command
2 = eyelids closed, but open to loud voice	
1 = eyelids closed, but open to pain	2 = eye opening to pain
0 = eyelids remain closed with pain	1 = no eye opening
Motor response	**Motor response**
4 = thumbs up, fist, or peace sign	6 = obeys commands
3 = localizing to pain	5 = localizing pain
2 = flexion response to pain	4 = withdrawal from pain
1 = extension response to pain	3 = flexion response to pain
0 = no response to pain or generalized myoclonus status	2 = extension response to pain
	1 = no motor response
Brain stem reflexes	**Verbal response**
4 = pupil and corneal reflexes present	5 = oriented
3 = one pupil wide and fixed	4 = confused
2 = pupil or corneal reflexes absent	3 = inappropriate words
1 = pupil and corneal reflexes absent	2 = incomprehensible sounds
0 = absent pupil, corneal and cough reflexes	
Respiration	
4 = not intubated, regular breathing pattern	
3 = not intubated, Cheyne-Stokes breathing pattern	
2 = not intubated, irregular breathing	
1 = breathes above ventilator rate	
0 = breathes at ventilator rate	

Adapted from Wijdicks et al. *Ann Neurol.* 2005;**58**:585–93.

Stupor: Patients appear asleep and can be aroused only by vigorous and repeated stimulation, but return to a sleep-like state as soon as stimulation ceases.[4]

Obtundation: This is a particularly vague term indicating moderate reduction in alertness. Patients require stimulation to arouse, but can be aroused enough to obey commands. Interest in the environment is minimal and there is increased sleep, especially when not stimulated.

Lethargy: This is also a vague term indicating a mild reduction is alertness. Patients prefer to sleep, but can interact appropriately with the environment upon stimulation.

Vegetative state: A vegetative state is one outcome after coma. Arousal and sleep–wake cycles return but unaccompanied by cognitive function. Patients are unable to interact with the environment, meaning there are no sustained, reproducible, purposeful, or voluntary behavioral responses to visual, auditory, tactile, or noxious stimuli. However, hypothalamic and brain stem autonomic functions are preserved as are cranial nerve and spinal reflexes to a variable degree.

- The term persistent vegetative state (PVS) can be applied after 1 month, and the state can be deemed permanent 3 months after nontraumatic injury and 12 months after traumatic injury in adults and children.
- Prognosis for recovery once the state is deemed permanent is extremely poor, and any recovery is to a state of severe disability.[5,6]
- The most common etiologies are head trauma and hypoxic–ischemic encephalopathy. These insults result in either neocortical or thalamic damage (hypoxic–ischemic insult) or diffuse axonal injury and subcortical white matter damage (trauma).[4,7,8]

  Minimally conscious state: This is a state similar to a vegetative state, with severely altered consciousness but in which there is minimal, but definite, evidence of self- or environmental awareness. A cognitively mediated behavior must be reproducible, even if inconsistent.[8]

  Akinetic mutism: In this syndrome, patients lie immobile with eyes open or closed and little or no vocalization. Sleep–wake cycles are intact, but there is an apparent absence of cognition or spontaneous motor activity. There may be minimal response to noxious stimuli. Etiologies can be quite varied, but include acute hydrocephalus, large bifrontal lesions, and severe cortical damage.[4]

  Locked-in syndrome: This syndrome is not actually a disorder of consciousness as patients are alert and fully aware of their surroundings; rather it is a state of complete paralysis. The etiology is most often a lesion of the ventral pons resulting in quadriplegia, anarthria, and paresis of horizontal eye movements. Blinking and vertical eye movements are preserved, as are hearing and brain stem autonomic functions. The preservation of the ascending reticular activating system allows for the maintenance of consciousness.

EMERGENT MANAGEMENT OF COMA

The management of a comatose patient largely depends on the etiology of the condition. However, there are some initial steps that must be taken in all patients with altered consciousness. These begin with the **ABC**s: **a**irway, **b**reathing, and **c**irculation of Basic Life Support (BLS).

- If a patient is not breathing spontaneously, bag mask ventilation should be initiated until the patient can be intubated.
- In cases of possible trauma, attention should be paid to the cervical spine and neck extension should be avoided.
- Often comatose patients are intubated for airway protection, especially in cases with impaired lower cranial nerve function. This often occurs before compromise of either oxygenation or ventilation.
- Circulation is assessed by palpating a pulse and then monitoring systemic blood pressure.
  - In cases of hypotension, fluid resuscitation and vasopressor support should be provided to maintain an adequate perfusing pressure.
  - However, hypertension is quite common in patients with acute brain injury.
  - The use of antihypertensives must be directed toward preventing further organ damage, while at the same time caution should be taken to avoid excessive drops of blood pressure that could lead to ischemia.
- Hyper- and hypothermia should be evaluated and reversed appropriately to normothermia with cooling and warming blankets, respectively.

INITIAL DIAGNOSTIC WORKUP OF COMA

Much of the treatment of coma is directed toward reversing the etiology. Therefore, once a patient is stabilized using the aforementioned techniques, the next step is to evaluate the patient with respect to possible causes of their altered consciousness. As soon as intravenous access is obtained, blood should be sent for laboratory studies to evaluate possible toxic and metabolic etiologies. Some of these laboratory studies can identify rapidly correctable causes of coma, such as hypoglycemia, diabetic ketoacidosis, electrolyte abnormalities, and drug overdoses. Table 18.2 lists the initial laboratory studies to be sent and the conditions that each will help to identify.

If any of the above causes of coma are identified, they should be treated emergently.

- Hypoglycemia should be treated by administering at least one ampule of D50 (50 mL of a 50% glucose solution) intravenously preceded

Table 18.2. Laboratory studies to identify causes of coma

Laboratory test	Coma etiology
Glucose	Hypoglycemia, nonketotic hyperglycemia, diabetic ketoacidosis
Complete blood count (CBC)	Infection/sepsis, anemia, thrombocytopenia
Electrolytes, including calcium	Hypo-/hypernatremia, hypo-/hypercalcemia
Liver function tests (AST, ALT, bilirubin, ammonia)	Hyperbilirubinemia, hyperammonemia, hepatic coma
Renal function tests (BUN, creatinine)	Uremia
Thyroid function tests (TSH)	Myxedema coma
Urinalysis, urine toxicology screen	Urosepsis, intoxication
Arterial blood gas (ABG)	Hypoxia, hypercapnia
Coagulation studies	Coagulopathy
Lactate	Lactic acidosis

by 100 mg of intravenous thiamine to avoid precipitating Wernicke's encephalopathy in a malnourished patient. In a patient in whom an insulin overdose is a possible cause of hypoglycemia, a continuous intravenous infusion of a glucose solution may be necessary.

- Hyperglycemia is treated with insulin, potassium and hydration with normal saline.
- Severe hyponatremia (serum sodium <125 mEq/L) can be treated with a hypertonic saline solution, although sodium should not be corrected above 130 mEq/L too quickly because rapid correction may lead to central pontine myelinolysis or other acute demyelination in brain.
- Hypercalcemia is corrected with normal saline infusion and intravenous bisphosphonate pamidronate.
- Drug ingestions are treated with activated charcoal and normal saline lavage. Hemodialysis may be necessary to clear some drugs.
- A narcotic overdose can be reversed with naloxone (0.4–2 mg IV q3min), although this should be done cautiously because acute reversal can result in an acute withdrawal syndrome. After administration of naloxone, patients should be monitored carefully, as the reversal is short-lived and patients can easily return to an opiate-induced coma and may require mechanical ventilatory support.
- Benzodiazepine overdoses can similarly be reversed with flumazenil (0.2 mg intravenously), although again it should be used cautiously because it can induce cardiac arrhythmias or

seizures. Flumazenil is contraindicated in patients with a possible ingestion of tricyclic antidepressants and in patients with active seizures.

- Broad-spectrum antibiotics should be initiated immediately in cases with high suspicion for meningitis. Cerebrospinal fluid (CSF) sampling is important but must not delay the administration of empiric antibiotics.
- Any evidence of ongoing seizure activity, for example tonic–clonic limb movements, nystagmoid beating of deviated eyes, should also be treated immediately with benzodiazepines and other intravenous antiepileptic medications.

EXAMINATION OF THE COMATOSE PATIENT

History

While the laboratory studies listed in the preceding text can identify many causes of coma, evaluation and management of the patient can proceed while awaiting the results. The roles of the history and physical examination cannot be underestimated. A history provided by family, friends, or witnesses can help to identify patients with histories of drug or alcohol use or preexisting medical conditions (diabetes, hypothyroidism) and medication noncompliance. Witnesses of an event can report seizure activity or trauma. Further, a history of the progression of the alteration of consciousness can be useful: Did the patient lose consciousness acutely? Was there a progression over hours or days? Sudden onset (within seconds to minutes) suggests a vascular etiology (brain stem stroke or subarachnoid hemorrhage), whereas rapid progression from hemispheric signs to coma within minutes to hours is more typical of intracerebral hemorrhage. Mass lesions such as tumor, abscess, and chronic subdural hematomas might progress toward coma over days to weeks. Preceding symptoms such as agitated delirium without any localizing neurologic signs suggests a metabolic etiology.

General Medical Exam

The physical examination of a comatose patient should begin with vital signs and a general medical exam.

- The triad of bradycardia, hypertension, and irregular respirations is known as the Cushing reflex and may suggest elevated intracranial pressure (ICP).
- Cardiac arrhythmias or murmurs that suggest valvular damage or vegetations, or distant sounds to suggest tamponade can also be identified on exam.
- Evidence of incontinence may suggest seizure, whereas presence of vomitus may indicate elevated ICP or toxin ingestion.
- As trauma is one of the leading causes of coma, a patient should be examined for signs of trauma: lacerations, hematomas, and fractures. Signs of head trauma, such as Battle's sign (postauricular ecchymosis), hemotympanum, or periorbital hematomas indicating a basilar skull fracture, are particularly important because they also may indicate brain trauma.
- Neck stiffness on exam is indicative of meningeal irritation that may be infectious, carcinomatous, inflammatory, or chemical (i.e., subarachnoid hemorrhage).
- A funduscopic exam can reveal subhyaloid hemorrhages indicative of subarachnoid hemorrhage, papilledema indicative of elevated ICP, or embolic material suggestive of carotid disease and stroke.

Neurologic Exam

The GCS and FOUR Score scales use elements of the neurologic examination to rate the severity of an alteration of consciousness, but both are rather superficial. Such an exam does not aid in identifying the etiology of coma or any but gross localization of a possible brain lesion. Table 18.3 lists some physical exam findings and their significance and localization.

Mental status: As with any neurologic exam, examination of a comatose patient should begin with the mental status, which includes careful observation for spontaneous motor movement or eye opening. Eye opening does not necessarily imply awareness, as in the case of a vegetative state where there may be spontaneous eye opening, but there is no meaningful interaction with environment. Next, there should be an attempt to elicit a response to loud voice and external stimulation. It is best to begin with less noxious stimuli before proceeding to painful or noxious stimuli such as nail bed pressure, pinching, supraorbital pressure, sternal rub, or intranasal swab. In patients with a coagulopathy or thrombocytopenia, attention should be paid to bruising with some stimuli. Carefully assess for a locked-in state by asking a patient to blink or look up before administering painful stimuli, as these patients can feel pain but will be unable to respond. Clear withdrawal or localization indicates more preserved function than reflexive responses such as posturing or triple flexion, or no response to a painful stimulus.

Cranial nerves: The cranial nerve examination should begin with an assessment of **eye movements**. First, are there spontaneous movements? If present, are the movements purposeful and do they track objects. Some spontaneous eye movements are pathological and suggest severe brainstem damage. Rhythmic eye movements may be subtle presentation of seizures. If there are no purposeful movements, are the eyes conjugate or disconjugate? Are the eyes deviated to one side? After evaluating spontaneous eye movements, the next part of the eye exam involves the pupillary size and reaction to light. Anisocoria is a difference in pupil size of >1 mm. Compression of third cranial nerve, such as in a transtentorial herniation, may lead to a unilateral dilated pupil with a loss of the pupillary light reflex. Many drugs, either systemic or applied directly

Table 18.3. Physical examination findings, their anatomic localization and common etiologies

Examination finding	Localization	Common etiologies
Neck stiffness	Meninges	Infectious or carcinomatous meningitis, subarachnoid hemorrhage
Battle's sign, periorbital hematoma	Basilar skull fracture	Trauma
Papilledema	Elevated intracranial pressure	Many
Eye Movements		
Horizontal gaze deviation	Frontal eye fields	Stroke (towards the lesion), Seizure (away from the focus)
	Pons, thalamus ("wrong way eyes")	Stroke, hemorrhage, central herniation
Ocular bobbing	Central Pons	Many
Reverse ocular bobbing	Midbrain/diencephalon	Metabolic or structural damage
Roving eye movements	Nonlocalizing, disappear with brain stem injury	
Pupillary Size and Reaction to Light		
Unilateral fixed dilated pupil	CN III compression	Uncal herniation, posterior communicating aneurysm
Unilateral miosis (Horner's syndrome)	Sympathetic denervation	Carotid dissection, Pancoast's tumor
Bilateral fixed dilated pupils	CN III compression	Herniation, massive overdoses, atropine (nebulizers), metabolic coma
Mid-position fixed pupils	Midbrain	Massive brain stem injury, end-stage herniation, brain death
Bilateral miosis (preserved light reflex)	Pons ("pontine pupils")	Narcotics, pontine hemorrhage, organophosphate poisoning
Oculocephalic and Vestibulo–Ocular reflexes		
Eyes remain fixed with head turn or cold calorics	Lower brain stem (pons, medulla)	Massive brain stem injury, brain death
Eyes deviate away from head turn or toward cold irrigated ear	Diffuse or bilateral hemispheres, normal brain stem response	Metabolic coma, elevated ICP without herniation
Nystagmus with fast phase away from irrigated ear	Normal	Psychogenic unresponsiveness
Neither eye deviates medially passed midline with head turn or cold calorics	Bilateral medial longitudinal fasciculus	Brain stem stroke or hemorrhage, demyelinating disease
Absent corneal reflex	CN V and VII	Brain stem injury, may be peripheral nerve damage if unilateral
Absent cough or gag reflex	CN IX and X	
Hemiplegia or paresis	Contralateral cerebral hemisphere or corticospinal tracts	Stroke, mass lesion
Flexor posturing	Thalamus	
Extensor posturing	Midbrain, upper pons	

to the eyes, can also cause pupillary abnormalities. Assessment of the internuclear pathways of the brain stem can be evaluated with the oculocephalic maneuver in patients in whom there is no concern for cervical spine injury. The head is moved rapidly in one direction; the normal response is for the eyes to move conjugately in the opposite direction in the same plane. In patients with possible cervical spine injury or in whom the oculocephalic maneuver produces unclear results, the vestibulo-ocular reflex can be tested. This provides a stronger stimulus of the same system. The ear canal is irrigated with cold water and the eyes should tonically deviate toward the irrigated ear in the unconscious patient with intact brain stem function. Disconjugate movements of the eyes will make any cranial nerve palsies apparent and absence of response suggests significant brain stem damage. In the conscious patient, nystagmus with the fast phase away from the irrigated ear is the normal response. Vertical eye movements should also be tested with the oculocephalic maneuver by moving the head vertically or with cold calorics by irrigating both ears simultaneously with cold water, which will produce tonic downward deviation of the eyes. The corneal reflex is assessed by touching a cotton swab to the cornea or using a drop of sterile saline and watching for the blink reflex. Tracheal suctioning assesses the cough reflex whereas stimulation of the posterior pharynx assesses the gag reflex, both of which assess cranial nerves IX and X. The gag reflex is difficult to assess in intubated patients.

Motor exam: In the comatose patient, the motor exam overlaps significantly with the mental status and sensory exams. If there is spontaneous movement, it should be observed for symmetry and rhythmicity. Is it purposeful, myoclonic, tonic–clonic in nature? Assessment of a patient's tone can help localize a lesion: a flaccid extremity might suggest a spinal cord lesion, whereas spasticity suggests damage to descending cortical spinal tracts. When assessing the motor response to pain, the stimulus should be applied to the inside of the upper arm or thigh so that a spinal reflex or triple flexion will not be confused with a true withdrawal. Painful stimulation may elicit a posturing response, referred to as flexor (decorticate) and extensor (decerebrate) posturing, although the localizing value of these responses is more limited than once believed. Flexor posturing involves flexion of the arms at the elbow, adduction of the shoulder and extension of the lower extremities. Extensor posturing is characterized by extension at the elbow with pronation of the arms and extension of the lower extremities. Classically, flexor (decorticate) posture is most commonly associated with damage to the thalamus or the upper midbrain above the level of the red nucleus and extensor (decerebrate) posture is associated with severe brain stem damage to the midbrain or upper pons. However, in the advent of better neuroimaging, these anatomical lesion demarcations are less clear. Severe metabolic disorders as well as bilateral deep hemispheric lesions can also result in extensor posturing. In clinical practice, extensor posturing compared to flexor posturing is regarded as a manifestation of worse injury.

Sensory exam: The sensory exam is performed in conjunction with the motor exam as described above. However, a patient with a hemi- or quadriparesis due to a structural lesion may have intact sensation but not be able to move or withdraw the extremity. Therefore, when applying a painful stimulus the face should be observed for grimacing and the vital signs should be monitored for physiologic responses to pain such as tachycardia and tachypnea. Locked-in patients are awake and aware of their surroundings and may be able to feel pain.

Respirations: Although not part of the traditional neurologic exam, there are some classical respiratory patterns in coma that can suggest specific pathological processes or localizations. Decreased tone of the upper airway can result in a failure to protect the airway and necessitate intubation. This can be associated with any reduced level of consciousness, but is particularly common in stroke.

■ Cheyne-Stokes respirations (alternating hyperpnea and apnea) are seen with bilateral cerebral dysfunction, increased ICP and metabolic disturbances.

- Central neurogenic hyperventilation, defined as sustained, rapid, deep breathing, results from damage to the midbrain tegmentum.
- Apneusis is alternating end-inspiratory and end-expiratory pauses and localizes to the mid- and caudal pons.
- Ataxic breathing is irregular, uneven breaths in no identifiable pattern and can be due to lesions in the reticular formation of the dorsomedial medulla.
- Kussmaul breathing is deep regular inspirations due to metabolic acidosis. While we provide these breathing patterns as part of our discussion, we emphasize that waiting for these breathing patterns to unfold may cause more injury to the patient. We encourage emergent airway protection and mechanical ventilation in appropriate patients.

ANCILLARY TESTING

While the initial laboratory studies, history and physical exam are often adequate to identify the etiology of a coma and to begin treatment, several other tests are critical to complete the evaluation. These are not all necessary for every patient and can be done in a stepwise manner according to the leading differential diagnoses. However, virtually every comatose patient, especially with focal neurologic findings, should receive a noncontrast computed tomography (CT) brain scan to assess for structural lesions and intracerebral bleeding. This should be done as soon as the patient is stable enough to undergo the procedure.

- A lumbar puncture should be performed rapidly in any patient in whom there is a suspicion of meningitis or CT-negative subarachnoid hemorrhage, as long as the head CT does not show a mass lesion. Signs and symptoms that should precipitate CSF analysis by lumbar puncture are fever, meningismus, a gradual course with delirium, and an elevated peripheral white blood cell count without other source of infection.
- An electroencephalogram (EEG) is critical for any patient who presents with seizure activity, even if the activity has stopped, or other patients with unexplained etiology for unresponsiveness as subclinical status epilepticus is otherwise difficult to diagnose.

  - Treatment of status epilepticus in a clearly seizing patient should not be delayed in order to obtain the EEG.
  - EEG can also be used to monitor patients receiving pharmacologic treatment for status epilepticus.
- Magnetic resonance imaging (MRI) can be useful in identifying strokes and characterizing mass lesions. However, it is not always readily available and because it is a time-consuming procedure should be performed only once a patient is hemodynamically and neurologically stable. MRI can be technically quite difficult in patients who are mechanically ventilated or who require continuous drug infusions. These challenges need to be considered when selecting an imaging modality.
- Cerebral angiography is an invasive procedure that can be used to identify the source of an aneurysmal subarachnoid hemorrhage or identify basilar thrombosis. Both conditions can also be treated endovascularly if identified on angiogram.
- A thorough systemic workup is necessary with an electrocardiogram (EKG), chest radiograph, and other related imaging modalities should be performed on all patients to identify systemic diseases that may be contributing to a patient's unresponsive state.

ETIOLOGY OF COMA

After the emergent management and initial workup, further management of coma is generally directed toward the specific etiology. Most of the workup described thus far has been geared toward deciding if there is a structural brain lesion that might require neurosurgical intervention. If there is a structural lesion, assignment of its localization to the supra- or infratentorial compartments will further guide management. Alternatively, in cases where there is no structural lesion, the cause may be a diffuse encephalopathy caused by a metabolic, infectious, or epileptic process that would commonly be managed medically. Table 18.4 lists common causes of coma classified by type and location.[9] Specific treatments geared toward various conditions are beyond the scope of this chapter and are addressed in other chapters of this text.

Table 18.4. Common etiologies of coma

Structural lesions	Metabolic derangements
Supratentorial	Hypoglycemia
Generalized/bilateral	Hyperglycemia (nonketotic hyperosmolar)
Infectious/postinfectious	Hyponatremia
Encephalitis	Hypercalcemia
Acute disseminated encephalomyelitis	Panhypopituitarism
Vascular	Hyperbilirubinemia
Anoxic–ischemic encephalopathy	Acute uremia
Multiple cortical infarctions	
Bilateral thalamic infarctions	
Traumatic	**Diffuse Physiologic Brain Dysfunction**
Diffuse axonal injury	Status epilepticus
Penetrating brain injury	Poisoning
Multiple contusions	Drug overdose
Neoplastic	Gas inhalation
Gliomatosis	Hypothermia
Leukoencephalopathy	Basilar migraine
Multiple brain metastases	Malignant neuroleptic syndrome
Lymphoma	Hypoxia
Acute hydrocephalus	
Focal (with mass effect)	
Intraparenchymal hematoma	**Psychogenic Unresponsiveness**
Large stroke with edema	Catatonia
Hemorrhagic contusion	Conversion disorder
Abscess	Malingering
Tumor	
Infratentorial	
Brain stem	
Pontine hemorrhage	
Basilar artery thrombosis	
Central pontine myelinolysis	
Cerebellum	
Infarction with edema	
Hematoma	
Abscess	
Tumor	

Adapted from Ziai WC. Coma and altered consciousness. In Bhardwaj A, Mirski MS, Ulatowski JA (eds), *Current Clinical Neurology: Handbook of Neurocritical Care*. Totowa, NJ: Humana Press, 2004, pp 1–18.

MANAGEMENT OF COMA

Despite the fact that most of the care should be directed toward reversing the etiology of the coma if possible, there are some elements of caring for a comatose patient that are common regardless of etiology. Comatose patients are particularly susceptible to infectious complications as they often intubated and immobile. Early tracheostomy for those without signs of early recovery should be considered to help minimize the risk of tracheal injury and further infections. The patient should be turned in bed frequently to prevent the development of decubitus ulcers. Attention should be paid to adequate nutrition with placement of a percutaneous endoscopic gastrostomy (PEG) tube with nutritional surveillance to assess ongoing needs. Deep vein thrombosis and pulmonary embolism are other complications of patients who are immobilized for long periods of time, and all comatose patients (with the exception of those with active, or high risk of, bleeding) should be prophylactically managed against these conditions with subcutaneous heparin or heparinoids and compression devices. Finally, physical and occupational therapy are important to prevent contractures of immobilized extremities. Patients should be monitored carefully to be maintained normothermic, euvolemic and normoglycemic.

PROGNOSIS OF COMA

The outcome from coma depends on multiple factors: primarily the underlying etiology, the severity, and the duration.

- Traumatic coma generally carries a better prognosis than nontraumatic coma in terms of both survival and probability of good (independent) outcome.
  - In a 2001 study of 248 patients with traumatic coma, there was 52% mortality, 27% of patients had a good outcome, and 19% had severe disability or vegetative state.[10] In this study, as in others, age is one of the strongest independent predictors of good outcome; the younger the patient, the better the outcome.
  - Interestingly, despite advances in imaging and treatment, these outcome data are not significantly changed from a 1975 study in which traumatic coma had a 49% mortality.[11]

- Poor prognostic factors in traumatic coma are low GCS on admission, hypoxia and hypotension in the first 24 hours and long delay before eye opening and spontaneous movement.
- Within the category of nontraumatic coma, prognosis is once again dependent on the underlying etiology.
  - Coma due to cerebrovascular disease – ischemic stroke, hemorrhagic stroke or subarachnoid hemorrhage – carry the worst prognosis, with mortality reported to exceed 70% and likelihood of good outcomes <5%.
  - Coma with a toxic or metabolic etiology tend to do somewhat better, with 25% of patients making a good recovery.[12] Table 18.5 summarizes outcomes based on etiology.

Many studies have reported clinical signs that may help to predict outcome in coma, but the study that remains the most widely cited and used clinically is that published by Levy and colleagues in 1985.[13] While the data from Levy's study are frequently used to predict outcome from coma due to multiple etiologies, it is important to recognize that the data were derived exclusively from patients with anoxic-ischemic coma after cardiac arrest. Since the publication of that paper, several other publications have evaluated the same and other predictors of poor outcome after cardiac arrest. These were reviewed and summarized in a Practice Parameter published by the American Academy of Neurology in 2006.[14] At 3 days, the most useful of the clinical indicators to predict poor outcome are absent pupillary response to light, absent corneal reflexes, and extensor or absent motor response to pain. In addition to the clinical exam, electrophysiology and biochemical markers were evaluated for their utility in prognostication.

- The bilateral absence of the cortical response on somatosensory evoked potentials (SSEP) predicts poor outcome after CPR, as does elevation of serum neuron-specific enolase >33 µg/L.[14]
- These ancillary tests may be useful, but the limited availability of expertise in SSEP, as well as the continued variability in cutoff values for neuron-specific enolase (NSE) limits the widespread application to date.
- While this practice parameter applies only to coma after cardiac arrest, SSEPs have also been

Table 18.5. Outcome of coma by etiology

	Death (%)	Persistent vegetative state (%)	Good recovery (%)
Hypoxic-Ischemic	58	20	8
Toxic-Metabolic	47	6	25
Cerebrovascular	74	7	3
Total	61	12	10

Adapted from Bates D. The prognosis of medical coma. *J Neurol Neurosurg Psychiatry*. 2001;**71**(Suppl 1): i20–3.

shown to be predictive of poor outcome in traumatic coma as well.[15] In summary, both the clinical exam and the electrophysiologic testing are quite accurate for predicting poor outcome; yet, there remains no optimal test to predict a good functional recovery.

BRAIN DEATH

Defining Death

Prior to the advent and routine use of mechanical ventilation and advanced cardiac care, death was determined by the cessation of cardiopulmonary function. However, with the advances in intensive care medicine, patients could be sustained despite a complete absence of brain function. In 1981, the Uniform Determination of Brain Death Act was written stating that death can be pronounced if the neurologic criteria for brain death, specifically the irreversible cessation of all brain function including the brainstem, are met. These criteria were published in JAMA in that same year (1981).[16]

- In adults, the most common causes of brain death are traumatic brain injury, subarachnoid hemorrhage, hypoxic–ischemic brain injury and fulminant hepatic failure.[17]
- In children, the most common causes are trauma secondary to abuse and motor vehicle accidents followed by asphyxia.[18]

Diagnosis of Brain Death

In 1995, the American Academy of Neurology published a practice parameter entitled "Determining Brain Death in Adults" (1995).[19] While this text provides guidelines for patients over 18 years of age, there is no legally proscribed way to determine brain death, and there are institutional variations. Further, the criteria are somewhat different for determining brain death in children. The pediatric brain death exam is beyond the scope of this text.

To confirm the irreversibility of the condition, a brain death exam should be performed at least twice for each patient. The interval is arbitrary, but at most institutions 6 hours is standard. (The interval is often longer in children.) The determination of brain death requires a specially trained clinician who is often a neurologist or neurosurgeon. The brain death exam can be broken into four parts. Part 1 is the meeting of prerequisite criteria. The other three parts of the exam reflect the cardinal findings in brain death: coma/unresponsiveness, absence of brainstem reflexes, and apnea. In addition to performing the brain death exam, the clinician should document each aspect of the exam in a standardized and detailed manner.

Part 1: Prerequisites for the brain death examination

- Evidence of a catastrophic brain injury with a known and irreversible proximate cause (should have clinical or neuroimaging evidence)
- Exclusion of confounding medical conditions (severe electrolyte, acid–base, endocrine disturbances, circulatory shock)
  - ▶ Blood glucose should be between 60 and 400 mg/dL
  - ▶ Blood pressure should be >90/40 mm Hg
- No drug intoxication or poisoning (ensure that all sedatives, anesthetics, and neuromuscular blockade agents are off and have had time to be metabolized or excreted).
- Core temperature >32°C (90°F)

Part 2: Evaluation of unresponsiveness

- No motor response to painful pressure applied to all extremities (nail bed pressure) or to core (supraorbital, clavicular pressure or sternal rub).
- No autonomic response to painful stimulation (listen to/watch cardiac monitor for changes in heart rate)
- Note: Some spontaneous limb movements are of spinal origin and *are consistent with* brain death.
- Note: Flexor and extensor posturing are brain stem reflexes are therefore *not consistent with* brain death.
- Note: Deep tendon reflexes and triple flexion are spinal reflexes and thus *are consistent with* brain death.

Part 3: Evaluation of brain stem reflexes

- Pupils
  - No constriction response to bright light
  - Size is midposition (4 mm) to dilated (9 mm)
- Ocular movement
  - Absent oculocephalic reflex (only test if there is no evidence of c-spine fracture or instability). Hold the eyes open and gently rotate the head from side to side and up and down. The reflex is absent if there is no movement of the eyes.
  - Absent vestibulo-ocular reflex. Ensure that the ear canals are unobstructed and the tympanic membrane is intact. Irrigate the ear with 50 mL of ice-cold water while holding the eyes open for 1 minute after injection completed. Wait 5 minutes before performing test on the other side. The reflex is absent if the eyes do not deviate.
- Facial sensation and facial motor response
  - No corneal reflex to touch with throat swab or drop of sterile saline
  - No grimacing to pressure on the supraorbital ridge, temporomandibular joint or nail beds (observe the face during part 1 of the exam to avoid repeating these painful stimuli). Intranasal stimulation with a cotton swab can also be used to elicit a facial grimace.
- Pharyngeal and tracheal reflexes (cough and gag reflexes)
  - No response to insertion of a suction catheter through the endotracheal tube (ET tube) and stimulation of the carina.

- No response to tongue blade stimulation of the posterior pharynx

Part 4: Apnea test. The purpose of the test is to validate the inability of the brain stem to trigger breathing in the presence of an elevated CO_2. Because the apnea test can result in hemodynamic instability, some institutions require it to be performed only once at the time of the second brain death exam.

- Prerequisites for the apnea test
  - Core temperature ≥36.5°C (97°F)
  - Systolic BP ≥90 mm Hg (may use fluids or vasopressors to maintain desired BP)
  - Euvolemia (option: positive fluid balance in the previous 6 hours)
  - Normal $Paco_2$ (option: arterial $Paco_2$ ≥40 mm Hg)
  - Normal Po_2 (option: preoxygenation to obtain arterial Pao_2 ≥200 mm Hg)
- To perform the apnea test
  - Send an ABG prior to testing to ensure $Paco_2$ 35–45 mm Hg, or to obtain a baseline $Paco_2$ in patients with chronic retention. It is ideal that the patient have an arterial line for easy access for repeated ABG testing.
  - Disconnect the ventilator.
  - Deliver 100% O_2 (6 L/min) at the level of the carina through a catheter inserted inside the ET tube.
  - Observe for respiratory movements (abdominal or chest excursions).
  - Monitor cardiac activity and pulse oximeter for evidence of cardiac instability or hypoxia. Vasopressors may be increased to maintain adequate blood pressure.
  - If patient remains hemodynamically stable, draw ABGs every 5–7 minutes until results reveal a rise in $Paco_2$ >20 mm Hg from pretest baseline
  - In the presence systemic instability, such as cardiac arrhythmias, hypotension, or significant oxygen desaturation, draw and ABG immediately and resume mechanical ventilation and oxygenation.
- The apnea test is consistent with brain death if there are no observed respiratory movements in the presence of $Paco_2$ ≥60 mm Hg or a rise in $Paco_2$ ≥20 mm Hg from baseline. If the test is concluded and the rise in $Paco_2$ is <20 mm Hg or the

Table 18.6. American Clinical Neurophysiology Society: Minimum Technical Standards for EEG Recording in Suspected Cerebral Death

1. A full set of scalp electrodes should be used.
2. Interelectrode impedances should be between 100 and 10,000 ohms.
3. The integrity of the entire recording system should be tested.
4. Interelectrode distances should be at least 10 centimeters.
5. Sensitivity must be increased from 7 μV/mm to at least 2 μV/mm for at least 30 minutes of the recording, with inclusion of appropriate calibrations.
6. Filter settings should be appropriate for the assessment of electrocerebral silence (ECS).
7. Additional monitoring techniques should be employed when necessary.
8. There should be no EEG reactivity to intense somatosensory, auditory or visual stimuli.
9. Recordings should only be made by a qualified technologist.
10. A repeat EEG should be performed if there is doubt about electrocerebral inactivity (ECI).

Adapted from www.acns.org/pdfs/Guideline%203.pdf

final $Paco_2$ is <60 mm Hg, the test is indeterminate and can either be repeated or confirmatory testing can be sought.

There are some conditions that may interfere with the clinical diagnosis of brain death, and therefore the testing described above will be inconclusive. In these cases, confirmatory tests are recommended. Situations that may require confirmatory testing include: severe facial trauma, preexisting pupillary abnormalities, toxic levels of sedative drugs (i.e., high dose of long-acting barbiturates), aminoglycosides, tricyclic antidepressants, anticholinergics, antiepileptic drugs, chemotherapeutic or neuromuscular blocking agents, sleep apnea, or pulmonary disease resulting in chronic retention of CO_2.

Confirmatory Testing

If any aspect of the clinical exam cannot be performed, then a confirmatory test is indicated. In some places, confirmatory testing is required before the pronouncement of brain death. Because of the variability in the use of confirmatory testing for brain death in different places, physicians should consult their local laws and guidelines governing this practice. The most commonly used ancillary tests include:

1. Radionuclide cerebral blood flow studies
2. Four-vessel cerebral angiography
3. Transcranial Doppler (TCD) sonography
4. SSEPs
5. EEG

The first three of these studies examine the intracerebral circulation and perfusion above the carotid bifurcation and at the level of the circle of Willis. In each of these, absent blood flow and/or perfusion is consistent with brain death. Because it can be done at bedside, a TCD examination is perhaps the most practical of these for routine use where there is appropriate expertise. An EEG is consistent with brain death if there is no electrical activity for at least 30 minutes of recording and meets the minimal technical criteria as set forth by the American Electroencephalographic Society (Table 18.6). Similarly, on SSEP examination the bilateral absence of N20/P22 response to median nerve stimulation is also consistent with brain death if the recording again meets the minimal technical criteria as set forth by the American Electroencephalographic Society.[20] Figure 18.1 shows examples of several confirmatory studies of brain death.

ORGAN DONATION

Organ donation has the potential to save many thousands of lives. However, this potential remains unrealized due to a lack of donated organs. In the United States, only about one half to one third of eligible organ donors (brain dead patients who meet medical eligibility) become organ donors. This unrealized potential is due to a variety of factors,

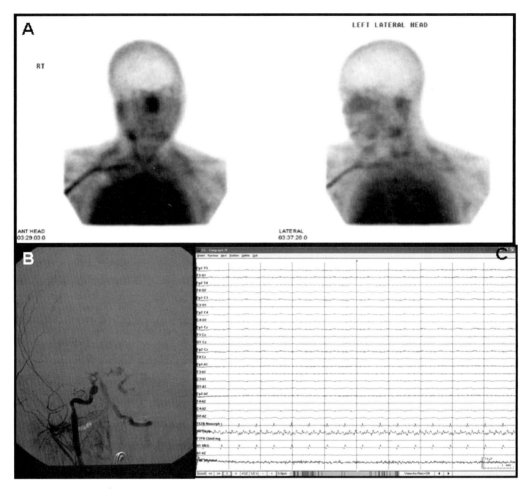

Figure 18.1. Confirmatory tests consistent with the diagnosis of brain death. **(A)** Radionuclide scan shows no perfusion of the brain, despite circulation in the neck and thorax. **(B)** Cerebral angiogram showing an AP view of a right carotid artery injection of contrast dye. The extracranial vessels are visualized with the injection, but there is no intracerebral perfusion beyond the circle of Willis. Contrast travels up the right carotid artery to the circle of Willis, then crosses to the left carotid and basilar arteries. (Courtesy of Phillipe Gailloud.) **(C)** EEG tracing shows electrocerebral silence. (Courtesy of Adam Hartman.) (See also figure in color plate section.)

including that an estimated 25% of families of eligible donors are not approached about organ donation, and there is a low consent rate among those who are presented with the option. Many states and institutions have instituted policies and procedures to increase the percentage of families who are approached about organ donation as well as to increase the consent rate.

The sequencing, timing and coordination of communications with a family can greatly influence their willingness to consent to organ donation. Nearly all hospitals in the United States work with the staff of an Organ Procurement Organization. These staff

members are specially trained to discuss transplantation with families and to coordinate between the family and the medical staff. One of the hallmarks of the current system is a "decoupled" approach. In this approach, the discussion notifying a family of a patient's brain death is performed separately from a discussion about organ donation. Often, the family is first informed of a patient's death and then the physician returns after an interval to introduce a member of the Organ Procurement Organization team.

In addition to obtaining consent for organ donation, there are medical issues that may arise in maintaining the organs in satisfactory condition for donation. The most common threats to organs are pulmonary edema necessitating additional ventilatory support, hypotension requiring fluid resuscitation and vasopressors, and diabetes insipidus requiring fluid and vasopressin repletion. Several studies have shown that aggressive management of organ donors to prevent cardiovascular collapse and with hormonal repletion increases the organs suitable for transplantation.[21]

REFERENCES

1. Plum F, Posner J. *The Diagnosis of Stupor and Coma, 3rd ed*. Philadelphia: F. A. Davis, 1982.

2. Teasdale G, Jennett B. Assessment of coma and impaired consciousness. A practical scale. *Lancet* 1974;**2**:81–4.

3. Wijdicks EF, Bamlet WR, Maramattom BV, Manno EM, McClelland RL. Validation of a new coma scale: the FOUR score. *Ann Neurol*. 2005;**58**:585–93.

4. Young GB, Ropper AH, Bolton CF. *Coma and Impaired Consciousness*. New York: McGraw-Hill, 1998.

5. The Multi-Society Task Force on PVS. Medical aspects of the persistent vegetative state (2). *N Engl J Med*. 1994;**330**:1572–9.

6. The Multi-Society Task Force on PVS. Medical aspects of the persistent vegetative state (1). *N Engl J Med*. 1994;**330**:1499–508.

7. Kinney HC, Korein J, Panigrahy A, Dikkes P, Goode R. Neuropathological findings in the brain of Karen Ann Quinlan. The role of the thalamus in the persistent vegetative state. *N Engl J Med*. 1994;**330**:1469–75.

8. Giacino JT, Ashwal S, Childs N, et al. The minimally conscious state: definition and diagnostic criteria. *Neurology*. 2002;**58**:349–53.

9. Ziai WC. Coma and Altered Consciousness. In: *Current Clinical Neurology: Handbook of Neurocritical Care* (Bhardwaj A, Mirski MS, Ulatowski JA, eds), pp 1–18. Totowa, NJ: Humana Press, 2004.

10. Masson F, Thicoipe M, Mokni T, Aye P, Erny P, Dabadie P. Epidemiology of traumatic comas: a prospective population-based study. *Brain Injury*. 2003;**17**:279.

11. Pazzaglia P, Frank G, Frank F, Gaist G. Clinical course and prognosis of acute post-traumatic coma. *J Neurol Neurosurg Psychiatry*. 1975;**38**:149–54.

12. Bates D. The prognosis of medical coma. *J Neurol Neurosurg Psychiatry*. 2001;**71**(Suppl 1):i20–3.

13. Levy DE, Caronna JJ, Singer BH, Lapinski RH, Frydman H, Plum F. Predicting outcome from hypoxic-ischemic coma. *Jama*. 1985;**253**:1420–6.

14. Wijdicks EF, Hijdra A, Young GB, Bassetti CL, Wiebe S (2006) Practice parameter: prediction of outcome in comatose survivors after cardiopulmonary resuscitation (an evidence-based review): report of the Quality Standards Subcommittee of the American Academy of Neurology. *Neurology*. 2006;**67**:203–10.

15. Sleigh JW, Havill JH, Frith R, Kersel D, Marsh N, Ulyatt D. Somatosensory evoked potentials in severe traumatic brain injury: a blinded study. *J Neurosurg*. 1999;**91**:577–80.

16. Report of the medical consultants on the diagnosis of death to the President's Commission for the Study of Ethical Problems in Medicine and Biomedical and Behavioral Research. Guidelines for the determination of death. *Jama*. 1981;**246**:2184–6.

17. Wijdicks EF. The diagnosis of brain death. *N Engl J Med*. 2001;**344**:1215–21.

18. Ashwal S, Schneider S. Brain death in children: Part I. *Pediatr Neurol*. 1987;**3**:5–11.

19. The Quality Standards Subcommittee of the American Academy of Neurology. Practice parameters for determining brain death in adults (summary statement). *Neurology*. 1995;**45**:1012–4.

20. Wijdicks EF. Determining brain death in fadults. *Neurology*. 1995;**45**:1003–11.

21. Salim A, Velmahos GC, Brown C, Belzberg H, Demetriades D. Aggressive organ donor management significantly increases the number of organs available for transplantation. *J Trauma*. 2005;**58**:991–4.

19 Neuroterrorism and Drug Overdose

Geoffrey S. F. Ling, MD, PhD, Scott Marshall, PharmD, and John J. Lewin III, PharmD, BCPS

Knowledge of proper clinical management of drug overdose and chemical and biological toxin exposure is important for the neurocritical care specialist. Many of the common offenders principally affect the central nervous system (CNS). Even those that do not will lead to a severely incapacitated state when overdosed such that the afflicted patient will require critical care in an intensive care unit (ICU).

Typically, drug overdose that occurs outside of the hospital is first managed in the emergency department and then, if critical care is needed, in the medical intensive care unit. However, there are medications that are used in the neurocritical care unit (NCCU) that may lead to toxic overdose either through inadvertent provider error or because of changes in a patient's drug elimination. The most common offending medications are analgesics, antipyretics, mood stabilizers, and sedative-hypnotics.

Sadly, there is another circumstance in which the neurointensivist may be called on to treat patients suffering from toxic overdose: a chemical or biological terrorist act. In this situation, emergency medicine and medical critical care physicians will be quickly overwhelmed, and it is certain that the neurocritical care specialist will be called upon to assist. Thus, a discussion of the clinical management of patients suffering from exposure to the leading known chemical weapons is warranted.

The opinions presented herein belong solely to those of the authors. They do not nor do they imply belonging to or endorsement by the Uniformed Services University of the Health Sciences, U.S. Army, Department of Defense, or U.S. government.

DRUG OVERDOSE

The most common medications leading to overdose are analgesics, antipyretics, sedative hypnotics, anticonvulsants, anticoagulants, antidepressants, bronchodilators, and antiarrhythmics. All are common medications used in the NCCU.

General clinical management always begins with the ABCs: airway, breathing, and circulation.

- For patients with compromised mental status, adequacy of the airway in terms of both patency and patient's ability to protect it must be determined.
- If the patient has a Glasgow Coma Scale (GCS) score <8, then an artificial airway should be placed such as by endotracheal intubation.
- Mechanical ventilation and supplemental oxygen in such circumstances is not always needed but may be if the patient has aspirated.
- Appropriate hemodynamic management, consisting of fluid resuscitation, vasopressors, and/or inotropes may also be required in cases resulting in myocardial depression and/or vasodilation.

After ensuring the above, the clinician will need first to recognize that the patient's condition is caused by a pharmacologic agent. The optimal way to identify the offending agent is to execute a careful and systematic approach beginning with taking a good history and culminating with laboratory tests.

- History and review of systems are especially useful. During overdose, the patient may not be able to provide details but the medical record and witness accounts may be illuminating.

- The physical exam may also reveal specific clinical clues such as pinpoint pupils in narcotic overdose or nystagmus in anticonvulsant excess.
- Laboratory testing may provide the critical evidence such as metabolic acidosis in aspirin toxicity or excessive drug levels in barbiturate overdose.

After ascertaining that the patient is suffering from toxic overdose, pharmacokinetic directed interventions should be initiated. Further drug absorption needs to be abated. Activated charcoal is the most commonly used agent for this purpose. Owing to its extensive surface area, activated charcoal binds many drugs that have not yet absorbed across the gastrointestinal tract. Once bound, the charcoal–drug mixture is excreted fecally. There is also evidence that activated charcoal interferes with enteroenteric, enterogastric, and enterohepatic recirculation of absorbed drug.

- A major benefit of activated charcoal is that it is nontoxic.
- The most common side effect is emesis, which has largely been controlled by removing sorbitol from preparations.
- However, it should be noted that rigorous scientific evidence is lacking that supports activated charcoal efficacy. In vitro adsorption studies are not always predictive of the drugs effects in vivo. Therefore, human studies are necessary to determine efficacy for any given drug or chemical.[1]

In accordance with recent American Academy of Clinical Toxicologists and the European Association of Poison Centres and Clinical Toxicologists (AACT/EAPCCT) guidelines, if the drug was ingested within 1 hour, then activated charcoal can be given. If not, activated charcoal will have minimal impact.

- Before treatment, it is critical that airway protection is established to minimize aspiration of charcoal or emesis.
- Once airway protection is accomplished, activated charcoal can be administered via a nasogastric tube. The recommended dose for adults is 25–100 grams in water.[1]

Drug exposure may need to be reduced, particularly to the site of action. For some agents, elimination may need to be enhanced through optimizing elimination conditions, such as alkalizing the urine. Urine alkalinization can be considered when the drug is a weak acid and is water soluble, such as barbiturates, salicylates, methotrexate, and lithium.

- Urinary alkalinization can be achieved in a number of ways. The suggested clinical approach is to dilute 150 mEq of sodium bicarbonate in 1 liter of D5W or sterile water.
- Addition of potassium chloride (20–40 mEq/L) to the sodium bicarbonate infusion can be considered in patients with intact renal function, so as to minimize development of hypokalemia.
- The infusion rate should be 2–4 times higher than the usual IV fluid maintenance rate, which results in 200–400 mL/h for most adults.
- The goal urine pH is 7.5–8.5 with additional boluses and/or adjustments to the infusion rate as needed.
- Urine pH should be monitored every 15–30 minutes until the goal urine pH is achieved and then every hour thereafter.
- At the beginning, baseline serum potassium and other electrolytes, creatinine, glucose, and arterial pH are needed. Abnormalities should be corrected.
- Although reported complications are rare, there is the potential for causing hypokalemia, hypocalcemia, reduced oxygen delivery to tissue as the oxyhemoglobin dissociation curve is shifted to the left, cerebral vasoconstriction, and fluid overload/pulmonary edema.
- Every hour thereafter, serum potassium, and arterial pH should be checked. Arterial pH should not exceed 7.50. Urine output should not exceed 200 mL/h.[2]

NARCOTIC ANALGESICS

Morphine is the prototypic drug of the opioid class of drugs. Derived from opium, it is an alkaloid. Most of the clinically used narcotic analgesics are derivatives of morphine or are chemically closely related. Collectively, these are known as opioids and include drugs such as codeine, oxycodone, meperidine, fentanyl, methadone, buprenorphine, heroin, hydromorphone, and so forth. As such, the therapeutic strategy in managing morphine overdose can be applied to these other opioids.[3]

The typical clinical presentation of narcotic analgesic overdose is a triad of "coma, respiratory depression, and pinpoint pupils." The primary mechanism leading to death from overdose is respiratory arrest. Although morphine and its congeners can lead to peripheral vascular dilation via histamine release, severe hypotension is not characteristic of opioid overdose. Thus, cardiac and cardiovascular compromise is uncommon until profound hypoxia occurs. Seizures are more typically related to meperidine and propoxyphene toxicity.[3,4]

- The therapy of choice for emergent reversal of opioid overdose is immediate administration of naloxone, an opioid antagonist, at 0.4 mg, IV or 0.8 mg, IM.
- In nonemergent situations, 0.4 mg can be diluted in 9 mL of 0.9% NaCl to make a 40 μg/mL solution.
- Give 40–80 μg (1–2 mL) IV every 2 minutes until the opioid effects are adequately reversed. Giving naloxone in this manner ensures the minimally effective reversal dose, to allow for better pain control and minimization of withdrawal phenomenon. This is particularly relevant for patients with chronic pain on long-term opioid therapy.
- The ideal route of administration is intravenous but it can be given by other parenteral routes and via an endotracheal tube as well.
- Naloxone should not be given orally because it is rapidly degraded via first-pass effect through the liver.
- Naloxone is effective for reversing all opioid effects. The response is within a minute or two and lasts for up to an hour.
- If recovery is incomplete, higher doses may be used but one should consider also the possibility that another class of drug may be contributing as well.[4,5]

An important aspect of naloxone therapy is the short duration of action. Thus, repeated doses of naloxone will be needed until the causative agent is completely eliminated. In the ICU setting, this can be via an IV infusion or periodic dosing.[5]

Untoward effects of naloxone are uncommon because naloxone does not have any agonist activity. However, naloxone can precipitate an acute opioid withdrawal syndrome because it causes agonists such as morphine to vacate opioid receptors.

Rarely, when given in very high doses, naloxone can result in pulmonary edema, agitation, and cardiac arrhythmia.[5]

Chronic use of opioids leads to physical dependence. Thus, abrupt cessation or reversal of dosing will lead to withdrawal. Controlled withdrawal from opioid dependence is managed differently from acute intoxication.

- Typically, a long-acting opioid such as methadone may be used. A dose of methadone equivalent to 25% of the daily narcotic dose is administered once per day to suppress withdrawal. This daily dose is gradually reduced, for example, 10%, over a week or more until the patient is fully tapered.
- Clonidine may be given in addition to methadone or another detoxification regimen. Symptoms of opioid withdrawal are due in part to increased noradrenergic activity in areas such as the locus ceruleus. Acting as a central α_2-adrenergic receptor agonist, clonidine may suppress this sympathetic outflow and abate some of the cardiovascular and other effects of withdrawal. However, clonidine does not typically resolve the subjective or autonomic signs and symptoms of opioid withdrawal. Thus, as the opioid is discontinued, clonidine is given in gradually smaller doses over 10 days to 2 weeks.[3]

Phenytoin

Phenytoin is one of the more commonly used drugs in the neurocritical care unit. Overdose is uncommon but has significant potential consequences should this occur.

- At the blood concentrations exceeding therapeutic levels, >20 μg/mL, the most common clinical findings are nystagmus, ataxia, diplopia, and vertigo. This is related to its excitatory effect in the cerebellum.
- As blood levels further increase, to >40 μg/mL, patients may experience hyperactivity, hallucinations, and confusion.
- At severely toxic levels, >40 μg/mL, patients become lethargic and, when >50 μg/mL, may progress to decerebrate rigidity and coma.
- Cardiac complications of arrhythmias and hypotension are more commonly associated with administering the drug intravenously too rapidly.

However, at toxic levels, these cardiovascular effects can be seen.[6]

Phenytoin is eliminated via a saturable hepatic microsomal enzyme system. Thus, elimination follows zero-order kinetics, which means a certain amount of drug is metabolized over time as opposed to a certain percentage. As the blood concentration becomes higher, the time to eliminate the drug fully becomes progressively longer.[6]

Medical care is primarily supportive. If the overdose was oral, then activated charcoal may be given. Hepatic function will need to be determined and carefully monitored as an untoward sequel may be hepatic failure.

Heparin

Unfractionated heparin (UFH) is a glycosaminoglycan with a molecular weight ranging from 3000 to 30,000 daltons. It is a drug with variable anticoagulant effects, as the different molecular weights have different affinities for clotting factors. In addition, molecular weight also affects clearance of the drug, as lower molecular weight molecules are cleared faster. UFH is an antithrombotic agent that acts indirectly through antithrombin (AT) to inhibit several clotting factors: XIIa XIa, IXa, Xa, IIa, and XIIIa. Blood clotting is fully inhibited in vitro at a concentration of 1 unit/mL of whole blood. A 10,000-unit bolus to a 70-kg male will lead to a blood concentration of 3 units/mL. The effects of this dose begin almost immediately and last about 1.5 hours.[7–9]

For UFH, partial thromboplastin times (PTT) are measured at regular intervals. If the PTT is excessively high or there has been inadvertent overdose, then further administration is stopped. Usually, no further intervention is needed. However, if there is evidence of excessive hemorrhage, then protamine sulfate, a heparin antagonist, may be given. Protamine acts by binding ionically to heparin to form an inactive complex.

- The dose of protamine sulfate needed to reverse heparin effects fully is 1 mg/100 units of retained heparin with a maximum of 100 mg. This is administered by slow IV bolus at a rate of dosing <20 mg/min.
- Side effects of protamine sulfate are related to histamine release and are thus dyspnea, flushing, bradycardia, and hypotension. These are largely avoided by slow administration. There have been reports of hypersensitivity and are usually associated with patients allergic to fish.[3,8,9]

Low molecular weight heparins (LMWHs) have an improved pharmacokinetic profile as compared to UFH. When compared to UFH, subcutaneous administration of LMWHs produces a more linear and reliable degree of anticoagulation. LMWH anticoagulation is due to preferentially binding to and inhibiting of factor Xa. This is highly relevant to toxicity as PTT cannot be used as a measure of LMWH anticoagulation. PTT is mediated via inhibition of thrombin (factor IIa). Antifactor Xa level can be used instead because this is a measure of the anticoagulant effects of LMWHs, but this test is not widely available. Another consideration is that many different LMWHs are available. Each possesses a different half-life, all of which are longer than UFH. The effects of UFH may last hours whereas LMWHs effects may last for hours to days. Also unlike UFH, LMWHs are primarily cleared via the kidneys, so renal dysfunction may prolong the half-life substantially.[8–10]

- There is no well-established method for reversing the effects of LMWH.
  - Protamine will only partially neutralize LMWH, about 60% of its effects.
  - The dose is 1 mg of protamine for every 100 units of antifactor Xa activity.
  - For enoxaparin, this is approximately 1 mg of protamine per milligram of enoxaparin to be reversed.[7,8]

Warfarin

Warfarin is a congener of dicumarol, which is derived from sweet clover. It is an antithrombotic agent that interferes with blood clotting by inhibiting the vitamin K dependent clotting cascade of factors II, VII, IX, and X. These factors are dependent on vitamin K to transition from inactive precursor proteins to their active form. Warfarin has an elimination half-life of about 36 hours. However, its pharmacologic antithrombotic effect is related to the degradation of the four target clotting factors. The degradation half-lives of VII, IX, X, and II are 6, 24, 40, and 60 hours, respectively. Thus, onset of action is about 8–12 hours after administration. To gain the full antithrombotic effect, there is a delay of about 3–5 days from peak drug concentration to allow degradation of circulating factors and warfarin's inhibition of further activation.[3,11]

Typically, the international normalized ratio (INR) of prothrombin time (PT) is used to monitor the antithrombotic effects of warfarin. The management of warfarin therapy and elevated INR in the absence of bleeding can be complex, and is beyond the scope of this chapter. The reader is referred to the American College of Chest Physicians' Guidelines for more information.[12]

- In the event of serious bleeding, further warfarin administration is stopped and fresh frozen plasma (FFP) or prothrombin complex concentrate (PCC) should be administered. In addition, one can consider giving 10 mg of vitamin K by slow IV infusion. If needed, vitamin K can be repeated every 12 hours.
- In the event of life-threatening bleeding, both PCC and 10 mg of vitamin K is given. In this setting, an alternative to PCC is recombinant factor VIIa. It should be noted that these high doses of vitamin K are reserved only for serious or life-threatening bleeds. Such dosing will render the patient warfarin-resistant for a prolonged period of time.
- If continued anticoagulation is needed after bleeding is stopped, UFH or LMWH may be used until the patient becomes responsive to warfarin. Of note, IV administration is associated with rare but serious anaphylactic reactions that do not appear to be dose-related.[3,11,12]

Direct Thrombin Inhibitors

Direct thrombin inhibitors, such as argatroban, lepirudin, and bivalirudin, are a newer class of anticoagulants used in the settings of heparin-induced thrombocytopenia, and acute coronary syndromes. There are no well-studied reversal agents for this class of drug. Aside from stopping the infusion, consideration may be given to recombinant factor VIIa or PCC.[13,14]

Acetaminophen

Acetaminophen is a commonly used antipyretic and mild analgesic. The mechanism of action is not fully understood but it is a weak cyclooxygenase (COX) 1 and 2 inhibitor. The predominant elimination pathways for acetaminophen are hepatic glucuronidation and conjugation with sulfate. The sulfate and glucuronide products are then excreted in the feces. However, about 10% is oxidized to N-acetyl-p-benzoquinone imine (NAPQI). NAPQI is hepatocyte toxic. NAPQI is conjugated with glutathione, which goes to cysteine and mercapturic acid. During acetaminophen overdose, glutathione stores are depleted, allowing NAPQI to accumulate and bind directly to hepatocytes. This results in hepatic necrosis.[3,15]

- Clinically, within the first 24 hours or phase 1, patients will complain of malaise, nausea and vomiting, and be diaphoretic.
- Phase 2 occurs 24–72 hours after ingestion. At this point, patients will have right upper quadrant tenderness, enlarged liver, elevated liver enzymes (aspartate aminotransferase [AST], alanine aminotransferase [ALT], bilirubin), prolonged prothrombin time and oliguria. Clinical symptoms of phase 1 resolve.
- Phase 3 occurs from 72 to 96 hours and is characterized by hepatic failure, renal failure, and cardiomyopathy. Patients will have recurrence of phase 1 symptoms.
- In phase 4, which occurs at 4 days to 2 weeks, patients will either recover or die. If this clinical condition should progress to fulminant hepatic failure, then prognosis becomes guarded, as only 50% of such patients will survive. The risk of developing fulminant hepatic failure is high when there is any one of the following: (1) metabolic acidosis of pH <7.3 in spite of fluid resuscitation, (2) creatinine >3.3, (3) PT >1.8, or (4) patient has reached phase 3 or 4.[16]

If the time of ingestion is known and a dose exceeding 150 mg/kg was taken, then intervention is necessary. If less than this, then a blood level should be obtained 4 hours after ingestion and plotted on an acetaminophen blood toxicity or Rumack–Matthew nomogram. Treatment should be started if in the toxicity range. If the time of ingestion is unknown, then a blood level should be obtained immediately. If >5 μg/mL, then treatment should be initiated. Of note, blood acetaminophen, transaminase, and ammonia levels are not prognostic.[16]

- If within 1 hour of ingestion, activated charcoal should be given, which will help reduce further absorption.
- The mainstay of acetaminophen toxicity therapy is *N*-acetylcysteine (NAC). NAC is administered PO beginning with a loading dose of 140 mg/kg. Thereafter, 70 mg/kg is given every 4 hours for a total of 17 doses or 72 hours.
  - ▷ NAC is a precursor to glutathione. Once given, NAC will bind to both NAPQI that is free and bound to hepatocytes. Thus, it both aborts ongoing hepatocyte toxicity and prevents further toxicity by facilitating elimination of NAPQI.[15]
  - ▷ The most common side effect from NAC is nausea and vomiting. If vomiting occurs, repeat dosing may be needed. This can be minimized by using an antiemetic agent.

Alcohol

Alcohol is a widely abused drug. It is rarely given in the NCCU for therapeutic purposes. However, patients are routinely admitted to the NCCU for non–alcohol-related problems but are concurrently in various stages of inebriation or withdrawal.

Alcohol is a sedative hypnotic drug. Like barbiturates, it is a global depressant. At low doses, inhibitory pathways are inhibited leading to net excitation. At progressively higher doses, drowsiness to lethargy to stupor and ultimately coma will ensue. Most inebriated patients can usually be managed conservatively and do not require intensive care monitoring. However, severely inebriated patients who present in stupor or coma, may need airway protection.

- All patients should be hydrated to maintain euvolemia.
- Thiamine, 100 mg, IV/IM is given to mitigate Wernicke–Korsakoff's syndrome. Wernicke's encephalopathy is due to acute thiamine deficiency whereas Korsakoff psychosis is the long-term sequel.
  - ▷ In Wernicke's encephalopathy, patients present with confusion, ataxia, ophthalmoplegia, and nystagmus.
  - ▷ This syndrome leads to Korsakoff's psychosis, which manifests as worsening confusion, confabulation, and amnesia. It is a result of lack of vitamin B_1, which is thiamine. The classic lesions are mammillary body and thalamic degeneration.[17]
- It is important to administer thiamine before glucose. During aerobic respiration, glucose is metabolized to pyruvate, which then enters the Krebs or citric acid cycle. However, this process requires thiamine.
  - ▷ If glucose is administered when thiamine is deficient, Wernicke's syndrome can be precipitated.
- As these patients are typically malnourished, they should also receive folate, magnesium, multiple vitamins and electrolyte replacement.[17]
- If there is concern of ethanol withdrawal, then a benzodiazepine should be given. This can be lorazepam or Serax. Longer acting benzodiazepines such as chlordiazepoxide or diazepam are effective but are used less often in the NCCU owing to their prolonged duration of action and potential for depressing mental status.

Barbiturates

The barbiturates are classic sedative-hypnotic drugs. All share common chemical features, for example, barbituric acid core. As such they have similar spectrums of action such as inducing drowsiness and suppressing central ventilatory control centers. Pentobarbital may be considered the prototype of this class of drugs. However, more commonly used agents are thiopental, phenobarbital, amobarbital, and secobarbital.[3]

All are global CNS depressants. At therapeutic doses, they have minimal effect on peripheral nervous system and tissue such as skeletal, cardiac, or smooth muscle. At toxic doses, these drugs can have a depressant effect on the medullary vasomotor area and thus lead to cardiovascular compromise. Clinically, patients become increasingly lethargic with increasing dosage. An electroencephalogram (EEG) will show slowing that progresses to burst suppression at high doses. Thus, at toxic doses, patients will be comatose, in respiratory arrest, hypotensive, and hypothermic.[3]

- Medical management is primarily supportive, involving airway, mechanical ventilation, and cardiovascular care.
- If the drug was administered orally, activated charcoal should be given.

- To facilitate elimination, the urine may be alkalinized.
  - This is more useful for long-acting agents such as phenobarbital. As phenobarbital has a pK_a of 7.2 and is water soluble, this approach can be effective.
- Hemodialysis, peritoneal dialysis, and hemoperfusion may be also considered. However, these are usually reserved for patients who are in extremis and are worsening in spite of conventional therapy.[2,18,19]

Benzodiazepines

Benzodiazepines are also sedative-hypnotics. However, they are chemically distinct from barbiturates. Benzodiazepines contain a benzene ring fused to a seven-member diazepine ring. Diazepam is the prototype of this class of drugs. Other commonly used congeners are midazolam, lorazepam, alprazolam, and clonazepam.[3]

These therapeutic agents share common clinical features. At low therapeutic doses, they cause sedation and muscle relaxation. They do not cause myocardial or ventilatory depression. As dosage increases, there is increasing CNS depression from hypnosis to stupor. However, even at very high doses, none of these agents will cause true general anesthesia. To achieve surgical anesthesia, these must be used in combination with other drugs.[3]

- Medical management is primarily supportive. If the only overdose drug is a benzodiazepine, then conservative management is best. Typically, even with very high doses, patients do not require airway protection, mechanical ventilation or cardiovascular support. If this is their only medical problem, they do not require ICU care.
- When combined with other CNS depressants, such as alcohol or opioids, high levels of benzodiazepine can contribute to a patient's comatose state. In such cases, more aggressive medical management is indicated, including advanced critical care.[3,20]
- Another therapeutic option is flumazenil, a benzodiazepine antagonist. For management of known or suspected benzodiazepine overdose, the initial dose of flumazenil is 0.2 mg given intravenously over 30 seconds. If the desired response

is not obtained after waiting 30 additional seconds, a dose of 0.3 mg can be administered over 30 seconds. Additional doses of 0.5 mg can be given over 30 seconds at 1-minute intervals up to a total cumulative dose of 3 mg.

- The onset of action is rapid, often within 1–2 minutes. It can reverse any effects of benzodiazepine.
- The duration of action is about 45 minutes. Thus, when treating overdose of long acting agonists, additional doses of flumazenil will be needed.
- There are untoward effects. As this drug blocks GABA/benzodiazepine receptors, it has the potential to lower seizure threshold. Also, flumazenil can precipitate withdrawal (including refractory seizures and status epilepticus) in patients who chronically take benzodiazepines.
- This agent is generally reserved for patients who are comatose and have ventilatory and cardiovascular compromise in whom benzodiazepine overdose is thought to contribute.[3,20]

Tricyclic Antidepressants

The tricyclic antidepressants (TCA) are widely used medications. The prototypes of this drug class are imipramine and amitriptyline. Other TCAs are nortriptyline, desipramine, doxepine, amoxapine and others. Their therapeutic mechanisms of action are serotonin and norepinephrine reuptake inhibition. These agents also have anticholinergic effects that contribute to their toxicity.[3]

The classic TCA triad of toxicity is *T*onic–clonic seizures, *C*ardiovascular and *A*nticholinergic. As TCA are centrally acting agents, it is not surprising that there are significant toxic CNS effects.

- In addition to seizures, patients can develop delirium, agitation and confusion but will progress with increasing doses to obtundation and coma.
- Cardiovascular effects are described as "quinidine-like" as conduction is slowed. EKG changes include widened QRS complexes, prolonged PR intervals, AV conduction blocks and, if severe, ventricular arrhythmias. Vasodilation and decreased myocardial contractility can lead to fatal hypotension and dysrhythmia. Electrocardiography (EKG) also has prognostic value. If QRS is >100 ms,

there is an increased risk of seizure and >160 ms, increased risk of dysrhythmia.

■ Anticholinergic effects are delirium, hyperthermia, flushing, anhydrosis, dry mouth, anuria, ileus and mydriasis. The clinical course of TCA toxicity is typically 48 hours.[21]

Therapy is mainly conservative. For seizures, lorazepam (1–4 mg, IV) can be used. Phenytoin should not be given as it can exacerbate TCA cardiovascular effects. If hypotension occur, fluid resuscitation and vasopressor therapy should be initiated.

■ Vasopressors that can be considered are epinephrine and norepinephrine.

■ Dopamine is not recommended as it requires release of endogenous norepinephrine to be effective, which may be blocked by TCA.

■ In the event of arrhythmias, sodium bicarbonate (1–2 mEq/kg) should be given with a goal of arterial pH 7.45–7.55. Class 1a and 1c antiarrhythmics are contraindicated.[21]

CHEMICAL AND BIOLOGICAL TERRORISM

Chemical and biological terrorism is a serious domestic concern. In 1984, a Salmonella attack was perpetuated in Oregon by the Rajneeshee cult and more recently, in 2001, the Amerithrax letter attacks. Outside of the United States, there have been many attacks on civilians. One particularly successive attack was the sarin attack in Tokyo. These and others underscore the importance of vigilance for both civilian and military medical systems world-wide. Awareness of this potential threat is important to the neurocritical care practitioner to ensure proper clinical management of attacked patients.[22]

In 1984, the Rajneeshee cult deposited a strain of *Salmonella typhimurium* on doorknobs, urinal handles, supermarket produce, and salad bars throughout an Oregon community. This resulted in the infection of 751 cases of severe gastroenteritis. Nearly 1,000 patients sought treatment, which overwhelmed the local medical care system. Fortunately, there were no fatalities. This attack had followed the Tylenol cyanide poisonings in the Chicago area in 1982, where 7 fatalities were reported related to product tampering and placement of potassium cyanide into medication capsules. Similar attacks, possibly related to the intense media coverage of the

Tylenol scare, occurred subsequent to the original Tylenol tampering case. The original case remains unsolved.[23]

Internationally, one of the most striking cases of biological warfare-related civilian disasters is the Sverdlovsk (now Yekaterinburg) anthrax infections beginning in April of 1979. An apparent accidental release of aerosol containing weapons grade *Bacillus anthracis* spores occurred in this region of the former Soviet Union. Exposed civilians over a 4-km area developed symptoms consistent with inhalation anthrax. There were 77 patients identified with inhalation anthrax, and of these, only 11 survived. To date, this is the most deadly anthrax event.[24,25]

Perhaps the most illustrative episode is the Tokyo subway sarin gas poisonings in 1995 perpetuated by the Aum Shinrikyo cult. This is a good example of what can happen to a modern medical care system when encountering a terrorist attack. Initially, within the first few hours, a few hundred patients were brought to the hospital. However, ultimately, more than 5,500 patients sought medical treatment, which was overwhelming. Among the casualties were unprotected healthcare providers who developed secondary contamination when treating victims. There were 12 deaths from the attacks, and at least 50 were seriously injured from organophosphate poisoning, including seizures. One important finding is that the vast majority of patients, about 80%, did not have evidence of nerve agent exposure. Instead, they had a wide variety of complaints that were largely not attributable to sarin exposure. This very large category of patients has been called "the worried well." However, their impact to significantly burden a very busy medical care system during a critical period cannot be underestimated. This attack serves as a case study for the potential for modern biological and chemical terrorism, and the medical, social, and political consequences of such.[22,26,27]

In a terrorist attack, the demands placed on the individual provider and local medical care system can be overwhelming. Traditional approaches to triage and care delivery will be inadequate. Thus, it is crucial that preparation for such events is done in advance and that the system as a whole practices. In the event of a terrorist attack in which many casualties result, neuro critical care specialists may find themselves assisting outside of the NCCU such as in a triage area, emergency department, or decontamination lane.

BIOLOGICAL AGENTS

Biological agents are attractive weapons to terrorists as these agents are inexpensive, relatively easy to procure, and present a time delay to onset of action that allows for successful deployment and escape from authorities. It was long held that these agents are difficult to refine to a weapons grade, that is, in a size and form that is easily disseminated to cause maximal effectiveness. In reality, weaponization of biological agents is within the ability of terrorists. From the Amerithrax letters case, FBI and other experts concluded that very high grade of refined anthrax spores was used. The terrorist was able to achieve a particle size of 1–5 μm in diameter, which is ideal to cause pulmonary anthrax, the most lethal manifestation of this disease.[24]

Anthrax

Bacillus anthracis is the bacteria responsible for anthrax. It has been manufactured in a weaponized form by the United States and several other nations, including the former USSR. Several days after the events of September 11, 2001, the anthrax mail attacks commenced, resulting in at least 22 cases of anthrax and 5 deaths. The historical potential for anthrax to present as a hemorrhagic meningoencephalitis makes this agent of particular interest to the neurocritical care physician.[28]

Inhalational anthrax is especially rare. Thus, it is advised that even a single case of inhalational anthrax should prompt local health officials to suspect a terrorist attack. Historically, this has been referred to as "wool sorter's disease," owing to its association with industrial mill's processing of hides, furs, and wool.

- Clinical symptoms present after an incubation period of 1–6 days, although there are reports of cases of inhalational anthrax that presented up to 6 weeks after exposure.
- Initial symptoms are nonspecific, such as fever, malaise, headache, and respiratory complaints.
- Patients with inhalational anthrax do not show typical signs of routine upper respiratory infections and pneumonia is uncommon.
- Physical examination findings are limited, but often patients present with tachycardia.
- The diagnosis is based on epidemiologic data and chest radiographic findings of widened

mediastinum and pleural effusions. This is likely due to a hemorrhagic mediastinitis.
  - ▸ Chest radiography or chest computed tomography (CT) should be performed in all suspected cases. In the 2001 attack, these were abnormal in every patient with inhalational anthrax.
- Organisms are not usually isolated from the sputum of patients. Instead, the majority of cases have been confirmed by blood culture, which can detect anthrax in its early stage.
- Other laboratory abnormalities include elevated transaminases, elevated white blood cell count with a polymorphonuclear leukocyte (PMN) predominance (average of 9800 cells/dL in the 2001 Amerithrax attacks).
- As the disease progresses, subsequent symptoms include respiratory distress and the development of septic shock. Death may follow severe pulmonary symptoms in 1–2 days unless intensive care support and proper antimicrobial management is instituted.
- Mortality reports vary widely from 45% to 99%, likely the result of modern intensive care management of the inhalation form of the disease. Evidence of this was taken from the Amerithrax letters of 2001 in the United States, which were associated with the lower end of this mortality spectrum owing to aggressive treatment and recognition of the disease.[24]

Cutaneous anthrax is the most common naturally occurring form of the disease. The most salient feature of cutaneous anthrax is a painless skin lesion that, over the course of days, can progress to a vesicle, ulcer, and then eschar with surrounding edema.

- These lesions can be cultured unless the patient has begun systemic antibiotic treatment.
- Gram stain will often show gram-positive bacilli.
- Mortality from the cutaneous form of anthrax is approximately 20%.

Gastrointestinal anthrax is another highly fatal form of this disease and occurs after eating of infected meat. This is another possible mode of terrorist attack.

- Gastrointestinal anthrax can present as an acute gastroenteritis, acute abdomen with peritoneal signs, or diarrheal illness.
- Stool culture is not very sensitive for anthrax.

- The diagnosis is usually made via polymerase chain reaction (PCR) and immunostaining of either peritoneal or ascetic fluid.
- Mortality from gastrointestinal anthrax ranges from 60% to 80%.[24,29]

Anthrax-associated hemorrhagic meningoencephalitis, seen in approximately 50% of cases of inhalational anthrax, can present after either the inhalational or cutaneous route of infection.

- This usually manifests as multifocal intracerebral hemorrhage well visualized on head CT.
- If the patient has severe pulmonary symptoms or cutaneous manifestations concerning for anthrax, prompt sampling of the cerebrospinal fluid (CSF) should be performed.
  - ▸ Often the organism can be seen on gram stain of the CSF, as *Bacillus anthracis* appears as large gram-positive bacilli singly or in short chains, with squared-off ends.
  - ▸ Other CSF findings are low glucose level, elevated protein, red blood cells, and a leukocytosis >500 cells/mL.
- Hemorrhagic meningoencephalitis from anthrax is an ominous condition as death usually ensues within 1 week of diagnosis.
- Other neurologic manifestations of anthrax include headache, mental status changes, visual field deficits, and changes in acuity. These symptoms can present with any mode of infection.[28,29]

Treatment of anthrax is dependent on the mode of bacterial inoculation. With inhalational anthrax, the emphasis is on ventilatory support and intravenous antimicrobials (Table 19.1). With early institution of antibiotics, survival may approach >50%.

- In adults, initial therapy should begin with ciprofloxacin 400 mg IV q12h or doxycycline 200 mg IV followed by 100 mg IV q12h.
- In children, the doses are ciprofloxacin 10–15 mg/ kg (maximum 400 mg) IV q12h, or doxycycline (100 mg IV q12h for children >8 years and >45 kg, and 2.2 mg/kg IV q12h for children <8 years or <45 kg).
  - ▸ The use of tetracyclines in children is generally discouraged.
- The addition of one or two other antibiotics with activity against *Bacillus anthracis* should also be used until susceptibilities return.

- The bacteria has shown genomic evidence for encoding of both constitutive and inducible β-lactamases and thus single agent use of a β-lactam antibiotics is not advised.
- Owing to poor penetration of the CNS with several of these antimicrobials, therapy of anthrax infection with any neurologic manifestation must include ciprofloxacin and rifampin.
- A preexposure vaccine is available, which is completed through a series of 6 doses over 18 months, followed by yearly booster vaccination.
- Patients with anthrax in any form of the disease require standard precautions. Person-to-person spread has not been documented.[24,29]

Botulinum Toxin

The toxin produced by the gram-positive bacillus *Clostridium botulinum* is widely known as the deadliest toxin. It is estimated that a gram of botulinum toxin could kill more than 1 million people. Ethical uses of botulinum toxin are for the treatment of spasticity, dystonia, blepharospasm, strabismus, cervical torticollis, and others.[29,30]

Botulism is most often acquired via the gastrointestinal route after ingestion of spores in contaminated food. Skin contact with botulinum toxin does not produce clinical infection or toxicity. There are three distinct forms of the disease: gastrointestinal, wound, and infant botulism. There are about 200 cases annually in the United States. An inhalational form of botulism has been produced experimentally in primates.[29,30]

The toxin has proven difficult to weaponize in an effective manner. Thus, it has not been developed as a conventional battlefield weapon. However, its potential use as a terrorist weapon is not inconceivable. Contamination of water supplies, food, and aerosol spraying are likely modes of dissemination for terrorist purposes. The Aum Shinrikyo cult attempted to deploy botulinum toxin without success. This was believed to be due to inadequate understanding of technical factors, as well as poor overall microbiology of *Clostridium botulinum*.[30]

Botulism as a disease is well known to neurologists, producing an acute, descending paralysis that begins in the bulbar musculature. The toxin acts via cleavage of the *N*-ethylmaleimide-sensitive factor attachment protein receptor (SNARE protein), which prevents fusion of the

Table 19.1. Antimicrobial treatment for various forms of *Bacillus anthracis* (adult doses)[24]

Manifestation of disease	Preferred therapy	Alternative therapy
Inhalational anthrax	Ciprofloxacin 400 mg IV q12h	Doxycycline 200 mg IV load followed by 100 mg IV q12h
Cutaneous anthrax	Ciprofloxacin 500 mg PO q12h	Doxycycline 100 mg PO q12h or amoxicillin 500 mg PO q8h
Gastrointestinal anthrax	Ciprofloxacin 400 mg IV q12h	Doxycycline 200 mg IV load followed by 100 mg IV q12hours
Anthrax-associated meningoencephalitis	Ciprofloxacin 400 mg IV q8h + rifampin (CNS penetration)	Doxycycline 200 mg IV load followed by 100 mg IV q12hours

acetylcholine-containing vesicles with the presynaptic membrane at the neuromuscular junction. This produces a paucity of acetylcholine in the synaptic cleft and results in clinical weakness. There are seven known types of botulinum toxin, all with similar clinical effects.[22,29,30]

The disease presentation is similar regardless of the type of toxin or the way in which it is contracted. An acute descending paralysis, beginning in the cranial nerves, precedes systemic weakness including respiratory musculature.

- The initial manifestations of clinical botulism are ptosis, poorly reactive dilated pupils, and the development of ocular misalignment with diplopia and disconjugate gaze. This can progress to facial weakness, dysarthria, and dysphagia.
- Some of these signs or symptoms may be confused with other forms of acute descending weakness with cranial nerve palsies, to include tick paralysis, Miller-Fisher variant of Guillain-Barré, myasthenia gravis, pontine infarction, or diphtheria infection.[31]
- One particular clinical clue to the diagnosis of botulism is the involvement of the pupils, which is unlikely in more common conditions such as myasthenia gravis.
- The diagnosis can be confirmed with serology available at the Centers for Disease Control and Prevention, but electrophysiologic studies including nerve conduction testing and repetitive stimulation at 50 Hz showing an incremental response is diagnostic. CSF analysis and neuroimaging studies are typically normal.
- This disease can be rapidly fatal unless patients are treated aggressively with botulinum antitoxin

and supportive measures including mechanical ventilator support.
  - ▶ Antitoxin is an equine immunoglobulin and is available from the Centers for Disease Control and Prevention.
  - ▶ This immunoglobulin can stabilize a deteriorating patient, but may not result in clinical improvement of motor weakness.
- Mechanical ventilation should be instituted when negative inspiratory flow declines below –30 to –20 cm of water or vital capacity falls below 15 mL/kg.
- Convalescence from botulinum intoxication can take up to 1 year for a complete recovery.[31]

Q Fever

Coxiella burnetii is the causative organism of Q fever. Its use as a terrorist weapon is based on the organism's ability to undergo a sporelike form. As a spore, it is resistant to inactivation from heat or desiccation, allowing it to survive in most environments for months. It is highly potent. This is a zoonotic illness, as the bacterial reservoirs are in sheep, cattle, cats, rodents, and goats. The organism is concentrated in the mammary glands and uteri of infected animals. Thus natural infection of humans usually occurs during contact with products of conception or by eating infected milk or cheese.

- It typically produces a self-limited respiratory infection, pneumonia, and/or hepatitis.
- Less frequently, meningoencephalitis can occur, along with cardiac manifestations including myocarditis and pericarditis.

- The hallmark of the disease is the onset of high fevers, up to 105°F, presenting a mean of 15 days after exposure.
- Chest radiographs typically show multifocal infiltrates.
- Serum studies show elevated transaminases, although fulminant hepatic failure is quite rare.
- Infections of pregnant women can lead to undesirable outcomes of pregnancy, such as abortion and low birth weight.[24,29]

Neurologic manifestations of Q fever occur in up to 23% of cases. These include psychosis, expressive aphasia, facial pain resembling tic douloureux, ocular misalignment with diplopia, and dysarthria. In the acute phase of this disease, optic neuritis can occur. In latter stages, if untreated, this condition can progress to encephalitis, encephalomyelitis, and myelopathy. The diagnosis is made via serology, as culturing this organism is difficult and dangerous to laboratory personnel.[32]

Infection control measures with known cases of Q fever involve standard precautions. Postmortem infections of healthcare workers during autopsy have been documented. The earlier treatment is initiated, the more effective antibiotics may be at preventing development of a chronic infection.

- Initial treatment is with doxycycline 100 mg every 12 hours for 15–21 days.
- Other options include fluoroquinolones such as ciprofloxacin for 3 weeks.
- For patients with neurologic symptoms, the quinolones are preferred because of better CNS penetration than doxycycline.[22,24]

Smallpox

Variola virus, the causative agent of smallpox, has been used to deliberately infect civilians since the British used this as a weapon against the Native Americans in the French and Indian War in the mid-1700s. The naturally occurring form of the disease was declared eradicated in 1980, and the last known case occurred in 1977.

Initial infection with variola virus occurs through the respiratory tract. Over the first 4 days, the virus is usually asymptomatic, but a blood-borne infection has begun. The characteristic skin lesion usually occurs on about day 6–8 of infection. The viral infectivity is high at this stage from exposure to droplets or environmental agents.[29,33,34]

- The clinical presentation of the virus begins with headache, backache, malaise, and in some cases, delirium. This can precede the emergence of the rash, which develops on the face and upper extremities before emergence of skin lesions on the trunk. This is helpful in distinguishing the rash from other more common viral exanthems such as varicella virus.
- There is currently a vaccine in use by the military and certain healthcare providers.

The virus is especially important to the NCCU physician because of an uncommon side effect of the renewed vaccination program. An estimated 1:300,000 of persons vaccinated with smallpox can develop post-vaccination encephalitis, which occurs 1–2 weeks after vaccine administration, and has a mortality of 25%. The encephalitis presents with headache, meningeal signs, fever, lethargy, vomiting, and rarely spastic paralysis that can progress to seizures, coma, and death. Treatment of the encephalitis is supportive.[33]

Venezuelan Equine Encephalitis

Venezuelan Equine Encephalitis (VEE) is the best characterized and studied member of the alphavirus family as a bioweapon owing to its place in the United States offensive biological weapons program in the 1950s and 1960s. This virus occurs naturally in the United States, and is often associated with horse outbreaks of encephalitis that usually precede human illness in the community. It is spread by infected mosquitoes, and is quite virulent in the equine population, resulting in a 30–90% mortality. The main cycle of transmission is via infected mosquitoes and wild birds. In humans, the mortality estimates are much lower, although an outbreak in Venezuela and Columbia in 1995 killed approximately 300 persons, with >75,000 cases reported.[24,35]

The most common presentation for VEE is that of an acute febrile, incapacitating illness which rarely results in clinical encephalitis in humans. Approximately 1 in 10 of those infected with VEE will require hospitalization.

- Symptoms occur within a week of inoculation, and include sudden complaints of high fever, malaise, chills, rigors, profound headache, photophobia, and lower extremity and back muscle soreness.
- The illness can take up to 2 weeks for convalescence, and often relapses can be seen clinically after apparent resolution.
- Pregnant females, children younger than 15 years of age, and the elderly population are more susceptible to serious neurologic manifestations of the illness with attack rates ranging from 1% to 4% of these populations and mortality ranging from 10% to 35%.
- Seizures, ataxia, and mental status changes can be seen, and the likelihood of such neurologic manifestations is theoretically greater after an intentional, likely aerosolized viral agent attack, via transmission of the virus directly into the CNS and the olfactory nerve.[24]

The diagnosis of VEE is based on epidemiologic data, sentinel herd data from equine surveillance, and serological studies and PCR analysis. IgM antibodies are produced within about 5 days after clinical symptoms appear. PCR is available commercially and at the Centers for Disease Control and Prevention. Treatment is supportive as no specific treatment is available for VEE.[35]

Tetrodotoxin

Tetrodotoxin (TTX) is produced by the puffer fish, or fugu, which is commonly found in the tropics. TTX is a sodium channel blocker. This can cause paralysis of respiratory musculature, generalized weakness, alteration of vasomotor tone, and sensory deficits. There have been three reported cases of toxicity since 1996, all of which were caused by eating poorly prepared fugu.[36]

Clinical manifestations of TTX toxicity can appear rapidly or up to 4 hours after ingestion of contaminated food or water, although delayed cases occurring up to 20 hours after ingestion have been reported. Facial or oral numbness and mild peripheral generalized weakness may be the initial complaint, but hypotension, seizures, generalized paralysis, cardiac arrhythmias, and respiratory failure may follow quickly. The patient may progress to a locked-in state, with preservation of consciousness

but no motor function. Eventual loss of all brain stem reflexes precedes death.[29,36]

The diagnosis is made clinically, especially a history of eating fugu. Other animal species, including amphibians are known to produce this toxin, but a vast majority of cases are due to ingestion of the puffer fish.

- Treatment currently is supportive. There are animal data to support the use of monoclonal antibodies to TTX to reverse the effects of this toxin. Other studies show benefit of 4-aminopyridine when used in guinea pigs. However, no human studies with TTX antitoxins are currently underway.
- Treatment with charcoal and gastric lavage may be helpful if given early in the course, and is a safe option in the case of suspected toxicity after eating exotic cooked or uncooked fish.[36]

Other Agents

There are many other agents that have either been weaponized for use as a biological weapon or have theoretical potential for use as such. However, many of these agents do not typically present with neurologic symptoms that would prompt admission to the NCCU. Familiarity with these organisms or agents is nevertheless prudent and has been advocated in the United States, given the current threat of bioterrorism that is prevalent for society as a whole. The United States Army Medical Research Institute of Infectious Diseases considers *Brucella* spp., *Burkholderia mallei* (glanders), *Burkholderia pseudomallei* (melioidosis), *Yersinia pestis* (plague), *Francisella tularensis* (tularemia), Yellow fever, and Filoviridae (Ebola and Marburg virus) as potential threats, in addition to those described above. Further information regarding these agents is readily available.[24,37]

Standard precautions practiced in the general care of ICU patients will provide adequate protection to the healthcare team for a majority of bioterrorism agents, which include the toxin-mediated diseases, anthrax, VEE, and Q fever. Suspected smallpox infection warrants special mention in that airborne transmission is likely. These patients should be isolated at the highest possible level, with airborne precautions requiring the wearing of a HEPA-filter mask by all members of the treatment team while caring for the patient.

CHEMICAL AGENTS

As a result of the wartime experience gained during World War I, and the subsequent development of more potent agents in World War II, more is known regarding the use of chemical agents than biological. Iranian military physicians serving during the Iran–Iraq war also provide first-hand accounts on the treatment of nerve agent casualties. The Aum Shinrikyo attack as described in the preceding text provides a good case study of terrorist use. In addition, the relevance of this threat is underscored by the likely ease of obtaining some of these chemicals, either through small laboratory production or diversion of some of the many tons of chemical agents used for legitimate industrial purposes. Accidental chemical spills or natural disaster are another source of casualties. In 1984, the accidental release of tons of methyl isocyanate into a large urban area in Bhopal, India is widely considered to be the world's worst industrial accident. It resulted in approximately 3800 deaths and subsequently 15,000 to 20,000 premature deaths. Those who were killed early were in close proximity to the chemical plant that released the gas, but adverse health effects from the exposure extended to populations who lived anywhere in the area. Other accidents with industrial chemical spills have occurred domestically, and in any Western city the likelihood of treating victims of a chemical exposure is possible. Thus, familiarity with the manifestations of the chemical or nerve agent civilian casualty is important for the neurocritical care physician.[38,39]

Organophosphates

Nerve agents, commonly referred to as organophosphates, are the most toxic of the weaponized chemical agents (Table 19.2). As a class, these agents act at the neuromuscular junction with inhibition of acetylcholinesterase, thereby producing clinical manifestations of cholinergic crisis, which can lead to incapacitation and death. They have a record of successful deployment, both on the battlefield, as well as in the civilian setting as discussed above. The only well documented use of nerve agents occurred during the Iran–Iraq, when as many as 45,000 casualties were inflicted on the Iranian army by Iraqi deployment of nerve agents sarin (GB), tabum (GA), and a mustard agent.[39]

These compounds were developed first in Germany in World War II, after more legitimate research on this material as a pesticide identified significant human toxicity. These agents were stockpiled by the Nazis during the war, but were never used. They are liquids at room temperature, but have variable volatility. There are two generations of nerve agents, commonly referred to as the "G" and "V" series. The G series were developed first and are more volatile than the V series, which are more refined, far more potent, and less volatile at room temperature.[40]

As stated in the preceding text, organophosphates anticholinesterases as they inhibit acetylcholinesterase preventing hydrolysis of acetylcholine leading to acetylcholine accumulate. This results in overstimulation and desensitization of both nicotinic and muscarinic receptor sites. These agents bind irreversibly to acetylcholinesterases. They are much more toxic than ethical preparations of anticholinesterases such as commercially available pesticides, for example, malathion and sarin, and medications, e.g., pyridostigmine, neostigmine, and physostigmine.

- Clinical manifestations of organophosphate toxicity are well characterized.
  - The earliest symptom may be the development of miosis and other eye complaints including eye pain and findings of hyperemia, which results from direct contact of vapor with the eye.
  - This is followed by excessive secretions, muscle fasciculations, involuntary urination and defecation, bronchoconstriction, mental status changes, confusion, seizures, changes in muscle tone, and eventually cardiopulmonary collapse and death if untreated.
  - The agent is readily absorbed by the skin or pulmonary system, and onset of symptoms after exposure is rapid.
- Physical signs are evident as discussed above, but other findings may include wheezing of bilateral lung fields, cardiac arrhythmias, and other abnormalities of the electrocardiogram, including heart block.
- The differential diagnosis of a patient with mild symptoms includes nonspecific upper respiratory

Table 19.2. Nerve agent and relative toxicity for LD_{50} from skin exposure[40]

Designator	Common name	LD_{50} (in mg)
GB	Sarin	1700
GA	Tabun	1000
GD	Soman	50
GF		30
VX		10

infection or allergic response. However, the presence of miosis should increase suspicion of nerve agent exposure. This distinction is more evident with severe intoxication, and these patients are of most concern and in need of prompt treatment.

- The diagnosis is likely to be made based on epidemiological data and presentation, although laboratory studies of acetylcholinesterase activity are available.[31,40,41]

Other neurologic manifestations of a large vaporized dose include rapid loss of consciousness, development of seizures, and apnea, likely of a central origin and not purely from motor weakness. Respiratory and circulatory support is crucial with severe exposures presenting with neurologic deficits. A concerning presentation is delayed development of the above symptoms after a mild bare skin exposure. There may be up to a 30-minute period of limited to no symptoms, but then an acute decompensation to neurologic compromise and death.[41]

Recognition of nerve agent exposure is vital, as it is paramount to begin decontamination and treatment early. Neurologic damage suffered by surviving organophosphate victims is due in large part to prolonged seizure activity, including status epilepticus. It is this complication that results in long-term cognitive and behavioral dysfunction. After exposure and seizures, lesions are found in cortex, hippocampus, and thalamus.[31,41,42]

Treatments recommended here are based on U.S. Army algorithms developed for battlefield exposure to nerve agent. However, it is reasonable to generalize this approach to any civilian population that has been similarly exposed. The management of the nerve agent casualty consists initially of decontamination. Depending on the severity of symptoms, patients with severe bronchoconstriction and

profuse pulmonary secretions will require early endotracheal intubation, ventilatory support, and aggressive pulmonary toilet. Once the airway is secured, the next step is institution of specific therapy for the cholinergic crisis and seizures.

- Atropine, an antimuscarinic medication, is the initial therapy of choice for nerve agent exposure. This will attenuate the effects of acetylcholine at muscarinic receptors, especially heart rate. Other ameliorative effects are to decrease secretions, reduce sweating, slow gastrointestinal motility, and pupillary dilation.
  - ▸ U.S. military use atropine auto injectors containing 2 mg of active drug and are trained to administer this medication intramuscularly in the case of a nerve agent attack.
  - ▸ Doses are administered until the patient is breathing comfortably.
  - ▸ Miosis and drying of secretions are not guidelines for therapy.
  - ▸ Toxicity from atropine, including delirium and hyperthermia, can occur at doses of 20 mg or more. Iranian physicians report several nerve agent patients required heroic atropine doses, up to 200 mg.[39,41]
- The second agent used in the U.S. Army's algorithm of nerve agent treatment is pralidoxime chloride, or 2-PAM. This oxime attaches to the organophosphate which has effectively bound the acetylcholinesterase and can restore normal activity to the enzyme. The most notable clinical effect of 2-PAM is stopping fasciculations in skeletal muscle and restoration of motor function.
  - ▸ Auto injectors of 600 mg of 2-PAM are packaged with atropine auto injector in the U.S. military's MARK-1 kit.
  - ▸ Other therapeutic approaches are 1–2 g of 2-PAM via intravenous delivery in 100 mL of normal saline over 15–30 minutes. Further dosing is based on ameliorating persistent weakness.
  - ▸ For severe toxicity, continuous infusions of 2-PAM can be given at a rate of 4–20 mg/kg per hour.
  - ▸ A continuous infusion might be useful for a number of reasons, including: slow absorption of organophosphates, unknown quantity ingested, and delayed nicotinic effects due to redistribution of lipid-soluble organophosphates.

▸ There is a lack of stability data for the infusion, and as such, it is recommended that the infusion be prepared immediately before administration, and changed every 4 hours.[31,41,43]

■ Diazepam should be used to treat seizures after nerve agent exposure. The U.S. Food Drug Administration has approved diazepam for this specific use.

  ▸ The U.S. military packages 10 mg of diazepam under the name Convulsive Antidote Nerve Agent, or CANA.

  ▸ Soldiers are taught that if the nerve agent casualty requires the use of the three MARK-1 kits then a single dose of CANA should be administered.

■ It is understood that, in civilian practice, diazepam is not the agent of choice for aborting seizure. Thus the NCCU physician can consider any appropriate benzodiazepine for this setting. If status epilepticus develops, treatment of the underlying condition should continue while separate, established algorithms for treatment of status are begun.

■ Pretreatment or prophylactic treatment with the acetylcholinesterase pyridostigmine bromide is also supported in the U.S. Army treatment algorithm. While this seems counterintuitive, the mechanism of such treatment is the temporary occupation of the cholinesterase with pyridostigmine, in order to deny access of the active site to a nonreversible organophosphate on subsequent exposure.[31,41]

Cyanide

Cyanide has been successfully used by terrorists domestically during the Tylenol incident in the Chicago area. It is reported that cyanide may have also been used on Iranian army units by Iraq during the Iran–Iraq war, although this remains unconfirmed. Cyanide is an unlikely agent for use on the battlefield due to the difficulties in deploying the high concentration of agent required to produce illness. However, terrorist use is considered possible with deployment of the agent indoors or in a confined space in a mass population setting. It is highly toxic agent with a very rapid time to incapacitation. This agent has been used historically on the battlefields of World War I, in German Nazi death camps during World War II, and by the Japanese on

Chinese civilians during the same period. It has also been used for mass suicides, such as the Jones' cult in Jonestown, Guyana in 1978, where more than 900 followers died after drinking cyanide.[39,40]

The ionic form of cyanide is the toxic moiety, which blocks electron transfer from cytochrome oxidase to molecular oxygen in the mitochondria, arresting oxidative phosphorylation. Lactic acidosis ensues, as well as loss of critical metabolic functions of the cardiovascular, respiratory, and CNS. Three different chemical agents that readily ionize to CN^- have been produced including hydrogen cyanide (AC), cyanogen bromide, and cyanogen chloride (CK). Cyanide is found naturally in many fruits including the pits of cherries, peaches, apricots, and apples. Poisoning by these food sources is possible. Other causes of cyanide poisoning are from residential and motor vehicle accident fires. Cyanide is relatively easy to procure because it is manufactured in large quantities for industrial use in production or processing of paper manufacturing, dying, printing, mineral extraction, photography, textiles, and is important in the plastics industry.[41]

Cyanide vapor is often described as having the particular odor of bitter almonds, although approximately one half of the population is unable to appreciate this odor, or the olfactory organs may accommodate to the odor rapidly on exposure.

■ Onset of symptoms is rapid and predictable after a large dose of cyanide.

■ Within 15 seconds after inhalation of concentrated cyanide, patients will begin to hyperventilate and quickly lose consciousness. This is followed in less than 1 minute with the onset of seizures, with cessation of all motor, respiratory, and cardiac activity approximately 6–8 minutes after exposure.

■ With lower concentrations, as might be encountered after smoke inhalation or via ingestion or percutaneous administration, the effects are much slower to develop, although the time period may still be on the order of minutes, during which time the patent is potentially treatable with antidote.[22,41,40]

The clinical presentation of a cyanide victim has classically been reported to show "cherry red" skin and fundus in the setting of respiratory distress. This is not specific for cyanide poisoning, however, and can also be seen with carbon monoxide poisoning. Other findings or complaints seen with cyanide toxicity include headache, anxiety, mental status changes, and agitation. There are specific laboratory tests for cyanide metabolites.

- Measurement of blood cyanide concentration is helpful in confirming the diagnosis, and can be used by forensic investigators to establish a cause of death.
  - Clinical effects are seen at concentrations of 0.5–1 µg/mL, and concentrations exceeding 2.5 µg/mL are often not consistent with survival.
- Arterial blood gases show an early decreased arteriovenous difference in P_{O_2} with a progressive lactic acidosis. A metabolic acidosis with a high anion gap can be present.
- Venous blood gas measurements show an elevated venous P_{O_2}, due to failure of the cellular respiratory chain and failure to off-load oxygen in the arterial circulation.[22,40]

Due to the rapid onset of action of this chemical, treatment of a suspected cyanide victim must begin as soon as possible, including by first responders.

- First, the victim should be removed from the source of exposure and administered 100% oxygen.
- If any liquid exposure is suspected, removal and decontamination must be performed before transport to avoid secondary contamination.
- Activated charcoal can be beneficial after cyanide ingestion.
- Mechanical ventilation, vasopressor support, intravenous hydration, seizure control with benzodiazepines, and correction of metabolic acidosis are vital measures.[40]

Specific cyanide poisoning antidote therapy is a two-step process consisting of methemoglobin formation and administration of a sulfur donor.

- The first step is administering sodium nitrite or a related drug. The goal of this methemoglobin therapy is to dissociate the bound cyanide from cytochrome *a*3, which frees this enzyme to participate again in production of ATP. Methemoglobin has a stronger affinity for cyanide than does cytochrome *a*3. Other than sodium nitrate, one can use amyl nitrite, 4-dimethylaminophenol (4-DMAP),

p-aminopropiophenone (PAPP), *p*-aminoheptanoylphenone (PAHP), or *p*-aminooctanoylphenone (PAOP) to form methemoglobin.
  - Because nitrites cause vasodilation, blood pressure and, if appropriate, intracranial pressure (ICP) must be monitored.
  - The dose of sodium nitrite, the preferred antidote used by the U.S. Army, is 300 mg or 10 mL of a 30 mg/mL solution intravenously over 5–15 minutes. This may raise the percentage of methemoglobin up to 20%, and a second dose of 5 mL or 150 mg can subsequently be given.
  - Pediatric dosing is 0.33 mL/kg, given over 10 minutes.
  - It is important to remember that methemoglobin is also toxic and can itself interfere with oxygen transport. Levels of methemoglobin should not exceed 40%.
  - Methemoglobin-forming compounds should not be given in smoke inhalation patients, due to the effects of carboxyhemoglobin, formed by carbon monoxide, on oxygen transport.
  - Smoke inhalation is not a contraindication to treatment with sulfur donor drugs.[22,40]
- Thiosulfate, a sulfur donor drug, should be given soon after sodium nitrate. The goal of thiosulfate administration is to provide substrate for the enzyme rhodanese, which catalyses the breakdown of cyanide to thiocyanate and sulfite. These breakdown products are then excreted by the kidneys.
  - The adult dose of sodium thiosulfate is 12.5 g IV, which is 50 mL of a 250 mg/mL solution.
  - The pediatric dose of is 1.65 mL/kg IV.
  - Two further treatments with half-doses of sodium thiosulfate can be given if needed.
- Other sulfur donors such as hydroxocobalamin appear to be useful under certain conditions as when treating smoke inhalation victims.[22,40,41]

Subsequent to the incident in Bhopal, India, it has become clear that delayed effects of cyanide toxicity exist. Post-cyanide exposure victims can develop clinical parkinsonism, dystonia, and other neurologic conditions, such as eye movement abnormalities, dysarthria, and ataxia. Delayed onset cognitive dysfunction after apparent convalescence has been reported. These may be related to hypoxic ischemic lesions in the brain, particularly in vulnerable areas of deep gray matter with symmetric bilateral basal ganglia lesions. Neuroimaging reveals findings similar to anoxia–ischemia or profound metabolic derangement. Magnetic resonance imaging (MRI) may show cavitations in the lentiform nucleus.[31,44]

Differentiating cyanide toxicity from organophosphate toxicity can be difficult initially. However, several of the signs seen with organophosphate poisoning are not seen clinically with cyanide toxicity.

- There can be some increase in secretions with cyanide; however, it is not as profound as the hypersecretion seen with a nerve agent.
- Miosis is a rare and late complication with cyanide, but an early finding following organophosphate poisoning.
- Fasciculations, a hallmark of organophosphate toxicity, are not seen with cyanide poisoning, although seizure activity may be confused with fasciculations by less experienced providers.
- Interestingly, cyanide victims are less likely to present cyanotic than organophosphate patients.[39,40]

Decontamination Principles After Known Chemical Agent Exposure

Decontamination should ensure patient safety as well as maintain a safe and contaminant-free treatment environment. This can be difficult early in the course of a suspected chemical exposure, but the concept can be generalized from current standard isolation procedures well known to hospital staff currently used for antibiotic-resistant organisms. This involves the separation of exposed and unexposed equipment, as well as an isolation line where those who have not yet been contaminated are initially treated before being declared safe to enter the definitive treatment facility. This process is most vital to patients exposed to a liquid, aerosol, or dry solid chemical agent. Vapor exposure is less likely to benefit from skin decontamination owing to the high volatility of vaporized agents.

The process begins with casualty isolation and demarcation of decontamination areas, with completed decontamination sites, in-progress decontamination sites, and contaminated triage areas. Windage must be taken into account in setting up these sites. Properly trained and equipped medical personnel begin by removing clothing from victims,

followed by removal of chemical agents from the skin with a solution of 0.5% hypochlorite solution, which is household bleach. The mixture used for skin decontamination is nine parts water to one part 0.5% hypochlorite solution. This can effectively decontaminate most chemical agents. An alternative is washing with nonfat-based soap and copious water irrigation. Thus, this latter method requires a good supply of water. If cases of eye contamination, eye flushes should be done with normal saline or water. The irrigation of abdominal or other cavity wounds with hypochlorite is contraindicated. Higher concentrations of hypochlorite can be used to decontaminate equipment, if needed.[40]

CONCLUSION

Toxins are ubiquitous in modern society. They may lead to patient injury from accidental, intentional, or malicious terrorist causes. The neurocritical care specialist should be familiar with these threats as he or she may be called on to care for afflicted patients. Also, vigilance for the index case of a biological or chemical attack, as well as institutional planning for civilian mass casualty occurrences, must be developed for both civilian and governmental agencies in all moderate to large-sized population centers.

REFERENCES

1. Chyka PA, Seger D, Krenzelok EP, Vale JA, American Academy of Clinical, Toxicology, European Association of Poisons Centres and Clinical, Toxicologists. Position paper: single-dose activated charcoal. *Clin Toxicol.* 2005;**43**:61–87.
2. Proudfoot AT, Krenzelok EP, Vale JA. Position paper on urine alkalinization. *J Toxicol Clin Toxicol.* 2004;**42**:1–26.
3. Hardman J, Limbird L, Gilman A. *Goodman & Gilmans: The Pharmacological Basis of Therapeutics*, 10th ed. New York: McGraw-Hill, 2005.
4. Haynes JF Jr. Medical management of adolescent drug overdoses. *Adolesc Med Clin.* 2006;**17**:353–79.
5. van Dorp EL, Yassen A, Dahan A. Naloxone treatment in opioid addiction: the risks and benefits. *Expert Opin Drug Safety.* 2007;**6**:125–32.
6. Treatment Guidelines. Pharmaceutical drug overdose. *Med Lett.* 2006;**4**:61–6.
7. Powner DJ, Hartwell EA, Hoots WK. Counteracting the effects of anticoagulants and antiplatelet agents

during neurosurgical emergencies. [see comment]. *Neurosurgery*. 2005;**57**:823–31.

8. Hirsh J, Raschke R. Heparin and low-molecular-weight heparin: the seventh ACCP conference on antithrombotic and thrombolytic therapy. *Chest*. 2004;**126**:188S–203S.

9. Hirsh J, Anand SS, Halperin JL, Fuster V, American Heart A. AHA scientific statement: guide to anticoagulant therapy: Heparin: a statement for healthcare professionals from the American Heart Association. *Arterioscl Thrombos Vasc Biol*. 2001;**21**:E9–9.

10. Laposata M, Green D, Van Cott EM, Barrowcliffe TW, Goodnight SH, Sosolik RC. College of American Pathologists conference XXXI on laboratory monitoring of anticoagulant therapy: the clinical use and laboratory monitoring of low-molecular-weight heparin, danaparoid, hirudin and related compounds, and argatroban. *Arch Pathol Lab Med*. 1998;**122**:799–807.

11. Hirsh J, Fuster V, Ansell J, Halperin JL. American Heart Association/American College of Cardiology Foundation. American Heart Association/American College of Cardiology foundation guide to warfarin therapy. *J Am Coll Cardiol*. 2003;**41**:1633–52.

12. Ansell J, Hirsh J, Poller L, Bussey H, Jacobson A, Hylek E. The pharmacology and management of the vitamin K antagonists: the seventh ACCP conference on antithrombotic and thrombolytic therapy. *Chest*. 2004;**126**:204S-33S.

13. Young G, Yonekawa KE, Nakagawa PA, Blain RC, Lovejoy AE, Nugent DJ. Recombinant activated factor VII effectively reverses the anticoagulant effects of heparin, enoxaparin, fondaparinux, argatroban, and bivalirudin ex vivo as measured using thromboelastography. *Blood Coagulat Fibrinol*. 2007;**18**:547–53.

14. Yee AJ, Kuter DJ. Successful recovery after an overdose of argatroban. *Ann Pharmacother*. 2006;**40**:336–9.

15. Draganov P, Durrence H, Cox C, Reuben A. Alcohol-acetaminophen syndrome. Even moderate social drinkers are at risk. *Postgrad Med*. 2000;**107**:189–95.

16. Lowell G. Acetaminophen toxicity. Available at: http://pediatrics.uchicago.edu/chiefs/documents/acetaminophentoxicity.pdf2005.

17. DeAngelo A, Halliday A. Wernicke-Korsakoff syndrome. Available at: eMedicine2005.

18. Greene T, Lafferty K, Khatiwala M. Toxicity, barbiturate. Available at: http://www.emedicine.com/emerg/topic52.htm (Accessed September 29, 2007).

19. Mohammed Ebid AH, Abdel-Rahman HM. Pharmacokinetics of phenobarbital during certain enhanced elimination modalities to evaluate their clinical efficacy in management of drug overdose. *Ther Drug Monit*. 2001;**23**:209–16.

20. Amrein R, Hetzel W, Hartmann D, Lorscheid T. Clinical pharmacology of flumazenil. *Eur J Anaesthesiol Suppl*. 1988;**2**:65–80.

21. Lowell G. TCA toxicity. Available at: http://pediatrics.uchicago.edu/chiefs/documents/TCA.pdf2005.

22. Office of the Surgeon General. *Textbook of Military Medicine*. Washington, DC: The Office of the Surgeon General, 1997.

23. Ayers S. Emergency film group. Available at: http://www.efilmgroup.com/News/Bioterrorism-in-Oregon.html (Accessed September 29, 2007).

24. Woods JB. *USAMRIID's Medical Management of Biological Casualties Handbook*. 6th ed. Frederick, MD: U.S. Army Medical Research Institute of Infectious Diseases, 2005.

25. Wampler RA, Blanton TS. The national security archive. Available at:http://www.gwu.edu/~nsarchiv/NSAEBB/NSAEBB61/ (Accessed September 7, 2007).

26. The University of Pittsburgh hospitalized patients supercourse. Available at: http://www.publichealth.pitt.edu/supercourse/SupercoursePPT/11011–12001/276,14,Hospitalized patients (AUM Shrinkyo). (Accessed September 29, 2007).

27. Kristof ND. Japanese cult said to have planned nerve gas attacks in U.S. Available at: http://query.nytimes.com/gst/fullpage.html?res=9905E1DF123BF930A15750C0A961958260. (Accessed 09/29, 2007).

28. Meyer MA. Neurologic complications of anthrax: a review of the literature. *Arch Neurol*. 2003;**60**:483–8.

29. Osterbauer PJ, Dobbs MR. Neurobiological weapons. *Neurol Clin*. 2005; **23**:599–621.

30. Arnon SS, Schechter R, Inglesby TV, et al. Botulinum toxin as a biological weapon: medical and public health management.[erratum appears in JAMA 2001;285(16):2081]. *JAMA*. 2001;**285**:1059–70.

31. Martin CO, Adams HP Jr. Neurological aspects of biological and chemical terrorism: a review for neurologists. *Arch Neurol*. 2003;**60**:21–5.

32. Smith DL, Ayres JG, Blair I, et al. A large Q fever outbreak in the west midlands: clinical aspects. *Respir Med*. 1993;**87**:509–16.

33. Henderson DA, Inglesby TV, Bartlett JG, et al. Smallpox as a biological weapon: medical and public health management. working group on civilian biodefense. *JAMA*. 1999;**281**:2127–37.

34. Pennington H. Smallpox and bioterrorism. *Bull WHO*. 2003;**81**:762–7.

35. Division of Vector-Borne Infectious Diseases. Arboviral encephalitis. Available at: http://www.cdc.gov/ncidod/dvbid/arbor/arbofact.htm (Accessed September 23, 2007).

36. Benzer TI. Toxicity, tetrodotoxin. Available at: http://www.emedicine.com/emerg/topic576.htm (Accessed September 29, 2007).

37. Pavlin JA. Epidemiology of bioterrorism. *Emerg Infect Dis*. 1999;**5**:528–30.

38. Broughton E. The Bhopal disaster and its aftermath: a review. *Environ Hlth*. 2005;**4**:6.

39. Newmark J. The birth of nerve agent warfare: lessons from Syed Abbas Foroutan. *Neurology*. 2004;**62**:1590–6.

40. Hurst G, Tuorinsky S. *Medical Management of Chemical Casualties Handbook*, 4th ed. Aberdeen Proving

Ground, MD: US Army Medical Research Institute of Chemical Defense, 2007.

41. Jett DA. Neurological aspects of chemical terrorism. *Ann Neurol.* 2007;**61**:9–13.

42. Shih TM, Duniho SM, McDonough JH. Control of nerve agent-induced seizures is critical for neuroprotection and survival. *Toxicol Appl Pharmacol.* 2003;**188**:69–80.

43. Singh S, Chaudhry D, Behera D, Gupta D, Jindal SK. Aggressive atropinisation and continuous pralidoxime (2-PAM) infusion in patients with severe organophosphate poisoning: experience of a northwest Indian hospital. *Hum Exp Toxicol.* 2001;**20**:15–8.

44. Hantson P, Duprez T. The value of morphological neuroimaging after acute exposure to toxic substances. *Toxicol Rev.* 2006;**25**:87–98.

45. Viral, and Rickettsial Zoonoses Branch. Q fever. Available at : http://www.cdc.gov/ncidod/dvrd/qfever/index.htm#treatment1 (Accessed September 29, 2007).

20 Central Nervous System Infections

Ricardo Carhuapoma, MD and H. Adrian Püttgen, MD

Central nervous system (CNS) infections are not uncommon in the neurocritical care unit (NCCU). This chapter reviews the most common causes of CNS infections and discusses the diagnosis and management of these life-threatening illnesses.

ENCEPHALITIS

Owing to the almost overwhelming number of possible etiologies involved, the care and diagnosis of a patient presenting with acute or subacute progressive encephalopathy poses a challenge particular to the neurocritical care environment. A clinical definition of the infectious encephalitis syndrome involves two criteria initially put forth by the California Encephalitis Project:

- Encephalopathy marked by >24 hours of depressed or altered metal status, lethargy, or personality change necessitating hospitalization.
- One or more of the following findings: fever, seizures, focal neurologic deficits, cerebrospinal fluid (CSF) pleocytosis, abnormal electroencephalogram (EEG), and abnormal CNS imaging.

In almost two-thirds of cases (62%), patients matching this description remain undiagnosed. Certainly, a confident diagnosis of an infectious cause is the exception rather than the rule, occurring in only 13% of cases.

VIRAL CAUSES OF ENCEPHALITIS

Herpes Simplex Virus Type 1

Background
HSV-1 is the most common cause of fatal sporadic viral encephalitis. Through mechanisms not completely understood and believed to involve host inflammatory reaction, primary invasion or reactivation of the virus quickly results in areas of hemorrhagic necrosis. Untreated, it has a fatality rate exceeding 70%. Morbidity and mortality of herpes simplex encephalitis (HSE) is greatly reduced by early treatment, defined as antiviral therapy initiated within 24 hours of symptom onset, or before the onset of coma (defined as a Glasgow Coma Scale [GCS] >8). The high efficacy and relatively innocuous side-effect profile of intravenous acyclovir, the mainstay of herpes encephalitis therapy, make early presumptive treatment for HSE a necessary early step in the treatment of patients with encephalopathy and fever.

Signs and Symptoms
- Patients with HSE will have some form of altered consciousness. Cases have been reported with presentations ranging from lethargy and coma to manic behavior.
- Fever is the most reliable physical finding in HSE, occurring in 95% of patients.
- Seizures are a common presenting symptom in HSE, although few patients present in convulsive status epilepticus.
- Due to the lesions involved, patients often have CNS dysfunction attributable to the frontal and temporal lobes such as aphasia, visual field cuts, or hallucinations.

Diagnostic Workup
LABORATORY
LUMBAR PUNCTURE
- CSF pressure is not characteristically elevated.

- CSF mononuclear pleocytosis is usually present, often with a neutrophil predominance early in the course.
- CSF erythrocytes are present in a majority of patients, but this finding is not a diagnostic criterion.
- CSF protein is usually elevated as well. CSF glucose should be normal.
- CSF HSV-1 polymerase chain reaction (PCR) has >95% sensitivity and specificity. It has replaced CNS biopsy as the gold standard diagnostic measure for HSE.

IMAGING

CT of the brain without contrast is often normal until several days into the course when hypodensities within the temporal lobes, usually asymmetric, appear. These signal a graver prognosis. Hemorrhages apparent on CT are possible, but unusual.

Magnetic resonance imaging (MRI, with and without contrast) is far more sensitive in detecting changes associated with HSE, but a normal MRI does not exclude the diagnosis. Lesions caused by HSV-1 will appear as hyperintensities on T_2-weighted sequences including DWI. These sequences are commonly misinterpreted as acute stroke. Gradient echo sequences may show evidence of hemorrhagic necrosis. Lesions of HSE will typically enhance with gadolinium.

OTHER TESTING

EEG is abnormal in a high proportion (up to 80%) of patients suffering from HSE. This modality is most important for selecting patients requiring adjunctive antiepileptic therapy.

Therapy

ANTIVIRALS

- A regimen of acyclovir 10–15 mg/kg IV q8H for 14–21 days should be used with attention to nephrotoxicity. Resistance to acyclovir has been reported, but only in immunocompromised patients.
- Foscarnet 40 mg/kg IV q8H for 14–21 days is available as a salvage regimen.
- Repeating a CSF PCR before ending antiviral therapy in patients with profound disease should be considered.

ADJUNCT THERAPIES

ANTIEPILEPTICS

- No recommendation exists for prophylactic administration.
- Patients presenting with seizures or having abnormal EEGs should be started on an AED.

OTHER THERAPIES

The risk of hemorrhage due to HSV-1 infection is not a contraindication for subcutaneous administration of heparin for prophylaxis of deep vein thrombosis.

PROGNOSIS

Prognosis of patients with HSE has been shown to depend on the extent of neurologic deficits at presentation and the amount of time between onset of symptoms and initiation of treatment. Even with treatment, six month mortality of 15% with long-term disability of 20% has been reported.

Varicella Zoster Virus

Background

Patients with neurologic symptoms due to VZV typically present with shingles. More dramatic presentations such as cranial neuropathies in the Ramsay Hunt syndrome have been also reported. Diagnosis in these patients is typically made from skin lesions, where scrapings can be examined for giant cells or a VZV EIA is available for biopsy specimens. VZV can also manifest as several diseases which may lead to ICU care needs.

Signs and Symptoms

- Patients with CNS involvement may present with encephalitis. VZV encephalitis has a high degree of variability with respect to the temporal association between VZV rash and the onset of CNS symptoms. The severity and distribution of CNS symptoms also varies. In the majority of cases, VZV encephalitis accompanies meningitis, which is normally benign and self-limiting.
- VZV can also cause myelitis. Immunocompromised patients are at greater risk for VZV myelitis. These patients present with paraparesis, sensory loss, or bowel and bladder dysfunction. An outbreak of VZV rash precedes these symptoms, but days or weeks may separate them.

- The gravest and most common cause of encephalitis attributable to VZV is vasculitis. VZV vasculitis has large and small vessel forms.
- A large vessel vasculitis occurs from 2 to 10 weeks after ophthalmic zoster. Patients present with acute, focal neurologic deficits in stroke distributions.
- The small vessel vasculitis has a more subacute presentation of encephalitis weeks or even months after a zoster outbreak. The small-vessel vasculitis is much more common in immunocompromised patients.

Diagnostic Workup
LABORATORY
LUMBAR PUNCTURE
- CSF mononuclear pleocytosis should be present.
- CSF protein may be elevated. CSF glucose should be normal.
- CSF PCR for VZV has a high sensitivity and specificity.

IMAGING
- CT of the brain with and without contrast is most often normal in VZV encephalitis.
- Subcortical infarcts ipsilateral to prior VZV infection sites (eye or rash) signal vasculitis.
- MRI of the brain with and without contrast should be performed with both magnetic resonance angiography (MRA) and diffusion weighted imaging (DWI) and an apparent diffusion coefficient map (ADC) to detect infarcts and large-vessel changes associated with vasculitis.

Cerebral angiography may be performed. Abnormal angiogram is more common in large vessel vasculitis and may demonstrate a diffuse vasculitis. Particularly severe cases with critical narrowing of the carotid artery at the level of the ganglion have been reported.

Therapy
ANTIVIRALS
- A regimen of acyclovir 10–15 mg/kg IV q8H for 14–21 days should be used with attention to nephrotoxicity.

ADJUNCT THERAPIES
- For suspected or established vasculitis, methylprednisolone 1000 mg IV per day or its equivalent should be administered for 3–5 days and tapered down thereafter.
- Prophylactic antiepileptics have not been shown to play an important role in management of patients with VZV.

Cytomegalovirus
Background
CMV encephalitis is primarily a disease of immunocompromised patients. It causes a rapidly progressive encephalopathy and is found in concurrence with other manifestations of CMV infection such as GI infection or retinitis.

Signs and Symptoms
Patients with CMV encephalitis may have a rapid onset of delirium progressing to coma, but a more subacute encephalopathy may also occur. Variability of presentation likely represents different levels of immunosuppression between patients.

Diagnostic Workup
LABORATORY
LUMBAR PUNCTURE
- A CSF pleocytosis will be present.
- CSF protein should be elevated. CSF glucose should be normal.
- CSF PCR for CMV has a sensitivity of 82% and a specificity of 99% in patients with AIDS.

IMAGING
On MRI periventricular T_2 hyperintensities are indicative of CMV infection, and accompany ependymal gadolinium enhancement on T_1 sequences.

Therapy
ANTIVIRALS
- Ganciclovir 5 mg/kg IV q12h for 14–21 days.
- This therapy is then followed by a daily maintenance regimen of 5 mg/kg per day.

Arboviruses

Arthropod-borne viral infections rarely cause severe clinical disease. However, two Flaviviridae have caused epidemic outbreaks of disease in increasing numbers during the last two decades. Outbreaks occur in the late summer and fall, when the mosquito vector population is at its peak, but climate changes have broadened this period and cases may present later in the season.

St. Louis Virus

Background
Though SLV is usually the source of a self-limiting illness characterized by headache and fever, elderly patients are susceptible to a more virulent encephalitis (SLE) marked by high fever and lethargy. Patients may also present with cranial nerve deficits or coma.

Signs and Symptoms
- Typically the course of disease is subacute and marked by generalized weakness rather than focal abnormalities.
- Although typically described as a meningoencephalitis, patients with SLE do not typically demonstrate meningeal signs or photophobia.

Diagnostic Workup
LABORATORY
LUMBAR PUNCTURE
- CSF pressure is normal or mildly elevated.
- CSF SLE antibody is elevated. The diagnostic level of antibody titer depends on the test used. Most often, final diagnosis rests on antibody trends.
- CSF IgM SLE antibody may become elevated early in the disease course and confirms the diagnosis.

SERUM
- SLV antibody testing can also be performed in serum, although the same limitations exist as for CSF testing.

Therapy
Therapy is purely supportive. Patients are at risk for cerebral edema as well as seizures.

West Nile Virus

Background
The natural history of West Nile virus infection passes through a series of phases. Most patients have no initial symptoms. After a period of 2 days to 2 weeks, a few patients, however, develop the brisk onset of nausea and vomiting, headache, fever, myalgias, and fatigue known as West Nile fever (WNF). West Nile fever may lead to aseptic meningitis from which the vast majority of patients recover without sequelae. Other patients, especially the elderly or the immunosuppressed, progress to an encephalitis (WNE) or a poliomyelitis with a much more dire prognosis.

Signs and Symptoms
No consistent cardinal features exist for the presentation of WNE. Patients may present confused or in coma. Patients can also have associated symptoms including myoclonus, tremor, and parkinsonism.

West Nile poliomyelitis occurs less frequently, and may prove the initial symptom rather than after WNF. West Nile poliomyelitis usually involves some extent of WNE. This condition is marked by weakness in a pattern characteristic of anterior horn cell dysfunction. Patients may also develop bulbar weakness with dysarthria and dysphagia ominous for impending respiratory failure.

Diagnostic Workup
LABORATORY
LUMBAR PUNCTURE
- CSF pressure is normal.
- A CSF pleocytosis is expected.
- A normal CSF glucose and mildly elevated CSF protein are also expected.
- CSF PCR for WNV is available, and although not sensitive enough to rule out disease, its specificity allows for diagnosis when positive.
- CSF WNV IgM antibodies also secure a firm diagnosis.

SERUM
- A rising titer of serum WNV IgG or IgM antibodies can also assist in securing a diagnosis.

IMAGING
MRI is most often normal in these patients, though gadolinium enhancement of the meninges and ependyma may occur.

Therapy
Treatment of patients with neurologic complications of West Nile virus is purely supportive at this time. Treatment with IVIg has been discussed in research literature.

Prognosis
West Nile encephalitis has a reported high mortality as high as 12–14%. Patients with West Nile poliomyelitis most often do not recover full motor function.

BACTERIAL CAUSES OF ENCEPHALITIS

Bartonella

Background

Bartonella henselae, a curved gram-negative rod, is commonly acquired from cats and leads to a systemic disease marked by high fever, painful adenopathy, and hyperpigmented plaques and ulcerated nodules known as cat scratch disease. Independent of this manifestation, however, some patients develop encephalitis with onset approximately 2–3 weeks after exposure.

Signs and Symptoms

- As with cat scratch disease, high fever marks *Bartonella* encephalitis.
- Seizures and status epilepticus occur in most patients with *Bartonella* encephalitis.
- Cranial nerve deficits such as Bell's palsy often presage the development of lethargy and coma.

Diagnostic Workup
LABORATORY
LUMBAR PUNCTURE
- CSF pleocytosis is expected, but CSF glucose and protein should be normal.
- Bacteria culture has proven difficult.
- CSF *Bartonella* PCR is available.

SERUM TESTING
- Rising titers of *Bartonella* antibody secures a diagnosis.

OTHER
- At times, diagnosis requires biopsy of an inflamed lymph node for silver staining.
- Due to the high rate and mortality associated with *Bartonella* endocarditis in patients with systemic disease, echocardiogram is recommended.

Therapy
ANTIBIOTICS
- Erythromycin 500 mg IV q6h for several months is required for full treatment

Prognosis
If supported through the acute illness, most patients with treated *Bartonella* encephalitis recover completely.

Legionella

Background

Mortality from pneumonia caused by *Legionella pneumophila* has been estimated as high as 1 in 4 in the elderly patients with a history of smoking and immunosuppression who are particularly at risk for the disease. A younger, healthier population is susceptible to encephalitis caused by the bacterium.

Signs and Symptoms

- Patients presenting with atypical pneumonia and encephalopathy merit testing for *Legionella*.
- Cerebral involvement manifests itself with headache and delirium or lethargy.
- More focal deficits such as ataxia or cranial nerve palsies have been reported.
- Syndrome of inappropriate antidiuretic hormone may also become evident.

Diagnostic Workup
LABORATORY
LUMBAR PUNCTURE
- CSF is usually normal.
- Legionella is not cultured or identified from CSF.

IMAGING
- CNS imaging is normal in patients suffering from *Legionella* encephalitis

OTHER TESTING
- Sputum or nasopharynx PCR swab is available with high specificity but inadequate sensitivity for ruling out disease.

Therapy
ANTIBIOTICS
- Usual therapy consists of high dose, intravenous fluoroquinolone such as levofloxacin 750 mg per day or moxifloxacin 400 mg per day.
- Rifampin 300 mg IV q12h should be added to the fluoroquinolone.
- Total length of therapy is 10 days.
- Patients able to tolerate PO medications may be converted to oral formulations once symptoms have resolved.

Mycoplasma

Background

Mycoplasma pneumoniae, which typically causes a systemic illness with high fever and a lengthy, unproductive cough, can also lead to a variety of neurologic diseases including transverse myelitis, Guillain-Barré syndrome (GBS), and a marked encephalitis.

Signs and Symptoms

- Seizures or nonconvulsive status epilepticus have been observed in up to 10% of cases.
- *Mycoplasma* more often causes a meningoencephalitis, and in more than 50% of patients, evidence of meningitis such as nuchal rigidity, Kernig's or Brudzinski's sign is present.
- Cases with cranial nerve palsies have also been reported.

Diagnostic Workup
LABORATORY
LUMBAR PUNCTURE
- CSF pressure is typically elevated.
- A heavy pleocytosis is evident. Neutrophils may predominate early, but a monocytic pleocytosis is expected.
- CSF PCR for *Mycoplasma* is available, though sensitivity limits its ability to rule out the disease.
- *Mycoplasma* antibodies, with attention to titer trends, are usually required for diagnosis.

SERUM
- Peripheral blood counts often have normal WBC counts, prompting consideration of atypical pneumonia in patients with a prodrome of cough and fever. Cold agglutinins, the classic finding of *Mycoplasma* pneumonia, will also be evident in encephalitis patients.
- Correspondingly, Mycoplasma IgM could secure a diagnosis, though this test is often negative for up to 2 weeks into the course of the disease.

IMAGING
CNS imaging is usually unremarkable in *Mycoplasma* encephalitis.

Therapy
ANTIBIOTICS
Standard therapy consists of erythromycin 500 mg IV q6h for 21 days. Patients with resolution of symptoms may be converted to oral erythromycin after 10 days.

Prognosis
Patients receiving adequate antibiotics and supportive care recover well.

MENINGITIS

In contrast to encephalitis, patients with meningitis do not have primary deficits of brain function. The disease is one of inflammation mainly of the leptomeninges. This does not preclude patients with meningitis from becoming lethargic or indeed gravely ill. However, the strict distinction between organisms causing meningitis or encephalitis becomes difficult to support as patients with overwhelming or progressing meningitis tend to develop a corresponding encephalitis. Indeed, patients requiring neurocritical care for meningitis usually require a high level of care to manage complications from ensuing encephalopathy.

VIRAL CAUSES OF MENINGITIS

Viruses typically cause a self-limiting meningitis. CSF from patients with viral meningitis usually has a relatively modest pleocytosis, normal to moderately elevated protein and normal glucose. Viruses involved include enteroviruses such as coxsackie and echovirus, HSV-2, Ebstein–Barr virus, CMV and VZV. These are typically self-limiting diseases often defying attempts at diagnosis and requiring little in the way of supportive care. Viruses such as HSV-2 may cause recurring meningitis, though these are again unlikely to require critical care. When viral CNS infection requires more acute care, the disease typically begins or rapidly progresses into encephalitis.

BACTERIAL CAUSES OF MENINGITIS

Background
The typical course of bacterial meningitis is one of a day or two of malaise, fever, and headache culminating in dramatic headache and neck stiffness, lethargy, fever, and even coma. Untreated, bacterial meningitis is considered a fatal disease, and outcomes of treated meningitis depend on the rapidity at which therapy is started. Thus, emphasis in the treatment of this disease is focused on rapid, empiric antibiotic coverage with little or no delay for diagnostic measures.

Signs and Symptoms
- Though authors argue the reliability of combinations of fever, nuchal rigidity, headache, and

altered mental status in diagnosing bacterial meningitis, all patients have at least two of these symptoms.

- Kernig's and Brudzinski's signs have only 50% sensitivity.
- A significant proportion (10%) of patients with bacterial meningitis present with seizures.
- Between 10% and 20% of patients also have cranial nerve palsies, especially III, VI, and VII.

Diagnostic Workup
LABORATORY
LUMBAR PUNCTURE
- CSF pressure is elevated.
- A heavy pleocytosis with neutrophil predominance is present.
- CSF glucose is <40 mg/dL or <40% of serum glucose.
- CSF protein is elevated >45 mg/dL.
- Gram stain often, but not always, gives an initial indication of pathogen.
- CSF culture is the source of final diagnosis.
- Performance of a lumbar puncture should not significantly delay administration of antibiotics. If the lumbar puncture proves difficult to perform, sensitivity of cultures should be sacrificed, and empiric antibiotics started first with the assurance that other CSF abnormalities will secure the diagnosis.

SERUM
Blood cultures are positive in a majority of patients, especially if drawn before the administration of antibiotics.

IMAGING
Debate as to whether CT of the brain should always precede lumbar puncture and therefore delay administration of antibiotics has to some measure been rendered moot by the broad availability of CT scanners.

- Patients who are more likely at baseline to have structural brain abnormalities and should therefore have a CT scan before lumbar puncture include patients who are older than 60 years, have prior brain disease, are immunocompromised, or who have had a seizure within a week of presentation.

- Outside of this group, patients presenting with abnormalities of consciousness or attention, patients with cranial nerve palsies or motor weakness, and patients with aphasia should all undergo CT before lumbar puncture.
- CT may show edema due to cerebritis or signs of abscess. CT without contrast is preferable to delaying imaging for administration of contrast.

MRI has also been used in the diagnosis of meningitis. Meningeal enhancement, especially apparent in coronal sections, is a key feature of the disease. MRI is also more sensitive for detecting abscesses that require an alternative therapeutic approach. In addition, MRI is also a sensitive means of discovering a source of bacterial invasion such as osteomyelitis or sinusitis.

Specific Pathogens
- *Streptococcus pneumoniae* is a gram-positive coccus responsible for approximately 60% of adult cases of bacterial meningitis and probably more in the elderly.
  - Asplenic patients are more susceptible to *S. pneumoniae* infection.
  - High rates of *S. pneumoniae* resistance in the United States to penicillin complicate selection of empiric antibiotics for bacterial meningitis.
  - Group B streptococci account for another 4% of bacterial meningitis cases.
- *Neisseria meningitides* is a gram-negative diplococcus responsible for another 20% of cases. This bacteria leads to disease marked by very rapid progression. In addition, this bacterium leads to a petechial rash or ecchymoses that signal onset of necrotizing vasculitis and gangrene of the extremities. Vasculitis may also manifest as profound adrenal insufficiency known as Waterhouse–Friderichsen syndrome.
  - Although a meningococcal vaccine is available, living contacts and healthcare providers exposed to a patient diagnosed with *N. meningitides* infection should take prophylactic antibiotics (four 600 mg doses of PO rifampin q12h or a single 500-mg dose of ciprofloxacin).
- *Listeria monocytogenes*, a gram-negative rod, accounts for about 6% of cases in adults, but up to 20% of cases in the elderly, the immunocompromised, or alcoholics. This bacterium may result in a rather benign CSF profile.

- *Hemophilus influenzae*, a gram-negative cocco-bacillus, is to be considered when patients present with bacterial meningitis after labyrinthitis or upper respiratory infection.
- *Staphylococcus aureus*, a gram-positive coccus, is most commonly introduced into the subarachnoid space by instrumentation or trauma.
- Other gram-negative bacteria, such as *Klebsiella*, *Pseudomonas*, and *Proteus*, usually occur in the context of bacteremia. *Pseudomonas* can occur after an instrumentation of the CSF space such as lumbar puncture, lumbar catheter placement, or spinal anesthesia.
- Anaerobic species, such as *Bacteroides*, *Actinomyces*, or anaerobic *Streptococci* species often occur in mixed infections associated with abscess, and diagnostic measures should be directed appropriately.

Therapy

Patient characteristics direct the coverage spectrum of empiric antibiotics. Therapy should only be narrowed on culture data and susceptibility data.

ANTIBIOTICS

- Patients 18–50 years of age
  - Vancomycin 1 g IV q12h for coverage of methicillin-resistant *Staphylococcus aureus* (MRSA)
  - Third-generation cephalosporin such as ceftriaxone 50 mg/kg IV q12h or cefotaxime 150 mg/kg IV q8h for broad coverage.
  - This regimen does not cover *Listeria* or *Pseudomonas*.
- Patients older than 50 years of age
  - Vancomycin 1 g IV q12h
  - Third-generation cephalosporin
  - Ampicillin 2 g IV q4h for coverage of *Listeria*
- Patients with a history of recent trauma
  - Vancomycin 1 g IV q12h
  - Ceftazidime 6 g IV q8h or cefepime 4 g IV q8h for broader gram-negative bacilli coverage
- Patients with trauma or recent surgery and a wound infection
  - Vancomycin 1 g IV q12h
  - Ceftazidime 6 g IV q8h or cefepime 4 g IV q8h
  - Metronidazole 500 mg IV q6h for coverage of anaerobes
- Patients with a CSF shunt or CSF leak
  - Vancomycin 1 g IV q12h
  - Ceftazidime 6 g IV q8h or cefepime 4 g IV q8h

ADJUNCT THERAPIES

CORTICOSTEROIDS

Use of corticosteroids is controversial. The use of dexamethasone has been shown to reduce morbidity and mortality. There exists some concern that steroids may stabilize the blood–brain barrier and reduce CNS penetration of antibiotics. If used, dexamethasone, 10 mg q6h should be given for 4 days and started before or with the first dose of antibiotics.

Prognosis

Mortality for bacterial meningitis depends on the pathogen. Meningococcal and *H. influenzae* meningitis carry a mortality of about 5%, although pneumococcal meningitis has a mortality around 15%. Meningococcal meningitis complicated by sepsis, gangrene, or adrenal failure also has a high mortality. Adults who survive do so without remnant deficits, although in up to 30% of complicated cases, hydrocephalus and cranial nerve deficits such as deafness and optic nerve dysfunction may result from the high CSF content of proteinaceous material during acute illness and well into recovery.

FUNGAL CAUSES OF MENINGITIS

Fungal meningitis is usually the result of seeding of the meninges due to fungemia resulting from systemic infection. Fungal meningitis may also occur as a result of direct invasion from adjacent infection. The usual course of disease is that of subacute or even chronic meningitis. Fungal meningitis is characteristically a disease of immunocompromised patients. Sources of immune dysfunction include HIV and medical immune suppression but also include lymphoma, leukemia, and systemic stress due to severe burns. In addition, diabetics are more prone to fungal infection, as are patients with collagen vascular disease. Finally, patients receiving total parenteral nutrition are also at heightened risk for fungemia and therefore fungal meningitis.

Cryptococcus

Background

Cryptococcus neoformans can cause meningitis in patients with or without immune suppression. Patients with normal immune systems have symptoms for several weeks before diagnosis.

Signs and Symptoms

- Increased intracranial pressure is a major complication of cryptococcal meningitis and may begin with headache and lethargy and lead to dysfunction of extraocular movements and blindness.
- Meningeal signs such as nuchal rigidity are common.
- Fever is a somewhat unreliable symptom in cryptococcal meningitis.
- Patients who are immunocompromised may have much more subtle presentation, but may also present with severe headache rapidly progressing to cranial nerve dysfunction and coma.

Diagnostic Workup

LABORATORY

LUMBAR PUNCTURE

- Highly elevated CSF pressure, sometimes beyond the range of manometers provided in sterile lumbar puncture kits is a distinctive finding.
- CSF pleocytosis, though expected, is often moderate.
- CSF protein is typically highly elevated and glucose is depressed.
- CSF India ink stain is rarely performed due to a high occurrence of false positives and negatives.
- A latex agglutination assay for cryptococcal antigen has high specificity and sensitivity.

IMAGING

CT of the brain without contrast is useful for evaluation of hydrocephalus. MRI of the brain with and without contrast is useful for detection of abscess formation. Elevated ICP and meningovascular disease are detectable by evaluating DWI and ADC sequences for new infarcts.

Therapy

ANTIFUNGALS

- Amphotericin B 0.7–1.0 mg/kg IV per day for 14 days.
  - ▸ Amphotericin requires close monitoring for nephrotoxicity.
- Some experts recommend addition of flucytosine 25 mg/kg PO q6h for the initial 14 course as well, although this is not universally required.

- Fluconazole 400 mg PO per day should follow IV medications for at least 10 weeks.
  - ▸ Immunocompromised patients require oral fluconazole until the resolution of immune suppression.

ADJUNCT THERAPIES

- Routine lumbar puncture is often required with a goal of normal closing CSF pressures.
- Some patients may require lumbar catheter to maintain acceptable cerebral perfusion pressures.
- Patients with persistently elevated pressures, especially those who presented with high CSF protein may require surgical placement of long-term CSF shunts.
- Patients with visual loss due to elevated ICP may benefit from optic nerve sheath fenestration.

Prognosis

- Mortality can reach up to 40% in patients with AIDS.
- Up to 50% of patients experience relapses.

Candida

Background

Meningitis due to *Candida* species is almost always due to *C. albicans*. Infections usually occur via hematogenous spread from a primary infection such as lung, bladder, skin, or heart. However, candidal meningitis may occur as a complication of surgery and may take several weeks to manifest. Patients at risk include patients with immune suppression, patients receiving parenteral nutrition, patients recently receiving broad-spectrum antibiotics and patients with severe burns. Meningitis is the most common result of CNS *Candida* infection. However, meningoencephalitis with microabscesses, vasculitis and mycotic aneurysms are common complications.

Signs and Symptoms

Candidal meningitis can cause either acute or chronic meningitis. Candidal endophthalmitis often leads to candidal meningitis. Patients with meningeal symptoms complaining of blurred vision or visual loss should undergo funduscopic examination which may reveal cotton exudates or small hemorrhages indicative of the disease.

Diagnostic Workup

LABORATORY

LUMBAR PUNCTURE

- CSF pressure is normal or modestly elevated.
- CSF protein is elevated and glucose moderately depressed.
- Isolation of budding yeasts in CSF secures diagnosis.
- CSF culture is often negative in candidal meningitis.

IMAGING

MRI

- MRI of the brain with and without contrast is particularly useful for detection of micro-abscesses.
- Candidal meningitis may also lead to vasculitis and the resultant infarcts are detectable with DWI and ADC sequences.
- Mycotic aneurysm rupture is detectable with gradient echo sequences.

Therapy

ANTIFUNGALS

- Amphotericin B 0.7–1 mg/kg IV per day
  ▹ Amphotericin requires close monitoring for nephrotoxicity.
- Flucytosine 25 mg PO q6h should be added for advanced cases.
  ▹ Therapy should continue for at least 4 weeks.
- *Candida lusitaniae*, though uncommon, is resistant to amphotericin.

ADJUNCT THERAPIES

Patients with candidal meningitis resulting from CSF shunt implantation require removal of hardware.

Histoplasmosis

Background

Patients susceptible to *Histoplasma capsulatum* meningitis live in the temperate climate of the Mississippi and Ohio River valleys. In addition, these patients are almost universally immune suppressed. Patients with disseminated pulmonary infections are at highest risk to develop CNS infection.

Signs and Symptoms

- *Histoplasma* presents as a chronic meningitis.

Diagnostic Workup

LABORATORY

LUMBAR PUNCTURE

- CSF pleocytosis with lymphocyte predominance is expected.
- CSF protein is elevated, CSF glucose is low.
- CSF culture is possible but demands high volumes for detection.
- Detection of *Histoplasma* antibody in CSF by complement fixation is diagnostic.
- A *Histoplasma* antigen enzyme-linked immunosorbent assay (ELISA) is also available.

SERUM

- Testing for antihistoplasmal antibodies is available although not entirely reliable.
- Serum culture for *Histoplasma* is time consuming but often diagnostic.

OTHER

  ▹ Urine antigen detection and antigen detection from alveolar lavage in patients with lung disease are other avenues of detection.

IMAGING

MRI with and without gadolinium may detect microabscess formation.

Therapy

ANTIFUNGALS

- Amphotericin B 0.7–1 mg/kg IV per day for 3 months
- Amphotericin requires close monitoring for nephrotoxicity.
- Intravenous therapy should be followed by fluconazole 800 mg per day for 8–12 months.
- Immunocompromised patients require ongoing fluconazole therapy.

Prognosis

- Mortality in *Histoplasma* meningitis is between 20% and 40%, although this may reflect the mortality of systemic disease.
- Almost half of patients will relapse.

MYCOBACTERIAL CAUSES OF MENINGITIS

Background

Meningitis caused by *Mycobacterium tuberculosis* (TB) is a disease marked by difficult diagnosis, dire complications, and lengthy therapy. Untreated, TB meningitis is fatal. Two-thirds of patients with TB meningitis have evidence of infection elsewhere. Patients with normal immune systems are prone to TB meningitis, though patients with AIDS have been shown to have accelerated courses.

Signs and Symptoms
Tuberculous meningitis moves through three clinical stages.

- In stage 1, patients are lucid but complain of fever, headache, and neck stiffness.
- In stage 2, patients exhibit cognitive impairment coupled with cranial nerve palsies and often seizures.
- In stage 3, patients have hydrocephalus leading to stupor and coma. Multiple cranial nerve palsies and motor deficits also define this stage.

Diagnostic Workup
LABORATORY
LUMBAR PUNCTURE
- Because TB meningitis can lead to tuberculoma formation, careful examination of CT images should precede lumbar puncture.
- Opening pressures are most often elevated.
- CSF protein is markedly elevated, with up to 75% having levels from 100 to 500 mg/dL. Higher protein indicates CSF blockage.
- CSF glucose is low, but rarely markedly so.
- CSF acid-fast bacillus culture often requires more time than is expedient for diagnosis, but offers much needed data regarding antibiotic sensitivities.
- CSF TB PCR offers a confirmation of diagnosis.

IMAGING
- TB typically leads to basilar meningitis readily observed as pachymeningeal enhancement on coronal sequences on MRI. Diagnosis of tuberculomas, which appear as space-occupying hyperintense lesions on T_2 sequences which enhance with gadolinium, is rarer in the United States, but affects management and prognosis.
- Chest radiography may also assist diagnosis, and designates patients who should be placed in respiratory isolation.

OTHER
- Purified protein derivative (PPD) is positive in patients without immune compromise, but

may give a false negative in immunosuppressed patients.
- When other measures fail, meningeal biopsy may be required.

Therapy
ANTIBIOTICS
Mycobacterium tuberculosis requires prolonged combination therapy including:

- Isoniazid 300 mg PO/IM per day
- Rifampin 600 mg PO/IV per day
- Pyrazinamide 15–30 PO mg/kg per day (2 g maximum)
- Ethambutol 15–25 PO mg/kg

Isoniazid is by far the most effective drug but carries risk of neuropathy (especially optic) and hepatotoxicity. Pyridoxine 50 mg PO per day is a necessary addition to drug regimens containing isoniazid.

Ethambutol has poor CNS penetration. If culture results become available showing good sensitivity to rifampin and isoniazid, this drug may be discontinued.

Multidrug-resistant TB requires alternate medications.

- Isoniazid 300 mg PO per day (with pyridoxine 50 mg PO per day)
- Three other drugs based on sensitivities
- Alternate medications include moxifloxacin and streptomycin

In TB and MDR-TB meningitis, antibiotic therapy usually lasts for 9–12 months.

ADJUNCT THERAPIES
- Patients presenting past stage 1 usually require corticosteroid therapy (dexamethasone 2-3 mg PO/IV q6h) for 1-2 months followed by a long taper.

Prognosis
- Mortality for immunocompetent patients is 21% for patients presenting past stage 1.
- For immunocompromised patients at the same stage, mortality reaches 33%.
- Chronic hydrocephalus is a common complication, often requiring CSF shunt placement.

CENTRAL NERVOUS SYSTEM ABSCESS

Treatment of CNS abscesses demands a multidisciplinary approach well suited to the neurocritical care unit. Although variable in onset and myriad in etiology, CNS abscess have a number of common features that lead to neurocritical care needs:

- Abscesses usually occur in patients in whom prior CNS has predisposed them to the disease.
- Abscesses are often a manifestation of systemic infection.
- The CNS has a fairly modest immune system to begin with, and patients with CNS abscesses often have superimposed immune compromise.
- Abscesses often evolve to include vasculitic disease resulting in ischemic or even hemorrhagic injuries.
- Abscesses may act as mass-occupying lesions requiring care management of intracranial pressure.
- Finally, treatment of a CNS abscess requires a combination of medical and surgical intervention.

Signs and Symptoms

Independent of etiology, cerebral abscesses present common collection of symptoms.

- Progressive headache
- Fever
- Altered mental status
- Seizures
- Focal neurologic deficit
- Increased ICP

BACTERIAL CAUSES OF CEREBRAL ABSCESS

Background
Bacterial cerebral abscesses go through four stages reflecting the process of infection and sequestration.

- Early cerebritis (day 1–3)
- Late cerebritis (day 4–9)
- Early encapsulation (day 10–13)
- Late encapsulation (day 14 and on)

Diagnostic Workup
LABORATORY
Lumbar puncture is contraindicated in cerebral abscess and in cases when the procedure was performed before diagnosis, CSF was unremarkable, and cultures were negative. In serum elevated peripheral white blood cell (WBC) count, erythrocyte sedimentation rate (ESR) and C-reactive protein (CRP) indicate infection, but cultures are usually negative.

IMAGING
CT
- CT with and without contrast should be performed as early as possible in the diagnosis of abscess as discovery of a mass-occupying lesion will determine therapeutic options.
- Cerebritis stages appear as hypodense areas with surrounding edema.
- Encapsulation stages appear as ring-enhancing lesions surrounded by hypodense edema.

MRI
- MRI with and without gadolinium is far more sensitive than CT in discovering areas of cerebritis and encephalitis.
- Cerebritis appears as hyperintensities in T_2 sequences.
- Encapsulation leads to ring enhancement of these lesions.

CHEST CT OR CHEST RADIOGRAPH
- Lung abscess, empyema and simple pneumonia are a common source of bacteremia leading to cerebral abscess.

OTHER TESTING
- Surgical specimens are available from a variety of interventions (see later), but cultures are negative in up to 25% of cases.

Specific Pathogens
Mixed infections are very common in bacterial abscess, and obtaining positive cultures can prove difficult. Hence, therapy most often centers on empiric antibiotic coverage. However, specific risk factors have been shown to predispose patients to particular pathogens.

In general, *Staphylococcus aureus, Streptococcus* species and anaerobes cause the majority of bacterial cerebral abscesses. Patients with a history of trauma or surgery tend to have abscesses composed of aerobic *Streptococci* species, *Staphylococcus aureus*, *Clostridium* species, and Enterobacteriaceae (such as *Proteus* and *E. coli*).

Abscess may form via direct invasion from an adjacent infection. Middle ear infections and mastoiditis can lead to cerebellar and temporal lobe abscesses. Nasal sinusitis can lead to frontal lobe abscess. The sphenoid sinus is rarely infected but carries a high risk of ensuing cerebral abscess. Bacteria involved in such cases are most often *Streptococci* species, *Staphylococcus aureus*, anaerobic gram-negative species (such as *Bacteroides*), and Enterobacteriaceae. Fungal abscesses are also suspected with such presentations.

Patients with bacteremia or endocarditis leading to cerebral abscess typically have aerobic *Staphylococcus aureus* or *Streptococcus* species infection. Patients with immune suppression (including patients after organ transplant, patients with leukemia or lymphoma, patients with AIDS, and patients on chronic corticosteroids) are susceptible to *Norcardia* species, *Actinomyces* species and *Listeria* abscess in addition to the species discussed above. These patients also have a greater risk for fungal abscess. Patients with AIDS with ring-enhancing lesions are a topic of particular interest, as more than 20% of these patients have more than one CNS opportunistic infection at a time.

Therapy
ANTIBIOTICS
Most initial antibiotic coverage is, by necessity, empiric and includes the following agents:

- Vancomycin 1 g IV q12h for coverage of MRSA.
- Third-generation cephalosporin such as ceftriaxone 50 mg/kg IV q12h or cefotaxime 150 mg/kg IV q8h for broad coverage.
- Metronidazole 500 mg IV q6h for coverage of anaerobes.
- Duration of therapy is uncertain, but general guidelines include a total of 6–8 weeks with 4 weeks of IV therapy.
- Imaging serves as a useful guide for terminating therapy.

ADJUNCT THERAPIES
- Dexamethasone is generally recommended for patients with a significant mass effect on imaging.
- Antiepileptic medications should certainly be prescribed for any patient presenting with seizure.

As 35–80% of patients with cerebral abscess eventually have a seizure, prophylactic antiepileptics are warranted.

SURGICAL INTERVENTION
- Surgical intervention is indicated for patients with lesions >2.5 cm or causing mass effect. Several interventions are available.
  - ▶ Aspiration serves as the mainstay of bacterial abscess management. It is best for deep abscesses or patients with multiple lesions. Repeated aspiration is often required.
  - ▶ Excision reduces the risk of recurrence and can reduce the length of required antibiotic coverage. It is performed for abscesses only in the late encapsulated phase that can be removed intact.

FUNGAL CAUSES OF CEREBRAL ABSCESS

As discussed in the preceding text, fungal meningitis can lead to abscess formation. In addition, direct invasion from infections of sinuses or mastoid air cells can result in fungal abscess as well.

Aspergillus
Background
Most patients with *Aspergillus* abscess initially had chronic sinusitis, mastoiditis or otitis from the same organism. Pulmonary aspergillosis can also lead to cerebral abscess formation.

Diagnostic Workup
LABORATORY
Lumbar puncture is contraindicated in most cases of cerebral abscess and rarely assists diagnosis.

IMAGING
MRI with and without contrast is best suited for detecting abscesses

OTHER TESTING
Fungal culture of biopsy specimens searching for hyphae with acute-angle branching often forms the basis of final diagnosis.

Therapy
ANTIFUNGAL
- Medical therapy alone is usually insufficient and surgical excision is required.

- Voriconazole 200 mg IV q12h can be replaced by PO administration of the same dose based on imaging. Length of therapy depends on observed response.

ADJUNCT THERAPIES
- Surgical excision and débridement of surrounding tissue is required for resolution of infections due to extension of local infection.

Zygomycosis
Background
Diabetics, alcoholics, and intravenous drug addicts are at greater risk of meningitis from fungi in the Zygomycetes class, as to immunocompromised patients. Presentation is typically infection of the turbinates or sinuses with spread along blood vessels to the frontal and temporal lobes. Spread may occur to the tissues of the orbits as well, resulting in proptosis and painful ophthalmoplegia. Infection of blood vessels can lead to hemorrhagic infarction. This path of infection can also lead to cavernous sinus thrombosis.

Diagnostic Workup
LABORATORY
- Biopsy cultures reveal nonseptate hyphae with 90-degree branching.

IMAGING
MRI
- Abscesses will appear hyperintense on T_2 sequences and will often contain central hypointensities signaling necrosis.
- Gradient echo (GRE) pulse sequences will detect hemorrhagic transformation of cerebritis.
- DWI and ADC sequences will detect new infarcts from vasculitis.

Therapy
SURGERY
Excision and débridement is the mainstay of therapy for zygomycosis infections, often necessitating broad removal of tissue for cure.

ANTIFUNGALS
- Liposomal amphotericin B 5 mg/kg IV per day.
- Amphotericin requires close monitoring for nephrotoxicity.

- The required length of therapy after surgery has not been defined, and should rest on clinical progression and imaging.

Subdural Empyema
Background
A collection of pus in the subdural space does not have anatomic barriers to spread, and patients with this disease suffer a rapid decline. Important correlations include cerebral abscess (25%), sinus infection (76%), chronic otitis (14%), and recent trauma or surgery (7%). Presentation is not specific to subdural empyema: headache, fever, altered mental status, and hemiparesis.

Diagnostic Workup
LABORATORY
Lumbar puncture is contraindicated because subdural empyema often causes a space-occupying mass. WBC count, ESR, and CRP in serum are elevated. Cultures are usually negative. Cultures of surgical specimens are often negative.

IMAGING
CT
- CT with and without contrast can show subdural empyema as a hypodensity along the falx or a hemispheric convexity.
- Bone windows may show sinusitis or osteomyelitis that could be the origin of disease.

MRI
- Empyema fluid appears hyperintense relative to CSF in T2 sequences.
- Empyema will also enhance with gadolinium.

Etiologies
- Aerobic *Streptococci* species
- *Staphylococci* species
- Gram-negative bacilli such as *Pseudomonas*
- Anaerobes such as *Bacteroides*

Therapy
SURGERY
- Burr-hole drainage may prove sufficient in early disease when the collection is fluid.
- Later in disease, craniotomy may prove necessary to fully relieve mass effect and the collection will develop loculations that defy burr-hole drainage.

ANTIBIOTICS

- Broad-spectrum coverage should be initiated.
- Vancomycin 1 g IV q12h.
- Ceftazidime 6 g IV q8h or cefepime 4 g IV q8h.
- Metronidazole 500 mg IV q6h for coverage of anaerobes.

ADJUNCT THERAPIES

- Antiepileptics are supported by the 40% seizure incidence for patients with subdural empyema.

Prognosis

- Mortality approaches 20%.
- Long term motor deficits, mostly hemiparesis, occur in 17% of patients.

Spinal Epidural Abscess

Background

Epidural abscess occurs most commonly in the thoracic or lumbar spine (70%), followed by the cervical spine. Patients at risk include patients with diabetes or a history of IV drug abuse or alcoholism. Not surprisingly, immunocompromised patients are also at heightened risk. Chronic renal failure is also a risk factor for epidural abscess. Interestingly, a significant portion of patients with epidural abscess report a history of trauma to the back, sometimes quite minor, at the level of abscess.

Mechanisms leading to epidural abscess include hematogenous spread from endocarditis, abscess elsewhere in the body, or contaminated venous injection. In addition, direct extension may lead to abscess formation, attributable to psoas abscess, perinephric abscess, decubitus ulcers, or penetrating injury.

Multiple organisms are commonly involved (in up to 10% of cases). In up to two-thirds of cases, *Staphylococcus aureus* is the causative pathogen, followed by aerobic *Streptococcus* species, *Pseudomonas*, and *E. coli*.

Signs and Symptoms

Cardinal symptoms of epidural abscess include
- Fever
- Neurologic deficits localizing to the spinal cord including
  - ▶ Distal weakness in extremities
  - ▶ Dysesthesia
  - ▶ Bowel and bladder dysfunction

- Signs of meningeal inflammation
- Excruciating, tender spine pain

Diagnostic Workup

LABORATORY

LUMBAR PUNCTURE
- Lumbar puncture is strongly contraindicated, as passage of a needle through the abscess may seed the previously sterile subarachnoid space with bacteria.
- Cultures of CSF are almost universally negative and of little diagnostic use.

SERUM
- Blood cultures are usually positive and can assist in narrowing antibiotic coverage.
- WBC count, CRP, and ESR are elevated.

IMAGING

CT
- CT myelogram of the whole spine is useful in detecting extradural cord compression, but the test requires lumbar puncture for administration of contrast.

MRI
- MRI of the spine with and without gadolinium should be ordered with levels directed by physical examination.
- Epidural abscesses appear as high-intensity lesions on T_2 sequences.
- The lesions will enhance with gadolinium.
- MRI images are also useful in detecting cord impingement.

OTHER TESTING
- Analysis of surgical specimens can also direct therapy, although patients often go to surgery after several doses of antibiotics, resulting in sterile cultures.

Therapy

SURGERY
- Most patients require surgical intervention to relieve cord compression.
- Contraindications to surgery include involvement of numerous spinal levels and cord dysfunction lasting more than 3 days.
- Goals of surgery include decompression of the cord, débridement of the abscess, and restabilization of the spine.

ANTIBIOTICS

- Empiric therapy covers the pathogens described above.
- Vancomycin 1 g IV q12h for coverage of MRSA.
- Third generation cephalosporin such as ceftriaxone 50 mg/kg IV q12h or cefotaxime 150 mg/kg IV q8h for broad coverage
- Intravenous antibiotics should be continued for 4 weeks, and then oral antibiotics started for another 4 weeks.

Prognosis

A portion of patients (5%) die from complications associated with sepsis. The determining factor for recovery of motor function is the amount of time weakness is present before surgery. Patients with more than 24 hours of symptoms are unlikely to recover fully.

PARASITIC INFECTIONS OF THE CNS

Malaria

Background

Malaria can cause enough intense systemic stress to yield encephalopathy, but only *Plasmodium falciparum* can cause the entity of cerebral malaria. This disease causes encephalopathy due to erythrocyte sludging and microvascular sequestration. Patients present with obtundation or coma. In addition, seizures are common. Symptoms of intracranial hypertension such as cranial nerve palsies appear.

Plasmodium species are not endemic to the United States, but humans may host the parasite for years. Regardless of when patients from endemic areas immigrated to the United States, they should be evaluated for malaria if the presentation is suspicious.

Patients with travel history to endemic areas should also be evaluated for malaria if symptoms support the diagnosis because prophylactic medications, even when taken correctly, do not provide absolute protection.

Signs and Symptoms

Diagnosis is based on clinical criteria:
- Deep unconsciousness
  - *Plasmodium falciparum* infection
- Exclusion of other etiologies of encephalopathy:

- Metabolic abnormalities from systemic malaria are corrected.
- Other infectious etiologies are excluded.
- More than 6 hours have passed since the last seizure.

Diagnostic Workup

LABORATORY

SERUM
- Anemia on peripheral cell count indicated malaria.
- Malaria can also cause marked hypoglycemia.
- An elevated WBC count contradicts the diagnosis of malaria
- Thick and thin blood smears are the standard diagnostic test for malaria, but depend on experienced laboratory staff.
- Several more modern staining methods exist that allow detection of the parasite, but only thin smear allows identification of the particular species.

IMAGING

- Imaging does not assist in the diagnosis of cerebral malaria.

Therapy

ANTIMALARIALS

- Quinine administered as follows:
  - Quinidine gluconate 10 mg/kg IV loading dose (maximum 600 mg) over 1–2 hours
  - Quinidine gluconate 0.02 mg/kg per minute IV drip until parasitemia drops below 1%
  - Quinine 650 mg PO q8h for 1 week
- Doxycycline 100 mg PO/IV bid

ADJUNCT THERAPIES

- Patients with parasitemia above 5% benefit from exchange transfusion.

Prognosis

- Mortality approaches 20%, usually within first 48 hours.
- Ventricular arrhythmias require telemetry monitoring.
- Neurologic deficits persist in 5–10% of patients.

Toxoplasmosis

Background

Though not impossible in patients with normal immune function, cerebral *Toxoplasma gondii* infection is now defined as a disease of immuno-compromised patients, specifically patients with AIDS.

Signs and Symptoms
- Patients initially experience vague constitutional symptoms and headache.
- As lesions progress, lethargy and confusion appear.
- When lesions generate enough mass effect, evidence of cortical dysfunction such as hemiparesis, aphasia, visual field cuts, or inattention appear.
- Without directed treatment, symptoms progress to coma.

Diagnostic Workup
LABORATORY
LUMBAR PUNCTURE
- Lumbar puncture is often contraindicated by mass effect of *Toxoplasma* lesions.
- When performed, CSF monocytic pleocytosis is found.

SERUM
- Diagnosis can be made on the basis of imaging and antibody titers.
- An IgG titer above 1:1024 is diagnostic as is a rise in IgG titer over time.
- A positive IgM antibody test also serves to confirm diagnosis
- In patients with severe immunocompromise, this immune response may not appear.

IMAGING
CT
- CT without contrast reveals periventricular calcifications are characteristic of toxoplasmosis.
- CT with contrast identifies *Toxoplasma* lesions by ring enhancement.

MRI
- MRI with and without lesions will often show multiple ring-enhancing lesions with surrounding T_2 hyperintensity.
- Lesions are most often located in the basal ganglia.
- Other Imaging[201] Thallium single-photon emission computed tomography ([201]Th SPECT) and 2-deoxy-2-[^{18}F]fluoro-D-glucose ([18]FDG).

- positron emission tomography (PET) are useful in differentiating toxoplasmosis and lymphoma, which otherwise appear similar to CT and MRI.

Therapy
ANTIPARASITICS
Initial therapy consists of three drugs:

- Pyrimethamine 50–100 mg PO per day
- Sulfadiazine 1000–1500 g PO q6h
- Clindamycin 600 mg PO q6h

After resolution of symptoms, therapy can be converted to the following:

- Pyrimethamine 25 mg PO per day
- Sulfadiazine 500 mg PO q6h

Therapy should continue for 3–6 weeks after resolution of symptoms. Patients with CD_4 counts below 100 cells/μL require lifelong therapy, as these medications only kill tachyzoites, leaving bradyzoites to cause recurrence. Patients may stop antiparasitics after CD_4 surpasses 200 cells/μL for more than 6 months.

Adjunct Therapies
Pyrimethamine therapy should be accompanied by leucovorin 10–20 mg PO per day to prevent profound bone marrow suppression.

Cysticercosis

Background
The etiology of cysticercosis is the larval stage of *Taenia solium*. These larvae escape host immune response by secreting complement protease inhibitor and form cysts within the brain. In Central and South America, cysticercosis is the leading cause of epilepsy, causing 50% of new seizures in patients older than age 25.

Cysts have a variety of natural histories. Parenchymal cysts are small, intraparenchymal cysts that contain larvae. These cysts may degenerate as the larvae die and form calcified granulomas and calcific cysts. Cysts may form in the subarachnoid space, where they may grow much larger than parenchymal cysts. Cysts forming in the ventricles may be free-floating or attach to choroid plexus. Cysts in the CSF space may progress to racemose cysts, which are disproportionately large, multilobulated cysts. Cysts in the CSF spaces are strongly inflammatory and can lead to arachnoiditis and basilar meningitis.

In the United States, the population of patients at risk is immigrants from Mexico, Guatemala, Bolivia, Peru, and Ecuador where prevalence for this disease approaches 25%. Onset of symptoms may be separated from exposure by years or even decades.

Signs and Symptoms
Definitive diagnosis of neurocysticercosis depends on identification of one minor criterion and extended contact with an endemic region and one absolute criterion or two major criteria.

- Absolute criteria
  - Histopathological evidence from brain or spine lesion
  - Consistent neuroimaging
  - Visualization of cysticerci in the anterior chamber of the eye
- Major criteria
  - Suggestive neuroimaging
  - Resolution of lesions with therapy
  - Spontaneous resolution
- Minor criteria
  - Compatible neuroimaging
  - Consistent clinical picture
  - Positive CSF ELISA
- Cysticercosis elsewhere in the body accompanied by encephalopathy is also sufficient to secure diagnosis.

Diagnostic Workup
LABORATORY
Lumbar puncture should be held until CT imaging shows no obstructive hydrocephalus.

- CSF shows pleocytosis, and the finding of eosinophils is indicative of parasite infection.
- CSF protein is elevated and glucose is normal.

SERUM
- Immunoelectrotransfer blot assay is very sensitive and specific for *Taenia solium*.
- WBC, ESR, and CRP are all elevated.

OTHER
Stool should be sent for ova and parasites, as 10–15% of patients have coexisting intestinal and cerebral cysticercosis. To increase chances for identification, samples from household contacts can also be sent.

IMAGING
CT
- CT without contrast can detect small calcified lesions left by dead larvae.
- CT with contrast reveals hypodense or isodense lesions with ring enhancement reflect immune response to a cyst.
- CT can also quickly provide evidence of noncommunicating hydrocephalus.

MRI
- MRI with and without contrast has the advantage of better detecting intraventricular lesions.
- Cysts are hyperintense on T_2 sequences.
- Meningeal enhancement provides evidence of arachnoiditis.

Therapy
ANTIPARASITICS
- Albendazole 7.5 mg/kg PO bid (maximum 800 mg/day) for 28 days

ADJUNCT THERAPIES
- Dexamethasone 4 mg PO/IV q6h with a taper after symptom resolution is to be considered to counteract expected increase in inflammation after initiation of therapy.
- Patients with neurocysticercosis should be started on prophylactic antiepileptics.

SURGERY
- Biopsy or excision is usually not required.
- Risk of cyst rupture makes surgery a high-risk procedure.
- Arachnoiditis or racemose cysts may cause intractable hydrocephalus requiring CSF shunt.

VENTRICULAR CATHETER INFECTIONS

Extraventricular Drain Infections

Background
Many conditions treated in the neurocritical care setting eventually require placement of an external ventricular drain (EVD) for measurement and

control of ICP. However, approximately 6% of these catheters result in infection such as ventriculitis. Several risk factors have been identified in the development of CNS infections after implantation of an EVD. Routes of infection include contamination of the catheter at the time of insertion and tracking of a biofilm from the entry point at the skin into the ventricular space. Factors leading to an increased risk for infection include:

- Intracranial hypertension
- Intraparenchymal hemorrhage, especially with intraventricular extension
- Repeated access or irrigation of the system
- The number of attempts needed to pass the catheter into the ventricular system
- Systemic infection

Other factors have previously been considered a source of increased risk have since been shown not to predict EVD infection. These include:

- EVD placement in the critical care unit rather than the operating room
- Administration of corticosteroids
- Length of catheterization beyond 5 days

The last factor remains somewhat controversial, but the vast majority of authors would agree that prophylactic replacement of an EVD is not warranted in trying to avoid infectious complications. Catheters impregnated with antibiotics (rifampin or minocycline) have been shown to significantly reduce bacterial colonization.

Signs and Symptoms
- Patients requiring EVD are often too ill to demonstrate new symptoms due to ventriculitis.

Diagnostic Workup
LABORATORY
CSF
- CSF collected from the EVD should periodically be sent for testing, as this is the working basis for diagnosis of EVD-related infections.
- CSF pleocytosis is not a reliable marker for infection.
- CSF glucose below 2.5 mmol/L or a ratio to serum glucose <0.4 strongly signals infection.
- CSF lactate may also rise in the face of infection.

- CSF Gram stain and culture are the standard means of diagnosis.

IMAGING
CT without contrast showing worsening hydrocephalus may also indicate an infectious complication.

Pathogens
The organisms typically responsible for EVD-related infections include

- Coagulate-negative *Staphylococcus* (47%)
- *Staphylococcus aureus* (14%)
- *Klebsiella*
- *Acinetobacter*

Therapy
SURGERY
The offending catheter should be removed as soon as possible. If and EVD is absolutely required, replacing the catheter should be considered.

ANTIBIOTICS
- Vancomycin 1 g IV q12h serves as adequate empiric therapy for most EVD infections.
- Third-generation cephalosporin such as ceftriaxone 50 mg/kg IV q12h or cefotaxime 150 mg/kg IV q8h for broad coverage.
- Attention to peak and trough vancomycin levels is required to reach adequate CNS penetration.
- Therapy should be tailored as soon as culture data and sensitivities are available.
- Guidelines for use of intrathecal vancomycin are not available.

CSF Shunt Infections

Background
Large population studies are not available, but the rate of CSF shunt infection for ventriculoperitoneal and ventriculoatrial shunts in adults is on the order of 2.5%. Shunt infections occur in two phases.

Early shunt infections are most likely the result of surgical contamination with bacteria from the skin of the patient. These are most commonly infections caused by *Staphylococcus epidermidis*, *S. aureus*, and gram-negative bacilli.

Late shunt infections are most often caused by *S. epidermidis* and are likely due to indolent infection or colonization of the hardware after meningitis.

These patients require careful scrutiny for the possibility of other etiologies of shunt malfunction or systemic symptoms.

Signs and Symptoms

- Shunt infection may present as shunt malfunction without headache or meningeal signs
- Shunt infection may also present with symptoms of acute bacterial meningitis

Diagnostic Workup

LABORATORY

CSF

- CSF pleocytosis is usually present but rarely above 100 cells/μL.
- CSF protein may be elevated and glucose low or normal.
- CSF Gram stain and culture are required, but negative in almost half of cases.

SERUM

- Peripheral blood cultures may also secure a diagnosis.
- ESR and CRP are elevated.

IMAGING

CT

- CT of the brain with contrast may demonstrate ependymal enhancement associated with ventriculitis.
- CT of the brain without contrast is also helpful in diagnosis shunt malfunction.

Therapy

SURGERY

- Removal or externalization of the distal portion of the shut is usually required.

ANTIBIOTICS

- Vancomycin 1 g IV q12h for coverage of MRSA
- Attention to peak and trough vancomycin levels is required to reach adequate CNS penetration.
- When culture and sensitivity data become available, antibiotic coverage should be narrowed, as these infections are not the result of multiple organisms.
- Antibiotics should be continued for 10–14 days after normalization of the CSF profile.

- After the full course of antibiotics, CSF shunt hardware may be replaced.

REFERENCES

Brain abscess and parameningeal infection. In Johnson RT, Griffin JW, McArthur JC. *Current Therapy in Neurologic Disease*, 7th ed. Philadelphia: C. V. Mosby, 2006.

Cerebral abscess. In Greeberg MS. *Handbook of Neurosurgery*, 5th ed. Lakeland, FL: Greenberg Graphics, 2001.

Cohen BA. Neurologic manifestations of toxoplasmosis in AIDS. *Semin Neurol*. 1999;**19**(2):201–11.

Cysticercosis. In Ropper AH, Brown RH. *Adams and Victor's Principles of Neurology*, 8th ed. New York: McGraw-Hill, 2005.

Darouiche RO. Spinal epidural abscess. *N Engl J Med*. 2006; **355**(19):2012–20.

de Gans J, van de Beek D, the European Dexamethasone in Adulthood Bacterial Meningitis Study I. Dexamethasone in adults with bacterial meningitis. *N Engl J Med*. 2002;**347**(20):1549–56.

Del Brutto OMD. Neurocysticercosis. *Semin Neurol*. 2005(03):243–51.

Gilden DH, Kleinschmidt-DeMasters BK, LaGuardia JJ, Mahalingam R, Cohrs RJ. Neurologic complications of the reactivation of varicella-zoster virus. *N Engl J Med*. 2000;**342**(9):635–45.

Glaser CA, Gilliam S, Schnurr D, et al. In search of encephalitis etiologies: diagnostic challenges in the California Encephalitis Project, 1998–2000. *Clin Infect Dis*. 2003;**36**(6):731–42.

Lam CH, Villemure JG. Comparison between ventriculoatrial and ventriculoperitoneal shunting in the adult population. *Br J Neurosurg*. 1997;**11**(1):43–8.

Lipton SA, Hickey WF, Morris JH, Loscalzo J. Candidal infection in the central nervous system. *Am J Med*. 1984;**76**(1):101–8.

Lo CH, Spelman D, Bailey M, Cooper DJ, Rosenfeld JV, Brecknell JE. External ventricular drain infections are independent of drain duration: an argument against elective revision. *J Neurosurg*. 2007;**106**(3):378–83.

Marra CM. Neurologic complications of Bartonella henselae infection. *Curr Opin Neurol*. 1995;**8**:164–9.

Nash D, Mostashari F, Fine A, et al. The outbreak of West Nile virus infection in the New York City area in 1999. *N Engl J Med*. 2001;**344**(24):1807–14.

Newton CRJC, Hien TT, White N. Neurological aspects of tropical disease: cerebral malaria. *J Neurol Neurosurg Psychiatry*. 2000;**69**(4):433–41.

Nussbaum ES, Rigamonti D, Standiford H, Numaguchi Y, Wolf AL, Robinson WL. Spinal epidural abscess: a report of 40 cases and review. *Surg Neurol*. 1992;**38**(3):225–31.

Petersen LR, Marfin AA, Gubler DJ. West Nile virus. *JAMA*. 2003;**290**(4):524–8.

Raschilas F, Wolff M, Delatour F, et al. Outcome of and prognostic factors for herpes simplex encephalitis in adult patients: results of a multicenter study. *Clin Infect Dis*. 2002;**35**(3):254–60.

Shunt infection in cerebral abscess. In Greeberg MS. *Handbook of Neurosurgery*, 5th ed. Lakeland, FL: Greenberg Graphics, 2001.

Tattevin P, Bruneel F, Clair B, et al. Bacterial brain abscesses: a retrospective study of 94 patients admitted to an intensive care unit (1980 to 1999). *Am J Med.* 2003; **115**(2):143–6.

Thwaites G, Chau TTH, Mai NTH, Drobniewski F, McAdam K, Farrar J. Neurological aspects of tropical disease: tuberculous meningitis. *J Neurol Neurosurg Psychiatry.* 2000;**68**(3):289–99.

van de Beek D, de Gans J, McIntyre P, Prasad K. Steroids in adults with acute bacterial meningitis: a systematic review. *Lancet Infect Dis.* 2004;**4**(3):139–43.

van de Beek D, de Gans J, Tunkel AR, Wijdicks Efm. Community-acquired bacterial meningitis in adults. *N Engl J Med.* 2006;**354**(1):44–53.

van der Horst CM, Saag MS, Cloud GA, et al. Treatment of cryptococcal meningitis associated with the acquired immunodeficiency syndrome. *N Engl J Med.* 1997; **337**(1):15–21.

Walker M, Zunt JR. Parasitic central nervous system infections in immunocompromised hosts. *Clin Infect Dis.* 2005;**40**(7):1005–15.

Wheat LJ, Musial CE, Jenny-Avital E. Diagnosis and management of central nervous system histoplasmosis. *Clin Infect Dis.* 2005;**40**(6):844–52.

Whitley RJ, Gnann JW. Viral encephalitis: familiar infections and emerging pathogens. *Lancet.* 2002;**359**(9305): 507–13.

Zabramski JM, Whiting D, Darouiche RO, et al. Efficacy of antimicrobial-impregnated external ventricular drain catheters: a prospective, randomized, controlled trial. *J Neurosurg.* 2003;**98**(4):725–30.

21 Spinal Cord Injury

Melissa Y. Macias, MD, PhD, and Dennis J. Maiman, MD, PhD

EPIDEMIOLOGY

Spinal cord injury (SCI) may be defined as disruption of the normal anatomy of the spinal cord with consequential neurologicdeficit. On average, 10,000 new cases of SCI occur in the United States annually; with an estimated 225,000–288,000 individuals currently living with paralysis.[1] The two most frequently injured regions are cervical C4–6 (39.4%) and thoracolumbar T12–L1 (11.6%). Correspondingly the most common levels of neurologic injury are:

- Cervical (51%)
- Thoracic (34.3%)
- Lumbosacral (10.7%)

In descending order of frequency, the majority of spine and spinal cord trauma are caused by:

- Motor vehicle crashes (MVCs)
- Falls
- Acts of violence (most commonly gunshot wounds)
- Recreational sporting activities (e.g., diving, contact sports, snowmobiling, etc.)

Since 2000, sports-related and violent spinal cord injuries have both decreased; however, those due to falls have increased – a trend that may reflect the continuing rise in the median age of the general population. Indeed, SCI in the elderly population (>60 years of age) has doubled since the 1980s and is most commonly caused by falls. The median age of persons with SCI is 37.6 years of age, an increase from the 1980s and early 1990s, also likely due to the aging population and proportion of injuries in the elderly. SCI in younger individuals continues to be caused primarily by motor vehicle accidents, violence, and sport related injuries.[1]

Immediate emergency and trauma management of SCI focuses on emergent immobilization, stabilization, and safe transport to a high-level care facility. Management of acute spinal cord injured patients should be undertaken in an intensive care unit (ICU) where multisystem monitoring can be optimized and a systemic approach implemented, with specific attention to cardiovascular, respiratory, gastrointestinal, urologic, and integument systems. ICU management goals encompass anticipation of acute complications and prevention of intermediate and long-term complications of SCI. Improved medical management after acute SCI has reduced both morbidity and mortality by 60–90%[2,3] translating to overall improvement in quality of life for SCI patients.[2-4]

The timing of surgical intervention for unstable spinal column injuries after acute SCI remains controversial. Instability due to undiagnosed associated traumatic injuries may be increased after early operative intervention.[5] Conversely, indications and benefits for early surgical stabilization in patients with either spinal column instability or cord compression from epidural hematoma or structural deformity[6,7] include:

- Progressive neurologic deficit
- Earlier mobilization
- Treatment of associated traumatic injuries
- Reduction of medical complications
- Decreased duration of ICU and overall hospitalization stays

This chapter identifies key medical considerations for neurocritical ICU management of acute spinal cord injured patients via a systems-based approach.

PHARMACOLOGIC CONSIDERATIONS

The main pharmacologic agent used in acute SCI is high-dose steroid infusion with methylprednisolone (MP). The decision to initiate treatment must be made within the first 8 hours following injury[8] according to the following protocol:

- Bolus dose of 30 mg/kg intravenous (IV) over 15 minutes followed by either
- 5.4 mg/kg/h IV for 23 hours if administered within 3 hours or
- 5.4 mg/kg/h IV for 47 hours if administered after 3 hours but before 8 hours of injury

High-dose MP may reduce vasogenic edema and inflammation, potentially limiting overall cord disruption. Although beneficial effects have been reported when given within 8 hours of injury,[8] treatment with high-dose MP is controversial. Recent studies advocate against high dose MP[3,9,10] due to the lack of reproducibility of the beneficial effects[11] and associated comorbidities [3,9-12] that include:

- Prolonged ventilator dependency
- Hyperglycemia
- Pneumonia
- Gastrointestinal (GI) hemorrhage
- Acute corticosteroid myopathy
- Increased risk of infection and sepsis

Though current medical evidence fails to support high-dose MP treatment after SCI, the possibility of even modest clinical benefit after SCI injury has led to its continued use by some clinicians. Treatment once initiated should be continued to completion in the ICU setting, with awareness and attention to its potential adverse systemic effects. Notable contraindications to high-dose MP usage include the following conditions[12]:

- Cauda equina syndrome
- Gunshot wounds to the spine
- Pregnancy
- Pediatric population <13 years of age

- Prior use of maintenance steroids
- Narcotic addiction

CARDIAC AND HEMODYNAMIC CONSIDERATIONS

Neurogenic shock, caused by disruption of the sympathetic nervous system coupled with unopposed vagal activity after acute SCI, is characterized by several hemodynamic irregularities [2,3,13,14] such as:

- Hypotension
- Dysrhythmias
- Reduced peripheral vascular resistance
- Reduced cardiac output

Vasodilatation causes third spacing of fluids and consequent intravascular depletion. Cardiac output must be increased and relies mostly on increased stroke volume rather than heart rate, which typically cannot be increased in the setting of sympathetic disruption.[2,14] Inevitably, this results in relative hypovolemia and hypotension.[2,13,15] Nearly 25% of SCI patients demonstrate hypotension (systolic blood pressure <90 mm Hg) and a decreased heart rate of (<90 beats/min)[13]; both often persist even after 4-6 liters of fluid resuscitation.[2] Pointedly, volume depletion is not the cause of hypotension. Fluids should be administered cautiously to prevent iatrogenic congestive heart failure, pulmonary edema, and hyponatremia in the absence of hemorrhagic hypovolemia from associated injuries.[2,3,15,16]

The ICU setting provides a necessary and ideal setting to for continuous electrocardiographic monitoring of hemodynamic parameters. Hemorrhagic hypovolemia must be either excluded or adequately addressed, after which a pulmonary artery catheter should be placed to monitor peripheral resistance (often <50%) and cardiac output.[2,13,16] Vasopressors are often required; an agent with both α- and β-adrenergic components is desired because of the vasoconstrictive effect to the peripheral vasculature and chronotropic/inotropic effects to the heart.[2,16] Commonly used vasopressors, their characteristics, and typical dosages are shown in Table 21.1.

- Dopamine is the pressor of choice, optimizing chronotropic cardiac and peripheral vascular improvement.
- Norepinephrine provides prominent increases in peripheral resistance and chronotropic/inotropic

Table 21.1. Vasopressors used in SCI

Rx	Typical dosing	Effects
Dopamine (***Agent of choice***-dose dependent α, β & dopaminergic effects)	0.5–2.0 µg/kg per minute	Dopaminergic with renal, mesenteric, coronary and cerebral vasodilatation; + inotropic cardiac effect
	2–10 µg/kg per minute	A and β_1 agonist; vasoconstriction with systolic and diastolic blood pressure; + inotropic cardiac effect
	> 10 µg/kg per minute	α, β and dopaminergic effects
Epinephrine (α and β agonist)	1–8 µg/min	Prominent vasoconstriction but also activates B_2 receptors causing vasodilatation and diastolic blood pressure; + chronotropic and inotropic cardiac effects
Norepinephrine (α and B_1 agonist)	1–20 µg/min	Minimal effect on B_2 receptors; prominent increase in peripheral resistance with increases in systolic and diastolic blood pressure but may get reflex bradycardia; + chronotropic and inotropic effects
Phenylephrine (purely α agonist)	40–100 µg/min	Noninotropic; *use in SCI is highly cautioned due to reflex bradycardia*
Dobutamine	2.5–10 µg/kg per minute (primarily β_1 selective)	Increasing cardiac output; + inotropic cardiac effect

support to the heart; however, it is also associated with undesired reflex bradycardia.

■ Dobutamine improves cardiac function but may also reduce systemic blood pressure and is **not recommended** for patients with SCI.

■ Pure α-adrenergics, such as phenylephrine, may increase peripheral vascular resistance; however, associated reflex bradycardia is detrimental to cardiac function and should be used judiciously in the SCI patient.

Maintenance of adequate organ perfusion is the goal of treatment, monitored by urine output (>0.5 mg/kg per hour), prevention of acid–base abnormalities, and appropriate mentation.[2,13,16] Optimal mean arterial pressure (MAP) to achieve this goal may vary among patients. In the acute phase of SCI, systemic hypotension may exacerbate already altered perfusion to the injured cord, potentially worsening secondary ischemic cord injury. Subsequently, maintenance of a MAP at >85–90 mm Hg for a minimum of 7 days after acute SCI has been suggested to optimize neurologic function and reduce morbidity and mortality.[3,13]

RESPIRATORY AND PULMONARY CONSIDERATIONS

Ventilation

Immediate airway protection must be ensured and adequate ventilation maintained. Respiratory insufficiency and pulmonary dysfunction are common, especially after cervical or thoracic SCI levels.[2,3,14,16] Key muscles of respiration, their functions, and consequence of injury[2,14,17,18] are described in Table 21.2.

Hypercarbia, hypoxemia, atelectasis, and inability to mobilize secretions are clear consequences of pulmonary dysfunction regardless of injury level.[2,18] Parameters for positive pressure ventilation include[2,14]:

■ Hypoxemia (PaO_2 <80 mm Hg)
■ Hypercarbia ($PaCO_2$ >50 mm Hg)
■ Elevated respiratory rate (>35 breaths/min)

Table 21.2. Muscles of respiration

Muscle group	Function	Injury sequelae
Intercostal muscles (T1–T12)	Stabilizes the chest during expiration	Functional flail chest phenomenon leading to inadequate tidal volume (V_t)
Diaphragm (C3–5)	Generates approximately 50–60% of forced vital capacity (FVC)	Dysfunction from fatigue following low cervical or high thoracic SCI it has assumed 100% of the workload of respiration leading to diminished lung volumes
Abdominal muscles (T7–L1)	Primary muscle of expiration	Increased end-tidal volumes and compromised lung capacity
Cervical accessory (C3–C8)	Augments respiratory mechanics	Compromised work of respiration

In alert, cooperative patients, evaluation of ventilation–perfusion abnormalities should be done using serial measurements of forced vital capacity (FVC), which includes tidal volume and inspiratory and expiratory reserve volumes (normally 65–75 mL/kg of ideal body weight). Impending respiratory failure occurs with FVC <15 mL/kg, necessitating intubation and mechanical ventilation.[2,18,19]

Standard ICU respiratory management of the SCI patient requires:

■ Continuous pulse oximetry monitoring
■ Supplemental oxygen
■ Frequent arterial blood gas measurements

Arterial blood gas values should be interpreted cautiously, as they may poorly reflect adequacy of ventilation, changing only after depletion of pulmonary and cardiovascular reserves.[2,14] In addition to a carotid chemoreceptor response to hypoxemia, early hypocapnia may be caused by dyspnea and increased ventilatory drive resulting from vagal mediated activation of primary pulmonary receptors.[2,18] Adequate respiratory reserve is a common misinterpretation of normal to low $PaCO_2$ in the setting of true respiratory distress. Further, supplemental oxygen may obscure ensuing hypoxemia leading to worsening respiratory pathophysiology. As fatigue with progressive tachypnea occurs, exacerbation of ventilation–perfusion abnormalities may lead to acute respiratory arrest. Keen awareness of the respiratory rate is essential because it may reflect impending respiratory failure.[2,18,19]

Altered pulmonary physiology may result in inadequate lung expansion. Positive pressure ventilation is therefore preferred and can be provided with volume-cycled mechanical ventilation using either[19]:

1. Synchronized intermittent mandatory ventilation (SIMV): sufficient respiratory effort but at risk for fatigue
▶ Pressure support (PS): minimizes fatigue from increased work of breathing
▶ Extrinsic positive end-expiratory pressure (PEEP): ceases expiratory flow at a preselected pressure, preventing alveolar collapse, improving lung compliance and gas exchange allowing inspired oxygen (FIO_2) to be reduced to less toxic levels (<60%)
2. Assist control ventilation (ACV): patients with minimal respiratory effort
▶ Fully assists all spontaneous breaths through a full cycle
▶ Provides breaths at a pre-selected rate
▶ Hyperinflation: undesirable result from decreased time for exhalation, accompanied by intrinsic or auto-PEEP, potentially causing hypercarbia, alkalosis, and tachypnea

A SCI patient may be weaned off ventilator support if the following criteria[14,20] are met:

■ Vital capacity >10 mL/kg
■ Tidal volume >5 mL/kg
■ Peak inspiratory pressure >20 cm H_2O
■ respiratory rate < 30 breaths/min

A gradual wean is generally preferred and may be accomplished by:

■ Slowly decreasing the rate of intermittent mandatory ventilation

- Continuous positive airway pressure support
- Extending periods off ventilator support utilizing T-piece trials

With clinical evidence that the diaphragm can be "trained,"[2,16] the latter is most commonly used in our institution. Patients unable to be weaned off ventilator support should be considered for a tracheostomy, such as quadriplegic patients from high cervical cord injury or any patient requiring prolonged mechanical ventilation >14 days.

Pneumonia

The most common cause of morbidity and mortality after SCI are pulmonary complications mostly due to pneumonia.[2,3,4,7,21] Aggressive respiratory therapy[20,22] aimed toward minimizing atelectasis and bronchial secretions include:

- Postural changes
- Sterile nasotracheal suctioning
- Aggressive chest physiotherapy

Despite these efforts, pneumonia occurs in 5–20% of cervical level SCI patients[21,22] and is most commonly caused by[2,14,21]:

- Poor secretion clearance
- Progressive bronchiole obstruction
- Ventilation–perfusion abnormalities
- Atelectasis

Combined with these factors and the acute angle of the left compared with the right bronchus, pneumonia is more frequently observed in the left lower lobe after SCI.[14,18] Prophylactic antibiotics are not recommended to avoid antibiotic-resistant infection.[18,21] Early removal of stomach contents by a nasogastric tube is advised to prevent aspiration pneumonia in the right lower lobe resulting from gastric atony with SCI.[23]

The microorganisms are polymicrobial, derived form the normal flora of the oropharynx; the most common isolates are gram-negative aerobic pathogens.[19] Development of ventilator-associated pneumonia (VAP) is usually caused by *Streptococcus pneumoniae* or *Hemophilus influenza* if within the first 4 days of ventilation or *Pseudomonas aeruginosa* or *Staphylococcus aureus* after 4 days.[19]

The clinical signs of pneumonia[21] in SCI patients include:

- Fever
- Leukocytosis
- Hypoxia
- Purulent sputum
- Infiltrates evident on chest radiographs

Cautious interpretation of these clinical signs is mandated because fever and leukocytosis may accompany atelectasis alone; and chest radiographic diagnosis is challenging in the likely presence of atelectasis.[2,3,21,22] If pneumonia is suspected, tracheal secretions should be sent for gram stain and culture analysis. Antibiotic therapy is directed at the most likely organisms while awaiting final culture results, after which treatment may be tailored accordingly. In patients in whom clinical improvement and radiographic clearance are noted, antibiotic treatment should not be changed based on subsequent culture results suggesting different or additional organisms.[2,21]

Thromboembolic Disease: Deep Vein Thrombosis and Pulmonary Embolism

The incidence of deep vein thrombosis (DVT) is significant in SCI patients, even as high as 100% based on radiolabeled fibrinogen scanning.[2,3] Thromboembolic disease after SCI occurs from venous stasis caused by both decreased vascular resistance and loss of muscle contraction.

The risk for catastrophic pulmonary embolism (PE) after DVT is elevated 2–10% above the general surgical population.[24] Interestingly, the incidence of clinically recognizable DVT in the SCI patient has been reported at 15% and for PE only 5%.[24] The risk of DVT and/or PE is greatest during the acute phase and up to the first 3 months of injury.[3,14,26] The significant morbidity and mortality associated with thromboembolic disease necessitates a high index of clinical suspicion coupled with aggressive prophylactic measures of 3 months' duration.[3,4,24]

Prophylactic treatment[3,12] in patients with severe motor deficits include:

- Mechanical devices: external pneumatic compression devices, compression stockings, rotating beds, or electrical stimulation

■ Anticoagulants: low-dose heparin, adjusted dose heparin, low molecular weight heparin (LMWH) or Coumadin

Mechanical devices carry minimal risk but do not provide sufficient prophylaxis alone. If started within the first 72 hours of injury, anticoagulation therapies may increase the risk of hemorrhage in the injured spinal cord. Like mechanical devices, when used alone anticoagulation modalities do not provide optimal thromboembolic prophylaxis.[3,12] Combined therapy appears to provide the greatest protection.[3,12] A reasonable ICU management strategy would employ mechanical devices within the first 72 hours followed by the addition of low-dose heparin (5000 units subcutaneously every 8 hours), adjusted dose heparin (titration of subcutaneous heparin every 12 hours to a partial thromboplastin time [PTT] of 1.5 times control) or LMWH.[3,24] Our strategy involves implementation of pneumatic compression devices in the acute phase of injury with the addition of Lovenox (LMWH) once the risk of hemorrhage in the injured cord is minimized.

DVT should be suspect in the SCI patient[2,3,14] with the development of:

■ Unexplained fever
■ Leg edema or redness
■ Increase in leg circumference and/or skin temperature

Mortality from DVT in SCI patients is 9%.[3,12] Diagnostic tests for DVT[2,3,12] include:

■ Duplex Doppler ultrasound: primary diagnostic test secondary to availability, low cost and accuracy of detection (sensitivity approximately 90%)
■ Venous occlusion plethysmography (VOP)
■ Fibrinogen scanning
■ D-dimer analysis: highly sensitive but not specific
■ Venography: considered the gold standard, but invasive and costly; reserved for patients with a negative ultrasound study but high clinical suspicion

Once diagnosis of DVT is made, full anticoagulation treatment with heparin followed by oral warfarin for 3–6 months with international normalized ratio (INR) levels of 1.5–2.5 is recommended.[3] In patients with contraindications to anticoagulation therapy or where therapy is ineffective, a vena cava filter should be placed.[2,3,15] Concern of PE must be raised in patients with confirmed DVT with development of the following symptoms:

■ Tachypnea
■ Tachycardia
■ Pleuritic pain (may be obfuscated from the underlying respiratory pathophysiology changes observed after SCI)

The diagnosis of PE can be made with the following diagnostic tests[2,3,14,16]:

■ Pulmonary angiography: considered the gold standard but invasive and costly
■ Chest radiography
■ Ventilation–perfusion scans
■ Spiral computed tomography (CT): most commonly used secondary to availability, cost, and noninvasiveness
■ Acute changes in arterial blood gases (ABG): decreases in oxygen saturation or arterial oxygen with a concomitant increase in arterial carbon dioxide should raise suspicion of PE but difficult to interpret with underlying pulmonary compromise
■ Electrocardiogram: may demonstrate signs of acute cor pulmonale; classic triad of a large S wave in lead I, large Q wave in lead III, and inverted T wave in lead III (S1Q3T3) is more commonly observed is sinus tachycardia than with PE.

Treatment of PE incorporates full anticoagulation, as described for DVT, and the placement of a vena cava filter is highly recommended to prevent further emboli.[3] With regard to vena cava filters, some centers recommend prophylactic placement in all SCI patients.[3] Significant complications, however, have been demonstrated with this strategy. SCI patients experience compromised abdominal muscle tone permitting distal migration, intraperitoneal erosion, and symptomatic IVC occlusion.[27] Caval filters, therefore, should be reserved for patients with persistent thromboembolic events despite anticoagulation or for those with contraindications to anticoagulation and/or pneumatic compression devices.[3,12]

GASTROINTESTINAL CONSIDERATIONS

Abdominal and Bowel Dysfunction

Acute life-threatening intra-abdominal problems such as splenic rupture or liver laceration should be identified by CT of the abdomen and pelvis during the early assessment phase and managed accordingly. More insidious and chronic gastrointestinal (GI) dysfunction[28,29] after sympathetic disruption from SCI includes:

- Gastric atony
- Stress ulcerations
- Bowel obstruction
- Constipation
- Abdominal bloating, pain
- Fecal incontinence

Despite intact vagal efferent innervation, loss of GI sympathetic outflow frequently results in impaired colonic transit.[2,29,30] Subsequent development of ileus with concomitant constipation is not uncommon. Left untreated, resultant fecal impaction may potentiate bowel obstruction with associated risks for distention and life-threatening bowel perforation. Thus, a daily bowel regimen is essential in the early phase of SCI. A standard regimen consists of agents that improve colonic motility and include a combination of stool softeners, rectal suppositories, and enemas.[2] Paradoxically, fecal incontinence already manifest secondary to loss of sphincter control may be aggravated by motility agents. Hence, dietary fiber and adequate hydration must be factored into the bowel regimen.[29] Functional bowel disorders persist beyond the ICU management period and are understandably a cause of anxiety and psychological distress. Timely bowel retraining should be incorporated into the early management of SCI patients.

Abdominal distention may cause diaphragmatic irritation manifest as referred pain to the shoulder regions, especially in injuries below C5.[2,28] Even so, possible mechanisms permitting the perception of visceral pain below the sensory level of injury include imbalance of sensory channels, loss of spinal inhibitory tone or the presence of a central pain generator. Significant anxiety from discomfort of visceral pain symptoms should be treated with anxiolytics as appropriate.[28]

Nutrition

Nutrition and timing of enteral feeding are important management considerations following SCI.[2,3,14] A nasogastric tube should be placed acutely to reduce the risk of vomiting and acute gastric dilatation, either of which may compromise pulmonary function through aspiration or decreased lung capacity, respectively.[2,3] Return of GI motility[14,31] is evidenced by:

- Decreased nasogastric output (typically 2–3 days after admission).
- Flatus
- Bowel movements

If not contraindicated, once GI motility has returned enteral nutrition should be started slowly, providing nutritional support and protection of stress ulceration.[32] Two complications of starting enteral feedings too early include high gastric residuals and recurrent GI ileus, both of which are associated with an increased aspiration risk.[31]

SCI patients are in a hypermetabolic and hypercatabolic state.[2,3,33] Significant nitrogen losses result from absent muscle tone and activity. Key nutritional goals are to meet caloric and nitrogen needs but not to restore nitrogen balance. In the early postinjury period the energy expenditure assessment method of choice is indirect calorimetry and not the Harris–Benedict equation, as the latter overestimates the caloric requirements.[2,3,33] Nutritional support should be provided within 7 days, to minimize hormonal alterations, which may lead to increased susceptibility to infection and delayed wound healing[2,3,33] and manifest as:

- Increased plasma cortisol and adrenocorticotropic levels
- Nutritional deficiencies
- Immune dysfunction

The preferred route of nutritional delivery is through enteral feedings, which maintain GI integrity and function. Parenteral nutrition should be used in patients with GI injury, prolonged ileus or mechanical obstruction.[2,3,14] Many commercial options are available for enteral feedings. In the critically ill patient, continual rather than bolus feeding is better tolerated (starting rate 10 to 30 mL/h, slowly increased to goal amount, typically

Table 21.3. GI prophylactic agents for stress ulceration

Category	Example Rx	Beneficial effects	Adverse effects
Antacids	Magnesium hydroxide (30 mL PO q24h) Aluminum hydroxide Aluminum-magnesium combinations	Maintains gastric pH >4.5 and inactivates pepsin	Diarrhea, constipation hypophosphatemia and metabolic alkalosis
H$_2$-antagonists	Ranitidine Famotidine Cimetidine (50 mg IV q6h)	Inhibits parietal cell histamine type 2 receptors; ↓ acid production	Hypotension, thrombocytopenia, inhibition of cytochrome P450 enzyme
Other	Sucralfate (1 g PO/NG q6H) (mixture of sucrose, sulfates, aluminum hydroxide)	Protects GI mucosa by increasing viscosity, mucin content and hydrophobicity	None

30 to 40 kcal/kg per day in the acute postinjury setting).[2,15] Nasogastric, orogastric, or small-bore nasoduodenal/nasojejunal tubes (in the presence of high gastric retention volumes) may be used to deliver enteral nutrition.[2,14,19]

GI Stress Ulceration and Hemorrhage

GI tract stress ulceration peaks at 4–10 days postinjury and are caused by the unopposed vagal tone after sympathectomy disruption from SCI.[2,14,34] Stress ulceration is most common in patients with cervical level injuries and high-dose steroid treatment may[11] or may not[30] increase the risk. Effective prophylactic treatment[3,30,34] against stress-related mucosal damage includes:

- Antacids
- H$_2$ receptor antagonists
- Sucralfate

The incidence of GI hemorrhage is decreased with maintenance of gastric pH > 4.[30,34] Example agents, beneficial and adverse effects of antacids, H$_2$ receptor antagonists, and sucralfate are summarized in Table 21.3. Antacids quickly neutralize gastric pH, however have several untoward side effects. Alternatively, IV H$_2$ antagonists have been shown to significantly reduce the risk of GI

hemorrhage from 43% to 17%, but interfere with the hepatic metabolism of other drugs including phenytoin, antibiotics and warfarin.[34] Sucralfate, on the other hand, stimulates prostaglandin production, which promotes mucosal regeneration and healing. With no known adverse effects and apparent increased efficaciousness compared to IV ranitidine[14,34] sucralfate is an appealing agent of choice for the prevention of stress ulceration.

GI hemorrhage should be suspected with declining hematocrit and platelet levels on serial cell blood counts, especially when no other etiology may account for these findings. Blood urea nitrogen (BUN) elevations despite adequate urine output and stable creatinine may be a flag for GI hemorrhage.[30,34] Endoscopic evaluation is the diagnostic tool of choice if GI ulceration/hemorrhage is suspected, and may provide hemostatic intervention. Urgent surgical intervention may be necessary with recurrent or refractory GI bleeding.[2,34]

UROLOGIC

Priapism

After acute SCI, priapism in men is nonischemic and likely a consequence of acute sympathectomy. Intracorporeal phenylephrine irrigation may be used; however, conservative management (observation) is preferred to preserve long-term erectile function.[35]

Urinary Tract Infection

Spinal shock accompanies acute SCI and usually lasts approximately 3 weeks postinjury. Bladder hypotonia is typical during this period and an indwelling Foley catheter should be placed emergently[2,3,14,16] for:

- Accurate volume monitoring during hemodynamic stabilization
- Bladder decompression

The length of catheterization is directly correlated to the risk of urinary tract infection (UTI).[36] Even so, prophylactic antibiotic treatment has not been proven effective because catheter bacteriuria is common. The signs and symptoms of a UTI[21,36] in SCI are difficult to identify secondary to sensation loss; however, clinical features may include:

- Fever
- Discomfort over the back or abdomen
- Increased urinary incontinence or spasticity
- Autonomic dysreflexia
- Malaise
- Urine cloudiness and/or odor

The causative microorganisms of UTIs[21,36] in SCI patients are:

- Gram-negative bacilli (*E. coli, Pseudomonas, Klebsiella*)
- Commensal organisms of the bowel (*Enterococcus*)

Confirmation of diagnosis must be made with a urine culture. Broad-spectrum antibiotics may be started for empiric treatment then tailored following identification and susceptibilities of the offending microorganism.

Bladder Dysfunction

The indwelling catheter should be removed and a bladder regimen initiated once the patient is medically stable. Typically, this is beyond the scope of initial ICU management and performed on transfer to SCI rehabilitation. With resolution of spinal shock, the return of bladder function is dependent on the level of SCI.

- Upper motor neuron injury above the sacral cord is most common with SCI and causes hypertonic bladder dysfunction.[14,37]
- Lower motor neuron dysfunction occurs with injuries that interrupt the local reflex arc and cause detrusor areflexia, or hypocontractility. Complications, manifestations and treatments of these conditions [2,14,37] are shown in Table 21.4.

Although urodynamic studies help guide treatment strategies, intermittent, clean, straight catheterization remains the treatment of choice because of decreased risk for UTI.[36,37] In bladder dysfunction from either upper or lower motor neuron injury, long-term indwelling catheters are the treatment of last resort, because of associated risk for abnormal intravenous pyelograms, calculi, urethral lesions, leakage, and previously mentioned UTIs.[2,21,36,37]

INTEGUMENT

Decubitus ulcers occur in SCI patients because of insensate integument, immobility, low blood pressure that decreases skin perfusion predisposing skin to necrosis and breakdown.[2,3,14] Decubiti may develop in patients left on a spine board for less than 6 hours.[2] Most common sites for decubiti include the ischial tuberosities, sacrum, lateral malleoli, greater trochanter, heels, and coccyx.[2,14,21]

- The primary goal of treatment remains frequent inspection of susceptible areas and hygienic care.
- Preventative measures incorporate pressure point padding, frequent turning with spine precautions, and utilizing air flotation beds.[2,3,14]

Once formed, pressure ulcer treatment involves immediate relief of pressure and wound débridement. Antibiotic therapy is reserved for confirmed wound infections and/or bacteremia.

- The most common pathogens associated with the necrotic tissue of decubitus ulcers are *Bacteroides, E. coli, Proteus, Enterococcus*, and anaerobic streptococci; whereas healing ulcers often demonstrate *P. aeruginosa* and *S. areus* isolates.[21]

Table 21.4. Categories of bladder dysfunction and treatments

Category	
Upper Motor Neuron Injury (Most Common In SCI Patients)	
Complications:	Ureteral reflux, hydronephrosis, pyelonephritis, renal dysfunction and autonomic dysreflexia*
Manifestations:	Treatments:
1. Detrusor-Sphincter Dyssynergia (Elevated bladder pressures and incomplete emptying)	anticholinergics, α- antagonists, antihypertonics, transurethral sphincterotomy, urethral stent placement and functional electrical stimulation
2. Detrusor Hyperreflexia (Urge incontinence)	anticholinergics, afferent desensitization agents and functional electrical stimulation

* Autonomic dysreflexia[22] is caused by massive sympathetic overdrive, may have life-threatening consequences.
Symptoms include sweating, headache, hypertension and bradycardia.

Lower Motor Neuron Dysfunction	
Complications:	Saddle anesthesia, reduced anal sphincter tone, loss of sphincter control and bulbocavernous reflex
Manifestations:	Treatments:
1. Detrusor Areflexia (Overdistention)	intermittent straight catheterization, chronic indwelling catheter – treatment of last resort

■ Complications from ulceration infection range from cellulites, abscess formation or osteomyelitis to potentially catastrophic bacteremia and sepsis. Clearly, vigilant attentiveness to patient positioning begins in the acute phase of injury and remains paramount in prevention of skin breakdown.

REFERENCES

1. The National SCI Statistical Center. *Spinal Cord Injury: Facts and Figures at a Glance.* University of Alabama at Birmingham National Spinal Cord Injury Center, June 2005.
2. Benzel EC. *Spine Surgery*, 2nd ed. Philadelphia: Elsevier Churchill Livingstone, 2005, pp 512–71.
3. Guidelines for the management of acute cervical spine and spinal cord injuries. *Neurosurgery.* 2002;**50**(3) (Suppl.).
4. DeVivo MJ, Kartus PL, Stover SL, et al. Cause of death for patients with spinal cord injuries. *Arch Intern Med.* 1989;**149**(8):1761–6.
5. Marshall LF, Knowlton S, Garfin SR, et al. Deterioration following spinal cord injury. A multicenter study. *J Neurosurgery.* 1987;**66**(3)400–4.
6. Albert TJ, Kim DH. Timing of surgical stabilization after cervical and thoracic trauma. *J Neurosurg Spine.* 2005;**3**:182–90.
7. Fehlings MF, Perrin, RG. The role and timing of early decompression for cervical spinal cord injury: update with a review of recent clinical evidence. *Injury Int J Care Injured.* 2005;36S-B13–26.
8. Bracken MB, Shepard MJ, Collins WF, et al. A randomized, controlled trial of methylprednisolone or naloxone in the treatment of acute spinal cord injury: results of the Second National Acute Spinal Cord Injury Study. *N Engl J Med.* 1990;**322**:1405–11.
9. Fehlings MG, Baptiste DC. Current status of clinical trials for acute spinal cord injury. *Injury Int J Care Injured.* 2005;**36**:S-B113–22.
10. Hugenholtz H, Cass DE, Dvorak MF, et al. High-dose methylprednisolone for acute spinal cord injury: only a treatment option. *Can. J. Neurol. Sci.* 2002;**29**:227–35.
11. Bracken MB, Shepard MJ, Holford TR, et al. Administration of methylprednisolone for 24 or 48 hours or tirilazad mesylate for 48 hours in the treatment of

acute spinal cord injury: results of the Third National Acute Spinal Cord Injury Randomized Controlled Trial. National Acute Spinal Cord Injury Study. *JAMA*. 1997;**277**:1597–1604.

12. Greenberg MS. *Handbook of Neurosurgery*, 6th ed. New York: Thieme, 2006, pp 702–7.

13. Levi L, Wolf A, Belzberg H. Hemodynamic parameters in patients with acute cervical cord trauma: description, intervention, and prediction of outcome. *Neurosurgery*. 1993;**33**:1007–17.

14. Andrews BT. *Intensive Care in Neurosurgery*. New York: Thieme, 2003, **137**–41.

15. Licina P, Nowitzke AM. Approach and considerations regarding the patient with spinal injury. *Injury Int J Care Injured*. 2005;**36**:S-B2–12.

16. Ball, PA. Critical care in spinal cord injury. *Spine*. 2001;**26**(245):S27–30.

17. Estenne M, Detroyer A. Respiratory muscle involvement in tetraplegia. *Prob Respir Care*. 1990;**3**:360–74.

18. Kocan MJ. Pulmonary considerations in the critical care phase. *Crit Care Clinic North Am*. 1990;**2**:369–74.

19. Marino PL. *The ICU Book*, 2nd ed. Philadelphia: Lippincott Williams and Wilkins, 1998, pp 421–48.

20. Schmitt J, Midha M, McKenzie N. Medical complications of spinal cord disease. *Neurol. Clin*. 1991;**9**:779–95.

21. Montgomerie JZ. Infections in patients with spinal cord injuries. *Clin Infect Dis*. 1997;**25**(6):1285–90.

22. Fishburn MJ, Marino RJ, Ditunno JF Jr. Atelectasis and pneumonia in acute spinal cord injury. *Arch Phys Med Rehabil*. 1990;**71**(3):197–200.

23. Gore, RM, Mintzer RA, Calenoff L. Gastrointestinal complications of spinal cord injury. *Spine*. 1981;**6**:538–44.

24. Green D, Sullivan S, Simpson J, et al. Evolving risk for thromboembolism in spinal cord injury (SPIRATE Study). *Am J Phys Med Rehab*. 2005;**84**(6)420–2.

25. Waring WP, Karuna RS. Acute spinal cord injuries and the incidence of clinically occurring thromboembolic disease. *Paraplegia*. 1991;**29**:8–16.

26. Lamb GC, Tomski MA, Kaufman J, et al. Is chronic spinal cord injury associated with increased risk of venous thromboembolism? *J Am Paraplegia Soc*. 1993;**16**:153–6.

27. Greenfield LJ. Does cervical spinal cord injury induce a higher incidence of complications after prophylactic after Greenfield usage? *J Vasc Interv Radiol*. 1997;**8**:719–20.

28. Ng C, Prott G, Rutkowski S, et al. Gastrointestinal symptoms in spinal cord injury: relationships with level of injury and psychologic factors. *Dis Colon Rectum*. 2005;**48**:1562–8.

29. Lynch AC, Wong C, Anthony A, et al. Bowel dysfunction following spinal cord injury: a description of bowel function in a spinal cord-injured population and comparison with age and gender matched controls. *Spinal Cord*. 2000;**38**:717–23.

30. Albert TJ, Levine MJ, Balderston RA, et al. Gastrointestinal complications in spinal cord injury. *Spine*. 1991;S522–5.

31. Rowan CJ, Gillanders LK, Paice RL, et al. Is early enteral feeding safe in patients who have suffered spinal cord injury? *Injury*. 2004;**35**(3)238–42.

32. Kuric J, Lucas CE, Ledgerwood AM, et al: Nutritional support: a prophylaxis against stress bleeding after spinal cord injury. *Paraplegia*. 1989;**27**:140–5.

33. Cruse JM, Lewis RE, Dilioglu S, et al. Review of immune function, healing of pressure ulcers, and nutritional status in patients with spinal cord injury. *J Spin Cord Med*. 2000;**23**:129–35.

34. Lu WY, Rhoney, DH, Boling WB, et al. A review of stress ulcer prophylaxis in the neurosurgical intensive care unit. *Neurosurgery*. 1997;**41**(2):416–26.

35. Gordon SA, Stage KH, Tansey KE, Lotan Y. Conservative management of priapism in acute spinal cord injury. *Urology*. 2005;**65**(6):1195–7.

36. Garcia Leoni ME, Esclarin De Ruz A. Management of urinary tract infection in patients with spinal cord injuries. *Clin Microbiol Infect*. 2003;**9**(8):780–5.

37. Burns AS, Rivas DA, Ditunno JF. The management of neurogenic bladder and sexual dysfunction after spinal cord injury. *Spine*. 2001;**26**(24 Suppl):S129–36.

22 Postoperative Management in the Neurosurgical Critical Care Unit

Andy J. Redmond, MD and Veronica L. Chiang, MD

Advances in neurosurgery and anesthesia have dramatically reduced intraoperative morbidity and mortality rates over the past several years. A significant part of the care of the neurosurgical patient, however, occurs postoperatively in the neurosurgical critical care unit (NCCU). The goal of care in a monitored environment during this time is to prevent and treat, in a timely fashion, potential early and often fatal complications of both surgery and anesthesia. This requires a team of highly trained specialists that may include neurosurgeons, anesthesiologists, neurointensivists, and nurses. Consultants and family members also play key roles in the management of the neurosurgical patient.

GENERAL CONSIDERATIONS

Greater than 90% of postoperative patients admitted to NCCUs pass through uneventfully and in general spend <24 hours in this monitored setting. Most complications occur within the first 24–48 hours after surgery and early detection can lead to quick and efficient remedies. Postoperative complications can be divided into those related to the effects of anesthesia in the context of the patient's premorbid medical conditions and those related to their neurosurgical disease. The most critical part of NCCU care is the ability to recognize and differentiate expected postoperative changes in clinical condition from those that are unexpected. To achieve this, there needs to be a clear understanding of the patient's baseline medical condition, neurosurgical disease, and operative procedure.

- A thorough medical and surgical history should be obtained by the admitting physician including a review of the medical record, especially if the patient is slow to recover from anesthesia. Many times family members are also a reliable source of information.
- Communication between the neurocritical care physician and the neurosurgeon and anesthesiologists involved in the operation is critical in clarifying perioperative details including which surgical approach was used, if there were unexpected or problematic events during surgery, and what postoperative expectations exist.
- Information regarding medications and fluids administered intraoperatively, estimated blood loss and urine output should also be conveyed.
- A baseline postoperative neurologic exam must then be obtained on arrival in the NCCU and any neurologic deficits clearly documented.
- Routine postoperative monitoring of electrocardiogram (EKG), oxygen saturation, blood pressure, and urine output should be implemented.
- A full set of baseline laboratory studies including an electrolyte panel, complete blood count (CBC) and platelet count, coagulation studies, cardiac enzymes, an arterial blood gas and relevant anticonvulsant levels should be obtained.
- In some cases, patients may require continued postoperative ventilatory support, intracranial monitoring, or continuous electroencephalography and there should be a clear discussion clarifying the goals of management.
- Additional tests such as computed tomography (CT) scans or chest radiographs may also need to be performed.

294

After completion of the initial baseline patient assessment, continued monitoring of the neurologic examination along with any detected physiologic abnormalities should be performed at regular intervals.

- As decreased level of consciousness, confusion, hyperreflexia, and some focal neurologic deficits may be accentuated by the persistence of halogenated anesthetic agents including isoflurane, neurologic examinations should ideally be repeated every hour, looking for progressive improvement in the deficits.
- In situations where this level of care is not feasible, a complete formal neurologic exam should be repeated within 2–4 hours after a standard anesthetic or within the time frame designated by the anesthesiologist in nonstandard situations.

Strict blood pressure control is recommended in all patients after intracranial surgery. The target blood pressure depends on the surgery that was performed, the patient's baseline blood pressure, and the patient's underlying cardiovascular and renal status.

- The indications for blood pressure control include a reduced risk of myocardial infarction, cerebral hemorrhage, and stroke.
- Concurrent with starting judicious medical therapy for hypertension, the physician should seek and treat other contributing causes such as pain, delirium, hypoxemia, and volume expansion.
- Intermittent doses of intravenous labetalol (5–20 mg IV q1h) or hydralazine (5–10 mg IV q1h) can then be used to treat the hypertension.
- Other medications available for treating hypertension include nitroprusside, nicardipine, esmolol, enalapril, and nitroglycerin.
- Nitroprusside used as an infusion is an extremely effective antihypertensive agent but as a vasodilator it is thought to worsen cerebral edema and therefore is not used as a first-line agent.

Maintenance of adequate fluid balance and normovolemia is also important. The general goal of postoperative fluid management is to provide maintenance fluids and to replete preoperative fluid deficits and insensible fluid losses. Neurosurgical patients may undergo significant fluid and electrolyte shifts as a consequence of intraoperative use of diuretics such as mannitol and lasix to reduce intraoperative brain swelling.

- As intraoperative urine output may not be a good indicator of intravascular volume status, some patients will have central venous catheters in place for monitoring.
- Postoperatively, while urine output tends to be a much more reliable indicator of fluid balance, total fluid intake and output, and hemodynamic parameters such as central venous pressure may need to be followed serially to guide intravenous fluid management.

Most patients who are not receiving oral nutrition should be started on intravenous fluids. Maintenance infusion of 0.9% NaCl at 75 mL/h can be started safely on the majority of patients.

- Brain tumor patients often receive steroids as well, which may affect their serum glucose levels. Hyperglycemic patients should receive normal saline only without dextrose.
- Hypo-osmolar fluids should not be used initially because of the tendency of many neurosurgical patients to develop hyponatremia, which could exacerbate cerebral edema or seizures.

Serum electrolytes including sodium, blood urea nitrogen (BUN) and creatinine and glucose should be checked before deciding on maintenance fluids for the next 24 hours. In the setting of persistent hyponatremia, the goals of management are both to restore normal serum sodium levels as well as to correct the cause of the metabolic abnormality.[3]

- Serum sodium levels of <130 mmol/L alone can account for focal neurologic deficits, alterations, and level of consciousness or postoperative seizures.
- The two most common neurosurgical causes of hyponatremia are syndrome of inappropriate antidiuretic hormone secretion (SIADH; common in most cases of tumor and trauma) and cerebral salt wasting (more common in vascular cases).
  - ▸ While urine electrolytes and osmolalities can help differentiate the two conditions, in the postoperative patient the predominant difference is the patient's intravascular volume.
  - ▸ Patients are usually intravascularly overloaded in SIADH and therefore the treatment for

hypervolemia is diuresis and fluid restriction to 1000–1800 mL of free water per 24 hours.

▶ In patients with cerebral salt wasting, patients are intravascularly depleted. 2% or 3% hypertonic saline solution is required to replete body sodium and water.

■ In patients with serum sodium levels <125 mmol/L it is important to raise serum sodium slowly to avoid central pontine myelinolysis.

As neurosurgical patients in general are prone to develop certain preventable complications, the timely use of several prophylactic agents has become standard. These include:

■ H_2 blockers or proton pump inhibitors for peptic ulcer disease[4]
■ Subcutaneous heparin[5] and intermittent pneumatic compression stockings[6] for deep venous thrombosis and pulmonary embolism
■ Prophylactic antibiotics for wound infections.

Antibiotics, ulcer prophylaxis, and pneumatic compression stockings should be implemented upon arrival in the NCCU. The routine use of antibiotics such as cefazolin for 24 hours postoperatively has been shown to reduce the incidence of wound infections in clean neurosurgical operations.[7,8] The timing of the introduction of subcutaneous heparin is somewhat controversial. The neurosurgical patient population as a whole has a much higher postoperative deep vein thrombosis (DVT)/pulmonary embolism (PE) rate than the average surgical patient. Unlike the orthopedic patient, however, the risk of postoperative bleeding into the surgical site carries far greater risk. While there are studies showing that it is safe to give prophylactic doses of heparin perioperatively, the majority of neurosurgical patients are started on SQ heparin 24 hours after surgery.

Lastly, postoperative fever is always a concern. Low-grade temperatures of less than 101.5°F arising within 24 hours of surgery are most commonly due to pulmonary atelectasis. Standard pulmonary therapy should be initiated in all possible extubated patients until they are independently ambulatory.

■ Fever of central origin is rare in our experience and therefore all cases of persistent or high-grade fever should be fully investigated.

■ The use of steroids significantly increases the risk of systemic infections and the usual suspects including sputum, urine, and blood should be cultured.
■ Evidence of wound infection or meningitis should also be sought via neurological exam, CT scans of the head with and without contrast and/or lumbar puncture for spinal fluid.
  ▶ Spinal fluid interpretation after intracranial surgery is often difficult as surgery itself can commonly result in pleocytosis and a low glucose level.
  ▶ Empiric antibiotics such as vancomycin and ceftazidime should be started after obtaining cerebrospinal fluid (CSF) if there are clinical indications of meningitis, such as CSF leak, meningismus or unexpected lethargy, until culture results are available.
■ The continuing workup or treatment of fever will not be detailed here with the exception of the one concern that persistent undetected or inadequately treated thromboembolic disease can also present as fever and occurs not infrequently in this postoperative population.

CAROTID ENDARTERECTOMY

Patients undergoing carotid endarterectomy (CEA) have had progressive occlusive disease of the internal carotid artery, which is most often due to atherosclerotic disease. The goal of surgery is to remove the atherosclerotic plaque and to restore blood flow to cerebral circulation, while reducing their lifelong risk of stroke. This procedure puts patients directly at risk for ischemic stroke and intracerebral hemorrhage secondary to cerebral hyperperfusion syndrome as well as being associated with a high rate of perioperative myocardial infarction (MI). Preoperative risk medical and neurologic risk factors that increase the risk of CEA include:

■ Angina
■ MI within 6 months
■ Congestive heart failure,
■ Severe hypertension defined as blood pressure >180/110
■ Chronic obstructive pulmonary disease
■ Age >70 years
■ Severe obesity

- Progressive neurologic deficit, frequent transient ischemic attacks (TIAs) not controlled by anticoagulants
- Recent CVA (within 7 days preoperatively).[9]

The postoperative examination in patients status post CEA should focus on the patient's cardiac function, neurologic examination, and include regular inspection of the surgical site.

Blood Pressure Management

CEA patients should be monitored postoperatively with telemetry and arterial catheter blood pressure tracings. Although some patients may continue to be persistently hypertensive, especially when exacerbated by anxiety and pain, many patients may in fact become hypotensive. This is due either to the persistence of iatrogenically induced intraoperative baroreceptor blockade or the exposure of the carotid receptor to markedly increased postoperative blood flow.

- Intravenous fluids should be used to keep patients euvolemic.
- The systolic blood pressure should be maintained between 110 and 150 mm Hg to ensure good cerebral perfusion.
- Mild hypotension may be treated with boluses of normal saline. Hypotension that is not responsive to fluid boluses may require pressors such as phenylephrine.

Myocardial Infarction

The incidence of myocardial infarction following CEA ranges from 0 to 2.1%.[2] It is important therefore to look for evidence of postoperative myocardial ischemia, especially in the elderly or diabetic patients who may not manifest any symptoms.

- An EKG should be performed on arrival in the NCCU.
- Cardiac enzymes should also be sent as part of the initial blood work and patients should be asked about symptoms of chest pain or discomfort.
  - ▸ Creatine kinase (CK), CK-MB, and troponin I should be sent every 6–8 hours during the first 24 hours after the operation.
  - ▸ Troponin I can detect myocardial infarction within 4–6 hours of the initial stress.
  - ▸ Three negative sets of enzymes over 24 hours rules out myocardial infarction.

If the EKG or cardiac enzymes suggest myocardial ischemia or infarction, the patient's pain should be adequately treated with narcotics, supplemental oxygen, and a beta-blocker should be used to control the heart rate and blood pressure. The cardiology consult service should be urgently notified to assist in further management. In our facility, aspirin is routinely started on all postoperative CEA patients within 24 hours of surgery both to decrease the rate of embolic complications as well as to continue cardiac protection.

Stroke

A decreased level of consciousness and/or evidence of motor asymmetry on physical examination in the postoperative patient raises concern for intracranial ischemia or hemorrhage. An emergent CT scan of the head will help differentiate between the two.

Cerebral thromboembolism accounts for the majority of stroke associated with CEA with an incidence of 5% in the perioperative period. Its management depends on the extent of the patient's deficit, whether it is progressing or resolving and the timing of the event post procedure. Some CVAs may be asymptomatic, but the majority of the major postoperative CVAs are caused by postoperative ICA occlusion or embolism from the surgical site.

- If the patient has a major neurologic deficit on awakening in the operating room and there is suspicion for an ischemic neurologic deficit, urgent surgical reexploration is recommended.
- If the neurologic deficit evolves in the early postoperative period while the patient is in the NCCU and an emergent CT scan of the brain rules out intracerebral hemorrhage, a diagnostic cerebral angiography should be arranged.
  - ▸ If the internal carotid artery is occluded on angiography, prompt surgical reexploration is required.
  - ▸ If, however, it is patent, examination of the major arterial branches may show occlusions or diffusion-weighted magnetic resonance

imaging (MRI) may show evidence of embolic phenomenon as illustrated in Figure 22.1. In these scenarios, there are few management options as anticoagulation and thrombolytic therapy are not feasible.

- In a patient has with recurrent embolic strokes, surgical reexploration may be required.

Intracerebral hemorrhage due to the cerebral hyperperfusion syndrome (CHS) occurs in 0–3% of patients after carotid endarterectomy. In addition to focal neurologic deficits it can cause throbbing unilateral headache, blurry vision, confusion, and seizures.

- CHS is defined as an increase in cerebral perfusion to >100% of the preoperative level.
- Hypertension subsequent to the restoration of normal perfusion to the previously chronically ischemic cerebral hemisphere is thought to be associated with the development of CHS.

It has been proposed that chronic stenosis of the internal carotid artery leads to a loss of autoregulation in the distal arterial system due to free radical mediated destruction of endothelial cells.[10] Restoration of blood flow leads to a hyperemic state. Many cases are mild but if untreated, some patients progress to intracerebral hemorrhage or death.

- A diagnosis of CHS can be confirmed by transcranial Doppler exam of the middle cerebral arteries.
- Tight blood pressure control using intravenous infusion of labetalol, nicardipine, or nitroprusside may be necessary for the prevention and treatment of CHS.[11]
- Evacuation of intracerebral hematomas is not usually indicated unless there is significant mass effect.

Nerve Injury

Most cranial nerve injuries after CEA are a result of traction and can be managed conservatively. Examples of these include:

1. Pupillary asymmetry due to injury to the sympathetic fibers surrounding the carotid artery causing visual blurriness

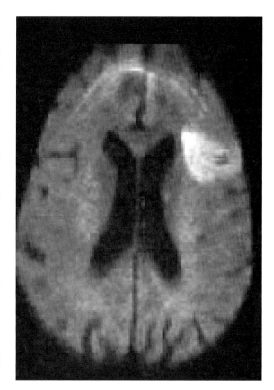

Figure 22.1. Diffusion-weighted MRI showing an acute ischemic stroke in the left frontal region.

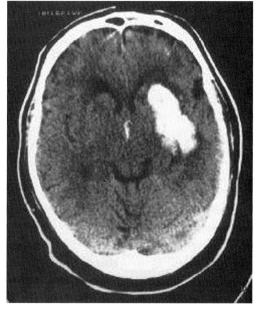

Figure 22.2. Noncontrast CT of the brain showing intracerebal hemorrhage in the left basal ganglia.

2. Asymmetry of the mouth suggesting retraction injury of the marginal mandibular branch of the facial nerve

3. Tongue deviation representing injury to the hypoglossal nerve causing speech difficulty

4. Shoulder weakness or pain due to spinal accessory nerve damage.

These findings, however, can indicate more serious situations and need to be closely monitored.

■ Pupillary asymmetry associated with blindness suggests the presence of an embolus lodging in the ophthalmic artery which likely is originating from the endarterectomy site. Radiological investigation using MRI diffusion studies along with carotid ultrasound is needed to determine if ongoing emboli are occurring requiring reoperation.

■ Facial droop associated with a decreased level of consciousness or evolving hemiparesis suggests and evolving stroke and an emergent CT scan and carotid ultrasound should be performed to determine if stroke etiology is hemorrhagic or ischemic and again whether reoperation is required.

■ Lastly, hoarseness can be a sign of recurrent laryngeal nerve injury. Unilateral injury is unlikely to cause significant morbidity but if the patient fails to recover after 12 weeks of conservative management, he or she can be referred to an otolaryngologist. The diagnosis can then be made definitively by laryngoscopic visualization of an immobile vocal cord. Laryngoscopy must be performed before considering performing surgery on the contralateral neck as bilateral vocal cord paralysis is not compatible with life.

Wound Hematoma

The development of a hematoma in the surgical wound can occur either from slow persistent oozing along the carotid endarterectomy line or acutely due to arterial rupture. The former is the more common scenario and often presents as increasing agitation in an otherwise neurologically intact patient associated with no output from the surgical drain.

■ As CEAs are being performed in older patients, the unwary house officer may mistake this agitation for sundowning and prescribe a sedative. This usually precipitates acute respiratory insufficiency

and it is only when a difficult intubation scenario is encountered due to a significantly deviated trachea that the diagnosis becomes obvious.

■ Should intubation not be possible, opening the wound cleanly at the bedside may be required to facilitate respiratory management. It is recommended that the most experienced team member secure the airway and the patient would then be taken emergently back to the operating room to explore the wound.

To avoid the above situation, serial hourly measurements of neck circumference along with serial examinations of the patient for stridor and tracheal deviation should be performed. Output from the surgical drain, respiratory rate and oxygen saturation should also be measured regularly.

New onset of respiratory difficulty after CEA always requires urgent attention. Respiratory obstruction in this patient population can also be due to mucosal edema or to lymphatic or venous obstruction.

■ Respiratory obstruction may be treated with steroids and moist steam inhalers.

■ Elevation of the head of bed to a sitting position and anxiolytics are also useful measures once wound hematoma has been excluded as the cause of the distress.

In the event that acute arterial rupture occurs, priority should be given to securing the airway while local pressure is applied to occlude the carotid. Carotid blowout causes rapid neck expansion and acute respiratory compromise. Airway control and exploration of the wound should proceed simultaneously at the bedside.[12]

■ The airway management team may intubate the patient or perform an emergent tracheostomy while the surgeon decompresses the hematoma compressing the trachea.

■ Once the disrupted arteriotomy site has been identified, the surgeon may compress the site of the arterial bleeding as the patient is being taken to the operating room for arteriotomy repair.

CRANIOTOMY FOR TUMOR

The mortality of brain tumor surgery depends on the size and location of the tumor, but overall it is <5%. The more common complications after brain tumor removal include hemorrhage, cerebral edema or infarction, seizures, and pneumocephalus.

- In our facility postoperative tumor patients are given a 4-day tapering dose of dexamethasone starting at 10 mg q6h to limit postoperative edema.
- Concurrent H2 blockers must also be started to prevent gastric ulceration.
- In addition, any preoperative anticonvulsants are continued into the postoperative period and maintained in the therapeutic range. The use of prophylactic anticonvulsants remains controversial. If there is a concern for perioperative seizures, phenytoin may be started intraoperatively and continued for 2–3 weeks postoperatively.
- If a patient is found to have a neurologic deficit that was not present preoperatively or was not expected from the neurosurgical procedure, an emergent CT scan should be obtained to rule out hemorrhage, edema, or hydrocephalus.

Hemorrhage

Postoperative hemorrhage occurs in 0.8–1.1% of cases, and represents the most severe and fatal complication of this procedure. While hemorrhage is more common with metastatic tumors such as renal cell carcinoma and melanoma and certain primary tumors such as gliomas, they can occur in the setting of unexpected coagulopathy or as part of an evolving cerebral infarction.

- Platelet counts and coagulation profiles need to be checked when postoperative hemorrhaging is discovered.
- MRI with diffusion may need to be performed in scenarios where infarction is suspected.
- In the NCCU, blood pressure can rise secondary to intracranial hemorrhage and should be normalized using standard antihypertensives. While there is no direct evidence to suggest that hypertension causes hemorrhage into the surgical bed, most surgeons believe that hemorrhage is less likely to occur or progress if the systolic blood pressure is maintained at less than 150 mm Hg for at least the first 24 hours after surgery.
- Evidence of epidural, subdural, or intraparenchymal hemorrhage causing significant neurologic

compromise is an indication for urgent surgical decompression. Smaller hematomas may be managed conservatively.

Cerebral Edema

The development of cerebral edema can also lead to worsening neurologic function. This finding may be demonstrated by a CT scan of the brain. Cerebral edema may occur as a consequence of the presence of residual tumor, especially in glioblastoma multiforme (Fig. 22.3). More commonly, however, edema occurring at 48–72 hours postoperatively is secondary to tissue retraction during surgery.

- In general maintaining or increasing steroid therapy along with judicious fluid management and serum sodium monitoring should allow most patients to recover without event.
- Cerebral edema is often associated with the onset of SIADH and diuresis is often required to attain mild hypovolemia.
  - Hyponatremia commonly occurs in this setting and should be treated with fluid intake restriction of around 2000 mL per 24 hours along with the intermittent mannitol or Lasix.
  - Hypertonic saline solutions are used only if serum sodium levels fall below 125 mEq/L to avoid seizure onset or if the hyponatremia is otherwise symptomatic.

A less common cause of cerebral edema is delayed venous infarction. This occurs especially in surgery where an inter-hemispheric approach is used or when surgery is performed on tumors adjacent to or involving large dural venous sinuses. Venous infarction can be a difficult diagnosis to make but an MR venogram should be performed to look for large venous sinus obstruction if suspected. Even if imaging is unable to demonstrate venous thrombosis, if this clinical entity is suspected, the management is different from the above in that fluid restriction must be avoided in order to assist in the development of venous collaterals. Mannitol has been used in these cases as it is thought to decrease the viscosity of the blood and therefore improve its rheology. It is important however to ensure that the patients is euvolemic and central venous monitoring is essential for this.

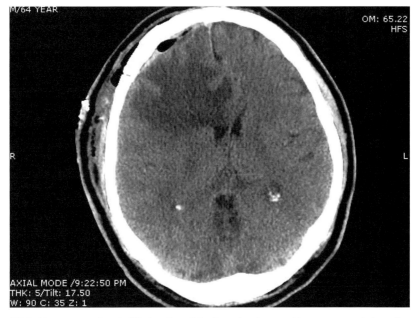

Figure 22.3. Noncontrast head CT showing right frontal edema with pneumocephalus after tumor resection.

Pneumocephalus

Air within the cranial vault may cause neurologic symptoms requiring treatment. Simple pneumocephalus, that is, the presence or air in the cranium that is not under tension, may cause lethargy, confusion, headache, nausea and vomiting, and seizures. Air may be located in the ventricles, over the convexities or in the posterior fossa.

■ Treatment is symptomatic along with the use of inhaled 100% oxygen by face mask.
■ It is thought that by allowing oxygen to replace nitrogen in the trapped air space, gaseous resorption can be accelerated.
■ Simple pneumocephalus usually resolves over 1–3 days.

Tension pneumocephalus rarely develops. It can occur if nitrous oxide anesthesia is not discontinued prior to closure of the dura; or if a "ball-valve" effect develops within the intracranial cavity such that soft tissue allows the entry of air, but prevents the exit of CSF or air; or in the presence of an infection from gas-producing organisms. The consequence is increased intracranial pressure that may be associated with mass effect on the brain.

■ Increased intracranial pressure can be diagnosed by CT scan which may show the Mt. Fuji sign in which the frontal poles are surrounded and separated by air. Skull films would also demonstrate pneumocephalus.
■ Treat noninfectious tension pneumocephalus with a twist drill or burr holes, or by insertion of a spinal needle through a preexisting burr hole to decompress the pneumocephalus.

Seizures

Postoperative seizures can be of any type and are due to direct surgical cortical irritation. They may be exacerbated by electrolyte imbalance, low anticonvulsant levels, or intracerebral hemorrhage. Airway management is paramount. If the patient fails to regain consciousness or has labored breathing, then the patient should be intubated to protect the airway.

■ Ativan 4 mg IV should be administered if seizures do not resolve spontaneously or occur repetitively.
■ If the patient is not on an anticonvulsant then they should be given a concurrent loading dose of 20 mg/kg of phenytoin.

- Electrolyte and anticonvulsant levels should be obtained and a CT scan of the head should be performed to rule out surgically amenable pathology.
- If the patient was previously on anticonvulsant therapy, it is safe to deliver a bolus dose of the patients' anticonvulsant medication before the return of the serum anticonvulsant levels.

POSTERIOR FOSSA CRANIECTOMY FOR TUMOR

Postoperative care for patients undergoing surgery for tumors in the posterior fossa requires an awareness of all the potential complications seen in supratentorial tumor surgery with two major differences.

- The first is that seizures are not known to arise from posterior fossa structures.
- The second is related to the specific contents of the region. The cerebellum, brain stem, and CSF outflow tracts are located in a confined space.
  - Therefore a minimal increase in edema or bleeding can significantly worsen brain stem function or hydrocephalus and can result in severe neurologic consequences including cranial neuropathies, long tract motor and sensory deficits, as well as coma and other altered states of consciousness.
  - Moreover, the centers for cardiac and respiratory function are located in this region and may be affected by the tumor or by the surgical procedure. Up to 50% of patients undergoing surgery for posterior fossa masses have cardiac arrhythmias.[2]
  - Irritation of the lower brain stem may cause unpredictable episodes of cardiac or respiratory arrest or distress in the first 72 hours after surgery.

Cranial Nerve Injuries

- Injury to the fifth or seventh cranial nerves may occur during posterior fossa surgery. Injury to the fifth cranial nerve can cause corneal anesthesia and injury to the seventh cranial nerve results in an inability of the patient to close the eyelid. Both of these predispose the patient to the development of corneal abrasions or desiccation and ulceration.

  - The cornea needs to be protected with isotonic saline eye drops during the day and Lubriderm ointment overnight.
  - Poor eyelid closure from cranial nerve VII injury can be treated with an eye patch or taping the eyelid shut.
- Many of the lower cranial nerves responsible for swallowing, speech and coughing are located in this region as well; therefore, inadvertent injury can cause severe morbidity. After surgery to this region, great care must be paid to watching for airway patency after extubation especially if there are, in addition, concurrent concerns about airway injury and edema, marginal pulmonary status, or decreased level of consciousness. If these issues are identified as extubation risks even before surgery then it is usually advised that patients be allowed to fully awake from the effects of anesthesia before considering extubation.
- If the patient is able to be extubated successfully, then it would also be advisable to examine the swallowing apparatus before feeding the patient, especially if there is a significant degree of speech hoarseness or difficulty with coughing effectively. Clearly if the patient fails extubation, tracheostomy and percutaneous enteral gastrostomy placement should be considered without delay.

Hydrocephalus

Critically located edema or hemorrhage in the posterior fossa near the CSF drainage pathways can be rapidly fatal due to the development of acute hydrocephalus. An abrupt increase in systolic blood pressure or change in respiratory pattern may signal increased pressure in the posterior fossa.

- Pupillary changes, increases in intracranial pressures, and decreasing levels of consciousness are late findings but this is most commonly when the diagnosis is in fact recognized.
- Rapid intubation is required in patients in this condition, followed by rapid placement of a ventricular catheter.
  - At this point the NCCU physician must decide usually clinically (or occasionally with the help of a CT scan of the head) whether the hydrocephalus is due to focal clot or edema around the drainage pathways or if the outflow obstruction is due to elevated pressure throughout the

posterior fossa, either due to massive hemor-rhaging or edema.

- In the first scenario of focal abnormality, standard drainage of CSF via the ventriculostomy is all that is required until the focal abnormality resolves or it is determined that permanent CSF diversion is required.
- In the second scenario, however, care must be taken to slowly drain a minimum amount of CSF from the ventriculostomy. Rapid decompression of supratentorial pressure could cause the contents of the posterior fossa to upwardly herniate through the tentorial incisura thus permanently injuring the midbrain. After intubation, the patient should be rushed STAT to the operating room where placement of the ventriculostomy should occur immediately before surgical decompression of the tight posterior fossa. Once surgical decompression has been achieved then CSF drainage can proceed as needed.

CSF Fistula

- The persistence of a CSF fistula resulting in the formation of a pseudomeningocele after posterior fossa tumor removal has an incidence of 5–17%. Unlike supratentorial surgery, dural defects may not be covered postoperatively with bone, especially in the setting of possible intracranial hypertension. In this situation, even in the face of immaculate dural closure, the risk of CSF fistula formation is high. Fistula formation is further facilitated by poor wound closure, for example in patient with prior whole brain radiation therapy (WBRT) or chemotherapy or by preexisting hydrocephalus.
- The leak of CSF comes from the skin incision and initial treatment includes oversewing the incision with 3–0 nylon suture in a running and interlocking fashion and elevation of the head of bed.
- If the leak persists beyond 3–5 days a lumbar drain should be placed. If this fails, then the defect should be closed surgically.
- Less commonly, mastoid air cells are entered during posterior fossa surgery and CSF may then leak through the middle ear into the nose and throat. Conservative management with a lumbar drain should again be tried first, but often surgical wound reexploration and closure of the air cells is ultimately required.

Craniotomy for Resection of Arteriovenous Malformation

Arteriovenous malformations (AVM) are developmental vascular anomalies in which there is direct shunting of blood from arterioles to dilated medium-sized veins without intervening capillaries causing ischemia in the surrounding brain. Prolonged ischemia results in persistent maximal dilatation and therefore loss of autoregulatory capacity of the vessels supplying these ischemic areas.

Surgical resection remains the definitive treatment of many of these lesions. Patients with AVMs may come to surgery with preexistent neurologic deficits either from cerebral ischemia, intracerebral hemorrhage, or complications from prior angioembolization.

- The predominant aim of postoperative care is to prevent normal perfusion pressure breakthrough bleeding.
  - ▶ Normal pressure breakthrough bleeding is thought to be due to the restoration of normal blood flow in the chronically dilated blood vessels supplying ischemic areas.
  - ▶ With the increased blood flow or the elevation of blood pressure above what is normally seen by the dysautoregulated vessels, cerebral edema and hemorrhage can result.
- Postoperative care in the NCCU consists of strict blood pressure control with an arterial catheter and maintenance of a euvolemic state.[13]
  - ▶ The systolic blood pressure should be maintained close to the patient's baseline range of blood pressures. In healthy young patients parenterally administered antihypertensives may be required to maintain the systolic blood pressure at <110 mm Hg.
- Patients should also be started on antiseizure medications such as phenytoin.
- Cerebral angiograms should be obtained during the postoperative period to assess the extent of resection of the AVM.

Any change in neurologic status should prompt an urgent CT scan to rule out cerebral hemorrhage or hydrocephalus. An MRI of the brain with diffusion weighted images should be obtained if cerebral infarctions are suspected. If good blood pressure control is achieved, intracerebral hemorrhage following AVM surgery is rare. Large bleeds may occur from both breakthrough bleeding as well as residual AVM, both of which may also require surgical evacuation.

TRANSSPHENOIDAL PITUITARY RESECTION

Pituitary tumors may be removed by several means. However, the transsphenoidal approach is most commonly used. This procedure is well tolerated and provides a good cosmetic outcome with mortality rates of 1% or less in experienced hands. Postoperative care involves the management and treatment of endocrine, surgical, and medical complications.

- The most common problems include diabetes insipidus and CSF rhinorrhea.
- The more concerning problems, however, include visual disturbances, cardiac dysfunction and complications arising from vascular injury.

Examination of the patient status post transsphenoidal pituitary resection should specifically include a thorough examination of the visual acuity, visual fields, and extraocular movements.

- At our institution, strict measurement of hourly fluid intake and output and urine specific gravities are recorded.
- Hydrocortisone 50 mg IV q6h is started and tapered at 10 mg/dose per day. After the hydrocortisone has been discontinued, a 6 A.M. cortisol level is drawn. If the cortisol level is low, hydrocortisone 50 mg PO q A.M. and 25 mg PO q P.M. should be given until adrenal reserve can be assessed by an endocrinologist as an outpatient.

Diabetes Insipidus

Diabetes insipidus (DI) is very common after transsphenoidal surgery. It develops after injury to the pituitary stalk or from manipulation of the posterior pituitary gland. A diagnosis of DI requires a triad of a high urine output exceeding 250 mL/h for 1–2 hours, a specific gravity of 1.005 or less, and a serum sodium level >145 mmol/L or a level that is progressively rising.

- After surgery the patient should be allowed to drink to thirst, and serum sodium levels, renal

profile, and serum osmolality should be obtained every 6 hours.
- Patients who have difficulty with oral fluid intake need to be supplemented with intravenous fluids.

In the first 24 hours after surgery, it is common for patients to demonstrate brisk urine output with borderline specific gravities and a normal or slightly low serum sodium level. The most common explanation of this is diuresis of intraoperative fluid load.

- In the patient who is not tolerating PO intake but whose urine outputs are persistently significantly >300 mL/h, it is suggested that the hourly urine output be replaced by 0.5 mL/mL of 0.45% normal saline so that if DI is subsequently diagnosed, the free water deficit is not so profound. The formula to estimate free water deficit is:
- $0.6 \times$ weight (kg) $\times$ [(serum Na/140) – 1]
- If the patient is unable to tolerate oral intake, D5W 0.45% or 0.225% NaCl solution may be used to correct the hypernatremia. If it becomes difficult to maintain a euvolemic state or normal serum sodium with PO intake and intravenous fluids, the patient should be given desmopressin (DDAVP) 0.5–1 ml (2–4 μg) on a PRN basis until the fluid balance status of the patient stabilizes over the ensuing 3–5 days. If long-term DDAVP therapy is needed, a daily dose of 10 mg intranasally can be prescribed.

CSF Rhinorrhea

CSF rhinorrhea is a common problem that occurs after transsphenoidal surgery. It is a result of a tear in the arachnoid above the diaphragma sella during tumor curettage and occurs in 0.5–9.6% of cases. Evidence of CSF leak is usually recognized at the time of surgery and either fat is packed into the sphenoid sinus or a watertight cement closure is performed to try to avoid further leakage. In cases where nasal splints are placed at the end of surgery, it is almost impossible to tell if there is a CSF leak postoperatively until the splints are removed. At this time, it is important to try to elicit evidence of a leak before allowing the patient to be discharged from medical care.

- CSF rhinorrhea increases the risk of meningitis and the development of intracranial abscesses.
- Lumbar drainage of 10 mL of CSF per hour over 3–5 days will stop CSF rhinorrhea in many cases.[14] Persistent CSF leakage will, however, require surgical repair of the defect.

Visual Deterioration and Ophthalmoplegia

Visual deficits that are noted to be new after surgery may be secondary to damage to the optic nerves, infarction, hematoma formation or herniation of the chiasm into the empty sella. A patient reporting a change in vision should be examined and taken to the CT scanner to rule out the presence of a hematoma at the surgical site. Urgent surgical decompression of a hematoma would be necessary to preserve vision. In cases of chiasmal herniation, a transsphenoidal chiasmaplexy and elevation of the diaphragm can rarely be performed to prevent further visual deterioration.[2]

During transsphenoidal surgery the third, fourth, and sixth cranial nerves may be injured as they course through the cavernous sinus lateral to the pituitary gland. Impaired ocular movement occurs in 0.3–1.2% of cases and about half of these improve with time.

Vascular Injury

Injury to the carotid artery or the cavernous sinus is a significant cause of morbidity and mortality in transsphenoidal surgery. Bleeding from overt rupture of the cavernous carotid artery during surgery is usually tamponaded by placing a significant amount of packing material into the sella to occlude the vessel. Once unilateral carotid occlusion has been demonstrated on emergent postoperative angiography, triple H therapy (hypertension, hypervolemia and hemodilution) needs to be instituted to try to maximize perfusion to the ischemic brain by increasing blood flow through existing collateral circulation thereby hopefully minimizing the size of the resulting infarct.

- At our facility, triple H therapy is initiated in the operating room and continued into the angiography suite and then the NCCU.
- As arterial and central venous monitoring lines are already in place from surgery, pressors and intravenous fluids are used to keep the systolic blood pressure at least 160–180 mm Hg and the CVP >10 mm Hg or a PCWP >14 mm Hg.
- The patient should be nursed with their head of bed flat and serial neurologic examinations as well as CT scans are used to monitor the patient's progress.
- Triple H therapy can be weaned off as the size of the stroke stabilizes over the next 3–5 days.

Very rarely, carotid artery bleeding manifests as severe epistaxis in the NCCU requiring angiography to identify the site of bleeding or to identify a pseudoaneurysm or carotid-cavernous fistula. Reoperation may then be required or therapeutic stenting or occlusion of the involved vessels angiographically may be possible to achieve hemostasis.

Complications Specific to ACTH-secreting Tumors

Patients with ACTH-secreting tumors have a high risk for perioperative cardiac instability whose presentation ranges from silent myocardial ischemia to full-blown cardiac arrest. During resuscitation of these patients, blood pressure can be both high or low and is usually difficult manage. It is particularly important in these patients to remember that high stress doses of hydrocortisone are essential in their postoperative care.

EPILEPSY SURGERY

There are many procedures for intractable epilepsy. These procedures include anterior temporal lobectomy (ATL), selective amygdalo-hippocampectomy, and corpus callosotomy, subtotal corpus callostomy, and hemispherectomy. Many of the surgical complications are similar to those outlined for craniotomy; however, there are numerous functional outcomes, some transient and others permanent, which need to be identified early.

- Postoperative epilepsy patients arriving to the NCCU should have their anticonvulsant levels and electrolytes measured, and any missed doses of anticonvulsants during surgery should be replaced to ensure that the full 24-hour dose of medication is received.

■ These patients should also be maintained on their antiepileptic medications throughout their hospital stay.

Anterior Temporal Lobectomy

Anterior temporal lobectomy (ATL) has a mortality rate <1%. Postoperative patients should be examined closely to rule out language and memory disorders, visual field deficits and hemiparesis.

■ Visual field deficits may occur in 2–3% of patients. The extent of resection of the temporal lobe, ischemia of the lateral geniculate body and manipulation of the anterior choroidal vessels may lead to visual field deficits.
■ Hemiparesis may occur secondary to manipulation[15] of the middle cerebral artery or the anterior choroidal artery.
■ Both transitory and permanent language deficits may occur after ATL. Cortical retraction and edema in essential language areas can cause anomic dysphasia which usually resolves within 1 week.[14] Permanent language disorders occur when more than 5–6 cm of the dominant temporal lobe is resected, in situations in which anatomical criteria alone are used to localize cortical language areas. Anatomical criteria for dominant temporal lobe resection leads to variable language outcomes post ATL. Therefore, preoperative Wada testing is helpful in localizing language function. Diminished postoperative, nondisabling, verbal memory performance has been noted in patients that had dominant temporal lobe lesions. These deficits correlate with both the extent of mesial and lateral resection of the temporal lobe.[14,16]

Functional Hemispherectomy

The mortality from functional hemispherectomy is approximately 6.6% and there is an elevated risk of developing acute hydrocephalus. Hemispherectomy patients need to be followed closely while in the NCCU. Symptoms such as headache, nausea, vomiting, confusion, and lethargy should prompt an emergent CT scan of the brain and possible CSF diversion.

Corpus Callosotomy

Immediately after surgical anterior callosotomy, patients usually develop an acute disconnection syndrome which is characterized by lethargy, difficulty with speech initiation or mutism, left leg and arm apraxia, nondominant forced grasping and Babinski reflexes, urge incontinence, and increase focal seizures. Sensory (posterior) disconnection syndrome may occur after splenial section.[14]

■ Generally these syndromes resolve over a 7–10-day period starting with speech and proximal limb motor recovery and within several weeks, patients mostly show full resolution of their deficits.
■ As these postoperative changes are transient, all efforts must be made to protect the patient from the complications of immobility.
■ At our institution, nasogastric feeding is initiated on postoperative day 1, patients undergo physical therapy daily and are started on aggressive DVT prophylaxis.

Rarely left hemiplegia and death associated with frontal lobe swelling after commissurotomies has been reported.[17] It is thought that the brain retraction during surgery compromises the parasagittal bridging veins during callosal exposure.

■ While treatment of venous infarction is not always successful, it is important to look for extension of venous thrombosis into the superior sagittal sinus by obtaining a magnetic resonance venography (MRV).
■ Even if the MRV shows no large venous thrombosis, if there is strong clinical suspicion the patient must be well hydrated to avoid worsening of venous thrombosis.
■ There is further evidence in the literature that a low-dose mannitol infusion is also useful in this setting in improving rheology and therefore blood flow through the compromised veins. The use of mannitol however must be counteracted by meticulous maintenance of euvolemia.

DEEP BRAIN STIMULATION

Deep brain stimulation (DBS) is an effective therapy for medication resistant Parkinson disease. DBS of the globus pallidus internus (GPi) and subthalamus can relieve Parkinson symptoms such as rigidity, bradykinesia, and levodopa-induced dyskinesia without irreversibly destroying tissue.[9] Patients with tremor as the predominant symptom may have stimulation of the ventralis intermedius (VIM) instead.

- Unilateral DBS of the VIM is associated with paresthesia and pain, while bilateral DBS may cause dysarthria and balance difficulty in some patients.[18]
- In DBS of the GPi, 2.5% of cases develop visual deficit due to the proximity of the optic tract to the globus pallidus.
- Hemiparesis may also occur as the internal capsule is also close to the globus pallidus.
- DBS of the subthalamic nucleus is associated with intracerebral hemorrhage (3.9%), seizures (1.5%), and infection (1.7%).[19] Stimulation-associated complications include dysarthria, weight gain, depression, and dyskinesia.

CONCLUSION

Postoperative care in the NCCU is aimed at avoiding secondary complications. Patients' comorbid conditions as well as the types of surgical procedures conducted predispose them to certain complications that must be anticipated. A clear understanding of the patients' past medical history and the expected outcomes from neurosurgical procedures would prepare the NCCU staff for optimally caring for their patients. Serial neurologic examinations are essential for early detection and treatment of problems that may arise. These guidelines provide a broad overview of management of patients in the NCCU after some of the more common procedures. The principles outlined here should serve as a foundation for the management of patients in situations other than those that were discussed here.

REFERENCES

1. Rosenberg H, Clofine R, Bialik O. Neurological changes during awakening from anesthesia. *Anesthesiology.* 1981;**45**:125–30.
2. Badjer HH, Loftus CM, eds. *Textbook of Neurological Surgery: Principles and Practice.* Philadelphia: Lipppincott Williams & Wilkins, 2003.
3. Diringer MN, Zazulia AR. Hyponatremia in neurologic patients: consequences and approaches to treatment. *Neurologist.* 2006;**12**(3):117–26.
4. Jung R, MacLaren R. Proton-pump inhibitors for stress ulcer prophylaxis in critically ill patients. *Ann Pharmacother.* 2002;**36**:1929–37.
5. Macdonald RL, et al. Safety of perioperative subcutaneous heparin for prophylaxis of venous thromboembolism in patients undergoing craniotomy. *Neurosurgery.* 1999;**45**(2):245–51
6. Bucci MN, Papadopoulos SM, Chen JC, Campbell JA, Hoff JT. Mechanical prophylaxis of venous thrombosis in patients undergoing craniotomy: a randomized trial. *Surg Neurol* 1989;**32**(4):285–8.
7. Haines SJ. Efficacy of antibiotic prophylaxis in clean neurosurgical operations. *Neurosurgery.* 1989;**24**:401–5.
8. Shapiro M. Prophylaxis in otolaryngologic surgery and neurosurgery: a critical review. *Rev Infect Dis.* 1991;**13**:S858–68.
9. Greenberg MS. *Handbook of Neurosurgery.* New York: Thieme, 2001.
10. van Mook WN, et al. Cerebral hyperperfusion syndrome. *Lancet Neurol.* 2005;**4**:877–88.
11. Beard JD, et al. Prevention of postoperative wound haematomas and hyperperfusion following carotid endarterectomy. *Eur J Vasc Endovasc Surg.* 2001;**21**:490–3.
12. Gunel M, Awad IA. Carotid endarterectomy prevention strategies and complications management. *Neurosurg Clin North Am.* 2000;**11**:351–64.
13. Ogilvy CS, et al. AHA Scientific Statement: recommendations for the management of intracranial arteriovenous malformations: a statement for healthcare professionals from a special writing group of the Stroke Council, American Stroke Association. *Stroke.* 2001;**32**:1458–71.
14. Post KD, Friedman ED, McCormick P, eds. *Postoperative Complications in Intracranial Neurosurgery.* New York: Thieme, 1993.
15. Penfield W, Lende R, Rasmusen T. Manipulation hemiplegia. *J Neurosurg.* 1961;**18**:760–76.
16. Katz A, et al. Extent of resection in temporal lobectomy for epilepsy. II. Memory changes and neurologic complications. *Epilepsia.* 1989;**30**:763–71.
17. Spencer SS. Corpus callosum section and other disconnection procedures for medically intractable epilepsy. *Epilepsia* 1988;**29**(Suppl 2):S85–99.
18. Pahwa R, et al. Long-term evaluation of deep brain stimulation of the thalamus. *J Neurosurg.* 2006;**104**:506–12.
19. Kleiner-Fisman G, et al. Subthalamic nucleus deep brain stimulation: summary and meta-analysis of outcomes. *Movement Disord.* 2006;**21**(Suppl 14):S290–304.

23 Ethical and Legal Considerations in Neuroscience Critical Care

Dan Larriviere, MD, JD and Michael A. Williams, MD, FAAN

Caring for patients in the neurosciences critical care unit (NCCU) requires consistent and conscientious application of important ethical principles and an understanding of the law concerning surrogate decision making. The vast majority of patients lack decision-making capacity due to coma, aphasia, delirium, or other alterations of consciousness, and therefore decisions regarding their treatment and care must be made by surrogates. In addition, many NCCU patients have uncertain prognoses that will influence the type of treatments offered by the NCCU team, and the types of decisions made by the surrogates.

COMPARISON OF ETHICS AND THE LAW

The terms morality and ethics are often used interchangeably, although some authors make the distinction that morality refers to "norms about right and wrong human conduct" and that ethics refers to ways of understanding or studying morality.[1] More plainly, morality answers the question of *what* should be done in a particular circumstance, and ethics answers the question *why* it should be done, or what justifies the action.[2] Bernat provides a practical combination of the two, defining clinical ethics as "the identification of morally correct actions and the resolution of ethical dilemmas in medical decision making through the application of moral concepts and rules to medical situations."[3]

Identification of morally correct actions can be guided by abstract principles such as autonomy, beneficence, nonmaleficence, and justice[4]; by virtues of the physician; or by various analytical methods such as utilitarianism or deontology. In the end,

ethics is about identifying the values relevant to a given situation and deciding how those values might guide our conduct. Ethical dilemmas represent a conflict of values, meaning that different persons may hold different values, but that does not necessarily mean that one is right or the other is wrong. It simply means that before a medical decision and course of action can be chosen, a decision must first be made as to which values will prevail. Sometimes this is easy, and sometimes it is extraordinarily challenging and results in an outcome in which no party involved feels completely satisfied.

Although important, the identification and application of values to a clinical situation is not the end of the inquiry that determines the appropriate course of action. In the United States, as in many other countries, there are federal and state statutes, court opinions, and regulations that also determine the legitimacy of a physician's actions, and these must be taken into account when making decisions with patients and their families.

In general, it is not a good idea to look to the law when trying to resolve clinical conflicts.

- First, the law is commonly a floor for behavior. That is, it outlines what society considers to be the minimally acceptable action in a given situation. As such, thoughtful physicians will need to look elsewhere for aspirational norms for their behavior.
- Second, law is dependent on legislative compromise, regulatory approvals, and multiyear lawsuits before it comes into existence. For this reason it tends to reflect established medical norms and rarely establishes new guidelines for

behavior and also tends to lag behind advances in clinical practice.

- Finally, when judging the actions of physicians, the law uses as its reference the customs of the profession. In other words, the medical profession determines the standards its members should follow. For all of these reasons, the law will rarely help physicians make a better decision than they would have made on their own or in consultation with their colleagues, and to focus on the law is to lose one's focus on patients.

Despite these limitations, however, in the area of surrogate decision making, state laws do provide physicians with a general structure within which end-of-life decisions must be made, and knowledge of those laws will be of use to the practicing physician.

DECISIONAL CAPACITY AND INFORMED CONSENT

Assessment of Decisional Capacity

- "Decisional capacity" refers to a patient's functional ability to consider the factors relevant to a specific decision and to arrive at and communicate an individually appropriate choice.
- Capacity refers specifically to a clinical judgment about patients' ability to participate meaningfully in decisions about their care. It is to be distinguished from "competency," which is a legal determination by a court concerning a person's ability generally to engage in many transactions of daily living (e.g., will-making, forming contracts, etc.).

As a general rule, decisional capacity is operationally defined and assessed. To have capacity, patients must:

- Be able to understand information that is relevant to the decision
- Be able to communicate a choice
- Be able to appreciate the nature of their situation and the consequences of their choice

In the NCCU, the ability to communicate a choice is often assumed to be absent for all intubated patients, but this is not necessarily so. Patients with neuromuscular diseases such as myasthenia

gravis or acute inflammatory demyelinating polyradiculoneuropathy may be able to communicate by attempting to mouth words, by writing, or by nodding the head.

In the NCCU, decisional capacity is definitely absent for all comatose patients and all patients with global aphasia. It is most likely absent for patients with dense expressive or receptive aphasia, it is probably absent for patients in delirium and with anosognosia, and it may or may not be absent for patients with dementia. In the United States, where English is the predominant language, patients who do not speak English fluently may lack decisional capacity unless an interpreter is present to help.

Decisional capacity can fluctuate, often with level of consciousness or stage of illness. In addition, a given patient may have decisional capacity for some choices, but not others. For example, a patient with "mild" alteration of consciousness or dementia may have decisional capacity for safe, low-risk procedures such as receiving an antibiotic for a urinary tract infection, but simultaneously may not have decisional capacity for riskier or invasive procedures that involve complex calculations of risk and benefit as applied to a background set of values and goals such as carotid endarterectomy for symptomatic carotid stenosis.

Because loss of decisional capacity is so common in the NCCU, physicians have a responsibility to assess it for virtually all patients, and if there is any question as to whether the patient may or may not have capacity, it is often wisest to involve family or surrogates, or to invite another physician to assess the patient's capacity.

Informed Consent for Treatment

In the NCCU setting, many patients require invasive procedures. With the exception for emergency treatment (outlined below), physicians are obligated to obtain valid informed consent from the patient or surrogate for the procedure.

- To perform a procedure on a patient without informed consent is considered battery, and regardless of the outcome of the procedure, physicians may be sued for doing so.

The key notion in informed consent is not the consent (i.e., permission), but rather that the patient be *informed* well enough to make a decision. Therefore, valid informed consent involves much more than simply getting a signature on a consent form. Informed consent is a process that involves providing information to patients in terms they can understand so that they can exercise their autonomy by making a decision that reflects their own values.

At a minimum, physicians must disclose the:

- Diagnosis
- Nature, purpose, benefits, and probability of success of the proposed treatment
- Relevant risks, including risks arising from the patient's particular health problems
- Alternatives to the proposed treatment (including no treatment), along with their risks, benefits, and probability of success.

Although there is often a question about *how* to quantify the risks and benefits of a procedure, there should be little question that there is an obligation to provide reasonable, factually based estimates of the risks and benefits. In the NCCU, perhaps the best example of this relates to carotid endarterectomy, where several studies have shown that the risks of the procedure are dependent on the degree of stenosis, the presence or absence of ischemic symptoms, and perhaps most importantly, the experience or track record of the physicians performing the procedure.[5] When possible, we would recommend a combination approach that describes the risks and benefits as generally understood in the medical literature, plus the experience by the team in the NCCU.

An important aspect of informed consent is that the patient's permission should be given voluntarily, and not coerced. While deliberate or overt coercion is rare, coercion may occur inadvertently due to the manner in which risks are presented to the patient. The framing of information can significantly affect decision making.[6,7] Framing bias, the sharing of information in such a way that it biases the family's decision, is an under-recognized communication phenomenon. An example of framing bias would be to say, "There's an 80–90% chance that treatment won't help."

- A communication goal is to share the content in a way that minimizes framing bias.
- One method to do so is called double-framing. The example above, if double-framed, would be restated, "There's an 80–90% chance that

treatment won't help, which also means there's a 10–20% chance that it will help." Double-framing helps patients and families see the risk:benefit analysis from both perspectives, and helps to prevent inadvertent coercion.

Informed Consent for Human Subjects Research

The standards for informed consent for research are stricter than the standards for treatment because the benefit of the research intervention is unknown until the research protocol is completed. The potential risks of research should not exceed the potential benefits of participation.[8]

- Valid informed consent for research requires that subjects be told pertinent information regarding the procedures, benefits and risks of participating in a study, and in the idealized model, they should be able to restate this in their own words to indicate their understanding.[9]

The therapeutic misconception, which is the research subject's belief that there is substantial benefit to them from participating in the research, even when the study is designed so that no benefit can be guaranteed, commonly influences the validity of informed consent. For example, patients may not understand randomization, and think that the physician-researcher can assign them to the study arm that is most beneficial to them, or they may not understand that in a placebo-controlled trial, there is a significant chance that they will not receive the investigational drug or treatment.[9,10]

The therapeutic misconception may be compounded in the ICU, because patients or their families may be desperate to find a "cure," even if it's an unproven therapy in a research protocol.[9] In addition, patients and families may be influenced by the ICU physician-researcher's endorsement of a research protocol.[11] As a safeguard against undue influence by the treating physician, it is often recommended that a researcher not involved with the patient's care present the research protocol to the patient or proxy.[12] Discussions of research protocols should describe whether treatments the patient would routinely receive will be influenced or altered.[13]

Criteria for Emergency Treatment Without Informed Consent

In the ICU, implied consent for treatment is permissible in emergency circumstances, especially for patients who lack decisional capacity, as they could be harmed by the delay needed to obtain informed consent from a proxy. One model that has been suggested for ICU practice is to obtain informed consent in advance for all procedures that have a reasonable chance of being performed on the patient (so-called universal consent) so that the discussion of the risks, benefits, and alternatives of the procedures does not need to be done under urgent circumstances.[14] This approach should be used only after careful planning and institutional approval, and is not advisable under ad hoc circumstances.

There is an important limitation to implied consent for emergency treatment, which is that it cannot be applied to other procedures or interventions performed on the same patient after the emergency circumstances have resolved.[15] For example, endotracheal intubation during resuscitation does not require informed consent, but the subsequent *elective* tracheostomy does.

SURROGATE DECISION MAKERS

Patients with Decisional Capacity Who Defer Decisions to Their Family

In a diverse world in which patients from many cultures and traditions travel long distances to receive health care, it is unwise to expect that all patients and families understand or will abide by the North American model of self-directed, autonomous decision making, especially for end-of-life decisions. In some cultures, the family assumes responsibility for such decisions, even for patients who have decisional capacity. Families may request that the patient not be informed of "bad diagnoses," such as cancer, an approach that can feel deceptive or paternalistic to physicians used to autonomy-based decision making.

One solution is that if there is an opportunity in advance (which there is likely to be because families often talk to the physician before the patient is seen), ask the patient and family how they would like information, including good news or bad news, to be communicated, and to whom. They can be given the choice of either making decisions the way they do in their own culture or country, or the way that is most common in North America. Providing patients these options is to respect their autonomy.

Because family are often unfamiliar with medical and hospital culture, and the large number of health professionals who interact with the patient, they can be reminded that while the physicians will do their best to respect the request not to disclose information to the patient, it may not possible to ensure that *everyone* will know of the agreement. Thus, despite good faith efforts, inadvertent disclosure of the information to the patient may occur.

Proxies Appointed by Durable Power of Attorney for Healthcare Decisions

Virtually all states allow patients to appoint a proxy to make decisions on their behalf by assigning durable power of attorney (DPOA) for healthcare decisions. Most of the time, the DPOA accompanies, or is part of the patient's advance directive. The authority of proxies appointed by DPOA to make decisions on the patient's behalf supersedes that of all other persons, including spouses and blood relatives, with the exception of court-appointed guardians.

Surrogates Appointed by Virtue of State Statutes in the Absence of DPOA

Almost all states have laws that delineate who is to make healthcare decisions for patients when a proxy with DPOA has not been appointed. In general, these laws designate an order for identifying surrogate decision makers based on the surrogate's relationship to the patient. Physicians are advised to check the laws in the states in which they practice; however, the usual hierarchy for selecting a surrogate is:

1. Spouse
2. Children of the patient who are above the age of majority
3. Parents of the patient
4. Adult siblings of the patient
5. Other relatives (e.g., Virginia Health Care Decisions Act).[16]

Some, but not all, states recognize a same-sex domestic partner as a decision maker, and some, but not all, states recognize common law marriage so that a common law spouse is a spouse for the purposes of the statute. Some state laws allow close friends who are not related to the patient but who may otherwise know the patient's preferences to serve as surrogate when no other persons are available or willing. The person with the highest position in the hierarchy is designated the surrogate, provided that person is willing to fulfill the responsibilities of that role.

Physicians should ask about the existence of other persons who are members of the same or higher level in the hierarchy as the surrogate who is present, and whether there are legal issues pending that could change a current designation (e.g., pending divorce). Keep in mind that surrogates at the "top" of the hierarchy may know less about the patient's preferences than someone "lower down." This means that the statutorily designated surrogate and the morally appropriate surrogate may not be the same person. Physicians in this circumstance should prepare to be flexible (e.g., if the primary surrogate cedes decision-making authority to another decision maker) and encourage family members and friends of the patients to thoroughly discuss the issues together before decisions are made. If there is concern that the statutorily designated surrogate is making decisions inconsistent with the patient's wishes (a circumstance usually identified by the morally appropriate surrogate), then an ethics consultation is most likely indicated to assist in the identification of the most appropriate surrogate.

Disputes Between Surrogates and Family or Friends

Disagreement and disputes between family and friends are regrettably common in end-of-life care. Most of the time, ICU teams strive for consensus in the decision-making process, but not all disputes can be resolved. In circumstances when there is one and only one surrogate of the highest rank (i.e., surrogate with DPOA or only one surrogate at the highest level of the hierarchy), then the decisions of the surrogate cannot be challenged or overturned by anyone else in the family, provided the surrogate is making decisions that are consistent with the patient's preferences.

If there are two or more surrogates at the same rank who are in disagreement, and if there are no surrogates above them in the hierarchy, the law generally does *not* give preference to one surrogate over the others. For example, the law does not generally give preference to "first-born" children, or to sons over daughters. Many state laws include dispute-resolution mechanisms. For example, Virginia law allows for a majority vote to resolve the conflict,[16] but we do not recommend this approach if at all possible. Instead, we recommend striving for consensus among decision makers whenever possible. This may require more discussion and education of family members. When disputes between surrogates of the same level occur and consensus cannot be reached despite reasonable attempts at doing so, or when a surrogate's decisions are alleged to be inconsistent with the patient's wishes or goals, then an ethics consultation is recommended.

Unbefriended Patients and Guardianship

All patients who lack decision-making capacity are entitled to have decisions made for them by a surrogate. If a surrogate cannot be found for a patient, as is often the case for homeless or unbefriended patients, then there is an obligation to ensure the patient's interests are represented in the process of making healthcare decisions. In most circumstances, this will require a court-appointed guardian. Therefore, as soon as the ICU team realizes a patient may be unbefriended, efforts should be initiated (1) to find friends or family and (2) to apply to the court for a guardian to be appointed should no surrogate be found.

■ A patient's unbefriended status does not entitle the ICU team to perform routine procedures that normally require consent (e.g., tracheostomy, percutaneous endoscopic gastrostomy) without consent from a guardian. Further, a guardian will be necessary for posthospital discharge planning and disposition.

EVIDENCE OF PATIENTS' WISHES OR BEST INTERESTS

Written Advance Directives

Advance directives (ADs) are legal instruments for patients to convey their treatment preferences in the event that illness or injury renders them unable to do so. ADs are thus considered autonomy-preserving instruments. In many states, decisions made in concordance with a valid AD do not need prior judicial approval.

- Almost all states have laws concerning the clinical conditions in which ADs apply and the treatment options allowed under an AD.[17]
- Most states limit the application of ADs to the clinical conditions of persistent vegetative state, "irreversible condition" or "terminal condition," although the terminology in the statute varies from state to state.
- In almost all states, patients may either refuse or request cardiopulmonary resuscitation and ventilation via an AD.
- States allow patients to request that artificial nutrition and hydration (ANH) be provided, but states also clearly allow patients to refuse ANH, although there is a lesser degree of uniformity on this issue among state laws.
- Most states allow patients to refuse ANH via an AD when their condition is "irreversible," "terminal," or persistent vegetative state.
- A few states restrict the withdrawal of ANH if the patient made no such request in an AD, and some states restrict the withdrawal of ANH in all cases.[17]

Oral Advance Directives

Patients who have decisional capacity may create an oral advance directive that will supersede an earlier, written AD. An oral AD may be made by the patient at any time – as long as the statement is witnessed – and it becomes a valid expression of current interests and should be followed instead of the written document.

Oral ADs may be made without a prior written AD. In the NCCU, one example for obtaining an oral AD would be a patient with aneurysmal subarachnoid hemorrhage who has decisional capacity but who lacks an AD. Considering that the clinical course of SAH carries high risk for neurologic complications or death, the opportunity to discuss with the patient both the goals of care and the patient's choice of surrogate is invaluable and respectful of the patient's autonomy. Such conversations should be witnessed, and should probably be discussed again with the patient and the surrogate as early in the hospital course as possible.

Substituted Judgment and Best Interest Standards

Frequently patients in the NCCU do not have ADs, especially if they are young. Thus, the process of determining the patient's wishes involves discussions between the HCP and the patient's family or proxy. As a general rule, they should make decisions that are consistent with the patient's previously stated wishes, if known. In the best circumstance, the family will recall a specific conversation the patient had about a health status that is close to the patient's current condition. If the patient never expressed any preferences, then a substituted judgment standard should be used. Under this standard, the decision maker attempts to integrate everything known about the patient: personal values, moral and religious outlook, prior conversations, and so forth to determine what the patient would have wanted in this circumstance.

If this information is not available or is unknown, then the surrogate is to make a decision using a best interest standard. Under this standard, the decision to be made is that which is in the patient's best interest, taking into account such factors as diagnosis, prognosis, risks and benefits of proposed treatment, and degree of discomfort. The best interests standard can be difficult to negotiate, as some persons may hold that a benefits/burdens analysis would justify withdrawal of life sustaining therapies if the patient's survival would be associated with pain or other burdens, whereas others may hold that it is always in a patient's best interests to remain alive. State statute may influence decisions made with the best interest standard.

Advance Directives and DNR Orders

While ADs are often used to guide the decision to write do not resuscitate (DNR) orders, the fact that a patient has and AD does not mean that a DNR order should be automatically written. Many healthy adults have valid ADs, and yet they would want resuscitation or transfer to an ICU if they became critically ill.

- The mere existence of an AD does not eliminate the positive duty to initiate resuscitation for all healthy persons.

When using ADs to decide whether to write DNR orders, it is important to remember that nearly all ADs describe specific conditions under which the person would want resuscitation or other interventions withheld or withdrawn. If those specific conditions are not present, then resuscitation should be attempted. Further, ADs become effective only if the patient lacks decisional capacity. If these conditions have not been met, then it is not appropriate to write a DNR order unless the patient or surrogate has requested it.

STRATEGIES FOR COMMUNICATION AND DECISION MAKING

Ends versus Means/ Goals of Care versus Treatments

As mentioned, when the patient's wishes are not well known, it falls to the ICU team to undertake conversations with patients and their families concerning the patient's values and preferences when making treatment decisions. In our view, a common mistake is for the ICU team to ask families which specific treatments or life-sustaining therapies the patient would want, such as cardiopulmonary resuscitation (CPR), intubation, antibiotics, and so forth. This approach inadvertently displaces to the family or proxy the responsibility for assessing the medical indications and likelihood of success of specific treatments, which is knowledge they're unlikely to possess, and therefore their decisions are likely to be uninformed. As a result, families may make requests that seem illogical to the ICU team, such as requesting CPR but not intubation if the patient has a cardiac arrest.

The flaw in this approach is that treatments are a means to an end, but the means to an end cannot be selected until the end is defined. Thus, if the ICU team and family have not discussed the desired ends of care – the goals of care – then it makes little sense to discuss or decide on the treatments because there will be no context in which to discuss them.

What's meant by goals of care? Patients and proxies tend to think in terms of acceptable or unacceptable medical conditions or outcomes of care, as best illustrated by the fact that most ADs become active if an outcome that's not acceptable to the patient is present (e.g., persistent vegetative state). Sometimes the goals of care are described in terms of *desired* outcomes, such as, "If he can be awake and interactive with the family, even though he may be unable to take care of himself, he would want treatment."

On the other hand, they are sometimes described in terms of *unacceptable* outcomes, such as, "If she's going to be in pain, unable to care for herself, or never wake up, then she wouldn't want treatment."

The goals of care are often to cure disease, often to alleviate symptoms and improve quality of life, and always to relieve suffering and provide comfort. Thus, interventions consistent with goals of care can be curative for the purpose of reversing disease, or palliative for the purpose of relieving suffering, promoting comfort, or even meeting a patient's last wishes and allowing final acts to be accomplished. The pursuit of curative and palliative goals of care can occur simultaneously, and often should.

Thus, the goals of care are the *end* to which the *means* of specific therapeutic interventions are considered and applied. Once the ends are clarified, then the means can be chosen. Stated more plainly, once the ICU team knows which outcomes are acceptable or unacceptable to the patient, then they can describe: (1) whether the ICU team thinks the outcomes can be reached and (2) which therapeutic interventions are necessary to reach the goal.

Using the goals of care approach allows the patient and family to participate in the decision making process by contributing what they know better than the ICU team:

■ the patient's values, wishes, and desired outcomes.

It also allows the ICU team to participate in the decision-making process by contributing what they know better than the family:

■ information about the patient's condition and prognosis, the risks and benefits of existing or proposed interventions, and an estimate of the likelihood that the interventions will achieve the desired goals of care.

Both sets of information are necessary to make informed decisions consistent with the patient's wishes.

By framing the decision in terms of the goals of care, it becomes easier to address misconceptions about therapeutic interventions the family might have. For example, even though the family might think the patient would *never* want to be on the ventilator, if the goal of care is to be treated for reversible conditions when the likelihood of successful treatment is high, then the ICU team can explain that use of the ventilator (e.g., for pneumonia) is consistent with the patient's goals of care.

At the same time, the goals of care framework should make it easier to address the limitation or withdrawal of therapy. If the family has described the goals of care, and if the ICU team's best estimate is that the goals are unlikely to be reached despite the available interventions, then the ICU team can explain that as much as they want to achieve the patient's goals of care, they cannot, and the palliative goals should be pursued more than the curative goals.

Iterative Interdisciplinary Approach to Family Conferences

These are high stakes decisions, and are best conducted by the physician on the healthcare team with the most experience in these conversations. Of course, ICU fellows must learn to conduct these conversations, and the degree of supervision by the ICU attending physician should be proportional to the fellow's experience and skills.

The decision-making process requires frequent conversations to identify and reassess the patient's condition, goals of care, response to therapies, and recommendations for further treatment. It is a profound mistake to believe that a single conversation will yield sufficient knowledge to make well-informed decisions for most patients in the ICU.

- Patients and families will usually not hear everything they are told in a family meeting because they are unfamiliar with ICUs and they are experiencing emotional distress. Therefore, if the family is crying or appears stressed, then stop talking and wait a few moments. They won't hear the discussion anyway.
- Do not presume the family is intellectually lacking or in denial simply because they may not understand everything after hearing it only once.
- Patience is vital, and information often has to be shared multiple times. ICU jargon and slang can be confusing to families, and should be avoided.
- It is helpful to ask if you can explain anything better or differently for them.
- It is especially helpful to take an interdisciplinary approach to family meetings, including physicians, nurses, hospital chaplains, or social workers who have complementary skills.

A major risk in ICUs is that multiple team members or consultants will speak with the patient and family independently, rather than coordinate their communication. The inevitable result is mixed messages to the family, with potential for confusion, anger, focus on minor details rather than the "big picture" and so-called splitting behaviors.

- The ICU team and consultants are responsible for reaching consensus when possible, and respectfully identifying differences of opinion when necessary, before speaking with the patient or family.

An important limitation of the perspective of many ICU team members in end-of-life decision making is that they do not usually see patients after they are discharged from the ICU. Thus, the ICU team may not have the experience of other healthcare personnel (e.g., surgeons and other physicians) who provide longitudinal care and often have seen the long-term outcomes of similar patients throughout their entire illness (i.e., after they leave the ICU). Such healthcare personnel may have a different perspective on the possibility of attaining the patient's desired outcomes, and their input is necessary to help families make informed decisions.

SPECIAL TOPICS

Limiting or Withdrawing Life-sustaining Interventions

The practice of withdrawal of life-sustaining interventions is widespread in ICUs, and is considered ethically permissible within the medical profession. The American Academy of Neurology[18],[19] and the Society of Critical Care Medicine-American College of Chest Physicians[20] have recognized the right of patients in specific situations to forego treatment, even if refusal may lead to death.

Brain Death Determination and Organ Donation

Brain death determination and participation in the process of organ donation are common in the NCCU. Although all 50 states in the United States and the District of Columbia have similar legal definitions of brain death (Uniform Determination of

Death Act), there are some state and hospital-based differences in the process for determining brain death. The American Academy of Neurology has published a practice parameter for the diagnosis of brain death in patients older than 18 years.[21]

NCCU physicians, due to their expertise and training, have an obligation to evaluate patients for brain death when indicated. Whether organ donation follows the determination of brain death depends on the status of the donor, which is evaluated by personnel from the organ procurement organization (OPO) assigned to the hospital.

- A timely examination is essential, as organ donation depends on adequate perfusion of the organs to be procured, and the hemodynamic status of brain dead potential organ donors can be unstable.
- There is specific language in the U.S. federal Health Insurance Portability and Accountability Act (HIPAA) regulations that allows physicians to share information with OPO coordinators,[22] and physicians should do so as part of their obligation to participate in the identification of potential organ donors.

Organ Donation After Cardiac Death

Organ donation may occur in circumstances other than brain death in the ICU. The process of organ donation after cardiac death (DCD), also known as "non-heart beating donation" has become more common in the last decade. Between 1995 and 2004, the number of DCD donors increased more than sixfold, from 64 to 391, or approximately 5% of donors in 2004.[23] The context for DCD is usually, but not always, a severe brain injury from which the patient is not expected to recover, followed by the proxy's decision to withdraw life-sustaining therapies. If it is reasonably likely that the patient will die less than 1 hour after the withdrawal of therapies, then the duration of warm ischemia is short enough that organs such as the kidneys or a portion of the liver can be procured and transplanted with a high rate of graft survival.[24] Many physicians are uncomfortable with requesting organ donation in this setting, and the procedures for doing so in a manner that is ethically permissible and simultaneously respectful and sensitive to the families needs have been outlined elsewhere.[25-27]

Ethics Consultation

An ethics case consultation (ECC) is "a service provided by an individual consultant, team, or committee to address the ethical issues involved in a specific clinical case. *Its central purpose is to improve the process and outcomes of patient care by helping to identify, analyze, and resolve ethical problems.*"[28,29])

- The first step in an ECC is when the healthcare team becomes aware that there may be an ethical dilemma or question.
- ECC may be called when an ethics-specific problem arises, when the requesting physicians feel they may not have adequate expertise, or when the patient care and ethics issues are so complex that input from multiple physicians and ethics consultants is warranted.

One barrier to ethics consultation is that a significant number of physicians believe ECC is too time consuming or makes things worse.[30] However, a multicenter randomized, controlled study of ethics consultations in the ICU setting found that 87% of physicians, nurses, and patients or surrogates found that ECC was helpful, and >90% of physicians and nurses would seek ECC again.[31] The same study found that there was no difference in survival between patients who had ECC and controls. In the authors' words, ECC was not "a subterfuge for 'pulling the plug,'" but the interval between randomization and death was 3 days less for patients who had ECC (8.66 ± 9.39 days for ECC vs. 11.62 ± 16.36 days for controls; $p = 0.01$).[16] Thus, it appears that physicians' apprehensions about ECC are not necessarily matched by the actual facts, and more likely than not, ECC will be beneficial. Most ethics committees and consultation teams would rather be consulted early in a case when the chances are higher that they'll be able to help. If they're called too late in a case, there may be little they can do to help resolve it.

Legal Consultation

There are times in the NCCU when, despite the HCT's best efforts, there exist irreconcilable differences between the HCT and the patient, or the patient's family or between surrogate decision makers. Some examples are (1) when surrogate decision makers want "everything done" but the ICU team considers continuation or escalation of medical care as futile; (2) when there is disagreement among the family or surrogates as to the type of care that should be provided or withheld; and lastly, (3) elective healthcare decisions, including DNR orders, that need to be made for unbefriended individuals who lack decisional capacity. When such issues cannot be resolved by ethics consultation, physicians should consider consulting with legal counsel for their institution. In fact, it is often wise to obtain simultaneous ethics and legal consultation.

There are many barriers to seeking legal consultation. One is the nature of the answers given by the law. Legal counsel is often sought for the purpose of determining 'what the law requires or allows' of everyone involved. For example, in the case of futile care, physicians seek legal counsel to determine whether the law "allows" them to stop treating a patient against the family's wishes. Attorneys may explain that while the law (depending on state statute) would allow them to do so after due process, and may even provide protection from liability (e.g., Maryland statute), this does not and will not prevent a family from initiating a lawsuit against the physician or the institution.

Physicians may feel as though the law offers little benefit or protection, thinking, "What's the point in legalizing the behavior if I am still subject to a lawsuit?" It should be kept in mind, however, that while the law represents society's collective opinion about acceptable behavior, it does not purport to represent a universal opinion. Persons who believe they have been harmed have a right to seek redress in a court, even if the odds are remote that they will recover. Protection from liability is the not the same as protection from lawsuit.

Another barrier to legal consultation is the amount of time that may be required of physicians. For example, the process of petitioning a court to appoint a guardian for a patient may require members of the healthcare team to testify in court. It will usually also require that the healthcare team continue to treat the patient while the guardian appointment process is carried out, which may take days or weeks, or rarely longer. A recent review of end-of-life care for homeless patients found that many physicians end up making decisions to limit or withdraw treatment without legal consultation.[32]

Despite these limitations, whenever there is a doubt about the propriety of a decision, or when substantial unresolved conflicts between the healthcare team and various decision makers remain despite an ethics consultation, it is prudent to seek legal counsel in order to bring into appropriate relief the permissible options available to all of the parties involved.

REFERENCES

1. Beauchamp TL, Childress JF. *Principles of Biomedical Ethics,* 5th ed. New York: Oxford University Press, 2001, pp 1–25.
2. Fletcher JC, Spencer EM. Clinical ethics: history, content, and resources. In Fletcher JC, Spencer EM, Lombard PA (eds), *Fletcher's Introduction to Clinical Ethics*, 3rd ed. Hagerstown: University Publishing Group, 2005, pp 3–18.
3. Bernat JL. *Ethical Issues in Neurology*. 2nd ed. Boston: Butterworth-Heinemann, 2002, pp 3–26.
4. Beauchamp TL, Childress JF. *Principles of Biomedical Ethics*, 5th ed. New York: Oxford University Press, 2001.
5. Halm EA, Tuhrim S, Wang JJ, Rojas M, Hannan EL, Chassin MR. Has evidence changed practice? Appropriateness of carotid endarterectomy after the clinical trials. *Neurology.* 2007; **68**:187–94.
6. Tversky A, Kahneman D. The framing of decisions and the psychology of choice. *Science.* 1981;**211**:453–8.
7. McNeil BJ, Pauker SG, Sox HC, Tversky A. On the elicitation of preferences for alternate therapies. *N Engl J Med.* 1982; **306**:1259–62.
8. National Commission for the Protection of Human Subjects of Biomedical and Behavioral Research. The Belmont Report: Ethical Principles and Guidelines for the Protection of Human Subjects of Research. Available at: http://ohsr.od.nih.gov/guidelines/belmont.html (Accessed April 8, 2007).
9. Luce JM. Research ethics and consent in the intensive care unit. *Curr Opin Crit Care.* 2003; **9**:540–4.
10. Schweickert W, Hall J. Informed consent in the intensive care unit: ensuring understanding in a complex environment. *Curr Opin Crit Care.* 2005;**11**:624–8.
11. Bigatello LM, George E, Hurford W. Ethical considerations for research in critically ill patients. *Crit Care Med.* 2003;**31**:S178–81.
12. Luce JM. Is the concept of informed consent applicable to clinical research involving critically ill patients? *Crit Care Med.* 2003;**31**:S153–6.
13. Chen DT, Miller FG, Rosenstein DL. Clinical research and the physician-patient relationship. *Ann Intern Med.* 2003;**138**:669–72.

14. Davis N, Pohlman A, Gehlbach B, Kress JP, McAtee J, Herlitz J, Hall J. Improving the process of informed consent in the critically ill. *JAMA*. 2003;**289**:1963–8.

15. Beauchamp TL, Childress JF. *Principles of Biomedical Ethics*, 5th ed. New York: Oxford University Press, 2001,165–224.

16. Virginia Health Care Decisions Act. at http://leg1.state.va.us/cgi-bin/legp504.exe?000+cod+54.1–2986 (Accessed April 8, 2007).

17. Larriviere D, Bonnie RJ. Terminating artificial nutrition and hydration in persistent vegetative state patients: current and proposed state laws. *Neurology*. 2006;**66**:1624–8.

18. Position of the American Academy of Neurology on certain aspects of the care and management of the persistent vegetative state patient. *Neurology*. 1989;**39**:125–6.

19. Bacon D, Williams MA, Gordon J. American Academy of Neurology position statement on laws and regulations concerning life-sustaining treatment, including artificial nutrition and hydration, for patients lacking decision-making capacity. *Neurology*. **68**:1097–100.

20. American College of Chest Physicians/Society of Critical Care Medicine Consensus Panel. Ethical and moral guidelines for the initiation, continuation, and withdrawal of intensive care. *Chest*. 1990;**97**:949–58.

21. Quality Standards Subcommittee of the American Academy of Neurology. Practice parameters for determining brain death in adults. *Neurology*. 1995;**45**:1012–14.

22. US Department of Health and Human Services, Office for Civil Rights. Summary of the HIPAA Privacy Rule [Internet]. Washington, DC: US Department of Health and Human Services; 2003. Available at: http://www.hhs.gov/ocr/privacysummary.pdf (Accessed February 13, 2007).

23. The Organ Procurement and Transplantation Network. OPTN/SRTR Annual Report: Chapter II: Organ Donation and Utilization. Available at: http://www.optn.org/AR2005/Chapter_II_AR_CD.htm?cp=3 (Accessed March 25, 2006).

24. Recommendations for nonheartbeating organ donation. A Position Paper by the Ethics Committee, American College of Critical Care Medicine, Society of Critical Care Medicine. *Crit Care Med*. 2001;**29**:1826–31.

25. Donatelli LA, Geocadin RG, Williams MA. Ethical issues in critical care and cardiac arrest: clinical research, brain death, and organ donation. *Semin Neurol*. 2006;**26**:452–60.

26. Herdman R, Potts JT. *Non-Heart-Beating Organ Transplantation: Medical and Ethical Issues in Procurement*. Washington, DC: National Academy Press, 1997.

27. Committee on Non-Heart-Beating Transplantation II: The Scientific and Ethical Basis for Practice and Protocols. Non-Heart-Beating Organ Transplantation: Practice and Protocols. Washington, DC: National Academy Press, 2000.

28. Fletcher JC, Siegler M. What are the goal of ethics consultations? A consensus statement. *J Clin Ethics*. 1996;**7**:122–6.

29. Schneiderman LJ. Ethics consultation in the intensive care unit. *Curr Opin Crit Care*. 2005; **11**:600–4.

30. DuVal G, Clarridge B, Gensler G, Danis M. A national survey of U.S. internists' experiences with ethical dilemmas and ethics consultation. *J Gen Intern Med*. 2004;**19**:251–8.

31. Schneiderman LJ, Gilmer T, Teetzel HD, et al., Effect of ethics consultations on nonbeneficial life-sustaining treatments in the intensive care setting. *JAMA*. 2003; **290**:1166–72.

32. Kushel MB, Miaskowski C. End of life care for homeless patients: "She says she is there to help me in any situation." *JAMA*. 2006;**296**:2959–66.

24   A Pulmonary Consult

Wendy Zouras, MD and Kenneth Presberg, MD

Neurocritical care patients are susceptible to a variety of pulmonary complications. Therefore the neurointensivist needs to be very familiar with the common pulmonary problems that are encountered in the neurointensive care unit (NICU). Almost all neurocritical care patients are at increased risk for nosocomial pneumonia and venous thromboembolic disease (VTE). Safe prevention remains the mainstay of therapy for VTE, but diagnosis and management of pulmonary embolism (PE) also need to be well understood.

Trauma patients who require neurocritical care may develop pulmonary contusion and acute lung injury (ALI). Many patients have neurologic problems that predispose them to aspiration of gastric contents putting them at increased risk for the development of acute respiratory distress syndrome (ARDS) in addition to aspiration pneumonia. Further, neurogenic pulmonary edema may occur in a variety of patients with neurocritical care problems, and the approach to these patients is similar to that of patients with ARDS. Management of patients with ALI/ARDS is particularly challenging in the NICU given the effects of hypercapnia on intracranial pressure (ICP) and more complex choices for sedation, analgesia, and neuromuscular blockade.

In addition, patients with common obstructive lung diseases, such as asthma or chronic obstructive pulmonary disease (COPD), often have exacerbations of their condition due to trauma, intubation, pneumonia, aspiration, or medications.

The discussion that follows is intended to assist the neurointensivist in the treatment of patients with common pulmonary problems in the context of their major neurologic comorbidities.

PULMONARY EMBOLISM

Background

Venous thromboembolic disease is a persistent and prevalent cause of morbidity and mortality responsible for an estimated 150,000 to 200,000 deaths each year in the United States. It remains the most common preventable cause of hospital death. VTE originates as systemic venous thrombosis. Conditions that favor thrombosis are venous stasis, injury to the venous intima, and alterations in the coagulation-fibrinolytic system. Deep vein thrombosis (DVT) of the lower extremities is the predominant source of clinically significant PE, accounting for >95% of events. The major risk factors for DVT include:

1. Surgery involving general anesthesia for more than 30 minutes
2. Injury or surgery involving the lower extremities or pelvis
3. Congestive heart failure
4. Any cause of prolonged immobility
5. Pregnancy, particularly during the postpartum period

Other factors that greatly increase the risk of DVT are cancer, obesity, advancing age, varicose veins, a prior episode of DVT, the use of estrogen-containing compounds, and dehydration. Risk factors are cumulative.

Prevention of VTE

The best way to reduce the morbidity and mortality associated with VTE disease is prevention. In general, all patients admitted to a critical care unit should be assessed for their risk of VTE. Most of these patients should receive thromboprophylaxis.

■ Subcutaneous low-dose unfractionated heparin (LDUH) or low molecular weight heparin (LMWH) is recommended in patients who do not have a contraindication such as active bleeding or coagulopathy.

■ In patients who cannot receive heparin, intermittent pneumatic compression (IPC), with or without graduated compression stockings (GCS), should be used.

A discussion of specific recommendations for the prevention of VTE in situations commonly encountered in the neurocritical care unit follows. In all patients, it is important to remember that appropriate prophylaxis significantly reduces the risk of VTE but does not eliminate it entirely.

■ Neurosurgery: Patients undergoing major neurosurgery are known to be at moderately increased risk of postoperative VTE and warrant the routine use of prophylaxis. Additional risk is associated with intracranial rather than spinal surgery, active malignancy, more lengthy procedures, the presence of leg weakness, and advanced age. Mechanical thromboprophylaxis is commonly used in neurosurgical patients because of concern for potential intracranial or spinal bleeding.
  ▸ Studies suggest that perioperative use of LDUH does not increase the risk of intracranial bleed and is more effective than IPC, with or without the use of GCS, for the prevention of DVT.
  ▸ LMWH, however, should be used with caution because some studies have seen a trend toward an increase in the incidence of bleeding in patients randomized to LMWH.
  ▸ Initiation of mechanical prophylaxis (IPC with or without GCS) is recommended at the time of surgery.
  ▸ Acceptable alternatives are prophylaxis with LDUH or postoperative LMWH.
  ▸ The combination of mechanical and pharmacologic prophylaxis is recommended in high-risk neurosurgery patients such as those with a malignant brain tumor.
■ Trauma: Patients recovering from major trauma have a DVT risk exceeding 50% without

prophylaxis. Factors that are independently associated with an increased risk include:
  ▸ Spinal cord injury
  ▸ Lower extremity or pelvic fracture
  ▸ Need for a surgical procedure
  ▸ Increasing age
  ▸ Femoral venous line insertion or major venous repair
  ▸ Prolonged immobility
  ▸ Longer duration of hospital stay

Mechanical prophylaxis with IPC is often used in trauma patients because it does not increase the risk of bleeding. However, studies have found inconsistent results as to the effectiveness of this modality in this group of patients. Aside from suboptimal protection, IPC cannot be used in up to one third of trauma patients due to lower extremity fractures, casts, or dressings.

■ IPC is not recommended as routine prophylaxis in trauma patients, but it may be beneficial when there is an active contraindication to anticoagulation.

Likewise, LDUH may prevent VTE in lower risk patients, but it is not particularly effective prophylaxis in trauma patients. LMWH has been shown to be superior to LDUH in a large study of major trauma patients without frank intracranial bleeding or ongoing bleeding at other sites.

■ LMWH is therefore the recommended prophylaxis for the majority of moderate-risk and high-risk trauma patients.
■ Current contraindications to the early initiation of LMWH prophylaxis include the presence of intracranial bleeding, ongoing and uncontrolled bleeding, an uncorrected major coagulopathy, and incomplete spinal cord injury (SCI) associated with suspected or proven perispinal hematoma.
■ Head injury without frank hemorrhage, lacerations or contusions of internal organs (lungs, liver, spleen, or kidneys), the presence of a retroperitoneal hematoma associated with pelvic fracture, or *complete* spinal cord injuries are not themselves contraindications to LMWH thromboprophylaxis, provided that there is no evidence of ongoing bleeding.

- Most trauma patients can be started on LMWH within 36 hours of injury.

For patients with contraindications to LMWH, mechanical modalities, such as IPC or GCS, should be considered despite evidence that they provide only limited protection. These devices should be applied to both legs as soon as possible, and their use should be continued around the clock until LMWH can be started.

- Screening Doppler ultrasound should be performed in high-risk patients who have received suboptimal or no thromboprophylaxis (especially before instituting IPC).
- Prophylaxis should be continued until hospital discharge, including the period of inpatient rehabilitation.
- Prophylaxis after hospital discharge should be considered in patients with major impaired mobility.
- Acute SCI: Without appropriate prophylaxis, patients with acute SCI have the highest incidence of DVT among all hospitalized groups (60–100% of SCI patients have asymptomatic DVT on routine screening). PE remains the third leading cause of death in these patients.
  - ▶ Factors that increase the risk of VTE even further include advanced age, concomitant lower extremity fracture, and delayed use of thromboprophylaxis.
  - ▶ Although the period of greatest risk for VTE after SCI is the acute care phase, symptomatic DVT or PE, and fatal PE also occur during the rehabilitation phase.

The very high risk of VTE after SCI supports the early use of thromboprophylaxis in all SCI patients.

- Several studies have shown that the use of LDUH alone or IPC alone is ineffective prophylaxis in SCI patients, while adjusted-dose unfractionated heparin and LMWH are substantially more efficacious.
- Once there is clinical evidence that primary hemostasis has been achieved, LMWH, or the combination of LMWH or LDUH plus IPC, are the recommended early options.
- If concern about bleeding at the injury site or elsewhere persists, mechanical prophylaxis should be initiated as soon as possible after hospital admission, and anticoagulant prophylaxis should be started once the bleeding risk has decreased.
- Screening Doppler ultrasound should be considered in SCI patients in whom effective prophylaxis has been delayed.
- After the acute injury phase, continuing prophylaxis with LMWH or conversion to warfarin with a target INR range of 2.0–3.0 for the duration of the rehabilitation phase is likely to be beneficial.

Diagnostic Strategies in PE/DVT

The mortality associated with PE can be reduced by prompt diagnosis and appropriate therapy. Unfortunately, the symptoms and signs may be subtle, atypical, or obscured by another coexisting disease. This is especially true of patients in the intensive care setting. The clinical presentation and standard tests such as electrocardiogram, chest radiograph, and arterial blood gases cannot be relied on to confirm or rule out the presence of PE. A well thought-out strategy for the evaluation of PE is crucial. We briefly discuss the available diagnostic tests and then present examples of algorithms that can be employed based on the particular clinical situation.

- Laboratory tests: Routine laboratory findings are nonspecific and include leukocytosis, an increase in the erythrocyte sedimentation rate, and elevations in serum LDH or AST.
  - ▶ Arterial blood gas analysis usually reveals hypoxemia, hypocapnia, and respiratory alkalosis, but in massive PE with hypotension and respiratory collapse, hypercapnia and a combined respiratory and metabolic acidosis is common.
  - ▶ Brain natriuretic peptide (BNP) levels are typically greater in patients with PE, but this finding is neither sensitive nor specific. An elevated BNP level may correlate with the risk of subsequent complications and may have a prognostic role in PE.
  - ▶ Troponin I and troponin T are elevated in 3–50% of patients with a moderate to large PE and although not useful for diagnosis, elevations are associated with marked increases in the incidence of prolonged hypotension and 30-day mortality.

- D-dimer is a degradation product of cross-linked fibrin. It can be detected in serum using a quantitative enzyme-linked immunosorbent assay (ELISA) or a semiquantitative latex agglutination assay. ELISA is more accurate, while latex agglutination is more rapid. D-dimer assays, particularly the ELISA test, for the diagnosis of PE have good sensitivity, but poor specificity. Thus a normal D-dimer by ELISA can be used to help exclude a diagnosis of PE. However, an elevated D-dimer is far too nonspecific to provide any useful clinical information. Hospitalized patients very commonly have elevations in the D-dimer level, severely limiting the usefulness of this test in these patients.
- Electrocardiography (ECG): ECG abnormalities exist in many patients with PE who do not have preexisting cardiovascular disease, but they are also common in patients without PE, limiting the diagnostic usefulness.
  - The most common abnormalities are nonspecific ST-segment and T-wave changes.
  - The classic abnormality most suggestive of PE is the S1Q3T3 pattern, with right ventricular strain, and a new incomplete right bundle branch block. This occurs infrequently with PE and is most common in patients with massive PE and cor pulmonale.
  - The ECG abnormalities associated with a poor prognosis include atrial arrhythmias, right bundle branch block, inferior Q-waves, and precordial T-wave inversions with ST-segment changes.
- Chest radiography: Radiographic abnormalities are common in patients with PE, but they are not diagnostically useful because they are similarly common in patients without PE. Atelectasis, infiltrates, pleural effusion, and cardiomegaly are all common but nonspecific findings.
- Ventilation–Perfusion (V/Q) scan: V/Q scanning has had a central role in the diagnosis of PE and is a valuable tool when the results are definitive. A normal V/Q scan essentially rules out the diagnosis, while a high probability scan is strong evidence for the presence of PE. Unfortunately, in the majority of patients with suspected embolism who undergo V/Q scanning, the findings are considered indeterminate, and additional testing is required.

- Lower extremity venous ultrasound: The rationale for using lower extremity venous ultrasound in the diagnostic evaluation of PE is that most pulmonary emboli arise from the deep veins of the legs and that venous thrombosis detected by ultrasound is treated in a similar manner (e.g., anticoagulation) as a confirmed PE.
  - Although ultrasonography can be very helpful and is particularly useful for critically ill patients who often cannot be safely moved from the intensive care unit for testing, many patients with PE (up to 71% in one study) have negative venous ultrasounds.
  - Performing a "complete" lower extremity venous ultrasound, which includes imaging the calf veins, may improve sensitivity, but the quality of such examinations is operator-dependent.
  - In addition, inability of the patient to cooperate fully with regard to positioning for the examination and/or intolerance of the pressure of the ultrasound probe on the skin, or inability of the examiner to obtain a complete examination secondary to the presence of bandages, casts, or extremity wounds may, in some cases, lead to a need for serial examinations or the performance of alternative diagnostic procedures.
- CT pulmonary angiography (CT-PA): Spiral or helical CT scanning with intravenous contrast, also referred to as CT pulmonary angiography, is being used increasingly for the diagnosis of PE. One of the most commonly cited benefits of CT-PA is the ability to detect alternative pulmonary abnormalities that may explain the patient's clinical presentation.
  - The specificity of CT-PA is excellent, and initial studies suggested that the sensitivity of CT-PA for the diagnosis of PE was very high. Subsequent studies, however, have not shown such promising results.
  - The diagnostic accuracy of CT-PA clearly varies widely from institution to institution due to differences in the experience of the person interpreting the images and to differences in image quality. Some centers perform CT venography as well, which uses the same contrast bolus as the CT-PA of the chest and can detect DVTs from the pelvis down to the calves, further improving sensitivity. Thus

clinicians need to consider their institution's experience when deciding whether to rely on CT-PA or to pursue additional diagnostic testing.

▶ CT-PA results that are discordant with clinical suspicion should be viewed with skepticism, and additional testing should be considered to confirm the findings.

Some major advantages to CT-PA include the high specificity, availability, safety, relative rapidity of procedure, and the ability to diagnose other pulmonary conditions. On the other hand, limitations include accuracy that is determined by the expertise of the reader, expense, lack of portability, need for contrast bolus, poor visualization of certain regions, inability to detect subsegmental emboli, and risk involved due to contrast-induced nephropathy and to contrast allergies.

■ Angiography: Pulmonary angiography is the definitive diagnostic test or "gold standard" in the diagnosis of acute PE. A negative pulmonary angiography excludes clinically relevant PE. It is generally safe and well tolerated in the absence of hemodynamic instability. Complications include those related to catheter insertion, contrast reactions, cardiac arrhythmia, or respiratory insufficiency.

■ Magnetic resonance angiography (MRA): The use of MRA for the diagnosis of PE is limited by respiratory and cardiac motion artifact, suboptimal resolution, complicated blood flow patterns, and magnetic susceptibility effects from the adjacent air-containing lung. However, technological advances offer promise for an expanded role of MRA in the future.

■ Echocardiography: Bedside echocardiography will demonstrate evidence of PE (increased right ventricular [RV] size, decreased RV function, and tricuspid regurgitation) in up to 80% of cases, especially in unstable patients when transesophageal echo is used. In cases of massive PE, these abnormalities are much more common, and echocardiography can be used to make a rapid presumptive diagnosis to justify the use of thrombolytic therapy in an unstable patient. It is especially useful for patients who cannot be safely transported for other diagnostic tests.

Recommended Diagnostic Strategy

An algorithm for the diagnosis of PE is shown in Figure 24.1. When PE is suspected on clinical grounds in a hospitalized patient, clinicians must determine which diagnostic modalities are readily available at their institution. If the institution has experience and expertise in performing and interpreting helical CT-PA, and the patient has no contraindication to the procedure, CT-PA is recommended because of its high predictive accuracy, ready availability, and ability to detect alternative diagnoses. In the rare instances that CT-PA is inconclusive or if the clinical suspicion is very high but the CT-PA is negative, additional testing should be obtained. This might include V/Q scanning, lower extremity ultrasound, or pulmonary angiography, as described below for CT-PA inexperienced institutions.

If, on the other hand, an institution is inexperienced with CT-PA, a V/Q scan is the recommended initial study since a normal exam will rule out PE and a high- probability exam confirms the diagnosis. The majority of V/Q scans, however, will be inconclusive, and even "low-probability" scans have sensitivities as low as 80% when clinical suspicion is high. Therefore, further testing is often required. Lower extremity venous ultrasound is used frequently in this situation because of its noninvasive nature. Although sensitivity is low (30–50% of ultrasounds are negative in patients with confirmed PE) and a negative test has limited utility, some studies have indicated that a negative ultrasound in conjunction with a "low-probability" V/Q scan has a 94% negative predictive value. When clinical suspicion remains high and further testing is necessary, pulmonary angiography would be the next step.

Management

Acute PE is often fatal, with a mortality rate of up to 30% without treatment. Most patients who die from PE do so because of recurrent PE within the first few hours of the event. Therapy with anticoagulants decreases the mortality rate to <8%. Therefore it is imperative that the diagnosis be considered and effective therapy be instituted as quickly as possible, often before confirmatory diagnostic tests can be done.

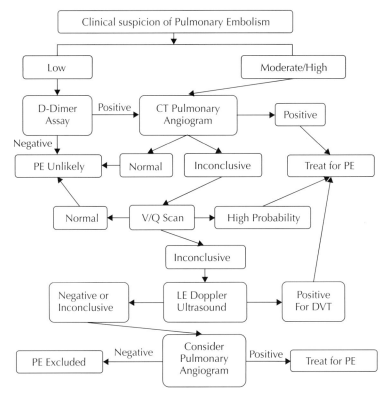

Figure 24.1. Clinical algorithm for evaluation of patients with suspected pulmonary embolism (PE). DVT = deep vein thrombosis, CT = computed tomography, V/Q = ventilation-perfusion, LE = lower extremity.

■ General supportive care: The initial care of the patient with PE should focus on stabilizing the patient.

▸ Supplemental oxygen should be administered if hypoxemia is present. Severe hypoxemia or respiratory failure requires immediate intubation and mechanical ventilation.

▸ If the patient has persistent hypotension, hemodynamic support, in the form of intravenous fluids, vasopressors, or inotropic agents, should be initiated promptly.

▷ Intravenous fluids can be beneficial but need to be administered with caution because the increased intravascular volume can precipitate RV failure, and the increase in RV wall stress due to the larger volume can decrease the RV oxygen supply/demand ratio and cause ischemia and deterioration in RV function. It is reasonable to provide an initial bolus of fluid while keeping these issues in mind.

▷ If the patient's hypotension does not resolve with fluid, vasopressor therapy should be initiated. Norepinephrine, phenylephrine, dopamine, and epinephrine are all effective. There is no evidence that one is better than the other; norepinephrine and phenylephrine are least likely to cause tachycardia. Dobutamine can be useful to increase myocardial contractility, but the associated vasodilation can worsen hypotension. Combination therapy with dobutamine and norepinephrine mitigates this problem.

■ Anticoagulation: Concomitantly to the supportive care, initiation of PE-directed therapy should be considered during the resuscitative period. Bedside diagnostic tests (lower extremity ultrasound, echocardiography, and at some institutions, V/Q scans) can be extremely helpful in these situations.

▸ When there is a high clinical suspicion of PE, empiric anticoagulant therapy should be started as soon as possible, with diagnostic evaluation postponed until after the patient is stabilized. The high risk of death due to recurrent PE in the untreated patient (about 30%) outweighs the risk of major bleeding due to anticoagulation (<3% overall, although this value is likely higher among patients in the NICU).

▸ If there is a high suspicion of PE in a patient with a strong contraindication to anticoagulation, diagnostic evaluation must be expedited so that an inferior vena caval filter could be placed, if necessary.

▸ Patients in whom anticoagulation was initiated during the resuscitative period should remain anticoagulated during the diagnostic evaluation.

▸ Long-term anticoagulation is indicated if PE is confirmed. If PE is excluded, anticoagulation can be stopped; adequate preventive treatment should be initiated at that time.

Full anticoagulation should be initiated using subcutaneous LMWH (enoxaparin) or intravenous unfractionated heparin (UFH) .

■ LMWH is usually preferred in hemodynamically stable patients.

■ In patients with renal failure or with persistent hypotension due to PE, UFH is appropriate. Also, UFH is often safer in critically ill patients who are at increased risk for significant bleeding complications.

■ The efficacy of anticoagulant therapy depends upon achieving a therapeutic level of heparin within the first 24 hours of treatment. This is best achieved using weight-based protocols for adjusting the heparin dose .

■ Thrombolytics: Persistent hypotension due to PE (i.e., massive PE) is a widely accepted indication for thrombolytic therapy (alteplase [TPA], streptokinase, urokinase). Use of thrombolytics for some other clinical circumstances including severe hypoxemia, large perfusion defects, right ventricular dysfunction, free floating right ventricular thrombus, and patent foramen ovale is controversial and should be considered on a case-by-case basis. Thrombolytic therapy accelerates the lysis of acute PE but may be associated with an increased likelihood of major hemorrhage and must be used with caution. Table 24.1

lists the absolute and relative contraindications for thrombolytic therapy.

■ IVC filters and embolectomy: Insertion of an inferior vena caval (IVC) filter is indicated if there is an absolute contraindication to anticoagulation, if PE reoccurs during adequate anticoagulant therapy, or if the patient has complications of anticoagulation such as severe bleeding. A recent retrospective study suggested that IVC filters may decrease mortality in the subset of patients with massive PE and persistent hypotension.

▸ Overall, IVC filters are associated with a decrease in the number of recurrent PEs; however, recurrent DVT is more common in patients with IVC filters.

▸ Other complications of IVC filters include those related to insertion (e.g., bleeding), filter misplacement, filter migration, filter erosion and perforation of the IVC wall, and IVC obstruction due to filter thrombosis.

▸ Because of the long-term complications, permanent IVC filter placement is discouraged in young patients with a long life expectancy. To address these concerns, retrievable IVC filters have been developed, but studies to evaluate their effectiveness and adverse effects are still lacking.

Embolectomy is the removal of the embolus either surgically or using catheters. It should be considered when there is persistent hypotension severe enough to warrant thrombolysis and thrombolysis either fails or is contraindicated. It is associated with a high mortality.

ACUTE RESPIRATORY DISTRESS SYNDROME

Background

The acute respiratory distress syndrome (ARDS) was first described in 1967 in 12 patients who presented with acute respiratory distress, cyanosis refractory to oxygen therapy, decreased lung compliance, and diffuse infiltrates evident on the chest radiograph. ARDS refers to the most severe form of "acute lung injury" (ALI). ALI refers to a syndrome of acute and persistent lung inflammation with increased permeability of the alveolar–capillary barrier leading to pulmonary edema with normal left heart filling

Table 24.1. Contraindications to thrombolytic therapy

Absolute:

Previous hemorrhagic stroke (ever)

Stroke or cerebrovascular event within 1 year

Known intracranial neoplasm

Active internal bleeding (other than menses)

Suspected aortic dissection

Relative:

Blood pressure >180/110 mm Hg or history of chronic severe hypertension

Prior stroke or known intracranial pathology other than the above

Bleeding diathesis, or warfarin and INR >1.7

Recent trauma or GI/GU bleeding (2–4 weeks)

Traumatic or prolonged CPR (>10 minutes)

Recent major surgery (within 2–3 weeks)

Noncompressible vascular punctures

Age >75 years or weight <67 kg (increased bleeding risk)

Pregnancy

Active peptic ulcer

pressures. The currently used simple definition of ALI/ARDS was recommended by the American–European Consensus Conference Committee (1994). The criteria set forth in this definition are:

1. Acute onset
2. Bilateral infiltrates on chest radiography
3. Pulmonary-artery wedge pressure <18 mm Hg if measured, or the absence of clinical evidence of left atrial hypertension
4. If $Pao_2:Fio_2$ <300, ALI is considered to be present
5. If $Pao_2:Fio_2$ <200, ARDS is considered to be present

This remains the preferred definition because it is simple to apply in the clinical setting and allows the clinician to compare their patients with those enrolled in clinical trials. Severity of ALI and ARDS has also been described by a "Lung Injury Score" (Murray, 1987).

- This score utilizes information from the (1) chest radiograph, (2) $Pao_2:Fio_2$ ratio, (3) lung compliance, and (4) level of positive end-expiratory pressure (PEEP).
- A value of 0–4 is given in each area and then averaged.
- A score of >2.5 indicates severe lung injury and has been used as an inclusion criterion for many studies.

ARDS is associated with numerous conditions, with varying incidence and prognosis. Some of the most common precipitants of ARDS are listed in Table 24.2. Neurogenic pulmonary edema (NPE) is a common problem seen in the neurocritical care unit. Although it is usually classified as a form of ARDS, its pathophysiology and prognosis are somewhat different and will be discussed in more detail below. In addition, it has been reported that ARDS develops frequently in patients treated with induced hypertension to manage cerebral pressure.

Pathogenesis

Clinical ARDS is primarily the result of inflammatory injury to the alveoli producing diffuse alveolar damage. Proinflammatory cytokines such as tumor necrosis factor, interleukin (IL)-1, IL-6, and IL-8 are released in response to any of a variety of precipitants. Neutrophils are recruited to the lungs, become activated, and release toxic mediators such as reactive oxygen species and proteases, which damage the capillary endothelium and alveolar epithelium Protein escapes from the vascular space, and the osmotic gradient favoring resorption of fluid is lost. Fluid pours into the interstitium and overwhelms the capacity of the lymphatics. Air spaces thus fill with bloody, proteinaceous edema fluid and debris from degenerating cells. Functional surfactant is lost, resulting in alveolar collapse. This results in:

- Hypoxemia from ventilation–perfusion (V/Q) mismatching and physiologic shunting;
- Increased physiologic dead space with impaired CO_2 elimination (particularly with the initiation of positive pressure ventilation);
- Decreased lung compliance due to the stiffness of poorly or nonaerated lung; the functional residual capacity of the lung is reduced, and ventilation occurs predominantly in the remaining unaffected portions of the lung. Therefore, even small tidal volumes result in a dramatic increase in airway pressures; and

Table 24.2. Common conditions associated with acute respiratory distress syndrome (ARDS)

Sepsis	Drug overdose
Aspiration	Near drowning
Infectious pneumonia	Smoke inhalation
Severe trauma	Cardiopulmonary bypass
Surface burns	Drug reaction
Multiple blood transfusions	Neurogenic pulmonary edema
Pancreatitis	Following upper airway obstruction

- Pulmonary hypertension due to a combination of hypoxic vasoconstriction, vascular compression by positive pressure ventilation, and microthrombosis.

Clinical Features

The mechanisms described above explain the hypoxemia, decreased lung compliance, and diffuse radiographic infiltrates seen in patients with ARDS. Despite many different clinical situations and precipitating causes, ARDS often follows a fairly stereotypical course characterized initially by severe hypoxemia and a prolonged need for mechanical ventilation. Patients tend to progress through three stages:

- The initial "exudative" stage is characterized by diffuse alveolar damage and pulmonary edema.
- This gives way to a "proliferative" stage characterized by proliferation of type II alveolar cells along the alveolar basement membrane, squamous metaplasia, interstitial infiltration by myofibroblasts, and early deposition of collagen.
- Some progress to a third "fibrotic" stage with obliteration of normal lung architecture, diffuse fibrosis, and cyst formation.
- Others enter a "recovery" stage characterized by the gradual resolution of hypoxemia and improved lung compliance.

The early clinical features reflect the precipitant of ARDS (e.g., sepsis, trauma, neurologic injury) in addition to the effects of diffuse alveolar damage.

Pulmonary dysfunction typically develops within 24–48 hours of the inciting event and is manifested by rapidly worsening tachypnea, dyspnea, and hypoxemia requiring high concentrations of supplemental oxygen and positive pressure ventilation to reduce shunt.

- Respiratory distress and diffuse lung crackles are observed on physical exam.
- Arterial blood gases usually show an acute respiratory alkalosis, an elevated alveolar–arterial oxygen gradient and severe hypoxemia.
- The chest radiograph typically shows diffuse, fluffy alveolar infiltrates in multiple lung zones with prominent air bronchograms.
- Computed tomography reveals patchy abnormalities with increased radiodensity in dependent lung zones.
- Mechanical ventilation is almost universally required, typically for prolonged periods, which may contribute to developing complications of major barotrauma (e.g., pneumothorax), nosocomial pneumonia, sepsis, and multiple organ failure.

Management

Few patients with ARDS die from respiratory failure alone. More commonly they succumb to their primary illness or to secondary complications such as sepsis or multiorgan system failure. The primary goals of treatment are, therefore, to treat the underlying cause that precipitated the development of ARDS and to provide meticulous supportive care to avoid potentially lethal complications.

- Sedation and paralysis: Most patients with ARDS require sedation and analgesia to provide comfort while on mechanical ventilation as well as to decrease oxygen consumption. A more thorough discussion of this topic appears in Chapter 5. In brief, a combination of a benzodiazepine or propofol and an opiate is usually used since it provides both sedation and analgesia and because when used in combination, there is a synergistic effect which decreases the required dose of each agent.
  - ‣ Propofol is particularly useful in the neurocritical care patient because its short half-life allows for more frequent evaluations of neurologic status.

▸ Sedation carries its own risks, however, and needs to be used thoughtfully. Strategies such as routine daily awakening of patients, using bolus doses rather than continuous infusion, and following a sedation and analgesia protocol may result in important benefits such as decreased time on the ventilator and fewer nosocomial infections.

Some patients may require neuromuscular blocking agents (NMBA) to facilitate mechanical ventilation. These agents have been associated with prolonged neuromuscular weakness after they have been discontinued. They should be used only when necessary and discontinued at the earliest appropriate time.

▪ Lung-protective ventilatory strategy: It is now recognized that although mechanical ventilation is required in most patients with ARDS to facilitate oxygenation and ventilation, it is not without risk. Lung protective ventilation is the only therapy that has been proven to decrease ARDS mortality. Its goals are to avoid lung overdistension to minimize volutrauma, provide adequate end-expiratory lung volume to avoid cyclical end-expiratory lung unit collapse and subsequent atelectrauma, and avoid high inspired oxygen concentrations.

  ▸ Studies have demonstrated a significant improvement in mortality using lung protective ventilatory strategies involving low tidal volumes and increased levels of positive end-expiratory pressure (PEEP). Interestingly, major barotrauma with pneumothorax was similar in both groups.

  ▸ The strategy used for the NIH ARDS Network Trial is outlined in Table 24.3. In general terms, initial tidal volumes (V_T) should approach 6 mL/kg *predicted* body weight. The inspiratory plateau pressure (P_{plat}) should be monitored and maintained at <30 cm H_2O by adjusting tidal volume and PEEP. Respiratory rate should be adjusted to provide adequate ventilation and maintain a pH of 7.30 to 7.45. Pao_2 is maintained at 55–80 mm Hg by adjusting the Fio_2 and PEEP. Fio_2 should be reduced to <0.6 as soon as possible after V_T and P_{plat} targets are met so as to minimize oxygen toxicity. PEEP levels may be limited by high airway pressure. However, a more recent ARDS network study comparing patients randomized to receive high or low levels of PEEP did not demonstrate any difference in outcomes.

Particular to patients in the neurocritical care unit, the effects of mechanical ventilation on intracranial pressure (ICP) and cerebral perfusion pressure (CPP) need to be considered.

▪ The use of smaller tidal volumes and higher levels of PEEP can potentially raise ICP through hypercapnia-mediated increases in cerebral blood flow or impaired venous drainage. In many patients with ARDS, however, maintaining a normal $Paco_2$ while avoiding overdistension injury can be challenging.

▪ A careful examination of the patient may uncover factors that could improve CO_2 clearance. These include removing any excess dead space from the ventilator circuit, ensuring adequate patient–ventilator synchrony, checking the endotracheal tube for partial obstruction, and considering maneuvers to improve respiratory system compliance such as draining large pleural effusions or massive ascites.

▪ If a high $Paco_2$ remains a problem then one must carefully weigh the risks and benefits of targeting eucapnia versus a limited tidal volume. Unfortunately there is no direct clinical evidence to guide these decisions.

In theory, PEEP may cause deleterious effects in the intracranial compartment by increasing intrathoracic pressure and, through retrograde transmission of central venous pressure (CVP), may interfere with cerebral venous outflow. PEEP can also reduce the cardiac output, resulting in a decrease in mean arterial pressure (MAP) and CPP. Although early studies showed conflicting results, more recent studies suggest that PEEP is safe in patients with subarachnoid hemorrhage, stroke, and traumatic brain injury as long as it is applied only in patients with poor lung compliance and adequate blood pressure is maintained. Most authors advise that the application of high levels of PEEP be done under monitoring of MAP, ICP, and CPP.

▪ Fluid management: Although increased vascular permeability is the primary cause of pulmonary edema in early ARDS, restricting fluids and thus

---

Table 24.3. NIH ARDS network: Lower-tidal volume ventilator strategy-

Calculate predicted body weight (PBW) in kg
- Men: 50 + 2.3 [(height in inches) – 60] or 50 + 0.91 [(height in cm) – 152.4]
- Women: 45.5 + 2.3[(height in inches) – 60] or 45.5 + 0.91[(height in cm) – 152.4]

Ventilator mode
Volume assist/control until weaning.

Tidal volume (V_T)
- Initial V_T : adjust V_T in steps of 1 mL/kg PBW every 1–2 hours until V_T = 6 mL/kg.
- Measure P_{plat} every 4 hours AND after each change in PEEP or V_T.
- If P_{plat} >30 cm H_2O, decrease V_T to 5 or to 4 mL/kg.
- If P_{plat} <25 cm H_2O and V_T <6 mL/kg PBW, increase V_T by 1 mL/kg PBW.

Respiratory rate (RR)
- With initial change in V_T , adjust RR to maintain minute ventilation.
- Make subsequent adjustments to RR to maintain pH of 7.30–7.45, but do not exceed an RR of 35/min and do not increase set rate if $Paco_2$ <25 mm Hg.

Ratio
Acceptable range = 1:1–1:3 (no inverse ratio)

Fio_2, PEEP, and arterial oxygenation
Maintain Pao_2 at 55–80 mm Hg or pulse oximetry oxygen saturation (Spo_2) at 88–95%. Use the following combinations of PEEP/ Fio_2:

Fio_2	0.3–0.4	0.4	0.5	0.5	0.6	0.7	0.7	0.7	0.8	0.9	0.9	1
PEEP	5		8	8	10	10	10	12	14	14	16	18	18–25

Acidosis management
- If pH <7.30, increase RR until pH = 7.30 or RR = 35/min.
- If pH remains <7.30 with RR = 35, consider bicarbonate infusion.
- If pH <7.15, V_T may be increased (P_{plat} may exceed 30 cm H_2O).

Alkalosis management
- If pH >7.45 and patient is not triggering ventilator, decrease set RR but not below 6 breaths/min.

Weaning:
Initiate weaning by pressure support when all of the following criteria are present:
1. Fio_2O_2 < 0.40 and PEEP <8 cm H_2O.
2. Patient is not receiving neuromuscular blocking agents.
3. Inspiratory efforts are apparent (ventilator rate may be decreased to 50% of baseline level for up to 5 minutes to detect inspiratory effort).
4. Systolic arterial pressure >90 mm Hg without vasopressor support.

---

reducing left atrial pressure reduces the hydrostatic pressure and limits the degree of edema formation. A very recent study by the ARDSnet investigators showed that a conservative strategy of fluid management can improve lung function and shorten duration of mechanical ventilation without increasing nonpulmonary organ failures.

However, this treatment strategy has not been shown to reduce mortality.
▶ Interestingly, pulmonary artery catheter-guided fluid therapy did not improve survival or organ function but was associated with more complications than central venous catheter-guided therapy.

▸ These results, when considered with those of previous studies, suggest that the pulmonary artery catheter should not be routinely used to guide fluid management for acute lung injury patients.

■ Other pharmacologic therapy: Unfortunately, no pharmacologic therapy has been shown to improve survival in patients specifically with ARDS. A recent large study by the ARDSnet investigators failed to show the benefit of corticosteroids in patients with persistent ARDS despite positive findings in previous smaller studies.

▸ Oxygenation, respiratory system compliance, and ventilator-free days improved over the first 28 days but survival at day 60 and 180 was not changed in the group who received corticosteroid treatment in addition to a lung protective strategy of mechanical ventilation.

▸ Furthermore, neuromuscular weakness was increased in the methylprednisolone group and mortality was increased in the patients who received corticosteroids later in the course of their ARDS (>14 days after the onset of ARDS).

A number of agents (surfactant, prostaglandins, ketoconazole, and others) have been studied without documented benefit.

■ Nosocomial pneumonia: it frequently complicates the course of ARDS and increases morbidity and mortality. It is often difficult to diagnose pneumonia in patients with ARDS because of the baseline radiographic abnormalities and frequent colonization of potential pathogens. Therefore, a high level of clinical suspicion must be maintained. On the other hand, inappropriate treatment of patients without pneumonia promotes the emergence of resistant organisms and should be avoided.

▸ Bronchoscopy with quantitative cultures of bronchoalveolar lavage (BAL) may permit more accurate diagnosis, with $>1 \times 10^4$ colonies of a single organism on BAL being a sensitive and specific criterion for pneumonia.

▸ Delayed, inappropriate, or inadequate antibiotic use is associated with poor outcome. Empiric treatment, therefore, should not be withheld when clinical suspicion of pneumonia

is high, and an initial antibiotic regimen taking local sensitivity profiles into account and sufficiently broad to cover likely infecting organisms is essential.

▸ Measures to prevent the development of nosocomial pneumonia should be implemented for all patients. These include maintaining the head of the bed at 30 degrees, avoiding the use of unnecessary antibiotics, careful attention to mouth care, use of weaning protocols to decrease the duration of mechanical ventilation, avoiding excessive sedation, avoiding ventilator circuit changes, and use of in-line suction catheters.

■ Prophylaxis for DVT and GI bleeding: Patients with ARDS, especially those requiring prolonged mechanical ventilation, are at high risk of developing deep vein thrombosis (DVT) and pulmonary embolism (PE) and are at increased risk for gastrointestinal (GI) bleeding.

▸ Unless there is a specific contraindication such as active bleeding or coagulopathy, all patients should receive DVT prophylaxis with low dose, subcutaneous heparin (either standard unfractionated or low molecular weight preparations).

▸ Patients who cannot receive heparin should receive prophylaxis with intermittent pneumatic compression boots.

▸ After tension pneumothorax has been expeditiously ruled out, PE should be considered in all patients who acutely develop shock or deterioration in oxygenation, including those who have been on prophylaxis.

The risk of GI bleeding can be decreased with a number of agents. Currently H_2 antagonists and proton pump inhibitors are the agents of choice.

■ Nutritional support: Patients with ARDS are catabolic and benefit from early and appropriate nutritional support.

▸ If the GI tract is functional, enteral feedings are preferred because they are associated with fewer intravascular infections, less GI bleeding, and preservation of the intestinal mucosal barrier, which may decrease bacterial translocation across the gut.

▸ Overfeeding should be avoided to prevent excessive carbon dioxide production.

Table 24.4. Prone position: contraindications and complications

Contraindications	Complications
Shock	Nerve compression
Acute bleeding	Crush injury
Multiple trauma	Venous stasis
Spinal instability	Airway security problems
Pregnancy	Diaphragm limitation
Raised intracranial pressure	Pressure sores
Abdominal surgery	Dislodging vascular catheters
	Retinal damage

▷ There is some evidence that an enteral diet enriched with the anti-oxidants eicosapentanoic acid and gamma-linolenic acid in ventilated patients with ALI may be beneficial for gas exchange, respiratory dynamics, and requirements for mechanical ventilation. A commercial preparation is available but is expensive. Further studies will be necessary to evaluate the cost-effectiveness of this therapy before it can be recommended routinely.

■ Prone positioning: Prone positioning of patients with ARDS and refractory hypoxemia improves V/Q matching by increasing blood flow to better ventilated lung and by promoting reexpansion of collapsed lung units. Benefits may also arise from an increase in functional residual capacity (FRC) and mobilization of secretions. In studies, prone positioning has improved oxygenation in patients with ARDS, but no survival advantage has been seen. Prone positioning is contraindicated in some patients and is associated with several potential complications (Table 24.4).

▷ While elevated ICP has long been considered a contraindication to prone positioning, a recent study has suggested that the beneficial effect on cerebral tissue oxygenation by increasing arterial oxygenation appears to outweigh the potential adverse effect of prone positioning on cerebral tissue oxygenation by decreasing cerebral perfusion pressure in patients with subarachnoid hemorrhage and ARDS.

Thus, prone positioning may be considered in patients with elevated ICP and refractory hypoxemia.

■ Nitric oxide (NO): Inhaled NO has been studied in patients with moderate to severe ARDS. Administration of NO at 5 ppm improves oxygenation by causing vasodilation in well-ventilated areas of lung and thus decreases V/Q mismatching. It can be helpful in patients with refractory hypoxemia, but studies have thus far failed to demonstrate improvement in patient survival with its use.

Neurogenic Pulmonary Edema (NPE)

NPE characteristically presents within minutes to hours of a severe central nervous system insult but may evolve over hours or days in patients with submassive brain injuries. The initial clinical features are indistinguishable from ARDS, but NPE carries a more favorable prognosis. Many cases are well tolerated and require nothing more than supplemental oxygen, and resolution typically occurs within 48 to 72 hours. The primary causes of NPE are listed in Table 24.5.

The pathophysiologic mechanisms responsible for NPE remain incompletely understood. Currently the medulla oblongata is believed to be the critical anatomic structure involved in the pathogenesis of NPE, probably acting via the sympathetic component of the autonomic nervous system. Additionally, NPE requires that a central nervous system event produce a dramatic change in the Starling's forces which govern the movement of fluid between the capillaries and the pulmonary interstitium, and/or increase the permeability of pulmonary capillaries. Changes in the Starling's forces may be due to left ventricular dysfunction secondary to excessive venous return to the heart, systemic hypertension, and the negative inotropic influences of excessive vagal tone producing passive elevation of left atrial and pulmonary capillary pressures. Also, pulmonary venoconstriction, which elevates capillary hydrostatic pressure, occurs in response to intracranial hypertension or sympathetic stimulation. The increase in pulmonary capillary permeability may be explained by alpha adrenergic agonists, either directly or by causing the release of second messengers, or by

Table 24.5. Causes of neurogenic pulmonary edema

Major causes

Epileptic seizures

Cerebral hemorrhage

Blunt or penetrating head injury
(including neurosurgical procedures)

Minor causes

Guillain-Barré syndrome	Multiple sclerosis with medullary involvement
Nonhemorrhagic strokes	Trigeminal nerve block
Bulbar poliomyelitis	Vertebral artery ligation
Ruptured spinal AVM	Air embolism to cerebral vasculature
Brain tumors	Electroconvulsive therapy
Induction of general anesthesia	Colloid cyst
Hydrocephalus	Reye's syndrome
Bacterial meningitis	Cervical spinal cord injury

pulmonary microvascular injury due to the initial rapid increase in pulmonary vascular pressure

Treatment of NPE is similar to that of ARDS and is mostly supportive. Supplemental oxygen is usually required, and mechanical ventilation (either non-invasive via face mask or via endotracheal tube) is sometimes necessary. Maintenance of low cardiac filling pressures through fluid restriction and diuresis may decrease edema formati on, but care must be taken to avoid compromise of cardiac output and cerebral perfusion. Pulmonary artery catheterization may be useful in select patients .

PULMONARY CONTUSION

Background

Pulmonary contusion involves traumatic extravasation of blood into the parenchyma of the lung accompanied by substantial tissue disruption. Pulmonary contusion is common and should be anticipated in any patient who has sustained a significant, high-energy blunt chest trauma. Physical findings of chest wall trauma, especially the presence of fractures or a flail segment, increase the likelihood of having an underlying contusion.

Radiologic Features

Focal or diffuse homogeneous opacification on chest radiograph is the mainstay of diagnosis. The opacification is irregular and does not conform to segments or lobes within the lung.

- Pulmonary contusion is not always immediately apparent radiographically, and one third of patients have no evidence of the diagnosis on initial chest radiograph.
- The mean time to opacification is 6 hours but may take up to 24 hours.

CT scans of the chest provide a more accurate means of detecting and quantifying pulmonary contusion. Quantification of the percentage of involved lung parenchyma has important prognostic implications.

- In one study, 82% of patients with a contusion of at least 20% of the lung developed acute respiratory distress syndrome (ARDS) versus only 22% of patients with a contusion <20%. There is also an increased risk of developing pneumonia in cases of greater contusion.
- In another study, all patients with pulmonary contusions >28% of total volume required intubation, compared with no patients with <18% contusion.

Clinical Features

Patients may complain of dyspnea, decreased exercise tolerance, and chest pain on the side of the injury, symptoms are typically masked by other

Table 24.6. Hospital management of exacerbations of chronic obstructive pulmonary disease (COPD)

Assess severity of symptoms, blood gases, chest radiograph

Administer controlled oxygen therapy and repeat arterial blood gas measurement after 30 minutes.

Bronchodilators: Increase doses or frequency; Combine ß$_2$-agonists and anticholinergics; Use spacers or air-driven nebulizers.

Add oral or intravenous glucocorticosteroids

Consider antibiotics if there are signs of bacterial infection or for severe exacerbations

Consider noninvasive or invasive ventilation.

Monitor fluid balance and nutrition

Consider subcutaneous heparin or alternative deep vein thrombosis (DVT) prophylaxis

Identify and treat associated conditions (e.g., heart failure, arrhythmias)

injuries. Hemoptysis may occur in up to half the patients, and there may be mild fever. Most pulmonary contusions heal within 14 days without complications. Many patients complain of dyspnea, chest tightness, and thoracic pain even years later. Persistent abnormalities in pulmonary function tests and an increased alveolar-arterial oxygen gradient are not uncommon.

Management

The primary treatment of pulmonary contusion is supportive.

- Initial efforts should address associated injuries with placement of thoracostomy tubes to relieve hemopneumothorax and pain control for chest wall injuries.
- Supplemental oxygen, aggressive pulmonary toilet with coughing, deep breathing, suctioning as needed, and postural changes have been shown to improve outcomes.
- Prophylactic intubation without signs of impending respiratory failure is not indicated.
- Despite the belief that aggressive fluid resuscitation may exacerbate the hypoxia of pulmonary contusion, studies have failed to substantiate the claim.
- The use of steroids has been shown to be of no benefit and may impair bacterial clearance within the pulmonary tissue.
- Empiric use of antibiotics is not warranted and fosters development of resistant organisms. Antibiotic use should be reserved for treatment of

specific organisms with the diagnosis of a superimposed pneumonia.

MANAGEMENT OF AN ACUTE COPD EXACERBATION

Background

Chronic obstructive pulmonary disease (COPD) is currently the fifth leading cause of death in the world and its prevalence and mortality rates are predicted to continue to increase in the coming decades. The Global Initiative for Chronic Obstructive Lung Disease (GOLD) guidelines define COPD as a progressive disease state associated with an abnormal inflammatory response of the lungs to noxious particles or gases that is characterized by airflow limitation which is not fully reversible. *Exacerbations,* defined as a sustained worsening of the patient's condition from the stable state beyond normal day-to-day variations that is acute in onset and necessitates a change in regular medication, occur commonly and are a major cause of morbidity in these patients. In the intensive care setting, exacerbations may be precipitated by such factors as infection, aspiration, traumatic intubations, and medications; beta blockers may induce bronchospasm and sedatives or narcotics can decrease respiratory drive and lead to early hypercapnic respiratory failure. The management of severe exacerbations is summarized in Table 24.6 and discussed in more detail below.

Assessment

The assessment of severity of a COPD exacerbation should include the following:

- Clinical assessment: The patient should be assessed for evidence of respiratory distress. Accessory muscle use, inability to talk in complete sentences, audible wheeze, cyanosis, inability to clear central airway secretions, and a decreased level of consciousness are signs of severe respiratory distress requiring immediate intervention.
- Arterial blood gas measurement:
  - PaO_2 <60 mm Hg and/or SaO_2 <90% with or without $PaCO_2$ > 50 mm Hg when breathing room air indicates hypoxemic respiratory failure
  - PaO_2 <50 mm Hg, $PaCO_2$ >70 mm Hg, and pH <7.30 suggest a life-threatening episode of respiratory failure with respiratory acidosis that needs close monitoring and immediate intervention.
- Chest radiograph: A Chest radiograph should be obtained to identify complications such as pneumonia and alternative diagnosis that can mimic the symptoms of an exacerbation.
- Electrocardiograph: EKG aids in the early diagnosis of ischemia; right ventricular hypertrophy, and arrhythmias may also be identified. For instance, multifocal atrial tachycardia, defined as at least three differently configured P waves, persistent irregularity with intact baseline P waves, and an atrial rate >100 beats/min, is well recognized to occur in patients with severe COPD and it requires different treatment than other SVT arrhythmias.
- Other laboratory tests: Sputum Gram stain, culture, and sensitivity data may be useful in cases that do not respond to initial antibiotic treatment. Careful replacement of electrolytes is particularly important for respiratory muscle function and in the presence of cardiac arrhythmias. Theophylline levels should be obtained especially in patients with suspected toxicity and in those with potential drug interactions that may increase the level during acute therapy.

Management

- Controlled oxygen therapy: Oxygen therapy should be initiated during COPD exacerbations to maintain adequate levels of oxygenation (PaO_2 >60 mm Hg or SaO_2 >90%). Excessive oxygen in patients with chronic respiratory failure can cause an increase in PCO_2 and a decrease in pH resulting in an increase in ICP. Oxygen should, therefore, be administered to maintain SaO_2 between 90% and 92%, and arterial blood gases should be checked 30 minutes later to ensure adequate oxygenation without development of CO_2 retention or acidosis.
- Bronchodilator therapy: Short-acting, inhaled ß$_2$-agonists (e.g., albuterol, salbutamol) are usually the preferred bronchodilators for the treatment of COPD exacerbations. If a prompt response does not occur, anticholinergics (e.g., ipratropium bromide) should be added.
- For severe exacerbations, addition of a methylxanthine (theophylline, aminophylline) can be considered but is generally not recommended due to cardiovascular and GI side effects and requires close monitoring of serum drug levels. The target therapeutic level is typically 10–20 µg/mL. Levels may be inadvertently increased into the toxic range by certain drug interactions, particularly with macrolide and quinolone antibiotics, propofol, and amiodarone. Minor side effects such as tremor, insomnia, irritability, and gastrointestinal upset can occur with levels well below 20 µg/mL. More serious side effects, including vomiting, dysrhythmias, hypotension, and seizures, generally develop at higher blood levels. Older patients are especially susceptible to toxicity.
- Glucocorticosteroids: Oral or intravenous glucocorticosteroids are recommended. The exact dose that should be given is not known.
  - Many clinicians treat with the equivalent of 100–125 mg of methylprednisolone intravenously at presentation, followed by about one half this dose every 6 hours and transitioned to 30–40 mg of oral prednisone when the patient has shown some improvement.
  - Steroids should be continued for 10–14 days, often with a tapered dose.
  - Prolonged treatment beyond 2 weeks does not improve efficacy but increases the risk of side effects. Hyperglycemia is the main side effect of this treatment.
- Antibiotics: Antibiotics should be used in patients with severe exacerbations or in those patients who have more typical signs of infection

---

Table 24.7. Indications and contraindications for noninvasive positive pressure ventilation (NIPPV)

Indications

- Moderate to severe dyspnea with use of accessory muscles and paradoxical abdominal movement.
- Moderate to severe acidosis (pH <7.35) and hypercapnia (Pa_{CO_2} >45 mm Hg).
- Respiratory frequency >25 breaths/min

Contraindications

• Respiratory arrest	• Inability to protect airway
• Cardiovascular instability	• Inability to clear secretions
• Impaired mental status	• High aspiration risk
• Upper airway obstruction	• Active upper gastrointestinal bleeding
• Extreme obesity	• Facial surgery, trauma, or deformity

Table 24.8. Indications for invasive mechanical ventilation

- Severe dyspnea with use of accessory muscles and paradoxical abdominal motion
- Respiratory frequency >35 breaths/min
- Life-threatening hypoxemia (Pa_{O_2} < 40 mm Hg or Pa_{O_2}/Fi_{O_2} < 200 mm Hg)
- Severe acidosis (pH <7.25) and hypercapnia (Pa_{CO_2} >60 mm Hg) not responsive to NIPPV within 2 hours.
- Respiratory arrest
- Somnolence, impaired mental status, inability to clear central airway secretions
- Cardiovascular instability
- Other complications (metabolic abnormalities, sepsis, pneumonia, pulmonary embolism, etc.)
- Noninvasive positive pressure ventilation (NIPPV) failure (or contraindicated)

---

with increased sputum production and purulence. The choice of antibiotic should cover *Streptococcus pneumoniae*, *Haemophilus influenzae*, and *Moraxella. catarrhalis* in patients who develop exacerbations shortly after admission. Hospital acquired organisms will need to be covered in patients with more prolonged hospitalizations.

■ Noninvasive intermittent positive pressure ventilation (NIPPV): NIPPV in severe COPD exacerbations has been shown to decrease the need for invasive mechanical ventilation and possibly decrease mortality. NIPPV increases pH, reduces Pco_2, reduces the severity of breathlessness, and decreases the length of hospital stay. However, NIPPV is not appropriate for all patients. Patients who do not show improvement within the first 2 hours should be assessed for intubation and mechanical ventilation. Indications

and contraindication for NIPPV are shown in Table 24.7. Many neurologic conditions may preclude the safe use of NIPPV.

■ Intubation and mechanical ventilation: Patients who show acute respiratory failure not responsive to NIPPV within the first 2 hours, and those with life-threatening acid–base disorders and/or altered mental status despite aggressive pharmacologic therapy require endotracheal intubation and mechanical ventilation. Table 24.8 lists the indications for initiation of mechanical ventilation during a COPD exacerbation. The most common modes of ventilation are assist-control ventilation, and pressure support ventilation either alone or in combination with intermittent mandatory ventilation. The mode is usually determined by clinician preference.

▸ One must remember that these patients are prone to developing excessive intrinsic PEEP

(PEEP$_i$) due to airflow limitation and increased lung compliance resulting in a prolonged expiratory phase. This can be detrimental to cardiac output and contributes to barotrauma.

▸ To avoid this complication, one should limit the total mandatory minute ventilation to just above normal to compensate for increased dead space; in addition, the inspiratory time to expiratory time ratio must be kept at a level that allows for adequate expiratory time (i.e., 1:3). This can be accomplished by limiting the respiratory rate and tidal volume and delivering the breath quickly to optimize expiratory time .

STATUS ASTHMATICUS

Background

Asthma is a chronic inflammatory disorder of the airways associated with hyperresponsiveness and, reversible airflow limitation. All patients with asthma are at risk of having exacerbations characterized by a progressive increase in shortness of breath, cough, wheezing, or chest tightness, and by a decrease in expiratory airflow that can be quantified by the peak expiratory flow rate and FEV$_1$. Triggers of asthma exacerbations are many and include: exposure to indoor and outdoor allergens or air pollutants, respiratory tract infections, exercise, weather changes, foods, additives, drugs, and extreme emotions. Asthmatics are at risk for respiratory complications during and after surgery, including acute bronchospasm triggered by intubation.

Assessment

Status asthmaticus is a medical emergency that requires immediate diagnosis and treatment. The assessment of an asthma exacerbation aims at determining the severity of the attack as well as evaluating the response to therapy.

■ Medical history: A brief history should be obtained to establish the proper diagnosis, identify possible triggers, and to determine time of onset and severity of symptoms, current medications, prior hospitalizations and episodes of respiratory failure.
■ Physical examination: Patients should be examined looking for signs of severe respiratory

distress and impending respiratory failure. These include:

▸ Accessory muscle use
▸ Sternocleidomastoid or suprasternal retractions
▸ Respiratory rate >30 breaths/min, tachycardia >120 beats/min
▸ Pulsus paradoxus >12 mm Hg

■ Pulse oximetry and arterial blood gases (ABGs): Measurement of oxygen saturation is necessary in all patients with an asthma exacerbation to exclude hypoxemia. Continuous Spo$_2$ monitoring should be performed with the goal of treatment being to maintain Spo$_2$ >92%. ABG measurements are not routinely needed during an asthma exacerbation but should usually be obtained for severe exacerbations, especially if Spo$_2$ remains low despite initiation of therapy and supplemental oxygen.

▸ Hypoxemia is usually responsive to supplemental oxygen because it is due to ventilation–perfusion inequality.
▸ If the hypoxemia is not readily responsive to supplemental oxygen then other causes, such as pneumonia, pneumothorax, or PE need to be considered.
▸ Some degree of hypoxemia and a respiratory alkalosis is commonly seen.
▸ With severe and prolonged exacerbations, the Pco$_2$ begins to rise as respiratory muscle fatigue sets in. An elevated or even normal Pco$_2$ in the midst of a severe asthma attack is an ominous sign, with an increased risk of respiratory failure.

■ Chest radiograph: In the absence of another underlying condition, the chest radiograph is usually normal or demonstrates only air-trapping during an acute asthma exacerbation. A radiograph is indicated in patients who present with signs of pneumothorax (pleuritic chest pain, mediastinal crunch, subcutaneous emphysema, cardiovascular instability, or asymmetric breath sounds) or signs of pneumonia (fever, sputum production, leukocytosis), or in a patient with a poor response to supplemental oxygen or initial asthma therapy.

Management

■ Oxygen: Hypoxemia is produced by V/Q mismatch and is easily correctable with modest amounts of supplemental oxygen. As in COPD, high concentrations of oxygen can lead to regional release of hypoxic pulmonary vasoconstriction and lead to an increase in P_{CO_2}, particularly when the P_{CO_2} before oxygen therapy is >40 mm Hg.

- Oxygen supplementation should therefore be administered in concentrations adequate enough to maintain S_{PO_2} >92%.
- Hyperoxia has *not* been shown to offer any additional benefits and may be harmful to some patients.
- There is limited evidence that humidification of the inspired oxygen may alleviate bronchoconstriction triggered by airway dehydration during an asthma attack.

- Bronchodilators: Short-acting inhaled ß$_2$-agonists (albuterol, salbutamol) are the mainstay of treatment for acute asthma.
  - The onset of action is 5 minutes, and their side effects are well tolerated.
  - Studies indicate that inhalation via metered-dose inhalers (MDI) with spacer (four puffs at 10-minute intervals) is at least as efficacious as administration of conventional doses (2.5 mg every 20 minutes) with a jet nebulizer. High doses can be administered more quickly with the MDI plus spacer.
  - Side effects are dose dependent and are more pronounced with oral and IV routes of administration than with inhalation delivery methods. The principal side effects include tachycardia, tachyarrhythmia, tremor, and hypokalemia.
  - Uncommon cases of *lactic acidosis* have been reported with high doses or continuous administration of beta agonists, and in patients with severe asthma exacerbations as well. Lactic acidosis should be investigated when metabolic acidosis also develops in the patient with an acute asthma exacerbation. This condition may worsen dyspnea and would warrant temporary discontinuation of ß$_2$-agonists rather than an increase in dose to treat the worsening symptoms.

Inhaled anticholinergics (ipratropium bromide) increase airway vagal tone. They are inferior to ß$_2$-agonists for the treatment of acute asthma, but they provide additional benefit when used in conjunction with them.

- Ipratropium bromide should be administered in combination with ß$_2$-agonists in doses of four puffs (80 μg) every 10 minutes by MDI with spacer or 500 μg nebulized every 20 minutes.
- One should be careful not to expose the eye(s) to these anticholinergic agents because they can cause pupillary dilation that may be misinterpreted as a sign of an acute neurologic event and lead to unnecessary testing.

- Corticosteroids: Systemic corticosteroids are effective in reducing the airway inflammation associated with asthma exacerbations.
  - They should be administered early but require 6–24 hours to improve pulmonary function.
  - IV and oral routes appear to have equivalent efficacy although the onset of action may be slightly less with the IV route.
  - The optimal dose of corticosteroids remains controversial. Methylprednisolone is commonly used initially in a dose of 1–2 mg/kg every 6 hours.
  - The side effects of high doses include hypokalemia, hyperglycemia, acute central nervous system alterations, hypertension, and peripheral edema.
  - Oral corticosteroids in a dose equivalent to 40–60 mg prednisone or prednisolone per day for a period of 7–14 days is effective in reducing the number of relapses following an acute asthma attack.

- Noninvasive positive pressure ventilation (NIPPV): The use of NIPPV in patients with acute asthma improves lung function, reduces P_{CO_2}, alleviates dyspnea and may avoid the need for intubation in some patients. NIPPV is warranted in patients at high risk for respiratory failure due to progressive fatigue.
  - Initial settings should be an expiratory positive airway pressure (EPAP) of 3–5 cm H$_2$O and an inspiratory pressure (IPAP) of 5–7 cm H$_2$O.
  - IPAP can be gradually increased (by 2 cm H$_2$O every 15 minutes to a maximum of 25 cm H$_2$O), the goal being to reduce respiratory rate below 25 breaths/min.
  - Close monitoring is crucial when initiating NIPPV.
  - If patients do not rapidly improve, are of marginal status, or cannot tolerate NIPPV, endotracheal intubation should not be delayed.

■ Intubation and ventilator strategies: When patients deteriorate despite pharmacologic intervention, with or without NIPPV, intubation should be performed.

▸ Nasal intubation should be avoided because of the increased risk of sinusitis in asthmatics and because of the increased incidence of nasal polyps.

▸ The largest possible endotracheal tube should be used to decrease the amount of additional resistance added by the tube. Also, it is common for asthmatic patients to develop large mucus plugs, which are more likely to obstruct small endotracheal tubes.

After intubation with Ambu-bag ventilation and initiation of mechanical ventilation, hypotension commonly occurs and is related to the decrease in systemic venous return caused by worsening hyperinflation and intrinsic PEEP. In this situation, a brief disconnection from the ventilator (30–60 seconds with close monitoring of SpO_2) will often lead to an increase in blood pressure. Ventilation should then be resumed with lower tidal volume and respiratory rate, and intravenous normal saline should be administered to increase intravascular volume. If these measures are not effective in improving blood pressure, one must suspect tension pneumothorax.

The primary focus of the mechanical ventilation strategy must be to avoid excessive airway pressure and minimize lung hyperinflation. This is done by allowing adequate time to exhale and by continued treatment of airflow obstruction.

▸ Expiratory time can be maximized by adjusting the respiratory rate and tidal volume to decrease minute ventilation and by decreasing inspiratory time by increasing inspiratory flow rate and using a square flow wave form.

▸ Appropriate initial settings are a tidal volume between 5 and 7 mL/kg and a respiratory rate of 11 to 14 breaths/min to achieve a minute ventilation between 6 and 8 L/min, combined with an inspiratory flow rate of 60–80 L/min.

▸ External PEEP should not be used. The level of PEEPi is difficult to measure accurately.

▸ The airway *plateau* pressure, P_{plat}, is likely the best and most practical variable for the monitoring of lung hyperinflation, with a reasonable target being to maintain end-inspiratory pressures <30 cm H_2O. High *peak* airway pressures are acceptable.

This strategy may result in hypoventilation and hypercapnia. This is often required to avoid hyperinflation. This appears to be well tolerated as long as $PaCO_2$ does not exceed 90 mm Hg and acute increases in $PaCO_2$ are avoided.

▸ It is particularly important to avoid acute hypercapnia in the neurocritical care setting because it may cause an increase in cerebral blood flow and further elevate ICP.

▸ To reduce hypercapnia, CO_2 production should be maximally reduced by the use of sedation, analgesia, and antipyretics.

▸ If these measures are insufficient, muscle relaxants must be considered.

▸ Although not supported by strong clinical data, blood alkalinization with a slow infusion of sodium bicarbonate may reduce the risk of increasing the ICP.

■ Sedatives and neuromuscular blockers: The ventilator settings described above tend not to be tolerated by the awake and alert patient, and high levels of sedation are often required. Midazolam, lorazepam, and propofol are commonly used.

▸ Propofol may be preferred because of its bronchodilating action but commonly causes hypotension, particularly in hypovolemic patients. Higher doses of propofol should be used with caution because of side effects that include the "Propofol infusion syndrome" and pancreatitis.

▸ Ketamine also has a favorable bronchodilating effect. However, this agent can stimulate tracheobronchial secretion and increase ICP and therefore has limited usefulness in the neurocritical care unit.

Concurrent administration of an opiate will alleviate the pain associated with intubation, may help suppress the ventilatory drive, and often decreases the dose of sedative needed. Synthetic opioids (e.g., fentanyl) are preferred over the natural opioid morphine because the latter can cause allergic reactions and bronchoconstriction. Often large doses and frequently multiple sedatives are necessary.

Despite the use of deep sedation, patient-ventilator asynchrony can persist that sometimes necessitates the use of neuromuscular-blocking agents (NMBA). Some nondepolarizing relaxants (atracurium, mivacurium, and tubocurarine, metacurium) are more commonly associated with histamine release, occasionally causing serious hypotension, tachycardia, and bronchospasm. The preferred paralytic agents are cisatracurium, pancuronium, and vecuronium.

However, NMBA have been implicated in an increased incidence of postparalytic myopathy in patients with asthma undergoing mechanical ventilation and should be avoided whenever possible.

▸ When NMBA must be used, they should be given as intermittent intravenous boluses rather than as a continuous infusion to reduce the dose and duration of administration.

▸ The decision to repeat a dose should only be made if patient-ventilator asynchrony reappears and cannot be suppressed by increasing the dose of sedative or opioid.

■ Magnesium sulfate: By inhibiting smooth-muscle cell calcium channels, magnesium blocks muscle contraction and therefore may be useful in the treatment of acute asthma. Recent studies have shown that administration of magnesium sulfate to nonintubated patients in an emergency department by aerosol (250 mmol/L) or IV (2 g in 30 minutes) had a powerful bronchodilating effect when used as an adjunct to aerosolized beta-agonists.

▸ Given the safety and low cost, it seems reasonable to give 2 g IV every 30 minutes, with a maximum cumulative dose of 10 g, in cases of refractory acute severe asthma.

■ Heliox: Heliox is a gas mixture of helium and oxygen with a lower density and higher viscosity than air that reduces turbulent airflow. This decreases airway resistance and allows for improved deposition of aerosolized bronchodilators. Studies have not demonstrated a significant benefit over standard therapy and do not support the role of Heliox in the initial treatment of acute asthma.

▸ It may be tried in very severe cases that are not rapidly responding to conventional treatment.

▸ Heliox is usually administered in a helium-to-oxygen ratio of 70:30 or 80:20.

▸ Increasing the percentage of oxygen diminishes the beneficial effect of low density gas inhalation, while increasing the amount of helium can worsen alveolar hypoxia.

■ Antibiotics: In the majority of cases antibiotics are not required in the treatment of acute asthma. They are indicated for patients with fever, sputum containing polymorphonuclear leukocytes, and clinical findings of pneumonia or acute sinusitis.

REFERENCES

Acute Respiratory Distress Syndrome Network. Ventilation with lower tidal volumes as compared with traditional tidal volumes for acute lung injury and the acute respiratory distress syndrome. *N Engl J Med.* 2000;**342**(18):1301–8.

Amato M, Barbas C, Medeiros D, et al. Effect of a protective-ventilation strategy on mortality in the acute respiratory distress syndrome. *N Engl J Med.* 1998;**338**(6): 347–54.

Ashbaugh D, Bigelow D, Petty T, Levine B. Acute respiratory distress in adults. *Lancet.* 1967; **2**(7511):319–23.

Bernard GR, Artigas A, Brigham K, et al. The American-European Consensus Conference on ARDS. Definitions, mechanisms, relevant outcomes, and clinical trial coordination. *Am J Respir Crit Care Med.* 1994;**149**: 818–24.

Brower RG, Lanken PN, MacIntyre N, et al. National Heart Lung and Blood Institute ARDS Clinical Trials Network: higher versus lower positive end-expiratory pressures in patients with the acute respiratory distress syndrome. *N Engl J Med.* 2004;**351**:327–36.

Büller HR, Agnelli G, Hull RD, et al. Antithrombotic therapy for venous thromboembolic disease; the seventh ACCP conference on antithrombotic and thrombolytic therapy. *Chest.* 2004;**126**:401S–428S.

Caricato A, Conti G, Cella CF, et al. Effect of PEEP on the intracranial system of patients with head injury and subarachnoid hemorrhage: the role of respiratory system compliance. *J Trauma.* 2005;**58**:571–6.

Cooper KR, Boswell PA, Choi SC. Safe use of PEEP in patients with severe head injury. *J Neurosurg.* 1985;**63**:552–5.

Davidson BL, Tomkowske WZ. Management of pulmonary embolism in 2005. *Dis Mon.* 2005;**51**:116–123.

Fedullo PF, Tapson VF. The evaluation of suspected pulmonary embolism. *N Engl J Med.* 2003;**349**:1247–56.

Fontes RB, Aguiar PH, Zanetti MV, et al. Acute neurogenic pulmonary edema: case reports and literature review. *J Neurosurg Anesthesiol.* 2003;**15**(2):144–50.

Frost EZ. Effects of positive end-expiratory pressure on intracranial pressure and compliance in brain-injured patients. *J Neurosurg.* 1977;**47**:195–200.

Geerts WH, Pineo GF, Heit JA, et al. Prevention of venous thromboembolism: the seventh ACCP conference on antithrombotic and thrombolytic therapy. *Chest.* 2004;**126**:338S–400S.

Leone M, Albanese J, Roussear S, et al. Pulmonary contusion in severe head trauma patients: impact on gas exchange and outcome. *Chest.* 2003;**124**(6):2261–6.

Lowe GJ, Ferguson ND. Lung-protective ventilation in neurosurgical patients. *Curr Opin Crit Care.* 2006;**12**:3–**7**.

Merli G. Diagnostic assessment of deep vein thrombosis and pulmonary embolism. *Am J Med.* 2005;**118**:3S–12S.

Murray JF, Matthay MA, Luce JM, et al. An expanded definition of the adult respiratory distress syndrome. *Am Rev Respir Dis.* 1988;**138**:720–3.

National Heart, Lung, and Blood Institute Acute Respiratory Distress Syndrome (ARDS) Clinical Trials Network. Comparison of two fluid-management strategies in acute lung injury. *N Engl J Med.* 2006;**354** (24):2564–75.

Oddo M, Feihl R, Sehaller MD, et al. Management of mechanical ventilation in acute severe asthma: practical aspects. *Int Care Med.* 2006;**32**:501–10.

Pauwels RA, Buist AS, Calverley PM, et al. Global strategy for the diagnosis, management, and prevention of chronic obstructive pulmonary disease. NHLBI/WHO Global Initiative for Chronic Obstructive Lung Disease (GOLD) Workshop summary. *Am J Respir Crit Care Med.* 2001;**163**(5):1256–76.

Perl M, Gebhard F, Bruckner UB, et al. Pulmonary contusion causes impairment of macrophage and lymphocyte immune functions and increases mortality associated with a subsequent septic challenge. *Crit Care Med.* 2005;**33**(6):1351–8.

Reinprecht A, Greher M, Wolfsberger S, et al. Prone position in subarachnoid hemorrhage patients with acute respiratory distress syndrome: effects on cerebral tissue oxygenation and intracranial pressure. *Crit Care Med.* 2003;**31**:1831–8.

Rodrigo GJ, Rodrigo C, Hall JB. Acute asthma in adults: a review. *Chest.* 2004;**125**:1081–1102.

Schumaker GL, Epstein SK. Managing acute respiratory failure during exacerbation of chronic obstructive pulmonary disease. *Respir Care.* 2004;**49**(7):766–82.

Shapiro JM. Intensive care management of status asthmaticus. *Chest* 2001;**120**:1439–41.

Simon, RP. Neurogenic pulmonary edema. *Neurol Clin.* 1993;**11**(2):309–23.

Singer P, Theilla M, Fisher H, et al. Benefit of an enteral diet enriched with eicosapentainoic acid and gamma-linolenic acid in ventilated patients with acute lung injury. *Crit Care Med.* 2006;**34**(4):1033–8.

Wanek S, Mayberry JC. Blunt thoracic trauma: flail chest, pulmonary contusion, and blast injury. *Crit Care Clin.* 2004;**20**:71–81.

Ware L, Matthay M. The acute respiratory distress syndrome. *N Engl J Med.* 2000;**342**(18):1334–49.

25 A Cardiology Consult

James Kleczka, MD, Timothy Woods, MD, and Lee Biblo, MD

ACUTE CORONARY SYNDROMES

Acute coronary syndromes are not uncommon in the neuro-intensive care unit (NICU). These syndromes include unstable angina, non-ST segment elevation myocardial infarction (NSTEMI), and ST segment elevation myocardial infarction (STEMI). The mechanism underlying the acute ischemic episode remains the key to effective therapy.

Ischemia can be the result of plaque rupture, which requires therapies directed at reperfusion. Ischemia can also result from the increased myocardial demand in the setting of fixed stable coronary disease. Hypertension, sepsis, blood loss, and pain can each increase myocardial workload precipitating ischemia in the setting of stable coronary disease.

Traditional guideline directed management strategies of cardiac ischemia in a NICU setting require a risk benefit analysis due to comorbid conditions. Patients with recent head trauma, stroke, or operative procedures may require conservative treatment due to neurologic priorities. Efforts to treat plaque rupture through reperfusion techniques can cause significant morbidity in the NICU. Efforts to decrease myocardial workload usually cause less morbidity but blood pressure or heart rate lowering strategies can be challenging in the NICU.

Unstable Angina and NSTEMI

Unstable angina and NSTEMI are usually caused by atherosclerotic coronary disease. Disruption of atherosclerotic plaque leads to formation of thrombus and partial or transient occlusion of an epicardial coronary vessel. Chest pain as a result of unstable angina or NSTEMI is due to an imbalance between myocardial oxygen supply and demand. The vast majority of cases are due to inadequate supply due to coronary atherosclerosis. The differential is usually acute plaque rupture leading to inadequate supply versus increased myocardial demand due to extrinsic stressors such as pain, extreme hypertension, fever, sepsis, or blood loss in the setting of fixed coronary disease.

DIAGNOSTIC CONSIDERATIONS

- Patient's symptoms are often atypical and may include neck, jaw, arm, or epigastric pain or even unexplained dyspnea.
- When a patient develops symptoms, decisions need to be made quickly.
- Several initial tests should be performed, including an evaluation to exclude secondary causes that can increase myocardial oxygen demand or decrease oxygen supply such as severe aortic valve stenosis, infection, fever, blood loss, tachycardia, hypoxia, hyperthyroidism, and sympathomimetic use (e.g., cocaine).
- A 12-lead electrocardiogram (EKG) should be obtained immediately.
  - ▸ Dynamic EKG changes are highly predictive of significant obstructive coronary artery disease.
  - ▸ Most commonly transient ST-segment depression or deep, symmetric T-wave inversion will occur during episodes of ischemic chest pain.
- Biochemical markers indicate myocardial necrosis.
  - ▸ Creatine kinase (CK-MB) is elevated with myocardial necrosis, but may also be elevated in

341

severe skeletal muscle injury. CK-MB levels begin to rise within 4 hours after cell damage and remain elevated for 2 days.

▷ Cardiac troponins have greater sensitivity and specificity than CK-MB for detecting myocardial infarction and begin to rise within 4 hours of the initial event and remain elevated for 2 weeks.

THERAPEUTIC CONSIDERATIONS

If the EKG or biochemical markers suggest ischemia, management decisions must weigh the benefits of addressing the cardiac substrate versus the risks that this management strategy will have to the neurologic substrate.

■ All patients with suspected cardiac chest pain should be placed on telemetry monitoring to evaluate for malignant arrhythmias associated with acute coronary syndromes.

■ Beta-blockers lower heart rate, reduce contractility, and reduce blood pressure, leading to a decrease in myocardial oxygen demand.

▷ These drugs are contraindicated in hypotension, severe bradycardia, or severe dynamic bronchoconstriction.

▷ Intravenous metoprolol, esmolol, or propranolol can be used in unstable patients, while oral formulations can be given in lower risk settings. Large studies have shown a significant mortality reduction with the use of beta-blockers in acute coronary syndromes. These studies excluded patients with acute brain injuries; thus caution should be exercised with their use in these settings. Nonetheless, beta-blocker use is recommended in all patients with acute coronary syndromes unless contraindicated.

If acute plaque rupture and thrombus formation are suspected, adequate antiplatelet and antithrombotic therapy should be considered. This decision requires a rapid multidisciplinary discussion weighing risks and benefits.

■ Aspirin is indicated in patients with acute coronary syndromes. If aspirin cannot be given due to allergy or intolerance, other antiplatelet agents such as clopidogrel should be given.

■ Studies have also shown reduced mortality when acute coronary syndrome patients are given unfractionated or low molecular weight heparin.

■ Glycoprotein IIb/IIIa inhibitors are indicated in those with unstable angina or NSTEMI who have ongoing symptoms or other high-risk characteristics such as increasing cardiac enzymes or worsening EKG changes.

■ Each of these strategies may not be appropriate in an acutely unstable neurologic syndrome; however, a discussion must ensue regarding consideration of each of these agents in each patient with an acute coronary syndrome.

Lipid-lowering agents should also be started in patients with suspected acute coronary syndromes. Preliminary data suggest the acute administration of statins is beneficial in patients with acute coronary syndromes.

Nitrates can be used to control symptoms. These agents have been studied in various settings and do not improve mortality.

■ Patients with ongoing cardiac chest pain are often started on intravenous nitroglycerin with dose titration until symptoms are relieved.

■ Morphine can be used for pain relief in those with continued symptoms.

■ An adverse reaction to both of these drugs is hypotension, which can worsen myocardial and neurologic perfusion. Therefore blood pressure management must be exquisite.

In patients with anginal symptoms but without cardiac enzyme elevations, medical management for several days seems prudent until the neurologic substrate is stable. In patients with cardiac enzyme elevations, a multidisciplinary discussion must ensue relative to the benefits and risks of an invasive strategy. Assuming coronary disease is found, the precatheterization multidisciplinary discussion must include how to proceed from that point. Therapeutic decisions including anticipated bleeding risks from necessary anticoagulation strategies for specific coronary interventions must be well delineated before entering the heart laboratory.

ST Elevation Myocardial Infarction

The key to treating STEMI is early recognition with reperfusion therapy to reestablish blood flow. Timely reperfusion decreases myocardial necrosis and reduces morbidity and mortality. The pathophysiologic substrate of a STEMI is the vulnerable plaque. When the fibrous cap ruptures an abrupt prothrombotic process ensues, and in the case of a STEMI, an occlusive thrombus results. The vulnerable plaque is typically a nonobstructive lesion and is therefore asymptomatic (and many times not recognized) before rupture.

DIAGNOSTIC CONSIDERATIONS

The patient with a STEMI experiences a pain syndrome similar to acute coronary syndrome (ACS). The chest pain is often associated with difficulty breathing, nausea, emesis, and diaphoresis.

- Problems arise when patients experience atypical symptoms not readily recognized as cardiac in etiology.
- Some patients will not experience any chest pain, but manifest only shortness of breath, or pain located in other areas such as the neck, jaw, or epigastric region.
- Consideration should also be given to aortic dissection as an etiology of the patient's symptoms, as this also represents a medical emergency. If dissection extends into the aortic root, the ostium of the right coronary artery is often compromised, thereby presenting as an inferior wall infarct.

The physical examination should focus on the stability of vital signs and clinical signs of hypoperfusion, evidence of heart failure (jugular venous distention, crackles on lung exam, left ventricular heave), assessment of heart murmurs or gallops, evidence of cerebrovascular disease (acute or chronic), and examination of peripheral pulses.

A 12-lead EKG should be performed immediately. When ST-segment elevation is present in multiple contiguous leads, the patient will benefit from reperfusion therapy, as opposed to those with unstable angina and NSTEMI, in whom reperfusion therapy is not acutely indicated.

Cardiac enzymes, a complete blood count, a basic metabolic panel, and a coagulation panel should be obtained.

THERAPEUTIC CONSIDERATIONS

In terms of medical therapy, aspirin at a dose of 162–325 mg should be given to all patients. Beta-blockers should be started unless a contraindication exists. Unfractionated heparin has also been shown to reduce mortality in STEMI regardless of which reperfusion therapy is utilized. Data also exist to support the use of statins, regardless of initial lipid levels. Each of these therapies may have contraindications in acute neurologic states. Again, a multidisciplinary discussion must ensue regarding therapeutic strategies.

Therapy to quickly and completely reestablish blood flow should be instituted if no contraindications exist with either the administration of fibrinolytic agents or coronary angiography with percutaneous intervention. Acute reperfusion therapy is often the most complex of the therapeutic decisions. Restoration of coronary perfusion is the key to improved mortality. The benefits of this strategy must be weighed against the potential risks in the setting of the acute neurologic process. In some instances, supportive care alone of the acute STEMI is appropriate. Acute echocardiography may give clinicians a better view of the cardiac future without reperfusion allowing more data to determine better a risk:benefit analysis of therapies.

STEMI engenders many life-threatening problems, including hypotension, pulmonary vascular congestion, or cardiogenic shock.

- Ventricular fibrillation is most common in the first 4 hours after symptoms and remains an important cause of mortality for the first 24 hours.
- Polymorphic ventricular tachycardia usually signals ongoing coronary ischemia. Many of these episodes are nonsustained (lasting <30 seconds).
- Significant bradycardia associated with inferior infarcts is due to increased vagal tone and can be treated with atropine.
- Heart block due to anterior wall infarctions requires acute temporary pacing.
- Acute stroke is usually associated with large myocardial infarcts and is embolic in nature.

Conclusions

Acute coronary syndromes outside the hospital are usually due to plaque rupture. In the ICU setting, numerous issues may lead to an increase in myocardial oxygen demand and despite stable coronary disease can result in an acute coronary syndrome without plaque rupture. When plaque rupture is present, the usual reperfusion strategies employed may be contraindicated in the NICU due to neurologic priorities. A multidisciplinary approach is essential to ensure optimal outcomes in these complex patients.

HEART FAILURE

Heart failure is the leading diagnosis in hospitalized patients in the United States. Systolic and diastolic heart dysfunctions are common and require different approaches. Further, acute neurologic disease can result in the release of catecholamines. Catecholamine excess can cause coronary vasospasm, myocardial dysfunction, and arrhythmias that can complicate heart failure.

Clinical Manifestation

- Patients complain of cough, dyspnea, orthopnea, paroxysmal nocturnal dyspnea, and chest discomfort.
- Physical examination can reveal tachypnea, tachycardia, and hypoxemia. Lungs examination can reveal basilar crackles.
- Cardiac auscultation may reveal an S3, S4, or both and a new or changed murmur.
- Elevated jugular venous pressure and peripheral edema can reflect elevated right-sided filling pressures.

Ancillary Studies

Laboratory data can confirm the diagnosis, evaluate the cause of decompensation and monitor for complications.

- Routine chemistries identify renal dysfunction and electrolyte abnormalities.
- A complete blood count can show anemia or suggest infection that may have precipitated the event.
- Cardiac enzymes (troponin and CK-MB) can be measured to rule out acute ischemia.
- B-type natriuretic peptide (BNP) can supplement the clinical diagnosis and is a strong predictor of cardiac prognosis.

The electrocardiogram may show myocardial ischemia, although patients with subarachnoid (SAH) and intracranial (ICH) hemorrhage may show similar changes of T-wave inversion, ST-segment elevation/depression, and Q-T interval prolongation.

Atrial fibrillation diagnosed by EKG may precipitate an acute decompensation of heart failure. A chest radiograph usually shows cardiomegaly and bilateral interstitial markings. Bilateral perihilar alveolar edema may give the butterfly appearance.

Transthoracic echocardiography can be used to evaluate left ventricular systolic and diastolic function, valvular abnormalities, and the cardiac source of embolism in patients with mural thrombus. Patients with ICH and SAH may demonstrate localized left ventricular apical hypokinesis or a ako-tsubo cardiomyopathy. This entity is frequently seen in conditions of extreme stress.

Differential Diagnosis

- Neurogenic pulmonary edema (NPE) is a rapid development of pulmonary edema after acute central nervous system (CNS) injury (epileptic seizures, head injury, cerebral hemorrhage) with normal left ventricular function.
- Aspiration pneumonia can occur in this setting of altered mentation and can be sometimes difficult to differentiate from heart failure; a serum BNP level may be very useful here .

Treatment

The immediate goals of treatment are to improve symptoms, congestion, and low-output symptoms. Possible precipitating comorbidities, both cardiac and noncardiac, such as atrial fibrillation, myocardial ischemia, valvular disease, hypertension, anemia, infection, and thyroid disease should be excluded and if present treated aggressively.

- Patients should receive supplemental oxygen to maintain arterial oxygen saturation above 90%.
- Noninvasive positive pressure ventilation can be used in patients with respiratory failure.
- Loop diuretics used intravenously are recommended to treat fluid overload.
  - ▹ Diuresis occurs 30 minutes after the administration.
  - ▹ Dose may be increased to produce a rate of diuresis sufficient to achieve optimal volume status.
  - ▹ In cases of persistent congestion, the loop diuretic can be administered as a continuous infusion.

- A second diuretic (metolazone or spironolactone) can be added in select situations.
- Strict intake and output, daily weights should be used to monitor the diuresis.
- Electrolyte abnormalities, renal dysfunction, and hypotension can result from diuresis.
- Ultrafiltration can be considered in patients refractory to the diuretics.
- Morphine can be used in patients with pulmonary edema and causes venodilation, mild arterial dilatation with reduction in dyspnea and anxiety.
- Intravenous vasodilators such as nitroglycerin and nitroprusside can be used in the absence of hypotension to treat congestive symptoms by decreasing left ventricular preload and afterload. Close monitoring of the blood pressure during therapy is warranted, especially in stroke patients. Nesiritide, recombinant human BNP, acts as vasodilator, diuretic and natriuretic and can be used for patients with acute decompensation who remain symptomatic despite intravenous loop diuretics. Hemodynamics, urine output, and renal function should be closely monitored during therapy.

Ionotropes (milrinone or dobutamine) may be used for symptom relief in patients with advanced heart failure (left ventricle dilatation with reduced ejection fraction) and decreased peripheral perfusion or target organ dysfunction. Cardiac rhythm and arterial blood pressure should be monitored continuously during inotropic therapy.

Intra-aortic balloon pump support can be considered as a temporizing measure in certain clinical scenarios.

Angiotensin-converting enzyme (ACE) inhibitors are not recommended in decompensated patients with hypotension, acute renal failure, and hyperkalemia. ACE inhibitors play an important role after the stabilization of the acute stage and are the mainstay of therapy for chronic heart failure.

Beta-blocking agents can usually be continued at home doses. In patients with primarily diastolic dysfunction – hyperdynamic left ventricle (LV) with a small cavity by echocardiography – beta-blockers and fluid resuscitation can reverse the symptoms of heart failure completely,

After the resolution of acute decompensated state, the patient can be transitioned to oral diuretics. Discharge plan should include optimizing medication (ACE inhibitors, beta-blockers), dietary instructions, weight monitoring at home, smoking cessation counseling, and referral to a disease management program.

ATRIAL FIBRILLATION

Atrial fibrillation occurs in 2–4% of the population in the United States. In the young adult, atrial fibrillation is uncommon, but the incidence doubles each decade of life such that atrial fibrillation is found in 13–15% of those older than age 80. Atrial fibrillation is associated with a high incidence of stroke, estimated at 5–6% per year. In the neurosurgic unit, atrial fibrillation is commonly seen in two clinical scenarios: (1) as the cause of a major embolic stroke or (2) as a complicating hemodynamic issue in a critically ill neurologic patient.

Etiology

The atria of most patients with atrial fibrillation have structural abnormalities, ranging from fibrosis to dilatation. Common cardiac syndromes such as hypertension, valve disorders, coronary disease, and ventricular dysfunction enhance changes in atrial tissue refractoriness that can support atrial fibrillation. In addition, several noncardiac conditions are associated with atrial fibrillation:

- Hyperthyroidism leads to a hyperadrenergic state.
- Holiday heart refers to atrial fibrillation that occurs 24 hours after an episode of binge drinking.
- Pulmonary diseases including pneumonia, pulmonary emboli, chronic lung diseases, and acute respiratory failure likely via hypoxia can lead to changes in atrial tissue refractoriness that may facilitate atrial fibrillation.

Clinical Manifestations

Patients with atrial fibrillation can present with a variety of symptoms, although many are asymptomatic or minimally symptomatic. In a single patient with paroxysmal atrial fibrillation, approximately two thirds of the episodes are asymptomatic. During atrial fibrillation, stasis can lead to thrombus formation in the left atrial appendage. The stroke risk in nonvalvular atrial fibrillation is about

6% per year. In a patient with stroke, the absence of cardiac symptoms does not exclude the possibility of an embolic stroke secondary to "asymptomatic" paroxysmal atrial fibrillation.

The loss of the atrial contraction during atrial fibrillation can lead to a variety of hemodynamic issues, particularly in patients with diastolic heart disease. Patients with diastolic heart disease (left ventricular hypertrophy, aortic stenosis, cardiac amyloid, etc.) can decompensate with the onset of atrial fibrillation as these conditions are very preload dependent. Thus, the onset of atrial fibrillation in a critically ill neurologic patient can facilitate a downward hemodynamic cascade.

Diagnosis

■ All patients with atrial fibrillation require a thorough history and physical examination. Classically, the heart beat is irregularly irregular. The pulse will vary in intensity due to the changes in preload and in the diastolic interval. An EKG documents no discrete atrial electrical activity.
■ An echocardiogram can determine the presence of valvular disease or LV dysfunction.
■ Laboratory work should include thyroid-stimulating hormone (TSH) to exclude hyperthyroidism.

Acute Treatment

The patient presenting with a stroke in the context of atrial fibrillation needs prompt evaluation to facilitate the best neurologic outcome. The assumption that the stroke is embolic in the setting of atrial fibrillation is logical but a definitive etiology is often difficult to make given the overlap of comorbidities in most patients with atrial fibrillation. Regardless, prompt imaging in the setting of an in-hospital care pathway is usually necessary to start thrombolytic therapy within the guideline-driven 3-hour window. This decision algorithm is discussed extensively elsewhere in the text.

A common scenario is the management of new onset or chronic atrial fibrillation in the context of an acute neurologic syndrome. The acute treatment is dictated by the clinical condition of the patient. The loss of atrial systole and the shortening of the diastole can lead to a decrease in cardiac output.

■ If the patient is hemodynamically unstable, acute cardioversion is often necessary.
■ In the absence of acute hemodynamic compromise, control of the rapid ventricular response is initially indicated. This strategy is called rate control.

Administration of an IV calcium channel blocker is commonly used for the acute control of the rapid ventricular response during atrial fibrillation.

■ IV diltiazem often successfully controls the ventricular response in atrial fibrillation.
■ The average time to a therapeutic response is <7 minutes from the beginning of the IV infusion.
■ Diltiazem may be associated with hypotension; however, usually blood pressure improves with the control of the rapid ventricular response.

Esmolol, an ultra fast acting beta-blocker, has also been used to acutely control the rapid ventricular response.

Classically, digoxin has been used acutely to control the rapid ventricular response. However, the therapeutic use of digoxin is inconsistent and often ineffective. The median time until adequate control of the ventricular response is 11.6 hours. Thus, the use of digoxin for the acute control of ventricular response in atrial fibrillation has been relegated to a secondary position. Digoxin may have a role as an adjunct to other AV node blocking agents, especially in patients with concomitant congestive heart failure.

Long-Term Treatment

When the patient's rapid ventricular response has been controlled, a decision must be made regarding the restoration of sinus rhythm versus simply continuing to control the ventricular response. The decision whether or not to cardiovert a patient with atrial fibrillation is complicated. If the onset of atrial fibrillation can be estimated at <48 hours, the usual clinical practice is to perform the cardioversion independent of the state of anticoagulation. This recommendation is based on the assumption that a thrombus usually takes >48 hours to form.

In patients with paroxysmal atrial fibrillation, asymptomatic episodes occur more frequently than symptomatic episodes. Thus, determining the onset of atrial fibrillation by using the patient's appreciation of symptoms may be hazardous. If the onset of atrial fibrillation cannot be determined, or is >48 hours, there are two strategies for attempting cardioversion to sinus rhythm.

■ The first strategy requires systemic anticoagulation for a 3-week period before elective electrical or pharmacologic cardioversion. This period of anticoagulation reduces the risk of embolization after cardioversion from 5% to 1%.
■ The second strategy permits cardioversion without an antecedent 3-week period of systemic anticoagulation if an atrial thrombus is not documented by transesophageal echocardiography.

Atrial stunning (evidence of sinus rhythm electrically but without effective mechanical contraction) can exist for several weeks after a cardioversion and predisposes to blood stasis in the atria; therefore systemic anticoagulation with heparin transitioning to warfarin must begin with and continue after the cardioversion for at least 4 weeks. In the second strategy, if an atrial thrombus is documented by transesophageal echocardiography, systemic anticoagulation should occur for 3 weeks before cardioversion. Cardioversion is then safe and the patient is treated for at least 4 more weeks after cardioversion with systemic anticoagulation therapy.

A high rate of recurrence occurs in patients' cardioverted without antiarrhythmic drug therapy. By 3 months, only 30% of patients who have undergone successful cardioversion remained in sinus rhythm. Thus, antiarrhythmic agents are usually initiated just before or just after cardioversion in most patients

The decision to use antiarrhythmic drug therapy is complex. The benefits of sinus rhythm with the restoration of atrial–ventricular synchrony; improved cardiac output, and physiologic heart rate control are clear. These benefits must be weighed against the risks of antiarrhythmic drug therapy. Class IA, Class IC, and Class III agents have been used to maintain sinus rhythm. Several studies have demonstrated an increase in mortality in patients who received antiarrhythmic drugs, presumably due to proarrhythmia. Seemingly paradoxical, the greatest risk of proarrhythmia appears immediately after cardioversion when sinus rhythm emerges.

■ Drugs such as quinidine and sotalol prolong repolarization to a greater extent at slower heart rates, thereby enhancing the possibility of Q-T interval prolongation and a ventricular arrhythmia.
■ In contrast, amiodarone, a Class III agent, has an extremely low proarrhythmic risk and remains the antiarrhythmic agent of choice in patients with structural heart disease. In patients with neurologic issues, amiodarone is likely safest in the short term.

Nonpharmacologic treatments such as catheter ablation, atrial fibrillation suppression by chronic pacing algorithms, and surgical Maze-like procedures are evolving. Consideration for these treatments may take place when the patient is able to leave the neurosurgical intensive care unit.

Treatment: Anticoagulation

A meta-analysis of clinical anticoagulation trials showed a 68% risk reduction in stroke when comparing warfarin adjusted to an INR between 2 and 3 versus placebo ($p < 0.001$). The benefits of aspirin compared to placebo were marginal. Risk stratification on the basis of this meta-analysis showed that patients with a history of hypertension, recent congestive heart failure, or previous thromboembolism were at the greatest risk for stroke. The incidence of stroke was highest (17.6% per year) if a patient had two or three risk factors. If only one of those risk factors was present, the risk was 7.3% per year. The low risk group comprised patients younger than 60 years in age and without any risk factors. These patients likely do not require systemic anticoagulation.

Summary

In a critically ill neurologic patient, atrial fibrillation can be the etiologic factor causing a stroke or can complicate the management of the critically ill patient. Therapy for stroke in the setting of atrial fibrillation should be algorithmically driven. The management of the hemodynamic issues is driven by the patient's clinical condition. Usually rate control with IV diltiazem or esmolol can acutely stabilize the patient and then allow thorough consideration of longer term issues such as chronic anticoagulation and the use of antiarrhythmic drugs. Nonpharmacologic therapies are evolving and are not at this time appropriate to employ in the ICU setting.

ECHOCARDIOGRAPHY IN THE EVALUATION OF CEREBRAL AND PERIPHERAL CARDIAC EMBOLISM

Cardiovascular ultrasound imaging is largely responsible for our current understanding of cardiac sources of embolism. Despite this technologic advance, there are relatively few cardiac abnormalities we can classify as cause-and-effect in relation to embolic stroke. This makes patient selection for this imaging modality critical, as assimilation of all patient data will be needed to use the imaging information appropriately.

Technique

Three ultrasound modalities are utilized to find cardiac source of embolism: transthoracic echocardiography (TTE), transcranial Doppler (TCD) ultrasound, and transesophageal echocardiography (TEE). The technique of saline contrast injection can be utilized with all three modalities with varying sensitivity and specificity for detection of right-to-left shunt.

TRANSTHORACIC ECHOCARDIOGRAPHY

Also known as a "surface echocardiogram," cardiac ultrasound images are obtained from various locations on the chest surface. Optimal images are obtained when patients are in the left lateral decubitus position and are able to cooperate with controlled breathing. Supine position, the use of mechanical ventilation and obesity, are a few examples of factors that limit the ability to obtain clinically useful images. When used in stroke patients, finding a cardiac source of embolism is more likely when underlying cardiac symptoms, heart disease, or an abnormal EKG or chest radiograph are present. When none of the above is present, the yield for identifying a potential source of embolism is low (2–9%).

SALINE CONTRAST ECHOCARDIOGRAPHY

A small amount of air mixed with saline is rapidly moved back and forth between two syringes using a three-way stopcock, and then injected into a large peripheral or central vein. The microbubble saline solution produces a contrast effect under ultrasound imaging. Saline bubbles large enough to be imaged cannot pass through pulmonary capillaries and enter left heart chambers. Based on this principle, any contrast appearing in the left heart is abnormal. The literature is confounded by a variance in the number of discrete left heart contrast bubbles required (1–5 bubbles) by investigators to define presence of a patent foramen ovale (PFO). Timing of left heart contrast appearance compared to opacification of the right heart is the primary method of distinguishing between right-to-left shunting from PFO or atrial septal defect (ASD), and a pulmonary arteriovenous malformation. The number of bubbles that appear in the left heart under cardiac ultrasound imaging has been used to grade the size of PFO as small (5–10 bubbles), moderate (10–20 bubbles), and large (>20 bubbles).

TRANSCRANIAL DOPPLER SONOGRAPHY

With this nonimaging technique, a Doppler ultrasound signal is focused along the middle cerebral artery (MCA) after peripheral intravenous injection of agitated saline contrast. Detection of microbubbles in the middle cerebral artery demonstrates the presence of right-to-left shunting. The right-to-left shunt size can be graded on the number of microbubbles detected. TCD is sensitive in identifying the presence of right-to-left shunt. The number of microbubbles recorded during TCD is used to estimate size (1–10 microbubbles is a small shunt, >10 without curtain effect is a medium size shunt, and hits too numerous to distinguish is a large shunt). Given the lack of imaging, there is poor specificity in determining the site of the intracardiac shunt and in excluding the presence of an extracardiac shunt. This makes TCD useful only as a screening test.

TRANSESOPHAGEAL ECHOCARDIOGRAPHY

TEE is an invasive technique requiring esophageal intubation with a gastroscope that has an ultrasound transducer mounted at the tip. TEE is typically done with conscious sedation, and often requiring paralytics in mechanically ventilated patients. Although the risk of death is remote, other serious injuries can include esophageal rupture, dental injury, methemoglobinemia, and the complications of conscious sedation. As the probe is blind (esophagus is not visualized), absolute contraindications to this study include esophageal obstruction (i.e., tumor mass or untreated stricture), high-grade varices, or swallowing difficulties that preceded the stroke. The diagnostic yield is much higher than TTE for identifying a cardiac source of embolism, particularly in that group with no known cardiac symptoms, cardiac disease, and EKG or chest radiograph abnormality. In this group, the yield for identifying a cardiac source of embolism is approximately 28%. TEE is also useful when aortic dissection is suspected. Sensitivity and specificity are similar to magnetic resonance imaging (MRI) and computed tomography (CT) without the required transportation issues of a critically ill patient.

CHOOSING AN APPROACH TO EVALUATION

Which patient to evaluate for cardiac source of embolism has been controversial. Figure 25.1 defines the approach followed by the Medical College of Wisconsin.

Cardiac Sources of Embolism

There have been many potential cardiac sources of embolism described, but relatively few have been proven as cause-and-effect. Most experts would agree the following are unequivocal sources of embolism when identified in patients with suspected ischemic events:

- Large or mobile left heart valvular vegetations
- Left heart tumor masses, such as atrial myxoma
- Thrombus, such as that in the left ventricle after infarction, or in the left atrial appendage with atrial fibrillation
- Presence of vegetation, thrombus, or mass in the right heart, with concomitant presence of PFO or ASD

There is increasing evidence that some abnormalities previously thought to be associated with stroke are probably not independently related. They include mitral valve prolapse, mitral annular calcification, and valve strands (Table 25.1). Patent foramen ovale and aortic atheroma have been studied most extensively over the past decade and are worthy of separate mention.

PATENT FORAMEN OVALE AND ATRIAL SEPTAL ANEURYSM

After birth, approximately 25% of the population do not obtain complete fusion of the atrial septum primum and secundum. This results in persistence of a potential one-way connection between the right and left atrium (Fig. 25.2). Although normal physiology should keep this flop-valve closed, transient increase in right atrial pressure from cough, Valsalva, or pulmonary hypertension can result in reversal of this gradient and an opening of this potential interatrial communication. This may result in transmission of embolic material to the systemic circulation that might have been otherwise degraded in the lungs. Atrial septal aneurysm is a thinned, mobile interatrial septum that must reach objective measures of mobility to be defined as an aneurysm. PFO literature is confounded by a variance between investigators in this definition.

- The most stringent criteria requires 15 mm in aneurysm length, and a total of 15 mm in deviation or excursion in septal motion.
- The "relaxed criteria" used by some investigators is 11 mm or more of aneurysm deviation from midline or total excursion.

Although atrial septal aneurysms are associated with PFO and ASD, in their absence, there is little evidence to suggest they are an independent risk factor for thromboembolism.

DETECTION BY ECHOCARDIOGRAPHY. Transthoracic echocardiography is the least sensitive technique for identifying the presence of a PFO, and typically requires saline contrast to identify the shunt. Although TEE can often identify a PFO by visualization and color Doppler flow characteristics, the addition of saline contrast is the most sensitive and specific way of confirming its presence. Transcranial Doppler is similarly sensitive, and also quantifies the amount of contrast reaching the brain. Significant controversy regarding the cause-and-effect of PFO and cerebral ischemic events exists. Clearly, the more scientifically rigorous the study, the less evidence there appears to be for a relationship. The Study by Mas et al., in patients younger than 55 years of age with cryptogenic stroke placed on aspirin therapy, suggests only patients with a PFO and an atrial septal aneurysm, regardless of PFO size, were at significantly increased risk of recurrent stroke (heart rate [HR]: 4.17, 95% CI: 1.47–11.84, $p = 0.007$).

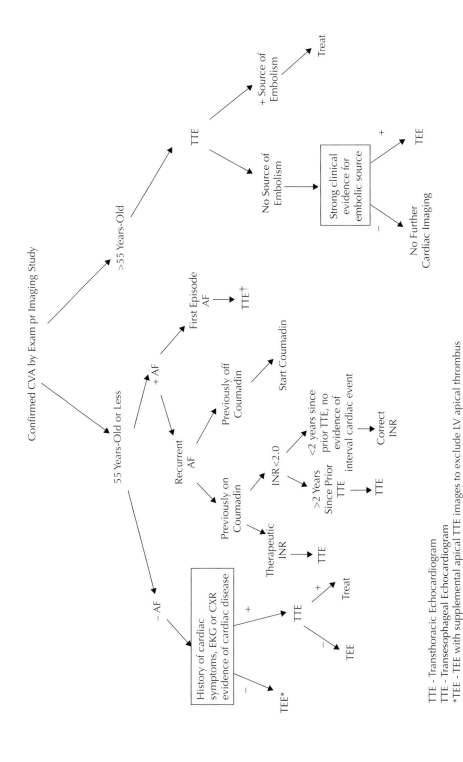

Figure 25.1. Approach to Evaluation of stroke patients.

TTE - Transthoracic Echocardiogram
TTE - Transesophageal Echocardiogram
*TEE - TEE with supplemental apical TTE images to exclude LV apical thrombus
†TTE - Complete TTE with saline contrast study

Table 25.1. Stroke risk and cardiac abnormalities

Cardiac abnormality	Relative strength of association with stroke	Sensitivity for detection improved by TEE
Atrial fibrillation (LAA thrombus)	****	+
Acute myocardial infarction	****	−
Spontaneous echo contrast	****	+
Aortic atheroma	***	+
Patent foramen ovale and atrial septal aneurysm	***	+
Valve strands	**	+
Nonbacterial thrombotic endocarditis (marantic endocarditis)	**	+
Rheumatic mitral stenosis (in the absence of atrial fibrillation)	**	−
Isolated atrial septal aneurysm	*	+
Mitral annular calcification	*	−
Mitral valve prolapse	*	−

LAA = left atrial appendage.
* Probably no independent associated risk with cerebral ischemia.
** Association based on case series, case reports, and/or inconsistent results between studies.
*** Moderate evidence: some prospective studies, but discrepancies persist.
**** Strong evidence of association, consistent between prospective, randomized studies.

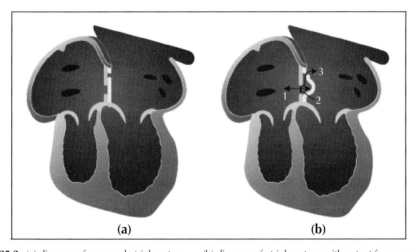

Figure 25.2. (a) diagram of a normal atrial septum …. (b) diagram of atrial septum with patent foramen ovale.

TREATMENT. The only randomized controlled study of treatment for PFO and atrial septal aneurysm was reported in a substudy of the Warfarin Aspirin Recurrent Stroke Study (WARSS) trial. The Patent Foramen Ovale in Cryptogenic Stroke Study (PICSS) evaluated 630 ischemic stroke patients with TEE entered in the WARSS trial, and prospectively followed them for up to 2 years for primary end points of recurrent CVA or death. Patients were randomized to warfarin or aspirin. In patients with cryptogenic stroke, there was no significant difference in the rate of recurrent events in those treated with warfarin versus aspirin. In the cohort of patients with PFO (34% of patients), the event rates were not significantly different for large or small PFO, as compared to no PFO. Similarly, PFO with or without a concomitant atrial septal aneurysm made no significant difference in development of end points. This study was unusual, however, in that it included patients older than 55 years of age (up to age 85), a group previously thought to be at less risk of stroke from PFO based on case-control studies.

Multiple percutaneous devices are currently being used under an FDA Humanitarian Device Exemption to close a PFO. Closure I (NMT Medical) and RESPECT (AGA Medical Corp) are currently underway and will help determine the efficacy and long term safety of such closure strategies. Until these large randomized treatment trials can further guide appropriate management in patients with PFO, AHA guidelines recommend antiplatelet therapy for patients with cerebral ischemic event and a PFO, and warfarin if other high-risk conditions are present. There are inadequate data to recommend surgical or percutaneous closure of a PFO after a first ischemic event, but this may be considered for patients with recurrent cryptogenic events refractory to medical treatment.

AORTIC ATHEROMA

Atherosclerotic plaques of the aorta include aortic atheroma, protruding aortic atheroma, and atherosclerotic aortic debris. These are manifestation of the systemic disease of atherosclerosis, sharing the same risk factors as coronary artery disease that includes age, tobacco abuse, hypertension, and dyslipidemia. Mobile densities visualized on or near a plaque usually represent attached thrombus.

CLINICAL SIGNIFICANCE. Numerous case-control studies have demonstrated an association between aortic atheroma and stroke. Amarenco et al. also suggested that the thickness of the plaque is a risk factor for stroke. After adjustment for other atherosclerotic risk factors and atrial fibrillation, the odds ratio for stroke was 9.1 compared to controls (95% CI 3.3–25.2, $p < 0.001$). Although some believe mobile plaques represent the fibrous cap of ruptured plaques, Karalis et al. suggested it is more likely thrombus. In their small study of 38 patients with aortic atheroma identified by TEE, the incidence of an embolic event was highest with pedunculated

and highly mobile lesions, as compared to layered or immobile plaques (ischemic events in 73% vs. 12% of patients, respectively, $p < 0.002$). Similarly, in patients with aortic atheroma who undergo cardiac catheterization, intra-aortic balloon pump placement, or coronary bypass surgery, cerebral and systemic embolic events are more likely.

DETECTION
- TEE is considered the imaging modality of choice for the detection of aortic atheroma, with excellent characterization of plaque morphology and thrombus motion. TEE provides portable and real-time aortic imaging, an advantage for both the neuro-intensive care unit, as well as the operating room.
- The use of CT scanning and MRI for detection of aortic atheroma has been limited by inferior motion resolution necessary to accurately detect thrombus.

TREATMENT
Primary Prevention. In absence of prospective randomized treatment trials, there is no consensus on therapy, and guidelines for management vary substantially by authoring bodies. All patients should receive aggressive risk factor modification for atherosclerosis, including attention to blood pressure, tobacco cessation, and good glycemic control for diabetics. Statin therapy is recommended. With a number of studies identifying aortic atheroma as a marker of concomitant coronary artery disease, targeted low-density lipoprotein (LDL) lowering based on secondary prevention goals should be considered (goal LDL about 70 mg/dL). The benefit of long-term antiplatelet therapy probably outweighs the risks for sessile plaques, but is still unproven. Neither ACCP conference on Antithrombotic and Thrombolytic therapy nor the American Heart Association makes recommendations for therapy in primary prevention. There are very limited data to guide primary prevention of ischemic events when mobile densities compatible with thrombus are identified. The SPAF-III trial suggested a significant risk reduction of ischemic events with adjusted dose warfarin as opposed to fixed low-dose warfarin and aspirin.

Secondary Prevention. When aortic atheroma is thought to be the proximate cause of an ischemic event all patients should receive aggressive risk factor modification for atherosclerosis as in primary prevention. Similarly, statin therapy is recommended, with aggressive pursuit of LDL lowering similar to that recommended with established coronary disease. Long-term antiplatelet therapy should be considered, but is of unproven benefit. Given the relative low risk of this therapy, most experts recommend antiplatelet therapy.

AORTIC ATHEROMA WITH THROMBUS

Two small, nonrandomized studies in stroke patients suggest anticoagulation may reduce the risk of a recurrent ischemic event when thrombus appears present. A prospective cohort study by Tunick et al., however, suggests that only statin therapy reduces chances of recurrent events. There are no agreed upon guidelines for treatment given the lack of prospective trials. The ACCP recommends either antiplatelet or anticoagulation therapy. Conspicuously absent from 2006 AHA guidelines are any recommendations or discussion of approach to aortic atheroma. Although there is fear that anticoagulation may result in plaque hemorrhage resulting in cholesterol emboli, this syndrome appears to be relatively rare. An alternate approach to management proposed by some experts is 2 months of adjusted dose warfarin with INR range 2–3, followed by long-term antiplatelet therapy.

Conclusion

Since the rigor of scientific evidence linking cardiac abnormalities and cerebral ischemia is highly variable, great care must be exercised in undertaking imaging for identifying potential embolic sources. Identifying a potential cardiac source of stroke must be carefully engaged with the clinical circumstances. The ACC/AHA have jointly developed guidelines for the appropriate use of echocardiography in the evaluation of patients suffering suspected cardiac embolic events. An algorithmic approach to undertaking an evaluation can be useful (Fig. 25.1).

In patients with potential cardiac and noncardiac sources of stroke, a neurologic event contralateral to the involved carotid artery or evidence of multiple or peripheral emboli are highly suspect of a cardiac or aortic source. Most importantly, the results of investigations should have reasonable chance of altering the course of patient management before being initiated.

ARRHYTHMIAS

The clinical presentation of patients with arrhythmias is quite variable. Palpitation, lightheadedness, and syncope are common symptoms. A nonspecific presentation may include fatigue, dyspnea, or exertional intolerance. The 12-lead EKG, 24-hour ambulatory EKG monitor, and EKG event recording can establish the diagnosis. The acute treatment of any arrhythmia consists of prompt restoration of stable hemodynamic parameters. If possible, sinus rhythm should be restored. A thorough characterization of the underlying cardiac substrate is usually indicated before embarking on long-term therapy. Generally, therapy directed toward improving the cardiac substrate will make management of the arrhythmia more effective.

Physiology

Under normal circumstances, the cardiac electrical system is controlled by the sinus node. The sinus node is the dominant cardiac pacemaker directing atrial depolarization across the atria from right to left and top to bottom. Thus during sinus rhythm on the 12-lead EKG: the P waves are always positive in leads II, II, and AVF and always negative in lead AVR. Electrical activity spreads to the ventricles via the AV node and HIS bundle and then through the right and left bundles generating a narrow QRS complex. Arrhythmias are classified as either supraventricular or ventricular based on their site of origin.

Specific Arrhythmias

SINUS TACHYCARDIA AND BRADYCARDIA

Sinus rhythm with a rate >100 beats/min is termed sinus tachycardia. A large number of stresses (both physiologic – exercise, anxiety, pregnancy – and pathologic – fever, infection, hypoxia, heart failure and sympathomimetic drugs) – can precipitate this arrhythmia.

Sinus rhythm with a rate <60 beats/min is termed sinus bradycardia. Sinus bradycardia can occur in well-conditioned athletes with enhanced vagal tone. Pharmacologic agents (e.g., beta-blockers, calcium channel blockers, and alpha-blockers), vagal maneuvers (e.g., eyeball manipulation, Valsalva maneuver, carotid sinus massage), and various disease states (e.g., hypothyroidism, sinus node dysfunction) may underlie sinus bradycardia. Augmented stroke

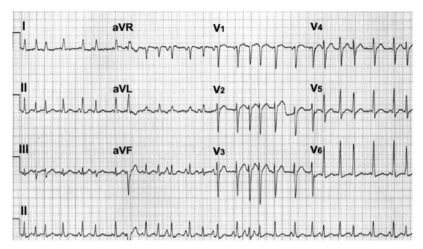

Figure 25.3. This 12-lead EKG documents MAT with different P wave morphologies and varying PR intervals.

volume often compensates for the bradycardia; thus, cardiac output remains normal. In nonreversible pathologic states the only durable solution to symptomatic sinus bradycardia is electrical pacing.

MULTIFOCAL ATRIAL TACHYCARDIA

Multifocal atrial tachycardia (MAT) remains a descriptive entity with a need for better characterization. MAT is diagnosed by ECG criteria: an atrial rate of >100 beats/min with P waves of at least three distinct morphologies. The chaotic nature of its P-wave morphology with varying AV intervals may cause confusion with atrial fibrillation (Fig. 25.3).

- MAT is usually observed in patients with acute pulmonary disorders and associated hypoxia.
- The basis for therapy should primarily be correction of the underlying pulmonary disorder.
- Neither cardioversion nor antiarrhythmic drugs have been successful in treating patients with MAT.

PREMATURE ATRIAL COMPLEXES

A premature atrial complex (PAC) appears on the ECG as a premature, morphologically abnormal P wave. Depending on the degree of prematurity, the PAC may not be conducted, aberrantly conducted (a right or left bundle branch block), or normally conducted (the HIS Purkinje network). The P-R interval of a PAC usually lengthens with increasing degrees of prematurity: the more premature the PAC, the longer the P-R interval.

- PACs are common, benign events and are associated with tobacco, caffeine, alcohol, emotional stress, atrial distension, or hypoxia.
- PACs may cause palpitation by triggering sustained reentrant tachycardias.

ATRIAL FLUTTER

Atrial flutter is a common arrhythmia and brief episodes may occur during an acute illness (e.g., thyrotoxicosis, acute pulmonary embolism, alcohol intoxication) and are common after open-heart surgery. In a few patients, no organic heart disease is evident.

- The ECG in typical atrial flutter demonstrates a "saw-tooth" flutter pattern with (F) waves occurring regularly at 300 beats/min.
- The undulating F waves are best appreciated in leads II, III, and aVF.
- Most commonly, 2:1 AV conduction occurs, resulting in a ventricular rate of 150 beats/min (Fig. 25.4). With 2:1 AV conduction, the QRS or T waves may obscure the alternate flutter waves. In these instances, carotid sinus massage or intravenous adenosine may help diagnostically by increasing the degree of AV block, unmasking the otherwise obscured F waves.

The durable treatment of atrial flutter is the return of sinus rhythm. Treating associated illnesses can evoke the spontaneous return of sinus rhythm.

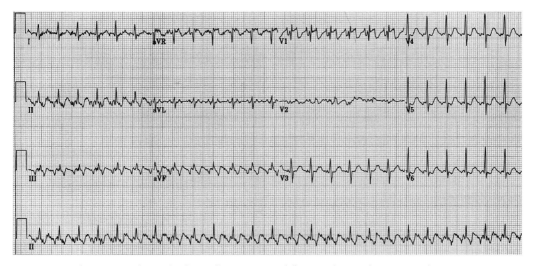

Figure 25.4. This 12-lead EKG documents atrial flutter with typical 2/1 AV conduction.

- Cardioversion at low energies (25–50 joules) usually restores sinus rhythm and is required if hemodynamic instability or acute ischemia are present.
- Rate control can be achieved with a variety of drugs: beta-blockers, calcium channel blockers, or digitalis. Control of the ventricular response, unlike in atrial fibrillation, is not durable. The ventricular response can be very unpredictable in atrial flutter. Small changes in AV nodal tone can result in inappropriately rapid or slow ventricular rates.
- Catheter ablation of a vulnerable portion of the flutter circuit in the right atria is curative; a lesion is placed from the tricuspid valve annulus to the ridge of the inferior vena cava or coronary sinus.

Anticoagulation is generally indicated in atrial flutter if structural heart disease is present. Most patients with atrial flutter, even after ablation, will have episodes of atrial fibrillation. Thus anticoagulation therapy should be addressed similarity to that in patients with atrial fibrillation.

ATRIAL TACHYCARDIA

Atrial tachycardia refers to an arrhythmia that is housed entirely in the atria and does not require participation of the AV node. The incidence of atrial tachycardia increases with age and the severity of the underlying heart disease. However, the tachycardia may occur in young otherwise healthy individuals. Most episodes of atrial tachycardia are paroxysmal but incessant episodes can lead to a tachycardia-mediated cardiomyopathy. This form of cardiomyopathy is reversible with control of the ventricular rate.

- The diagnosis of atrial tachycardia is made by analyzing the EKG.
- The standard way to determine the presence of an atrial tachycardia is to demonstrate that with AV block the arrhythmia continues.

Catheter ablation has become the primary therapy for symptomatic patients.

NONPAROXYSMAL AV JUNCTIONAL TACHYCARDIA

In nonparoxysmal AV junctional tachycardia, the AV junction, rather than remaining the default pacemaker, usurps control from the SA node. The mechanism is thought to be automatic. The usual rate is 100–130 beats/min. Retrograde P waves may be present or AV dissociation may occur. Digitalis toxicity, myocardial ischemia or myocarditis usually underlies this arrhythmia. Treatment is directed at the underlying cause.

AV NODAL REENTRY TACHYCARDIA

AV nodal reentry tachycardia (AVNRT) is characterized by a regular, narrow-complex tachycardia at a rate of 150–250 beats/min. Dual AV nodal pathways are necessary. A second pathway in the AV node is present in approximately 1/100 people. Retrograde conduction to the atria commonly results in the P wave being buried in the QRS complex. The terminal portion of the QRS complex can house the retrograde P wave producing a "pseudo r pattern".

■ Vagal maneuvers or IV adenosine can terminate AVNRT, as this arrhythmia is AV node dependent.
■ Catheter ablation of the slow pathway in the AV node is the preferred treatment in symptomatic patients.

ORTHODROMIC AVRT

A bypass tract (also termed an accessory AV connection) consists of aberrant muscle fibers that cross the fibrous AV annulus and can electrically connect the atrium and the ventricle. This provides the necessary substrate for a reentrant tachycardia, orthodromic AVRT. The reentrant circuit in orthodromic AVRT consists of normal antegrade conduction through the AV node (resulting in a normal-appearing QRS complex) and retrograde conduction from the ventricle to the atria via the bypass tract. In this instance, the retrograde P wave usually distorts the ST segments. With orthodromic AVRT, the tachycardia is terminated by blocking conduction in one of the limbs of the circuits.

■ Vagal maneuvers, such as carotid sinus massage, or a Valsalva maneuver, may be successful by blocking conduction through the AV node and should be tried initially.
■ If these maneuvers fail, adenosine (6–12 mg IV) virtually always results in transient AV node block and will terminate this arrhythmia.
■ Catheter ablation of the bypass tract has become the preferred therapy for orthodromic AVRT.

WOLFF–PARKINSON–WHITE SYNDROME

Wolff–Parkinson–White (WPW) syndrome is seen when patients have palpitation usually from orthodromic AVRT and also have a delta wave on their ECG during sinus rhythm. The prevalence of WPW syndrome in the general population is about 0.15%, with a 2:1 preponderance for men. Patients are at risk for developing very rapid ventricular rates, when atrial arrhythmias, such as atrial fibrillation or flutter, occur because the bypass tract can conduct also in an antegrade fashion. Rapid ventricular

rates, faster than 200 beats/min, during atrial fibrillation can cascade to ischemia, ventricular fibrillation, and death. Sudden cardiac death can rarely be the presenting symptom in patients with the WPW syndrome.

■ First-line therapy for symptomatic patients (WPW syndrome) is radiofrequency catheter ablation of the bypass tract.
■ Patients with hemodynamic compromise during atrial fibrillation require immediate cardioversion.

Digitalis, beta-blockers, and calcium channel blockers are contraindicated during atrial fibrillation in patients with the WPW syndrome. These agents block conduction of AF impulses down the AV node which indirectly facilitates conduction of AF impulses down the bypass tract. This facilitation is indirect as elimination of impulse conduction down the AV node eliminates the subsequent retrograde penetration of these impulses into the bypass tract. This occasional retrograde penetration into the bypass tract resulted in collision with other AF impulses conducting in an antegrade fashion down the bypass tract. These ongoing collisions resulted in fewer antegrade impulses depolarizing the ventricles and therefore a slower ventricular response during atrial fibrillation.

During a narrow QRS tachycardia, ventricular depolarization occurs via the AV node-His Purkinje network. Key considerations are summarized as follows.

■ 12-lead EKG tracings, rather than single-lead tracings, are preferable for the analysis of an arrhythmia.
■ If there is a 1:1 AV conduction, the location of the P wave relative to the QRS complex (before, within, or after) should be determined. In general, atrial tachycardia – P wave before the QRS; AV nodal reentrant tachycardia – P wave within the QRS; orthodromic-AV reentrant tachycardia – P wave follows the QRS.
■ AV block terminates AV nodal-dependent rhythms, such as AV nodal reentrant tachycardia, or orthodromic-AV reentrant tachycardia. AV block in general does not terminate an atrial tachycardia.

- Vagal maneuvers can help in the differential diagnosis of tachyarrhythmias. By increasing vagal tone, (1) a slight transient decrease of rates will occur in sinus tachycardia; (2) abrupt termination of AV nodal reentrant tachycardia or orthodromic-AV reentrant tachycardia can occur if AV block is noted.
- Adenosine can be used to produce brief, high-grade block of the AV node, which will terminate AV nodal reentrant tachycardia or orthodromic-AV reentrant tachycardia. By producing transient AV nodal block, adenosine can "unmask" atrial fibrillation, atrial flutter, or atrial tachycardia.

VENTRICULAR ARRHYTHMIAS

PREMATURE VENTRICULAR COMPLEXES. Premature ventricular complexes (PVCs) are a common ventricular rhythm disturbance. PVCs are single wide QRS complexes that originate in the ventricles.

- Two successive PVCs are termed a couplet and three successive PVCs at a rate of >100 beats/min are termed ventricular tachycardia.
- PVCs of similar morphology are termed monomorphic, but if the morphology varies, PVCs are multifocal or polymorphic.
- If PVCs successively alternate with a sinus beat, the rhythm is termed bigeminy.

PVCs may become manifest or exacerbated with alcohol, emotional stress, sympathomimetic agents, hypoxia, or other conditions, including any type of heart disease. Antiarrhythmic therapy of PVCs has never been shown to improve outcome and can increase mortality owing to proarrhythmic mechanisms. Thus, in patients with PVCs, reversible factors should be sought and corrected. Underlying heart disease requires evidence-based therapy.

VENTRICULAR TACHYCARDIA. Ventricular tachycardia arises from the ventricular myocardium. In ventricular tachycardia, the QRS complex is >120 milliseconds in duration, as depolarization is slow due to cell-to-cell propagation. AV dissociation is often present, but retrograde activation of the atria from the ventricles (ventricular–atrial association) can be present.

- If, the QRS complexes do not vary in morphology, the ventricular tachycardia is monomorphic; if the QRS complexes vary in morphology, the ventricular tachycardia is polymorphic.
- Ventricular tachycardia is further classified as sustained (lasting >30 seconds or associated with hemodynamic compromise) or nonsustained (>3 consecutive beats but lasting <30 seconds).

The spectrum of symptoms observed in patients with ventricular tachycardia can range from none to hemodynamic collapse. Monomorphic ventricular tachycardia usually implies structural heart disease. Polymorphic ventricular tachycardia usually results from proarrhythmia due to Q-T interval prolongation or from ischemia.

The differential diagnosis in a wide QRS complex tachycardia is either ventricular tachycardia or a supraventricular tachycardia conducted to the ventricles with aberration: a right or left bundle branch block. Historical, clinical, and EKG variables are helpful diagnostically to determine if the arrhythmia is ventricular or supraventricular with aberration. Any wide QRS complex tachycardia should be assumed to be ventricular in origin in the presence of structural heart disease.

Management of Ventricular Tachycardia

- For acute treatment, IV lidocaine or IV amiodarone are usually the initial agents of choice.
- If the patient is hemodynamically unstable, prompt restoration of sinus rhythm by electrical cardioversion is necessary.
- Patients with the potential for recurrent sustained ventricular tachycardia often require an implantable cardioverter defibrillator (ICD).
- Underlying cardiac conditions must always be optimized.

TORSADES DE POINTES. Torsades de pointe (twisting of points) refers to a polymorphic ventricular tachycardia that occurs in the presence of a prolonged Q-T interval. Morphologically, this ventricular tachycardia is characterized by the gradual oscillation of the peaks of successive QRS complexes around the baseline. Torsades de pointe occurs at a rapid rate and is usually self-terminating. Patients often present with recurrent dizziness or syncope.

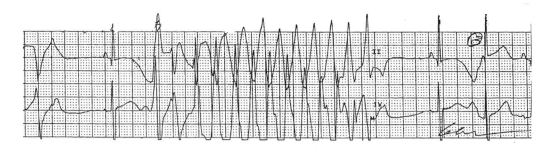

Figure 25.5. This is a telemetry tracing of torsades de pointes. Note the markedly prolonged Q-T interval just before the first beat of tachycardia.

Deterioration to ventricular fibrillation is not uncommon (Fig. 25.5).

The syndrome may be congenital or acquired. The acquired form may be caused by a variety of medications that can lengthen action potential duration by blocking potassium current (Table 25.2).

- Often combinations of drugs are "partners" in the acquired syndrome, one typically a weak potassium current blocker, and one that interferes with the metabolism of the first drug resulting in higher systemic concentrations and enhanced potassium current blocking effects. Treatment of this arrhythmia involves removing causative drug.
- Electrolyte abnormalities specifically low potassium and low calcium, and low magnesium can also lengthen the action potential duration leading to Q-T prolongation. Intravenous magnesium (regardless of the actual serum magnesium levels) may suppress the arrhythmia.

In the congenital form, at least seven culprit gene abnormalities have been identified. Chronic treatment may involve oral beta-blockers, cervicothoracic sympathetic ganglionectomy, or ICD implantation.

ACCELERATED IDIOVENTRICULAR RHYTHM. Three or more ventricular complexes occurring at a rate of 60–100 beats/min constitute an accelerated idioventricular rhythm. This is commonly observed in spontaneous coronary reperfusion or after percutaneous coronary interventions. Episodes of AIVR are brief and often asymptomatic. Treatment is not necessary; however, this arrhythmia usually requires an evaluation to exclude ischemia (Fig. 25.6).

VENTRICULAR FIBRILLATION. Ventricular fibrillation (VF) is characterized electrocardiographically by baseline undulations of variable amplitude and periodicity. No definitive QRS complexes or T waves are evident. Effective cardiac contraction is absent. Loss of consciousness ensues followed by death within 3–5 minutes unless a durable rhythm is restored. VF is usually seen after active ischemia, after VT causing ischemia, or after atrial fibrillation with a rapid ventricular response causing ischemia.

The risk of ventricular tachycardia or ventricular fibrillation in patients is predicted by the extent of LV dysfunction. Primary prevention with an ICD is now advocated in patients with LV dysfunction with an EF <35%.

Conduction Disorders

HEART BLOCK

Optimal cardiac performance depends on an orderly sequence of events occurring in the cardiac conduction system: pacemaker impulses arising in the SA node initially depolarize the atrial myocardium, propagate slowly through the AV node, and finally spread through the His-Purkinje network to the ventricular myocardium. Failure of the conduction can occur anywhere in this electrical network but is most common and readily recognized in the AV node, His bundle, and the bundle branches.

FIRST-DEGREE AV BLOCK. First-degree AV block is a misnomer as block is not present. Delay in conduction from the sinus node to the ventricles results in a P-R interval longer than 0.20 seconds. Slow conduction through the AV node is usually due to high vagal tone, to intrinsic AV nodal disease or to drug effect.

Table 25.2. Drugs that have a risk of causing torsades de pointes

Generic name	Brand name	Class/clinical use	Comments
Amiodarone	Cordarone	Anti-arrhythmic/abnormal heart rhythm	Females > males, TdP risk regarded as low
Amiodarone	Pacerone	Anti-arrhythmic/abnormal heart rhythm	Females > males, TdP risk regarded as low
Arsenic trioxide	Trisenox	Anti-cancer/leukemia	
Astemizole	Hismanal	Anti-histamine/allergic rhinitis	No longer available in the United States
Bepridil	Vascor	Anti-anginal/heart pain	Females > males
Chloroquine	Aralen	Anti-malarial/malaria infection	
Chlorpromazine	Thorazine	Anti-psychotic/anti-emetic/ schizophrenia/nausea	
Cisapride	Propulsid	GI stimulant / heartburn	Restricted availability; females > males.
Clarithromycin	Biaxin	Antibiotic/bacterial infection	
Disopyramide	Norpace	Anti-arrhythmic/abnormal heart rhythm	Females > males
Dofetilide	Tikosyn	Anti-arrhythmic/abnormal heart rhythm	
Domperidone	Motilium	Anti-nausea/nausea	Not available in the United States
Droperidol	Inapsine	Sedative; antinausea/anesthesia adjunct, nausea	
Erythromycin	Erythrocin	Antibiotic; GI stimulant/bacterial infection; increase GI motility	Females > males
Erythromycin	E.E.S.	Antibiotic; GI stimulant/bacterial infection; increase GI motility	Females > males
Halofantrine	Halfan	Anti-malarial/malaria infection	Females > males
Haloperidol	Haldol	Anti-psychotic/schizophrenia, agitation	When given intravenously or at higher-than-recommended doses, risk of sudden death, Q-T prolongation and torsades increases.
Ibutilide	Corvert	Anti-arrhythmic/abnormal heart rhythm	Females > males
Levomethadyl	Orlaam	Opiate agonist /pain control, narcotic dependence	
Mesoridazine	Serentil	Anti-psychotic/schizophrenia	
Methadone	Methadose	Opiate agonist/pain control, narcotic dependence	Females>Males
Methadone	Dolophine	Opiate agonist/pain control, narcotic dependence	Females > males
Pentamidine	NebuPent	Anti-infective /Pneumocystis pneumonia	Females > males
Pentamidine	Pentam	Anti-infective /Pneumocystis pneumonia	Females > males

(continued)

Table 25.2 (*continued*)

Generic name	Brand name	Class/clinical use	Comments
Pimozide	Orap	Anti-psychotic/Tourette's tics	Females > males
Probucol	Lorelco	Anti-lipemic hypercholesterolemia	No longer available in the United States
Procainamide	Pronestyl	Anti-arrhythmic/abnormal heart rhythm	
Procainamide	Procan	Anti-arrhythmic/abnormal heart rhythm	
Quinidine	Cardioquin	Anti-arrhythmic/abnormal heart rhythm	Females > males
Quinidine	Quinaglute	Anti-arrhythmic/abnormal heart rhythm	Females > males
Sotalol	Betapace	Anti-arrhythmic/abnormal heart rhythm	Females > males
Sparfloxacin	Zagam	Antibiotic/bacterial infection	
Terfenadine	Seldane	Anti-histamine/allergic rhinitis	No longer available in the United States
Thioridazine	Mellaril	Anti-psychotic/schizophrenia	

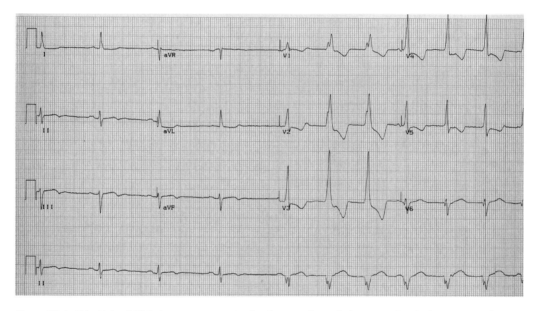

Figure 25.6. This 12-lead EKG documents an episode of an accelerated idioventricular rhythm (AIVR). Clear AV dissociation is seen on the rhythm strip at the bottom of the tracing.

SECOND-DEGREE AV BLOCK. Second-degree AV block is characterized by intermittent failure of AV conduction. Type I second-degree AV block (also termed Mobitz type I or Wenckebach) is the more common type and is characterized by a progressive lengthening of the P-R interval and shortening of the R-R interval until a P wave fails to conduct. Typically, the P wave following the nonconducted P wave has the shortest P-R interval.

The most common site of type I second-degree AV block is the AV node. In such patients, the QRS complex is narrow and the prognosis is benign. Type I block may occur in normal individuals as a manifestation of enhanced vagal tone, but it also occurs in a wide variety of medical conditions, such as acute inferior wall myocardial infarction and congenital or acquired diseases of the AV node, or with medications that slow AV conduction.

- In most cases, type I second-degree AV block requires no specific therapy. However, in patients who develop type I second-degree block in the absence of an identifiable acute process, particularly the elderly with severe coronary artery disease or calcific aortic disease, electrophysiologic testing should be considered to identify the site of the block.
- If the block is not the AV node but within or below the His bundle, permanent pacing is indicated.

Type II second-degree AV block (Mobitz type II) differs from type I second-degree block in that abrupt failure of AV conduction occurs without the preceding gradual P-R prolongation. The location of type II second-degree block is always within or below the His bundle.

Most patients with type second-degree block II block have broad QRS complexes indicative of conduction system disease and are commonly symptomatic (dizziness and syncope). Causes include degenerative diseases of the conduction system, anterior wall myocardial infarction, calcific aortic valve disease, hypertensive heart disease, and cardiomyopathy. Permanent pacing is indicated in all patients with type II second-degree AV block.

COMPLETE AV BLOCK. Complete or third-degree AV block features total independence of the atria and ventricles, due to the complete failure of the atrial impulses to be conduced to the ventricles. The atrial rate exceeds the ventricular rate. Third-degree AV block exhibits total dissociation between P waves and QRS complexes; with the ventricles being controlled by a subsidiary pacemaker site. The site of the conduction defect may be at the AV node or infranodal (within or below the His bundle). The site of the block has prognostic value.

- If the QRS complexes are narrow and the ventricular rate exceeds 50 beats/min, then the block is likely at the AV node, with a usually favorable prognosis. These patients are usually asymptomatic, and their heart rate can increase with exercise.
- If the QRS complexes are wide and the ventricular rate is 30–40 beats/min, then the site of the block is likely infranodal. Such blocks account for the vast majority of episodes of complete heart block, causing slow heart rates that are unresponsive to autonomic influence. Symptoms are frequent.

Reversible causes being infrequent, permanent pacing is usually indicated.

PERMANENT PACEMAKERS. A permanent pacemaker consists of an electrode lead (or leads) and a pulse generator. In most circumstances two electrode leads are inserted transvenously, one into the right atrial appendage and one into the RV apex. The generator is placed in a subcutaneous pocket below the clavicle. The power source is a lithium battery with a life expectancy of 5–10 years.

A letter code designation is used to describe the complex function of pacemakers. The first letter indicates the chamber paced; the second letter, the sensed chamber; the third, the mode of the pacemaker response to a spontaneous cardiac impulse; and the fourth letter indicates that the pacemaker has the property of rate modulation (i.e., the unit can increase its pacing rate in response to increased physiologic need).

Common indications for permanent pacing include symptomatic bradycardia experienced in patients with sinus node dysfunction and or with heart block. Most patients requiring a permanent pacemaker should be considered for dual-chamber pacing. Pacemaker systems that include atrial pacing, as opposed to a simple VVI system which paces and senses only the ventricle; have the advantage of maintaining AV synchrony.

Complications of permanent pacing include infection and erosion at the site of the generator implant, failure to pace the ventricular or atrial myocardium, and failure to appropriately sense underlying cardiac electrical activity.

Patients with permanent pacemakers should be monitored regularly. The need for battery replacement is often heralded by a spontaneous, automatic slowing of the pacing rate, a property built into the pacemaker to alert the physician to the need for battery replacement.

Summary

Cardiac arrhythmias are ubiquitous and range in clinical spectrum from benign to lethal. Characterization of the arrhythmia prior to treatment is important to a successful outcome. Initial characterization via electrocardiography is preferred. Clinical risk stratification is often accomplished by examining the underlying cardiac substrate. With LV dysfunction, cardiac arrhythmias carry a more ominous prognosis.

REFERENCES

Abraham WT, Adams KF, Fonarow GC, et al.; ADHERE Scientific Advisory Committee and Investigators; ADHERE Study Group. In-hospital mortality in patients with acute decompensated heart failure requiring intravenous vasoactive medications: an analysis from the Acute Decompensated Heart Failure National Registry (ADHERE) *J Am Coll Cardiol.* 2005;**46**(1):57–64.

ACC/AHA/ASE 2003 Guideline Update for the Clinical Application of Echocardiography. *J Am Coll Cardiol.* 2003;**42**:954–70.

Adjusted-dose warfarin versus low-intensity, fixed-dose warfarin pous aspirin for high-risk patients with atrial fibrillation: Stroke Prevention in Atrial Fibrillation III randomized Clinical Trial. *Lancet.* 1996;**348**:633.

Albers GW, Amarenco P, Easton JD, Sacco RL, Teal P. Antithrombotic and thrombolytic therapy for ischemic stroke: the Seventh ACCP Conference on Antithrombotic and Thrombolytic Therapy. *Chest.* 2004;**126**:483–512.

Amarenco P, Cohen A, Tzourio C, et. al. Atherosclerotic disease of the aortic arch and the risk of ischemic stroke. *N Engl J Med.* 1994;**331**:1474–9.

Antithrombotic Trialists' Collaboration. Collaborative meta-analysis of randomised trials of antiplatelet therapy for prevention of death, myocardial infarction, and stroke in high-risk patients. *BMJ.* 2002;**324**:71–86.

Antman E, Braunwald E. Acute myocardial infarction. In Braunwald E, Zipes DP, Libby P, eds. *Heart disease: a textbook of cardiovascular medicine,* 6th ed. Philadelphia: WB Saunders, 2001, pp 1114–231.

Antman et al., Management of Patients with STEMI: Executive Summary. *J Am Coll Cardiol.* 2004;**44**:671–719.

Beta-Blocker Heart Attack Study Group. The beta-blocker heart attack trial. *JAMA.* 1981;**246**:2073–4.

Binanay C, Califf RM, Hasselblad V, et al.; ESCAPE Investigators and ESCAPE Study Coordinators. Evaluation study of congestive heart failure and pulmonary artery catheterization effectiveness: the ESCAPE trial. *JAMA.* 2005;**294**(13):1625–33.

Boersma E, Mercado N, Poldermans D, Gardien M, Vos J, Simoons ML. Acute myocardial infarction. *Lancet.* 2003;**361**:847–58.

Canto JG, Shlipak MG, Rogers WJ, et al. Prevalence, clinical characteristics, and mortality among patients with myocardial infarction presenting without chest pain. *JAMA.* 2000;**283**:3223–9.

Colucci WS, Elkayam U, Horton DP, et al. Intravenous nesiritide, a natriuretic peptide, in the treatment of decompensated congestive heart failure. *Nesiritide Study Group. N Engl J Med.* 2000;**343**(4):246–53.

Dressler FA Craig WR, Castello R, et al. Mobile aortic atheroma and systemic emboli: efficacy of anticoagulation and influence of plaque morphology on recurrent stroke. *J Am Coll Cardiol.* 1998;**31**(1):134–8.

Ferrari E, Vidal R, Chevallier T, Baudouy M. Atherosclerosis of the thoracic aorta and aortic debris as a marker of poor prognosis: benefit of oral anticoagulants. *J Am Coll Cardiol.* 1999;**33**(5):1317–22.

Freemantle N, Cleland J, Young P, Mason J, Harrison J. Beta blockade after myocardial infarction: systematic review and meta regression analysis. *BMJ.* 1999;**318**:1730–7.

French Study of Aortic Plaques in Stroke Group. Atherosclerotic disease of the aortic arch as a risk factor for recurrent ischemic stroke. *N Eng J Med.* 1996;**334**:1216–21.

Fuster V, Rydén LE, Cannom DS, et al. ACC/AHA/ESC Guidelines for the management of patients with atrial fibrillation: executive summary: a report of the American College of Cardiology / American Heart Association Task Force on Practice Guidelines and the European Society of Cardiology Committee for Practice Guidelines and Policy Conferences. (Writing Committee to Revise the 2001 Guidelines for the Management of Patients With Atrial Fibrillation). *J Am Coll Cardiol.* 2006;**48**:854–906.

Heart Failure Society of America. Evaluation and management of patients with acute decompensated heart failure. *J Card Fail.* 2006;**12**(1):e86–e103.

Hirsh J, Fuster V, Ansell J, Halperin JL. AHA/ACC Scientific Statement: American Heart Association; American College of Cardiology Foundation Guide to Warfarin Therapy. *J Am Coll Cardiol.* 2003;**41**:1633–52.

Homma S, Sacco RL, Di Tullio MR, for the PFO in Cryptogenic Stroke Study (PICSS) Investigators: Effect of medical treatment in stroke patients with patent foramen ovale: Patent Foramen Ovale in Cryptogenic Stroke Study. *Circulation.* 2002;**105**(22):2625–31.

Hunt SA; American College of Cardiology; American Heart Association Task Force on Practice Guidelines (Writing Committee to Update the 2001 Guidelines for the Evaluation and Management of Heart Failure). *J Am Coll Cardiol.* 2005;46(6):e1–82.

Kannel WB. Silent myocardial ischemia and infarction: insights from the Framingham Study. *Cardiol Clin.* 1986;**4**:583–91.

Karalis DG, Chanddrasekaran K, Victor MF, et al. Recognition and embolic potential of intraaortic atherosclerotic debris. *J Am Coll Cardiol.* 1991;**17**:73.

Markides V, Schilling RJ. Atrial fibrillation: classification, pathophysiology, mechanisms and drug treatment. *Heart.* 2003;**89**:939–43.

Mas JL, Arquizan C, Lamy C, et al. Recurrent cerebrovascular events associated with patent foramen ovale, atrial septal aneurysms, or both. *N Engl J Med.* 2001;**345**:1740–6.

Petty GW, Khanderia BK, Meissner I, et al. Population-based study of the relationship between patent foramen ovale and cerebrovascular ischemic events. *Mayo Clin Proc.* 2006;**81**(5):602–8.

Sacco RL, Adams R, Albers G, et al. Guidelines for prevention of stroke in patients with ischemic stroke or transient ischemic attack. *Stroke.* 2006;**37**:577–617.

Scheinman MM, Morady F. Nonpharmacological approaches to atrial fibrillation. *Circulation.* 2001;**103**:2120–5.

Sheifer SE, Gersh BJ, Yanez ND, Ades PA, Burke GL, Manolio TA. Prevalence, predisposing factors, and prognosis of clinically unrecognized myocardial infarction in the elderly. *J Am Coll Cardiol.* 2000;**35**:119–26.

Tunick PA, Nayar AC, Goodkin GM, et al. Effect of treatment on the incidence of stroke and other emboli in 519 patients with severe thoracic aortic plaque. *Am J Cardiol.* 2002;**90**:1320–5.

Ware LB, Matthay MA. Clinical practice. Acute pulmonary edema. *N Engl J Med.* 2005; **353**:2788–96.

Wyse DG, Waldo AL, DiMarco JP, et al.; The AFFIRM Writing Group. A comparison of rate control and rhythm control in patients with atrial fibrillation. *N Engl J Med.* 2002;**347**:1825–33.

Yancy CW, Lopatin M, Stevenson LW. Clinical presentation, management, and in-hospital outcomes of patients admitted with acute decompensated heart failure with preserved systolic function: a report from the Acute Decompensated Heart Failure National Registry (ADHERE) Database. *Am Coll Cardiol.* 2006;**47**(1): 76–84.

Yusuf S, Peto R, Lewis J, Collins R, Sleight P. Beta blockade during and after myocardial infarction: an overview of the randomized trials. *Prog Cardiovasc Dis.* 1985;**27**:335–71.

Zimetbaum PJ, Josephson ME. Use of the electrocardiogram in acute myocardial infarction. *N Engl J Med.* 2003;**348**:933–40.

26 An Infectious Diseases Consult

Michael Frank, MD and Mary Beth Graham, MD

Intensive care unit (ICU) patients represent 5–10% of all hospitalized patients, yet the incidence of infections in this patient population is 5- to 10-fold higher than in general hospital wards and some studies estimate that up to 25% of all nosocomial infections occur in the ICU setting.[1,2] The majority of infections in critically ill patients are related to device utilization including catheter-related urinary tract infections (UTI), ventilator-associated pneumonia (VAP), and catheter-related bloodstream infections. Many studies have shown that these nosocomial infections not only increase morbidity and mortality but also add significantly to the cost and duration of hospitalization.[3,4] In this chapter we review the workup of fever in the ICU, management of common infections encountered in the ICU, and infection control guidelines to prevent the spread of nosocomial infections among patients and caregivers.

WORKUP OF FEVER IN THE ICU

The definition of fever is variable, but it is generally agreed on that a temperature >38.3°C warrants investigation in a hospitalized patient.[5,6] In patients in the neurosurgical ICU (NICU), fever can be an important sign of a potential complication or can be a consequence of the primary process requiring admission to the unit as seen with subarachnoid hemorrhage.

■ The development of fever is associated with a worse prognosis in the NICU, as is hypothermia.[7-10]
■ Fever is often a physiologic and appropriate response, and the fever itself should not

necessarily be treated except in cases of primary ischemic or traumatic brain injury.[11-13]
■ Finally, it is important to remember that many patients in the NICU are on high-dose steroids that will suppress the normal febrile response, so a normal temperature should not be taken as evidence of lack of infection.

The potential causes of fever in the ICU are listed in Table 26.1. The most significant noninfectious causes include drug fever (usually presenting without rash or eosinophilia,[14] deep venous thrombosis, blood products, adrenal insufficiency, "central" fever, subarachnoid hemorrhage, alcohol withdrawal, malignancy, thyroid storm, neuroleptic malignant syndrome, and malignant hyperthermia secondary to anesthetics. The most significant infectious causes include infections of the lung, bloodstream, urinary tract, sinuses, abdomen, and wounds.

The workup of fever in the ICU can be broken down into historical factors, physical examination considerations, and diagnostic testing[10]:

■ A thorough history should also include careful review of past and current medical records, noting past infections, past interventions including surgery (note, benign postoperative fever usually occurs within 48 hours of surgery and patient evaluation is otherwise negative), intravascular and other catheters placed, medications and allergies, changes in sputum production, bowel movements, or wound drainage, and changes in ventilator requirements.
■ Complete physical examination should be performed with special attention to the vital signs,

Table 26.1. Causes of fever in the ICU

Noninfectious	Infectious
Drug fever	Pneumonia/lung abscess/empyema
Reaction to blood products	Bloodstream infection with either bacteria or fungi
DVT/PE	IV line-related infection
Hemorrhage, especially CNS	Other prosthetic device infection, e.g., CNS shunt infection
Alcohol withdrawal	*Clostridium difficile* colitis
Pancreatitis	Intraabdominal abscess
Autoimmune/inflammatory diseases	Cholangitis/cholecystitis
Adrenal insufficiency	Sinusitis
Hyperthyroidism	Pyelonephritis
Heat stroke	Surgical or traumatic wound infection
Malignant hyperthermia	Cellulitis
Neuroleptic malignant syndrome	
Malignancy, especially lymphoma	

Table 26.2. Laboratory and radiologic testing for fever in the ICU

CBC with differential, looking for left shift or eosinophilia

Urinalysis and urine culture

Blood culture: two to three draws initially (one through line) with another pair in 24 hours

Sputum/endotracheal suction/bronchoalveolar lavage gram stain and culture: if evidence for pneumonia (new infiltrate, worsening pulmonary status); including pneuomocystic carini pneumonia and acid fast bacilli PCP, AFB, and fungal stains and cultures if immunocompromised

Clostridium difficile toxin testing if diarrhea is present, × at least 2

Quantitative/semiquantitative cultures of any lines removed

Cultures of other fluids as indicated: CSF, pleural, joint, ascites, abscess

Chest radiograph and/or chest CT

Lower extremity ultrasound/helical chest CT or ventilation–perfusion scan

CT or MRI of head, spine, or sinuses if indicated by clinical suspicion

ventilator settings and oxygenation, skin, IV and other catheter sites, wounds, fundi, oral cavity, heart murmurs or rubs, lung percussion and auscultation, abdomen for rigidity, mass, tenderness, or peritoneal signs, and any focality or change in neuro exam.

- Laboratory and radiologic testing is shown in Table 26.2. Because ICU patients are usually colonized with hospital flora, sputum, or other respiratory cultures should be obtained only if there is evidence for pneumonia because they are otherwise meaningless. Likewise, chronic wounds should not be cultured because they will only show colonization, which is unimportant.

MANAGEMENT OF COMMON INFECTIONS

Pneumonia

Nosocomial pneumonia, whether ventilator-associated (VAP) or not, is extremely common in the ICU, comprising about 25% of all ICU infections. In fact, up to one quarter of intubated patients will develop VAP. An algorithm for management is

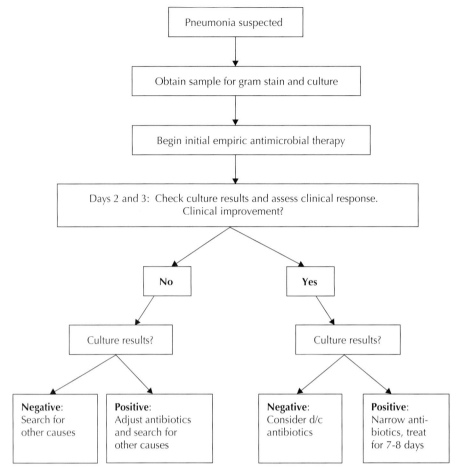

Figure 26.1. Management of pneumonia in the ICU. (Adapted from the American Thoracic Society and the Infectious Diseases Society of America guidelines[11].)

shown in Figure 26.1. Principles of management include[15]:

- Diagnosis is based on the presence of fever or other changes in vital signs, worsening in ventilation or oxygenation parameters, and new or worsening infiltrate on chest radiograph or CT.
- If pneumonia is present, samples for gram stain and culture should be sent from sputum, endotracheal suction, or bronchoalveolar lavage. Sputum gram stain results are more specific than cultures, and quantitative bronchoalveolar lavage cultures are more helpful than qualitative. Blood cultures should also be sent before antibiotics are started.
- Empiric antibiotic therapy should be started pending these results. The choice of specific

drug(s) should take into account local unit flora and that VAP is usually caused by gram-negative bacilli such as *Pseudomonas* or methicillin-resistant *Staphylococcus aureus*, and not anaerobes. Thus, appropriate initial empiric therapy usually consists of linezolid or vancomycin, plus either cefepime or imipenem or piperacillin-tazobactam, plus a quinolone such as ciprofloxacin.
- Therapy should be adjusted within 48–72 hours, based on results of Gram stains and cultures, and antibiotics should either be discontinued or modified to the most narrow-spectrum agents that will cover the microorganisms of concern.
- The duration of antibiotics should be limited to 7–8 days for uncomplicated, non-*Pseudomonas* or *Acinetobacter* VAP.

Intravascular Catheter-Related Infections

Because almost all ICU patients have central venous access, catheter-related infections are a common complication. The key principles in management are[16]:

- Line infection needs to be considered in all patients with fever, because localizing evidence for infection at the line site is often absent. Empiric changes of lines should be part of the management of continued fever without a source in the ICU patient.
- If exit site pus is present, it can be cultured. Blood cultures drawn both through the line and peripherally are crucial, and differential time to positivity can be an important clue to the presence of a line infection. Cultures of catheters should be quantitative or semiquantitative.
- Central venous catheter infections are most often due to staphylococci, gram-negative bacilli or candida. In patients with blood cultures positive for *S. aureus*, a transesophageal echocardiogram (TEE) should be performed, if not contraindicated, to rule out vegetations, due to the high rates of complicating endocarditis.
- Follow-up blood cultures should be obtained to assess clearance.
- Infected peripheral venous catheters should be removed.
- Central venous catheters should be removed and placed in a new site if there is evidence of exit site infection or sepsis, or if positive blood cultures or fever persist after initiation of antibiotics. If the catheter was exchanged over a guidewire and the catheter culture shows significant colonization, the line should be removed and a new line inserted in a new site. If blood cultures still remain positive even after removal of the line, a thorough search for another source should be performed.
- The duration of antibiotic therapy is dependent on the situation and is pathogen-specific. After catheter removal in uncomplicated cases, coagulase-negative staphylococcal infections should be treated 5-7 days, *S. aureus* infections for 14 days ONLY IF a TEE is performed and is negative for endocarditis and for 4-6 weeks otherwise, most gram-negative bacilli for 10-14 days, and candida for 14 days after the last positive blood culture.

Clostridium difficile Colitis

With the widespread use of antibiotics in hospitals and especially in ICUs, *C. difficile* infection is an increasingly common complication; recently identified strains are associated with especially severe disease.[17] The key principles of management include[18],[19]:

- Diarrhea is a common side effect of antibiotics; only 10-20% of antibiotic-associated diarrhea is actually due to *C. difficile*. In addition, ICU patients often have other reasons for diarrhea such as tube feedings and other drugs.
- Additional manifestations of *C. difficile* disease include fever, abdominal pain and cramping, and leukocytosis.
- Diagnosis depends on detection of the *C. difficile* toxin. The gold standard cell culture toxin assay has been replaced by faster and less expensive enzyme immunoassay toxin assays; although the specificity of these tests remains excellent, the sensitivity may be lower (75-90%), so that up to three specimens should be sent to improve the yield of testing. Because 10–30% of asymptomatic hospital patients are colonized with *C. difficile*, cultures of stool are not helpful.
- Antibiotics should be stopped if at all possible. This may be the only treatment that is necessary for mild cases. Rehydration, correction of electrolytes, and proper infection control also should be addressed.
- The preferred specific treatment is oral metronidazole 500 mg tid or 250 mg qid for 10 days. An alternative is oral vancomycin 125 mg qid.
- Improvement should be seen by 2-3 days, with resolution by 6 days. Lack of improvement should prompt a search for complications, such as toxic megacolon. The above regimens are both associated with success rates of 90–97%, although about 20% of patients will relapse later. Relapses usually respond to a repeat course of the same treatment regimen.

Urinary Tract Infections

UTIs are the most common nosocomial infections, representing 40% of all such infections.[20] Most nosocomial UTIs are related to bladder catheterization. Multiple risk factors for catheter-associated UTIs have been identified, including the duration of catheterization, lack of systemic antibiotic therapy, female sex, age older than 50 years, and azotemia. To decrease UTIs in a cost-efficient manner, efts should be concentrated in areas that have been shown to be beneficial.[21]

- Have an established infection control program.
- Catheterize patients only when necessary, by using aseptic technique, sterile equipment, and trained personnel.
- Maintain a closed sterile drainage system; do not disconnect the catheter and drainage tubing unless absolutely necessary.
- Remove the catheter as soon as possible.
- Follow and reince good handwashing technique.
- Changing indwelling catheters at arbitrary fixed intervals and regular bacteriologic monitoring of catheterized patients are not cost-effective practices and should not be permed.

Studies on catheter related UTIs suggest that most episodes of low colony count bacteriuria (10^2–10^4 cfu/mL) rapidly progress to high ($\geq 10^5$/mL) colony counts within 24–48 hours.[22] Treatment of catheter-associated UTI depends on the clinical circumstances. In an asymptomatic patient, therapy should be postponed until the catheter can be removed. Symptomatic patients (e.g., those with fever, chills, dyspnea, and hypotension) require immediate antibiotic therapy with broad-spectrum antibiotics covering nosocomial gram-positive and gram-negative organisms. *Candida albicans* and other *Candida* species account for up to a third of all ICU-acquired UTIs.[23] The clinical presentation can vary from an asymptomatic laboratory finding to sepsis. In asymptomatic patients, removal of the urethral catheter results in resolution of the candiduria in as many as one third of cases. For patients with symptomatic candiduria (fever with or without cystitis symptoms), oral fluconazole, 200 mg/day for 7–14 days, has been shown to be highly effective. This regimen was even effective for non-*albicans* species of *Candida* that had reduced susceptibility to fluconazole, possibly because of the high concentrations achieved in the urine.[24]

Sepsis

In the United States, sepsis is a leading cause of death in non-coronary ICU patients, and the tenth most common cause of death overall, killing 20–50% of severely affected patients.[25] Sepsis is considered present if infection is highly suspected or proven and two or more of the following systemic inflammatory response syndrome (SIRS) criteria are met[26]:

- Heart rate >90 beats/min
- Body temperature <36ºC or >38ºC (<96.8ºF or >100.4ºF)
- Respiratory rate >20 breaths/min; or $PaCO_2$ <32 mm Hg
- White blood cell (WBC) count <4000 cells/mm^3 or >12,000 cells/mm^3; or >10% band forms

The therapy of sepsis rests on antibiotics, surgical drainage of infected fluid collections, fluid replacement and appropriate support for organ dysfunction (e.g., hemodialysis, mechanical ventilation, transfusion of blood products, and vasoactive agents for hypotension).

Before 1987, gram-negative bacteria were the predominant pathogens in severe sepsis. Among the organisms reported to have caused sepsis in 2000, gram-positive bacteria accounted for 52.1% of cases, with gram-negative bacteria accounting for 37.6%, polymicrobial infections for 4.7%, anaerobes for 1.0%, and fungi for 4.6%.[27] Combination antimicrobial therapy is indicated in the initial empiric therapy of severe sepsis. Empiric antimicrobial combinations should include vancomycin or linezolid to cover potentially resistant gram-positive organisms and an antipseudomonal β-lactam (e.g., cefepime, ceftazidime, piperacillin-tazobactam) combined with either an aminoglycoside (e.g., gentamicin or tobramycin) or antipseudomonal fluoroquinolone (e.g., levofloxacin or ciprofloxacin) to cover gram-negative pathogens. Additional coverage for anaerobic organisms should be included when the sepsis source is an intra-abdominal/pelvic infection or a necrotizing skin and soft tissue infection.[28]

Studies have demonstrated that the administration of recombinant human activated protein C (drotrecogin alfa [activated]) results in significant improvements in organ function and has shown a mortality benefit in patients with severe sepsis. Criteria for treatment with drotrecogin alfa include[29]:

- Severe sepsis or septic shock
- APACHE II score of 25 or greater
- Low risk of bleeding

Table 26.3. Organisms requiring isolation precautions in hospitals

Contact isolation	MRSA: methicillin-resistant *Staphylococcus aureus* VRE: vancomycin-resistant enterococcus multidrug resistant gram negative bacteria *Clostridium difficile Herpes simplex*: severe mucocutaneous or disseminated potentially infectious diarrhea of unknown cause Draining abscesses (if dressing does not contain drainage adequately Pediculosis
Droplet isolation	Influenza *Neisseria meningitidis:* pneumonia or meningitis Pertussis Parvovirus B19 *Haemophilus influenzae:* pneumonia or meningitis (infants and children) *Mycoplasma* pneumonia
Airborne isolation	Mycobacterium tuberculosis: pulmonary or laryngeal disease Varicella: primary or reactivation* Rubeola Rubella SARS* Smallpox*

* Also requires contact isolation.
Adapted from Refs. 30 and 31.

INFECTION CONTROL IN THE ICU

Infection control is the discipline concerned with preventing the spread of infections within the healthcare setting. Transmission of infection within a hospital requires three elements[30],[31]:

- A source of infecting microorganisms
  - ▸ Human sources include patients, staff, or visitors
- A susceptible host
  - ▸ Host factors include age; comorbid diseases; degree of immunosuppression; and breaks in the first line of defense mechanisms (e.g., indwelling catheters or other devices, breaks in skin)
- A means of transmission for the microorganism
  - ▸ Five main routes of transmission: contact, droplet, airborne, common vehicle, and vector-borne.

There are two tiers of isolation precautions: Standard Precautions and Transmission Based Precautions Standard precautions are used for all patients regardless of diagnosis or presumed infection and stress the need for hand hygiene and use of personal protective equipment (e.g., gloves, gowns, masks, face shields, and eye protection)

when contact with blood or body fluids is expected. CDC has recommended three specific categories of transmission based precautions which are always to be used in addition to standard precautions: Contact, Droplet, and Airborne. There are a number of infectious agents included in each category with a brief listing outlined in Table 26.3.

Contact Precautions are designed to prevent transmission of infectious agents, including epidemiologically important microorganisms by direct or indirect contact with the patient or the patient's environment.

- CDC recommends implementation of contact precautions for all patients infected with multidrug-resistant organisms (MDROs) and for patients that have previously identified as being colonized with target MDROs.

Duration of isolation is reasonable for the duration of hospital stay, but potentially can be discontinued after surveillance cultures for the target organism are repeatedly negative over the course of a week or two in a patient who has not been received antimicrobial therapy.[32] Practitioners should consult their local infection control practitioners for policies and procedures specific to their institution regarding institution and discontinuation of isolation.

Droplet precautions are used for patients known or suspected to have serious illnesses transmitted by large particle droplets (>5 μm in size). Duration of isolation for the organisms included in this group varies.

- For bacterial pathogens, isolation can usually be discontinued after 24 hours of appropriate antibiotic therapy.
- For the viral pathogens listed, the duration of isolation is less defined but the usual recommendation is to maintain isolation for the duration of illness.[30],[31]

Airborne precautions are used for patients known or suspected to have illnesses transmitted by small particle droplets (<5 μm in size). Patients should be placed in a private room with negative pressure and HEPA filtration. Everyone entering the room should wear an N95 respirator or equivalent.

- Patients presenting with an unknown generalized rash or exanthema should be placed in airborne and contact isolation while the evaluation for the specific cause ensues.
- For the majority of infections listed in Table 26.3, isolation is continued for the duration of hospitalization.
- Isolation for varicella can be discontinued when all lesions are crusted. For *Mycobacterium tuberculosis*, only pulmonary and laryngeal disease requires airborne precautions.
- Patients with extrapulmonary tuberculous disease, including meningitis, require only standard precautions.

All healthcare personnel should know how to contact the infection control practitioners and policies for their institution. The ultimate goal of an Infection Control program is the prevention and control of infections and communicable diseases, through surveillance, interventions, and education.

REFERENCES

1. Singh N, Yu V. Rational empiric antibiotic prescription in the ICU. *Chest.* 2000;**117**:1496–9.
2. Kollef MH, Faser VJ. Antibiotic Resistance in the Intensive Care Unit. *Ann Intern Med.* 2001;**134**:298–314.
3. Chastre J, Fagon JY. Ventilator-associated pneumonia *Am J Respir & Crit Care Med.* 2002;**165**(7):867–903.
4. CDC NNIS System National Nosocomial Infections Surveillance (NNIS) System Report, data summary from January 1992 through June 2004, issued October 2004. *Am J Infect Control.* 2004;**32**:470–85.
5. Mackowiak PA, Bartlett JG, Borden EC, et al. Concepts of fever: recent advances and lingering dogma. *Clin Infect Dis.* 1997;**25**:119–38.
6. O'Grady NP, Barie PS, Bartlett JG, et al. Practice guidelines for evaluating new fever in critically ill adult patients. *Clin Infect Dis.* 1998;**26**:1042–59. Also available at http://www.idsociety.org/Content/Navigation Menu/Practice_Guidelines/Standards_Practice_Guidelines_Statements/Standards,_Practice_Guidelines,_and_Statements.htm.
7. Commichau C, Scarmeas N, Mayer SA. Risk factors for fever in the neurologic intensive care unit. *Neurology.* 2003;**60**:837–41.
8. Wartenberg KE, Schmidt JM, Claasen J, et al. Impact of medical complications on outcome after subarachnoid hemorrhage. *Crit Care Med.* 2006;**34**:617–23.
9. Diringer MN, Reaven NL, Funk SE, Uman GC. Elevated body temperature independently contributes to increased length of stay in neurologic intensive care units. *Crit Care Med.* 2004;**32**:1489–95.
10. Peres Bota D, Lopes Ferreira F, Melot C, Vincent JL. Body temperature alterations in the critically ill. *Intens Care Med.* 2004;**30**:811–6.
11. Gozzoli V, Schottker P, Suter PM, Ricou B. Is it worth treating fever in intensive care unit patients? Preliminary results from a randomized trial of the effect of external cooling. *Arch Intern Med.* 2001;**161**:121–3.
12. Kilpatrick MM, Lowry DW, Firlik AD, Yonas H, Marion DW. Hyperthermia in the neurosurgical intensive care unit. *Neurosurgery.* 2000;**47**:850–5.
13. Ryan M, Levy MM. Clinical review: fever in intensive care unit patients. *Crit Care.* 2003;**7**:221–5.
14. Mackowiak PA, LeMaistre CF. Drug fever: a critical appraisal of conventional concepts. *Ann Intern Med.* 1987;**106**:728–33.
15. The American Thoracic Society, and the Infectious Diseases Society of America. Guidelines for the management of adults with hospital-acquired, ventilator-associated, and healthcare-associated pneumonia. *Am J Respir Crit Care Med.* 2005;**171**:388–416. Also available at http://www.idsociety.org/Content/Navigation Menu/Practice_Guidelines/Standards_Practice_Guidelines_Statements/Standards,_Practice_Guidelines,_and_Statements.htm.
16. Mermel LA, Farr BM, Sheretz RJ, et al. Guidelines for the management of intravascular catheter-related infections. *Clin Infect Dis.* 2001;**32**:1249–72. Also available at http://www.idsociety.org/Content/NavigationMenu/Practice_Guidelines/Standards_Practice_Guidelines_Statements/Standards,_Practice_Guidelines,_and_Statements.htm.
17. Bartlett JG. Narrative review: the new epidemic of *Clostridium difficile*-associated enteric disease. *Ann Intern Med.* 2006;**145**:758–64.
18. Bartlett JG. Antibiotic-associated diarrhea. *N Engl J Med.* 2002;**346**:334–9.

19. Gerding DN, Johnson S, Peterson LR, Mulligan ME, Silva J. SHEA position paper. *Clostridium difficile-associated diarrhea and colitis. Infect Control Hosp Epidemiol.* 1995;**16**:459–77.

20. Wong ES. Guideline for prevention of catheter-associated urinary tract infections *Am J Infect Control.* 1983;**11**(1):28–36.

21. Epstein SE. Cost-effective application of the Centers for Disease Control Guideline for Prevention of Catheter-associated Urinary Tract Infections *Am J Infect Control.* 1985;**13**(6):272–5.

22. Stamm WE. Catheter-associated urinary tract infections: epidemiology, pathogenesis, and prevention. *Am J Med.* 1991;**91**(3B):65S–71S.

23. Bagshaw SM, Laupland KB. Epidemiology of intensive care unit-acquired urinary tract infections. *Curr Opin Infect Dis.* 2006;**19**:67–71.

24. Gupta K, Stamm WE. Urinary tract infections. ACP Medicine Online, Dale DC; Federman DD, Eds. WebMD Inc., New York, 2000.

25. Martin GS, Mannino DM, Eaton S, Moss M. The epidemiology of sepsis in the United States from 1979 through 2000. *N Engl J Med.* 2003;**348**(16):1546–54.

26. Bone RC, Balk RA, Cerra FB, et al. Definitions for sepsis and organ failure and guidelines for the use of innovative therapies in sepsis. The ACCP/SCCM Consensus Conference Committee. *American College of Chest Physicians/Society of Critical Care Medicine. Chest.* 1992;**101**(6):1644–55.

27. Martin GS, Mannino DM, Eaton S, Moss M. The epidemiology of sepsis in the United States from 1979 through 2000. *N Engl J Med.* 2003;**348**(16):1546–54.

28. Nguyen HB, Rivers EP, Abrahamian FM, et. al. Severe sepsis and septic shock: review of the literature and emergency department management guidelines. *Ann Emerg Med.* 2006;**48**(1):28–54.

29. Bernard GR, Vincent JL, Laterre PF, et al. Recombinant human protein C Worldwide Evaluation in Severe Sepsis (PROWESS) study group. Efficacy and safety of recombinant human activated protein C for severe sepsis. *N Engl J Med.* 2001;**344**(10):699–709.

30. Garner JS; Hospital Infection Control Practices Advisory Committee. Guideline for isolation precautions in hospitals. *Infect Control Hosp Epidemiol.* 1996;**17**:53–80.

31. Garner JS; Hospital Infection Control Practices Advisory Committee. Guideline for isolation precautions in hospitals. Part 1: Evolution of isolation practices. *Am J Infect Control.* 1996;**24**:24–52.

32. Siegel JD, Rhinehart E, Jackson M, Chiarello L; the Healthcare Infection Control Practices Advisory Committee. Multidrug-resistant organisms in Healthcare settings, 2006. Found at: http://www.cdc.gov/ncidod/dhqp/pdf/ar/mdroGuideline2006.pdf

27 A Gastroenterology Consult

Yume Nguyen, MD, Thomas Kerr, MD, PhD, and Riad Azar, MD

Diseases that affect the gastrointestinal tract, liver, and pancreas are a diverse and vast group of disorders that encompass a wide array of pathology. Topics covered in this chapter focus mainly on gastrointestinal issues that affect patients in the intensive care unit setting. The chapter is organized by disorders commonly encountered in this patient population and outlines the appropriate approach to diagnosis and management.

GASTROINTESTINAL BLEEDING

Gastrointestinal bleeding (GIB) can present with hematemesis, coffee-ground emesis, blood from a nasogastric tube, hematochezia, maroon stool, or melena. Risk factors include a prior history of GI bleeding, liver disease, colon cancer, diverticulosis, prior abdominal surgery, angiodysplasia, and nonsteroidal anti-inflammatory drug (NSAID) and anticoagulant use. It is important to determine the location of bleeding, as this will guide subsequent management. Massive GI hemorrhage is potentially life-threatening and prompt diagnosis and treatment is imperative.

Location of Bleeding

- Upper GI bleeding by definition occurs proximal to the ligament of Treitz. It may present as hematemesis, blood observed from the nasogastric tube, melena (present in 70% of upper GI bleeds), or heme-positive stools.
  - If rectal blood is melenic, it is from a source proximal to the ligament of Treitz. However,

a briskly bleeding upper GI bleed can lead to hematochezia in up to 15% of cases.[1]
- Etiologies of upper GI bleeding: peptic ulcer disease (50% of upper GI bleeds), gastritis, Mallory–Weiss tears, varices, erosive esophagitis, vascular malformations
- *H. pylori* infection has not been associated with increased risk of gastrointestinal bleeding in the ICU setting.[2]
- Lower GI bleeding (distal to the ligament of Treitz): Etiologies include diverticular disease, angiodysplasia, colitis (infectious, ischemic, inflammatory), neoplastic disease, or hemorrhoids.

Initial Evaluation/Management

- Obtain adequate intravenous access; two large-bore (16- or 18-gauge) peripheral IV lines are usually sufficient. If this is not obtainable central venous access should be placed.
- Fluid resuscitation: Tachycardia or orthostatic hypotension signifies significant blood loss and should be treated with aggressive fluid resuscitation with isotonic crystalloid and blood products as appropriate.
- Placement of a nasogastric tube with lavage of the stomach and duodenum is the next step in diagnosis. A bloody or coffee grounds–appearing nasogastric aspirate suggests a high-risk lesion on endoscopic examination.[3] It is useful to note whether bile is obtained from the lavage, as this indicates that the duodenum was sampled. This may also clear stomach contents to facilitate upper endoscopy.[4]

- Endotracheal intubation: Often an endotracheal tube is necessary to prevent aspiration of blood and protect the airway especially if the patient is obtunded.
- Laboratory tests: Type and screen, complete blood count (CBC), comprehensive metabolic panel (CMP), coagulation studies. It may take up to 24 hours for the blood counts to reflect the degree of blood loss. Blood transfusion may be necessary with significant blood loss. Any coagulopathies or thrombocytopenia should be corrected.
- High-dose intravenous proton pump inhibitor or histamine$_2$ blocker initiation is warranted when an upper GI source is determined.

Treatment

- After the appropriate initial measures have been performed, a gastroenterologist should be notified as soon as possible.
- Upper GIB: Endoscopic gastroduodenoscopy (EGD) is the mainstay of treatment in UGIB. It can be both diagnostic and therapeutic because endoscopic interventions including cautery or injection therapy may be performed.
- LGIB: Lower GI bleeding is more likely than upper GI bleeding to spontaneously stop. If a patient is stable enough to undergo bowel prep, a colonoscopy is the procedure of choice. Diverticular disease or bleeding due to arteriovenous malformation may be amenable to endoscopic epinephrine injections, cauterization, embolization, or surgery.
  - In brisk LGIB when the patient may be hemodynamically unstable, a tagged red cell scan can localize bleeding at rates as low as 0.1 mL/min. If the patient remains unstable and continues to bleed, arteriography may locate the site of bleeding. This can localize bleeding as low as 0.5 mL/min, and can lead to therapeutic interventions such as coil embolization.
  - If bleeding continues despite the above therapeutic interventions, surgery may be the only remaining option.

Special Cases

- Variceal bleeds are more common in patients with end stage liver disease due to portal hypertension. Acute variceal bleeding warrants urgent upper GI endoscopy.

- Every attempt should be made to correct coagulopathy or thrombocytopenia. Octreotide infusion has a high rate of controlling bleeding.[5] Endoscopic band ligation is the preferred intervention and has a high likelihood of controlling bleeding.[6] Sclerotherapy, balloon tamponade, surgery, and transjugular intrahepatic portosystemic shunt (TIPS) are reserved for refractory bleeding.

ACUTE MESENTERIC ISCHEMIA

Acute mesenteric ischemia (AMI) is typically divided into three categories: arterial thrombus, nonocclusive mesenteric ischemia, and venous thrombosis. Risk factors include cardiovascular disease, embolic disease (i.e., atrial fibrillation, endocarditis), and hypercoagulable state.

Diagnosis

- Clinical history may include postprandial pain ("intestinal angina"), early satiety, and food avoidance with resultant weight loss. Patients may present nausea, vomiting, diarrhea, bloody stool, or acute or subacute onset of abdominal pain which is usually diffuse and poorly localized. Notably, abdominal pain may be absent in 15–25% of cases.
  - Physical examination
    - Abdominal pain out of proportion to exam
    - May have peritoneal signs, abdominal distension, hypoactive bowel sounds, ileus, fecal occult blood test positive or frankly bloody stool, or shock.
- Laboratory tests
  - Check lipase to rule out pancreatitis. Amylase is frequently elevated in ischemic bowel.
  - Check for elevated white blood cell count (WBC) (typically >15,000 cells/μL), lactate dehydrogenase (LDH), creatine phosphokinase (CPK), lactic acid (late), metabolic acidosis.
  - Check for blood urea nitrogen (BUN)/creatinine elevation from prerenal azotemia/hypovolemia.
- Diagnostic tests
  - Abdominal computed tomography (CT) to evaluate for pneumatosis; abdominal ultrasound with Doppler is used to evaluate blood

flow and plain radiograph may show "thumb-printing," pneumatosis intestinalis, adynamic ileus.

▶ Angiography is the gold standard.

Treatment

■ Early recognition and treatment are critical to optimize survival.

■ IV fluid resuscitation, nasogastric tube decompression, broad-spectrum antibiotics

■ For acute arterial embolus, consider thrombolytics or surgery.

■ For venous thrombosis; consider anticoagulation therapy.

■ Nonocclusive mesenteric ischemia: Intra-arterial infusion of papaverine and hemodynamic optimization

■ Surgical intervention: Thromboembolectomy for acute arterial embolism, bypass grafting, endarterectomy, angioplasty ± bowel resection for mesenteric infarction

ACUTE INTESTINAL PSEUDO-OBSTRUCTION (ILEUS)

An ileus involves dilatation or signs of obstruction without any indication of mechanical obstruction. Risk factors include acute or chronic illness, electrolyte imbalance, and medications. On physical examination, particular attention should be paid to any signs of perforation.

■ Laboratory evaluation: basic metabolic panel (BMP), Mg, CBC, amylase, lipase

■ Diagnostic tests: Obstructive series radiograph of the abdomen; CT scanning may be necessary to distinguish obstruction from ileus.

■ Treatment: Bowel rest/nothing by mouth, intravenous fluids, and correction of any electrolyte disturbances. Encourage increasing ambulation and general physical activity if the patient is able.

▶ In refractory cases, it is sometimes necessary to initiate total parenteral nutrition (TPN). Turn the patient from side to side. Implement intermittent suction from the nasogastric tube. Distal decompression with a rectal tube or colonoscopic decompression especially when the cecal diameter approaches 9–10 centimeters. Neostigmine may result in colonic decompression but may be contraindicated

if there remains a possibility of mechanical obstruction. Surgery has little role in ileus and is reserved for cases where perforation or intestinal ischemia has occurred.

NAUSEA AND VOMITING

The causes of acute nausea and vomiting are vast, and in the ICU setting most commonly include bowel obstruction, side effect of medications, central nervous system (CNS) disorders, systemic illness, infection, and delayed gastric emptying. Initial management should focus on supportive care as most cases are self-limiting. This includes treating the underlying cause of the vomiting and correcting volume deficits and electrolyte abnormalities. Nasogastric tube decompression is warranted when bowel obstruction is present. Typically per oral intake is withheld while investigating the source of nausea and vomiting or allowing bland foods such as clears and crackers is acceptable.

■ Antiemetics

▶ Dopamine antagonists: Prochlorperazine (Compazine) 5–10 mg PO, IM, IV q4–6h or 25 mg suppository q6h; promethazine (Phenergan) 12.5–25 mg PO, IM, PR q4–6h; metoclopramide (Reglan) 10–20 mg PO q6h or 0.5–2 mg/kg IV q6–8h. Antiemetic property of the phenothiazines and related agents are due to the dopaminergic blockade and sedation. Acute dystonic reactions and other extrapyramidal effects may occur.

▶ Antihistamines/anticholinergics: Diphenhydramine (Benadryl) 25–50 mg PO, IV, IM q4–6h; dimenhydrinate (Dramamine) 50–100 mg PO q4h; meclizine (Antivert) 12.5–25 mg PO q24h) are most useful in motion sickness and postoperatively.

▶ Serotonin 5-HT$_3$ receptor antagonists (Odansetron or Zofran 0.15 mg/kg IV q8h): Receptors are found in the GI tract and central and peripheral nervous system. Especially effective in chemotherapy-related nausea or refractory nausea.

▶ Sedatives/CNS altering agents: Benzodiazepines (diazepam 2–5 mg PO, IV q4–6h; lorazepam 1–2 mg PO, IV q4–6h) can be useful in nausea with a psychological or anticipatory component.

DIARRHEA

Diarrhea is defined as an increase in frequency or change in stool volume.[7] The etiology of diarrhea is typically classified as acute (<14 days) versus chronic (>14 days).

Classification of Acute Diarrhea

- Infectious: Viral, parasitic (*Entamoeba*), bacterial (*E. coli, Shigella, Salmonella, Campylobacter, Clostridium difficile*). Prolonged hospitalization, elderly age, nursing home residence, and ICU admission increase the risk of developing *C. difficile* colitis.[8,9]
- Inflammatory
- Malabsorptive
- Osmotic
- Secretory
- Motility-related

Evaluation

Particular attention should be paid to travel, ingestions, medications especially antibiotics, recent institution of tube feedings, recent hospitalization, sick contacts, and HIV status in the history. On physical examination the general appearance, vital signs, orthostatics, and abdominal examination can provide important clues. If dehydration, fever, mucus, pus, blood, abdominal pain is present or if the patient recently used antibiotics, diagnostic tests may be warranted:

- Fecal leukocytes, fecal occult blood, and *C. difficile* toxin may differentiate inflammatory from noninflammatory diarrhea.
- Noninflammatory diarrhea: Stool ova and parasite
- Inflammatory diarrhea: Obtain stool cultures; consider irritable bowel disease.
- A stool osmolar gap, the difference between calculated and measured stool osmolarity >70 mOsmol suggests osmotic causes such as enteral feeding.[10]
- Endoscopy may be necessary to evaluate for inflammatory bowel disease or microscopic colitis

Treatment/Management

Treatment focuses on supportive therapy with hydration and electrolyte management.

- Empiric treatment (metronidazole 500 mg PO/IV tid/qid) may be warranted in the setting of recent antibiotic use or when there is a high suspicion for pseudomembranous colitis.
- Discontinuation of tube feeding for enteral feeding-associated diarrhea is generally not necessary if the patient's fluid and electrolyte status remain in acceptable ranges.
- Antidiarrheals such as opiates (loperamide 2–4 mg up to 16 mg/day), anticholinergics (Lomotil), and bismuth subsalicylate.
- In bile acid–associated diarrhea, cholestyramine may be useful.
- In cases of hormone-mediated secretory diarrhea such as with neuroendocrine tumors, octreotide may be effective.

STRESS GI PROPHYLAXIS

Stress-related mucosal disease (SRMD) is a common source of gastrointestinal bleeding in the ICU setting; however, clinically important upper GI bleeding occurs in fewer than 2% of patients.[11] Risk factors include renal failure, pharmacologic damage to the gut mucosa, coagulopathy, mechanical ventilation, sepsis, hypotension, and severe burns. The cause of SRMD is usually due to mucosal hypoperfusion, elevated gastric acid, and bile salts. Current recommendations suggest that stress ulcer prophylaxis be reserved for patients with risk factors for GI bleeding.[12]

PHARMACOTHERAPY

- Proton pump inhibitors prevent stress gastritis and ulceration by directly inhibiting the proton pumps that acidify the stomach.
- Histamine$_2$ blockers are very effective at reducing the rate of clinically significant GI bleeding, although tachyphylaxis may develop.
- Antacids are infrequently used because of the necessity to administer these agents every 1–2 hours.

ACUTE LIVER INJURY/ABNORMAL LIVER CHEMISTRIES

The two general patterns of liver injury are (1) hepatocellular injury, which typically presents with elevated transaminases and (2) cholestatic liver injury, the hallmark being elevated alkaline phosphatase and γ-glutamyl transpeptidase (GGT). There is often overlap between these two patterns but it provides a framework by which to proceed.

Diagnosis

- History
  - Abdominal pain, right upper quadrant pain, diarrhea, pale stools, dark urine, or yellow skin.
  - Make an assessment of risk factors for liver disease such as intravenous drug abuse, blood transfusions, sexual promiscuity, homosexual contact, tattoos, history of malignancy, family history of liver disease and autoimmune disorders.
- Physical examination: Evaluate for stigmata of chronic liver disease and jaundice.
- Laboratory evaluation
  - Aspartate aminotransferase (AST)/alanine aminotransferase (ALT): Elevations indicate hepatocellular damage
  - Alkaline phosphatase: Elevations suggest biliary process.
  - Bilirubin is the product of heme protein breakdown and may be elevated in intra- or extrahepatic biliary obstruction.
  - Markers of liver disease: Albumin, prothrombin time (PT), international normalized ratio (INR), serum cholesterol
  - Acute viral hepatitis panel, γ-glutamyl transpeptidase (GGT) or 5′-nucleotidase (5′NT) if alkaline phosphatase is elevated and if there is any uncertainty regarding its etiology, CBC, PT/PTT
  - Antimitochondrial or antismooth muscle antibodies: Depending on clinical suspicion.
  - Acetaminophen level should be checked in all cases of acute liver failure.
- Diagnostic tests
  - Right upper quadrant ultrasound: May detect biliary dilation, stones, or inflammation and evaluate liver echotexture and vasculature.
  - Contrast-enhanced CT and magnetic resonance imaging (MRI) may characterize the liver parenchyma and assess vascular and ductal structures.
  - Endoscopic retrograde cholangiopancreatography (ERCP), magnetic resonance cholangiopancreatography, and percutaneous transhepatic cholangiography allow direct visualization of the biliary tree.

Treatment

Treatment focuses on withdrawal of the offending agent and supportive care.

- Immunoglobulin and/or vaccination as appropriate.
- Acute viral hepatitis C: Interferon-α therapy may decrease the likelihood of progressing to chronic hepatitis.[13]
- Acetaminophen overdose: N-acetylcysteine therapy if initiated promptly after acetaminophen ingestion.[14]

Complications of End-Stage Liver Disease

PORTAL HYPERTENSION AND ASCITES

Once ascites occurs, the 1-year mortality rate increases substantially, as well as the risk of developing spontaneous bacterial peritonitis (SBP), hepatic hydrothorax (typically occurs in the right hemithorax), and hepatorenal syndrome.[15]

- Physical examination
  - Shifting dullness and a fluid wave, spider angiomas, caput medusa, ecchymosis.
- Paracentesis
  - Perform diagnostic paracentesis if there is new-onset ascites, clinical deterioration, new-onset encephalopathy, abdominal pain or signs of infections.
  - Fluid should be routinely sent for Gram stain and culture (inoculate two culture bottles at the bedside with 10 mL of ascites fluid to increase the yield of culturing a specific organism), cell count with differential, albumin, and total protein.
  - Serum-ascites albumin gradient (SAAG) can be done to determine the cause of ascites. SAAG >1.1 g/dL = portal hypertension-related; SAAG <1.2 g/dL = nonportal-hypertension related.
  - If there is suspicion for a chylous effusion, check peritoneal fluid triglyceride levels. Other labs may include cytology, mycobacterial smear for acid fast bacilli and culture, amylase/lipase if complicated pancreatitis is suspected.

- Therapy
  - Sodium restriction, diuretic therapy for uninfected ascites.
  - If diuretic therapy fails at maximum tolerated doses, large-volume paracentesis or TIPS may be required. List patients for liver transplantation if they meet transplant criteria.
- Spontaneous bacterial peritonitis (SBP) is defined as ascitic fluid with polymorphonuclear cell count >250 cells/μL. Treat with antibiotics (usually third-generation cephalosporin such as ceftriaxone 2 g IV qd, cefotaxime 2 g IV q12h, or quinolones such as ciprofloxacin 500 mg IV q12h) and albumin to prevent renal impairment.[16]
- Gastroesophageal varices
  - Gastroesophageal varices occur in approximately 40% of patients with well compensated cirrhosis and in up to 85% of those with decompensated cirrhosis.[17] Hemorrhage usually occurs when the portal to hepatic pressure gradient exceeds 12 mm Hg.
  - In active variceal hemorrhage, IV octreotide, antibiotics, and endoscopic band ligation may be used. TIPS may be required in patients who have failed primary and secondary treatment options. (see gastrointestinal bleeding section).
- Hepatic encephalopathy (HE)
  - The cause of HE is likely multifactorial, but accumulation of ammonia and other toxic substances that cause excitation of γ-aminobutyric acid (GABA) and inhibit glutamate plays a central role.
  - Conditions that commonly precipitate hepatic encephalopathy include gastrointestinal bleeding, infections, and constipation.
  - Diagnosis: Clinical suspicion in combination with elevated blood ammonia level determines the diagnosis.
  - Treatment: Treat the underlying condition and use lactulose and antibiotics.
- Fulminant hepatic failure (FHF)
  - Defined as encephalopathy that occurs within 8 weeks of acute liver injury.
  - Encephalopathy that occurs between 8 and 24 weeks after the initial injury is considered sub-fulminant or late-onset hepatic failure.
  - Development of cerebral edema is the most serious complication and is the cause of death in 30–50% of patients with FHF.

- In the United States, the majority of FHF is due to drugs and toxins, with acetaminophen being the most common cause. The remainder of acute liver failure is mostly due to viral infections. Other sequela of FHF involve other organ systems and include pulmonary disease (acute respiratory distress syndrome [ARDS], respiratory alkalosis), renal (hepatorenal syndrome, acute tubular necrosis, electrolyte disturbances), cardiovascular collapse, hematologic (disseminated intravascular coagulation, coagulopathy), infectious complications and endocrine (hypoglycemia).
- Hepatorenal syndrome (HRS)
  - Vasoconstriction of renal vessels that manifests as progressive oliguria and azotemia. Fluid challenge is useful in determining the etiology. Precipitants include large-volume paracentesis, SBP, GIB, and aminoglycosides. The only definitive treatment is liver transplantation.[18]

ACUTE PANCREATITIS

The etiology of pancreatitis is most commonly alcohol and gallstones. Less common causes include medications (thiazide diuretics, furosemide, sulfa drugs, estrogen, azathioprine, antiretrovirals), metabolic problems (hypertriglyceridemia, hypercalcemia), trauma, obstruction, and infection.

Diagnosis

- Clinical presentation: Nausea/vomiting, mid-epigastric abdominal pain with radiation to back (relieved by leaning forward), and fever.
- Physical examination: Mid-epigastric abdominal tenderness on palpation, hypoactive bowel sounds (adynamic ileus is common); if severe, hypotension and shock may ensue.
- Laboratory/imaging studies: Elevated amylase and lipase, elevated hematocrit (indicating volume contraction; may be low in setting of hemorrhage), WBC, BUN/creatinine, glucose (indicating pancreatic synthetic dysfunction), CRP, ± liver enzymes, low Ca.
- Diagnostic tests: Abdominal CT with IV contrast and pancreas protocol is modality of choice but may be normal in up to 28% of mild cases. It is not necessary to pursue a CT exam unless the patient is clinically worsening.

Treatment

- Supportive care: Early and aggressive volume resuscitation and electrolyte repletion.
- Analgesia: Demerol has been recommended to prevent sphincter of Oddi contraction which may occur with other analgesics.
- NPO, nasogastric suction if refractory nausea and vomiting
- Antibiotics if clinically deteriorates or fails to improve over next few days and persistently febrile.[19]
- Therapeutic interventions: CT-guided abscess drainage or fine-needle aspiration of necrotic mass or ERCP in the setting of gallstone pancreatitis causing obstruction

BILIARY DISEASE

Disorders of the pancreas and biliary tree can range from asymptomatic gallstones to serious and potentially life-threatening infection. In this section we reserve discussion of the most commonly encountered pancreaticobiliary disorders seen in the ICU setting.

Acute Cholecystitis

Cholecystitis is inflammation or infection of the gallbladder usually caused by obstruction by gallstones. Acalculous cystitis can be seen in critically ill patients and can result in significant morbidity and mortality.[20]

Acute Cholangitis

Cholangitis is an infection superimposed upon an obstruction of the biliary tree usually secondary to gallstones but strictures and neoplasms may be other causes. Recent manipulation of the biliary tree is also a risk factor. Clinical manifestations include fever, abdominal pain and, occasionally, jaundice. Laboratory abnormalities include elevated transaminases, bilirubin, or alkaline phosphatase.

Gallstone Pancreatitis

Often results from biliary stone disease causing disruption of the pancreatic ducts. Stone passage or impaction at the ampulla is responsible for gallstone pancreatitis.

DIAGNOSIS

- Physical examination may reveal icterus, hepatomegaly, ascites, or focal tenderness over the liver or gallbladder. Findings range from acute abdomen to nonspecific fever and ileus.
- Laboratory tests
  - The bilirubin is usually elevated, and although serum transaminase elevations are the hallmark of hepatocellular injury, elevated levels can also be seen with biliary disease, especially inflammatory and infectious conditions and acute biliary obstruction.
- Imaging
  - Ultrasonography is very sensitive for detecting biliary ductal dilatation and cholelithiasis with an accuracy exceeding 95%.
    - Does not exclude the presence of stones in the distal common bile duct (CBD) due to overlying bowel gas.
  - CT is highly accurate for the detection of the level and cause of biliary obstruction, especially in the pancreatic head region.
  - MRI techniques that incorporate cholangiopancreatography also provide highly useful images of the liver and entire biliary tree without requiring invasive procedures.[21]
  - Radionuclide scanning
  - ERCP and percutaneous transhepatic cholangiogram (PTC)
    - Both can be performed emergently when necessary, both for diagnosis and therapy of biliary disorders (see below).

MANAGEMENT

- Ascending cholangitis and biliary obstruction:
  - If cholangitis is suspected, broad-spectrum antibiotics should be started promptly. Extended-spectrum penicillins, cephalosporins, and fluoroquinolones are usually recommended.[22]
  - Aggressive supportive measures should be started with IV fluids and pressors if needed.
  - Patients should undergo emergent biliary decompression by either ERCP or PTC. With ERCP a biliary sphincterotomy and stone extraction can be achieved but placement of a biliary stent can be sufficient for decompression. If ERCP is not available, PTC is a safe alternative and also provides adequate drainage of the biliary tree.[23–25]

- Acute cholecystitis
  - Percutaneous cholecystostomy under ultrasonographic guidance has become the therapy of choice in patients too unstable for operative cholecystectomy or when acute cholecystitis does not respond to antibiotics. This can be performed at the bedside in the ICU.
    - The cholecystostomy drainage catheter is left in place until acute symptoms resolve, at which time an elective surgical cholecystectomy can be scheduled. In patients with severe comorbid medical conditions, the tube may simply be removed with or without percutaneous stone extraction.
- Acute gallstone pancreatitis (see also acute pancreatitis section):
  - Although most patients with acute gallstone pancreatitis improve with conservative therapy for pancreatitis, early ERCP may be indicated for removal of impacted or retained common bile duct stones, limiting further pancreatic inflammation and preventing cholangitis.[26]
  - Definitive therapy with elective cholecystectomy (or percutaneous cholecystotomy or endoscopic sphincterotomy in nonoperative candidates) is indicated to prevent recurrences.

NUTRITION

Basal energy expenditure (in kcal/day) is approximately 25 times the weight of the patient in kilograms. Stress may increase basal energy expenditures up to 1.6-fold. Disorders may stem from decreased intake, decreased absorption, or increased utilization. The goal is to maintain nitrogen balance and keep up with metabolic requirements in order to promote healing and prevent infection. If the patient is without nutrition for up to a week, intestinal mucosal atrophy may occur, leading to bacterial translocation and sepsis.[27] Diets may be chosen based on the specific needs of the patient (diabetic, low sodium, renal, low fat, low cholesterol, etc.).

- Enteral nutrition is preferred over parenteral nutrition when feasible due to reduction in risk of infection, need for frequent electrolyte monitoring, and cost. Contraindications to enteral feeds include circulatory shock, intestinal ischemia, ileus, or complete intestinal obstruction.
  - Enteric feeding formulas may be selected with the assistance of a nutritionist. The typical caloric density is 1 kcal/L.
    - Gastric feedings are typically done in a bolus fashion, whereas postpyloric feeding is typically continuous.
    - Postpyloric enteral feeding has not been consistently shown to decrease the risk of aspiration pneumonia.[28]
    - When gastric feeding is initiated, gastric residuals should be checked to ensure that the stomach is emptying properly. Residual values >200 mL should prompt further evaluation and suspension of tube feeds.
    - Complications of tube feeding include tube occlusion, aspiration, and diarrhea.
- Parenteral nutrition: When a special situation occurs that precludes enteric feeding, total parenteral nutrition (TPN) may be initiated. This is best done through a central vein and the assistance of a nutritionist. Close attention should be made to blood glucose monitoring as patients can develop significantly elevated blood sugar levels during initiation of TPN, and electrolyte monitoring.
- PEG/PEJ: Nasogastric and nasojejunal tubes can be used for periods of up to 1 month. The drawbacks include patient discomfort and the increased risk of infection such as sinusitis. Percutaneous enterogastrostomy (PEG) or enterojejunal (PEJ) tubes may prevent long-term infectious and structural complications of nasally placed tubes.
  - If postpyloric feeding is required, options include a jejunal extension placed through an existing PEG or an endoscopically placed percutaneous enterojejunostomy tube. Long-term patency appears to be better in direct percutaneous jejunostomy tubes than in PEG tubes with jejunal extensions.[29]
  - Aspiration risk may be decreased by elevating the head of the bed and checking gastric residuals.

REFERENCES

1. Esrailian E, Gralnek IM. Nonvariceal upper gastrointestinal bleeding: epidemiology and diagnosis. *Gastroenterol Clin North Am.* 2005;**34**:589-605.

2. Robert R, Gissot V, Pierrot M, et al. Helicobacter pylori infection is not associated with an increased hemorrhagic risk in patients in the intensive care unit. *Crit Care.* 2006;**10**:R77.

3. Aljebreen AM, Fallone CA, Barkun AN. Nasogastric aspirate predicts high-risk endoscopic lesions in patients with acute upper-gi bleeding. *Gastrointest Endosc.* 2004;**59**:172–8.

4. Lee SD, Kearney DJ. A randomized controlled trial of gastric lavage prior to endoscopy for acute upper gastrointestinal bleeding. *J Clin Gastroenterol.* 2004; **38**:861–5.

5. Sung JJ, Chung SC, Lai CW, et al. Octreotide infusion or emergency sclerotherapy for variceal haemorrhage. *Lancet.* 1993;**342**:637–41.

6. Laine L, Cook D. Endoscopic ligation compared with sclerotherapy for treatment of esophageal variceal bleeding. *A meta-analysis. Ann Intern Med.* 1995; **123**:280–7.

7. Thielman NM, Guerrant RL. Clinical practice. Acute infectious diarrhea. *N Engl J Med.* 2004;**350**:38–47.

8. Modena S, Bearelly D, Swartz K, Friedenberg FK. *Clostridium difficile* among hospitalized patients receiving antibiotics: a case-control study. *Infect Control Hosp Epidemiol.* 2005;**26**:685–90.

9. Raveh D, Rabinowitz B, Breuer GS, Rudensky B, Yinnon AM. Risk factors for Clostridium difficile toxin-positive nosocomial diarrhoea. *Int J Antimicrob Agents.* 2006;**28**:231–7.

10. Irwin RS, Rippe JM. *Manual of Intensive Care Medicine: With Annotated Key References*, 3rd ed. Philadelphia: Lippincott Williams & Wilkins, 2000.

11. Cook DJ, Fuller HD, Guyatt GH, et al. Risk factors for gastrointestinal bleeding in critically ill patients. Canadian Critical Care Trials Group. *N Engl J Med.* 1994;**330**:377–81.

12. Stollman N, Metz DC. Pathophysiology and prophylaxis of stress ulcer in intensive care unit patients. *J Crit Care.* 2005;**20**:35–45.

13. Jaeckel E, Cornberg M, Wedemeyer H, et al. Treatment of acute hepatitis c with interferon alfa-2b. *N Engl J Med.* 2001;**345**:1452–7.

14. Smilkstein MJ, Knapp GL, Kulig KW, Rumack BH. Efficacy of oral n-acetylcysteine in the treatment of acetaminophen overdose. Analysis of the national multicenter study (1976 to 1985). *N Engl J Med.* 1988; **319**:1557–62.

15. Garcia-Tsao G. Current management of the complications of cirrhosis and portal hypertension: variceal hemorrhage, ascites, and spontaneous bacterial peritonitis. *Gastroenterology.* 2001;**120**:726–48.

16. Bass NM. Intravenous albumin for spontaneous bacterial peritonitis in patients with cirrhosis. *N Engl J Med.* 1999;**341**:443–4.

17. Sharara AI, Rockey DC. Gastroesophageal variceal hemorrhage. *N Engl J Med.* 2001;**345**:669–81.

18. Gonwa TA, Mai ML, Melton LB, Hays SR, Goldstein RM, Levy MF, Klintmalm GB. Renal replacement therapy and orthotopic liver transplantation: the role of continuous veno-venous hemodialysis. *Transplantation.* 2001;**71**:1424–8.

19. Isenmann R, Runzi M, Kron M, et al. Prophylactic antibiotic treatment in patients with predicted severe acute pancreatitis: a placebo-controlled, double-blind trial. *Gastroenterology.* 2004;**126**:997–1004.

20. Kalliafas S, Ziegler DW, Flancbaum L, Choban PS. Acute acalculous cholecystitis: Incidence, risk factors, diagnosis, and outcome. *Am Surg.* 1998;**64**:471–5.

21. Fulcher AS, Turner MA, Zfass AM. Magnetic resonance cholangiopancreatography: a new technique for evaluating the biliary tract and pancreatic duct. *Gastroenterologist.* 1998;**6**:82–7.

22. Leung JW, Ling TK, Chan RC, et al. Antibiotics, biliary sepsis, and bile duct stones. *Gastrointest Endosc.* 1994;**40**:716–21.

23. Kavanagh PV, vanSonnenberg E, Wittich GR, Goodacre BW, Walser EM. Interventional radiology of the biliary tract. *Endoscopy.* 1997;**29**:570–6.

24. Stage JG, Moesgaard F, Gronvall S, Stage P, Kehlet H. Percutaneous transhepatic cholelithotripsy for difficult common bile duct stones. *Endoscopy.* 1998;**30**:289–92.

25. Sugiyama M, Tokuhara M, Atomi Y. Is percutaneous cholecystostomy the optimal treatment for acute cholecystitis in the very elderly? *World J Surg.* 1998;**22**:459–63.

26. Ramirez FC, McIntosh AS, Dennert B, Harlan JR. Emergency endoscopic retrograde cholangiopancreatography in critically ill patients. *Gastrointest Endosc.* 1998;**47**:368–71.

27. De-Souza DA, Greene LJ. Intestinal permeability and systemic infections in critically ill patients: effect of glutamine. *Crit Care Med.* 2005;**33**:1125–35.

28. Jabbar A, McClave SA. Pre-pyloric versus post-pyloric feeding. *Clin Nutr.* 2005;**24**:719–26.

29. Fan AC, Baron TH, Rumalla A, Harewood GC. Comparison of direct percutaneous endoscopic jejunostomy and peg with jejunal extension. *Gastrointest Endosc.* 2002;**56**:890–4.

Jeffrey Wesson, MD, PhD and Aaron Dall, MD

A nephrology consult could be requested for numerous reasons, many of which are beyond the scope of this chapter, but only the relatively small list that bears on the urgent and emergent issues related to patient management in the neuro-intensive care unit (NICU) is addressed in this chapter. These include diagnosis and management of renal failure (both acute and chronic), electrolyte disorders, and acid–base disorders. In particular, it is important to note that early involvement of a nephrologist has been shown to improve morbidity and mortality in acute kidney injury (also known as acute renal failure) in intensive care unit (ICU) patients, even when dialysis was not required. The following sections briefly summarize the critical issues associated with each of these categories of disease and the key features in initial management.

RENAL FAILURE

The majority of nephrology consults in any ICU setting are for acute kidney injury (AKI). Although it is usually caused by physiologic disturbances related to other medical conditions, AKI is associated with mortality in excess of 50% in ICU patients (depending on concurrent illnesses), and it carries an independent risk for death in those afflicted. Early recognition and appropriate treatment of contributing factors are important in improving outcomes. In contrast, chronic kidney disease (CKD) in the ICU setting is an important modifier of patient management decisions, but does not have nearly as great an impact on outcomes as AKI. Most CKD cases are caused by diabetes mellitus and hypertension, but it not useful to review the myriad factors involved

because the cause of CKD has little influence on management.

Diagnosis

Recognition of reduced renal function, routinely characterized as a reduction in glomerular filtration rate (GFR), is the critical first step. Distinguishing AKI from CKD clearly requires knowledge of renal function at some recent prior baseline date, although it can frequently be inferred from a combination of other lab tests and history of the current illness.

- Of primary importance is the demonstration of ongoing urine production because the absence of urine production indicates a complete functional failure of filtration (a GFR of 0 mL/min).
  - Urine production should be continuous, and rates <400 mL/day are defined as oliguria, with anuria defined as 24-hour volumes of <75 mL.
- Serum levels of creatinine and urea are also critical to the assessment, and are generally used to define renal function in all patients.
  - The serum creatinine can be used to approximate the true GFR, using various formulas, including modification of diet in renal disease. Modification of Diet in Renal Disease 1 (MDRD1), Modification of Diet in Renal Disease 2 (MDRD2), or the simpler expression by Cockroft and Gault (Table 28.1), but all of these formulas truly apply only to a steady-state condition, which cannot exist without adequate urine production and consistent concentrations of waste products over a period of days.

Table 28.1. Methods for estimating GFR from endogenous parameters

Creatinine	
	$GFR = 100/S_{cr}$
Cockroft and Gault	$GFR = (140 - Age)Wt/(72 * S_{cr})$; {* 0.85 for females}
MDRD1[A]	$GFR = 170 * S_{cr}^{-0.999} * Age^{-0.176} * S_{urea}^{-0.170} * Alb^{0.318}$; *{0.762 if female}, *{1.180 if black race}
MDRD2	$GFR = 186 * S_{cr}^{-1.154} * Age^{-0.203}$; *{0.742 if female}, * {1.210 if black race}
Creatinine clearance	$GFR = U_{cr} * V/(S_{cr} * t)$
Urea	
Urea clearance	$GFR = U_{urea} * V/(S_{urea} * t)$

S_{cr} is the serum creatinine concentration (mg/dL), Wt is the lean body mass (kg), S_{urea} is the blood urea nitrogen concentration (mg/dL), U_{cr} is the urine creatinine concentration (mg/dL), V is the volume of urine collected in time t, and U_{urea} is the urine urea nitrogen concentration (mg/dL).
[A] MDRD1: Modification of Diet in Renal Disease 1.

▷ These formulas are less accurate for patients at the extremes of age or physiologic health.

▷ Also, it should be noted that steady-state serum values for urea and creatinine are normally achieved only after several days at constant filtration, even in the presence of severe acute injury to the kidneys, so it should always be assumed that the serum values will overestimate the true GFR in the face of recent acute injury.

■ Other tests for measuring renal clearance, typically nuclear medicine tracer studies, are required only in rare or unusual circumstances to define renal function in an ICU setting, and are not discussed here.

Acute Kidney Injury

The approach to a patient with AKI should focus on distinguishing between prerenal, renal, and postrenal causes (Table 28.2), as rapid correction of precipitating causes can limit the extent of renal injury and facilitate recovery.

■ The initial evaluation should include a careful review of the patient's history, paying particular attention to any history of renal disease, recent changes in urine characteristics (symptoms such as dysuria, hematuria, incontinence, or difficulty initiating micturition) or total output, and other factors that could contribute to kidney injury, such as changes in hemodynamic stability preceding the recognition of AKI, new medications, or large changes in input/output balance.

■ The physical examination should focus on current hemodynamic parameters, including vascular integrity (bruits or other evidence of occluded vascular structures), volume status, and an assessment of current urine production (particularly signs of urinary retention such as bladder distension). Volume assessment needs to focus on parameters related to altered intravascular volume, such as hypotension or orthostatic blood pressure drops in low-volume states or elevated jugular venous pressures, pulmonary edema, and to a lesser extent peripheral edema and ascites in high-volume states. Other important findings include assessment of bladder emptying (observation of normal urine flow rates through micturition or indwelling catheter output, along with palpation of the lower abdomen for bladder distension), palpation for abdominal or rectal masses, and assessment of kidneys by palpation and percussion to detect enlargement or inflammation in either kidney.

■ Laboratory studies should include a complete blood count, blood chemistry panel (typically including sodium, potassium, calcium, magnesium, chloride, bicarbonate, phosphate, albumin, glucose, creatinine, and urea), and urinalysis with microscopic examination of the urine sediment.

Table 28.2. Acute renal failure: Categories and contributing factors

- Prerenal – loss of blood delivery to kidney
  - Hypovolemia (decreased intake, increased losses of blood or fluid)
  - Decreased cardiac output (CHF, PE, redistribution, shock)
  - Renal vascular occlusion (thrombotic, embolic, vasculitis, dissection, compression)
- Renal – injury to renal parenchyma
  - Glomerular
    - Acute postinfectious GN
    - Goodpasture's syndrome
    - Rapidly progressive GN
    - Lupus nephritis
    - IgA nephropathy
  - Tubular
    - Ischemic
    - Nephrotoxic
    - Exogenous (aminoglycosides, contrast agents, cisplatin)
    - Endogenous (pigments-myoglobin, protein-myeloma, crystals)
  - Interstitial
    - Infectious (staphylococcus, gram-negative bacteria, AFB, viruses, ...)
    - Infiltrative (leukemia, lymphoma, sarcoidosis)
    - Drugs (penicillins, NSAIDs, diuretics, ...)
  - Vascular
    - Malignant hypertension
    - Vasculitis (medium or small vessel)
    - HUS/TTP
    - Preeclampsia
    - Cholesterol emboli
- Postrenal – blockage of urine discharge
  - Internal (clots, stones, papillary necrosis, fungus balls)
  - External
    - Ureteral (ligation, scarring, tumors, aberrant vessels)
    - Urethral (stricture, BPH or CA, bladder CA, neurogenic bladder)

BPH = benign prostatic hypertrophy; CA = cancer; AFB = acid-fast bacillus; CHF = congestive heart failure; GN = glomerulonephritis; HUS = hemolytic-uremic syndrome; NSAIDs = non steroidal anti-inflammatory drugs; PE = pulmonary embolism; TTP = thrombotic thrombocytopenic purpura.

- Imaging of the kidneys and lower urinary tract by ultrasound or noncontrast computed tomography (CT) scanning is frequently required to fully assess possible obstruction of urine outflow above the level of the bladder and to verify renal anatomy, but it may not be necessary when a clear cause for AKI has been identified and the patient continues to demonstrate adequate urine output.
- Other studies may be indicated according to possible factors uncovered in the history of present illness that might pertain to specific

possible injuries to the kidneys, and these are best understood by reviewing the categories of injury.

Prerenal causes include all processes that can lead to reduced blood flow and blood pressure at the kidney, specifically at the glomerulus. The most common causes of pre-renal AKI in the ICU are decreased effective intravascular volume (including volume depletion, acute bleeding, or the loss of effective vascular volume due to sepsis or low oncotic pressure in the blood) and cardiac failure (such as myocardial infarction, cardiac arrhythmias, valvular disease, or cardiomyopathy).

The history and physical examination findings are generally adequate to define these parameters, although some complicated cases may require direct measurements of cardiac output, central venous pressures, or pulmonary capillary wedge pressures to define the true volume state of the patient. Rarely, prerenal causes will include acutely restricted flow in the renal arteries, due to dissection, vasculitis, thrombosis (renal vein or artery), embolism, or traumatic injury.

In addition to the tests enumerated in the preceding text, the fractional excretion of sodium (FeNa) may be helpful in identifying a prerenal cause in ambiguous cases. FeNa is defined as:

$$FeNa = \frac{(U_{Na}/S_{Na})}{U_{Cr}/S_{Cr}} \times 100\%,$$

where U_{Na} and S_{Na} are the urine and serum sodium concentrations, and U_{Cr} and S_{Cr} are the urine and serum creatinine concentrations, respectively. As the renal response to low blood flow or blood pressure states is to concentrate the urine maximally to maintain blood volume, the urine specific gravity will be high (generally >1.020, although typically it will be >1.030 with good renal function at baseline), leading to a large ratio of U_{Cr} to S_{Cr} and consequently a low FeNa (generally <1% in near normal baseline renal function). The use of diuretics at the time of measurement may override the concentrating mechanisms for sodium within the kidney, but the fractional excretion of urea (FeUrea, calculated in a manner similar to FeNa) would still be reduced (<30% defining the prerenal condition).

In the face of acute tubular necrosis (ATN), the kidneys are no longer able to concentrate the urine appropriately, and normal values for either FeNa or FeUrea are not reliable indicators of effective renal blood flow. These cases are usually easily recognized by the presence of very coarse granular casts (also called "muddy brown" or ATN casts) in the urine sediment. Many patients with ATN will have a recent history of marked hypotension resulting in ischemic injury to the kidney, but ATN can also be caused by toxic chemical exposures. Microscopic quantities of blood and non-nephrotic proteinuria can frequently be seen in more severe cases of pre-renal AKI.

Renal causes are the most diverse and complicated in their diagnosis and management, and the diagnostic evaluation can usually sort conditions between the four major categories of injury: glomerular, tubular, interstitial, or vascular (Table 28.2).

The most common causes of renal AKI in the NICU are related to drug and chemical exposures, typically leading to tubular or interstitial lesions, which can progress rapidly to anuria in severe cases.

- The radiocontrast dyes used during arteriography or CT imaging studies are among the most common causes of renal tubular AKI, leading to ATN through a pathway that is thought to involve either direct toxic injury or ischemia.
- Previously, the use of gadolinium in magnetic resonance imaging (MRI) was thought to be completely safe, but some case reports have suggested that gadolinium can also cause AKI in patients with significant underlying chronic kidney disease.
- Many chemotherapeutic agents and some antibiotics (particularly aminoglycosides and amphotericin B) can also cause direct tubular injury and ATN.

Interstitial AKI or acute interstitial nephritis is the result of an infiltration of white blood cells in the interstitial tissues of the kidney, which can either be allergic in origin or related to direct infection of the kidney (pyelonephritis), usually from upstream extension of a lower urinary tract infection.

- The most common drugs to cause allergic interstitial nephritis (AIN) are various antibiotics in the ICU setting; however, nonsteroidal anti-inflammatory drugs (NSAIDs) are frequently implicated, and many other medications are known to cause AIN.

The only vascular conditions categorized as "renal AKI" are the small and medium vessel vasculitides (including conditions such as Wegener's granulomatosis, microscopic polyarteritis, Churg–Strauss syndrome, and Henoch–Schönlein purpura), and these conditions will typically have other systemic manifestations, including neurologic processes, and only rarely present as a rapidly evolving AKI.

Similarly, glomerular lesions, while being more common in general terms, rarely present as a rapidly evolving AKI syndrome in an ICU setting. In most cases, acute glomerular nephritis will have other systemic symptoms and signs, and the myriad causes are beyond the scope of this chapter.

Since drug and chemical exposures are important causes of renal AKI, a careful review of the recent history, including medication changes, is critical to identifying the offending agent.

Laboratory tests can help determine the etiology by categorizing the type of injury.

- Glomerular lesions characteristically lead to hematuria and nephrotic range proteinuria (>2000 mg of protein per gram of creatinine in a random urine or > 3000 mg of protein in a 24-hour urine sample).
- The finding of red blood cell casts or hemoglobin casts in the urine sediment is pathognomonic of glomerular lesions.
- Serologic studies and renal biopsy help to distinguish individual disease processes.
- "Muddy brown" casts in the urine sediment confirm the diagnosis of ATN, but it cannot distinguish between ischemic and toxic tubular injury; that distinction is usually drawn from the clinical history. Mild to moderate proteinuria and microscopic hematuria is usually also present.
- The finding of white blood cell casts in the urine is diagnostic for AIN. The pyelonephritis cases are characteristically septic, due to the severity of this deep tissue infection, whereas the drug-related AIN patients can be otherwise quite stable.
- Urine eosinophils are found only in about one quarter of patients with AIN.
- Elevated serum eosinophil count is suggestive of AIN, but can be due to other causes.
- Vasculitides routinely have serologic markers of disease, but many of these tests are typically sent out to specialized laboratories and therefore are not immediately available for diagnosis at the time of consultation.

Postrenal causes of AKI include any condition affecting the flow of urine through the ureters, bladder, or urethra, and can result from either external compression or internal blockage of any of these structures by a variety of processes. Acute obstruction at any level usually creates a colicky pain in the affected portion of the urinary tract, but chronic obstruction is more insidious in onset and can be completely asymptomatic. In a patient with evidence of systemic infection or sepsis and AKI, the possibility of postobstructive infection must be definitively ruled out because infection in the obstructed portion of the urinary tract is effectively an abscess and potentially life threatening. Efforts to drain that space surgically should be made immediately on identification of this condition. A record of continuously normal urine production does not rule out unilateral obstructive processes because one kidney can normally maintain the appropriate fluid balance. It should be noted, however, that complete unilateral obstruction should reduce the GFR only by half (increase the serum creatinine by a factor of 2) in people with normal renal anatomy.

Possible causes of internal upper tract or ureteral obstruction include kidney stones, blood clots, tumors, papillary necrosis with sloughing, or rarely aggressive fungal infections. The urinalysis will likely show blood with any of these conditions, and typically normal or modest elevations in urine protein. Obviously, evidence for urinary tract infection (leucocyte esterase or nitrates on dipstick, with elevated white blood cell counts or bacterial or fungal elements on microscopic examination) necessitates a workup for internal obstruction. External compression of the ureters is also common, as they are a low-pressure system, and are easily compressed by masses in any adjacent structure, including lymph nodes, gastrointestinal organs, ovaries, uterus, adjacent musculoskeletal structures, or other retroperitoneal masses (e.g., hematomas). The urinalysis is normally bland with external compression at any level. Similarly, the bladder can be obstructed internally by stones, clots, or tumor processes. These conditions are relatively rare because the bladder is normally

Table 28.3. Stages of chronic kidney disease

Stage	GFR (mL/min)
1	>90
2	61–90
3	31–60
4	15–30
5	<15
ESRD	On dialysis

GFR = glomerular filtration rate; ESRD = end-stage renal disease.

emptied by muscular contraction clearing smaller objects. Loss of the normal contractile function, as in neurogenic bladder, is a functional obstruction, as the urine is not emptied properly from the body. The urethra is seldom obstructed internally, especially in women, unless it is with an externally placed device (i.e., an improperly placed indwelling catheter). The most common external obstruction is from prostatic enlargement or cancer in middle-aged or elderly men, although other tumor masses can occur in this area of the body. Patients who have undergone arteriography can occasionally develop hematomas that track into the groin (retroperitoneal or perineal) and cause external compression of the bladder and/or urethra.

- In most clinical circumstances, an abdominal ultrasound focused on the kidneys and lower urinary tract is used as the definitive laboratory study to assess patency of the urinary tract and characterize the renal anatomy. It is simple, essentially risk free, and readily available.
- A noncontrast CT scan may be an appropriate alternative depending on patient characteristics and suspected cause of AKI, particularly if kidney stones or other internal ureteral obstruction processes are suspected.
- MRI may also be suitable, but MR scans are generally more expensive and less readily available.
- Plain radiographs have a very low diagnostic yield without the use of contrast enhancing agents and are not recommended. Contrast-enhanced studies are generally avoided, because of the risk of inducing renal injury; however, they may be

appropriate when required to diagnose other related disease processes concurrently with the renal assessment.

Chronic Kidney Disease

Chronic kidney disease or chronic renal failure encompasses the full range of reduced renal function from near normal to patients on chronic dialysis (see Table 28.3), and obviously describes those patients with preexisting renal failure.

- Generally, patients with CKD stages 1–3 (ranging from almost no loss to moderate loss of function) will require no special attention to be managed safely, although their medications should be checked for possible dose adjustments when the GFR is below 50 mL/min.
- Patients in stages 4 or 5 (severe reduction to impending need for dialysis) need to be monitored closely for changes in fluid status or electrolyte concentrations, as they are very susceptible to changes in their homeostatic balance with alterations of their inputs and outputs that might occur during acute illnesses and many medications require dose adjustments for GFR values <30 mL/min.
- Patients with mild to severe loss of kidney function are also at greater risk for AKI from a variety of causes. A nephrology consult should be considered more strongly in these patients as the severity of their condition rises.
- Finally, those patients already on dialysis (true end-stage renal disease [ESRD]) or with functional kidney transplants require nephrology management for their ongoing need for renal replacement with dialysis (either hemodialysis or peritoneal dialysis) in the former or management of their transplant related issues in the latter.

The diagnosis is known in these patients, but the stability of their condition compared to baseline needs to be assessed by examination of their hemodynamic parameters, volume status, presence of urine output, and laboratory testing to confirm the stability of their renal clearance and electrolyte concentrations. Urinalysis is typically bland and unrevealing, and there is no role for renal imaging in stable CKD or ESRD. A previously undiagnosed case of CKD or ESRD should be approached as if they have AKI, so that any correctable component can be rapidly identified and treated .

TREATMENT

The principal patient management issues of fluid and electrolyte balance, as well as avoidance of drug toxicities and uremia are addressed in the same manner, regardless of whether the renal injury is acute or chronic in nature. Decisions will depend on the ability of the residual kidney function to adjust for existing or anticipated imbalances in fluids or electrolytes. Consequently, a mild acute injury and stage 2 CKD are managed in essentially the same manner, and likewise, a severe acute renal injury, which can lead to an anuric condition (effectively a GFR of 0), requires the same management as in ESRD. The lone difference in AKI management is to remove or correct the condition or agent causing renal damage, which in most instances will allow the kidneys to heal, recovering some or all of their baseline function. Treatment needs to be based on an estimate of the existing level of clearance on a day-by-day basis until the kidneys return to normal function. Electrolyte imbalances is covered in the next section. Most drugs have documented dose adjustments for CKD patients in standard drug compendia, such as the *Physicians' Desk Reference* (PDR), so the remainder of this section addresses adjustments for fluid imbalances and the need for dialysis.

Indications for Dialysis

There are only four indications for emergent dialysis: intractable fluid overload, intractable hyperkalemia, uremia, or toxic overdoses. Chronic or maintenance dialysis is simply the application of a pattern of scheduled dialysis treatments at a dose and frequency that will prevent any of these four conditions from developing in the patient. Consequently, the timing of the next required dialysis treatment in a patient with ESRD or severe AKI is somewhat flexible for any patient, in the absence of a clinical indication for emergent dialysis, at least within the timeframe of a few days. It is important to remember, however, that the time to death after stopping dialysis in an otherwise stable ESRD patient is typically about 1 week.

The determination that any of the 4 indications for dialysis has reached an emergent state is largely a matter of clinical judgment, but can be loosely defined as follows.

- Fluid overload is gauged principally in terms of respiratory status. It becomes intractable when florid pulmonary edema with current or impending respiratory failure is present, coupled with the inability to induce significant urine production despite large doses of intravenous diuretics.
- ESRD patients infrequently retain the ability to produce large volumes of urine, though they may require dialysis for clearance or electrolyte regulation, but many cases of AKI can also present with greatly reduced ability to excrete salt and water.
- Hyperkalemia becomes life-threatening when it begins to affect nerve conduction, as evidenced by electrocardiogram (EKG) changes (typically for serum potassium values above 7 mEq/L). Although this condition can be temporarily stabilized with medical interventions (see next section) and some clearance can be obtained with the use of polystyrene sulfonate resins (Kayexalate) in the gut, there is no effective way to clear large quantities of potassium without dialysis in ESRD or severe AKI patients.
- Uremia is purely a clinical diagnosis, and it can occur at quite widely variable levels of azotemia (elevations of serum urea and creatinine levels above normal ranges), but typically not until the GFR falls below 10 mL/min.
  ▸ Mild symptoms, such as nausea, vomiting, itching, and decreased appetite, do not require emergent intervention, but severe levels of uremia, characterized by encephalopathy, seizures, or coma, can be addressed only with emergent dialysis.
  ▸ Finding a pericardial effusion (pericardial rub) in a patient with azotemia is presumed to be a manifestation of uremic pericarditis and also requires emergent dialysis .
- Toxic chemical levels requiring emergent dialysis or hemofiltration occur rarely during hospitalizations from pharmaceutical agents, but they are seen on admission with some regularity in most major hospitals.
  ▸ The most commonly found toxic chemical agents are usually lower alcohols, other than

Table 28.4. Equations for Fe_K^+ and TTKG

a. Fractional excretion of potassium (Fe_K^+) $\frac{\text{(Urine [K}^+\text{]/plasma [K}^+\text{])}}{\text{(Urine [Cr]/plasma [Cr])}} \times 100\%$	In hyperkalemia <10% Renal cause >10% Extrarenal cause In hypokalemia n/a
b. Transtubular potassium gradient (TTKG) $\frac{\text{(Urine [K}^+\text{]/Plasma [K}^+\text{])}}{\text{(Urine Osmol/plasma Osmol)}}$	In hyperkalemia <6 Renal with decreased aldosterone effect >10 Nonrenal cause In hypokalemia <2 Gastrointestinal losses >4 Renal losses, excess aldosterone

ethanol (e.g., ethylene glycol, isopropyl alcohol, or methanol), ingested either by accident or intent (suicide attempts), and lithium in bipolar patients.

Modes of Dialysis

Dialysis describes the process of the diffusive exchange of chemical agents (ions and small organic molecules) across a semipermeable membrane between blood and an "external" fluid, called the dialysate. In general, the dialysate is an aqueous solution that is pH balanced and nearly isotonic with serum, containing appropriate quantities of essential mineral ions, such as sodium, calcium, and magnesium, but none of the toxic waste products and little or no potassium and phosphate that accumulate in renal failure. The diffusive process tends to equalize the concentrations of small ions and organic molecules between the blood and dialysate, and therefore leads to the net transport of waste products, potassium, and phosphate to the dialysis fluid, so that they can be removed from the body. In addition, a net transport of fluid from the blood space to the dialysate is engineered into the system, depending on the modality of dialysis. There are only two options for the semipermeable membrane, which define the two major modalities of dialysis.

- In peritoneal dialysis, the peritoneal membrane is used as the semipermeable membrane. Provision must be made to insert the dialysate into the peritoneal space, typically with a single-lumen plastic catheter inserted below the umbilicus. Although the catheter insertion can be done

on an emergent basis in the face of AKI, some healing time is required before this modality can be fully utilized, so peritoneal dialysis is routinely performed only on patients dialyzed using this modality before hospitalization.

- The other dialysis modality is called hemodialysis, and in this case, the semipermeable membrane is a hollow synthetic polymer fiber. Typically, a cartridge containing a bundle of such fibers is constructed so that blood can be pumped through the center of each fiber, while dialysate is circulated around the outside of the fibers. With current fiber technology, the transport of small ions and molecules can be accomplished very efficiently, making hemodialysis far superior to peritoneal dialysis for rapid clearance of any component. Consequently, about 90% of ESRD patients in the United States opt for this modality for their chronic treatment. For the most efficient operation, large volumes of blood must be circulated through the cartridge (dialyzer), typically 300–500 mL/min, so access to the patient's blood is critical. For newly diagnosed ESRD or AKI patients requiring dialysis, access to the blood is obtained by placement of a special double-lumen central catheter (Mahurkur catheter) into preferably the jugular vein, though femoral and subclavian placements are also used. In chronic hemodialysis treatments, time on the machine is minimized requiring rapid changes in body chemistry and volume status, with removal of as much as 5 or 6 liters of fluid in a 4-hour period. Many ICU patients are hemodynamically unstable, and do not tolerate such rapid adjustments to their fluid status. For these patients, machine settings allowing for slow continuous removal of fluid and solutes throughout the course of the entire day may be used. These techniques are known by various acronyms (CVVH, CVVHD, SCUF, etc.) and are chosen depending on the balance between the fluid removal and the solute removal needs of the patient.

ELECTROLYTE DISORDERS

Disorders of fluids and electrolytes are very common in the intensive care setting. In this section we discuss the general diagnosis and management of commonly seen disorders including hyperkalemia, hypokalemia, hypercalcemia, hypocalcemia, hypomagnesemia, and hypophosphatemia. Certainly, the discussion of each of these entities in full would be exhaustive and beyond the scope of this section. Therefore, it is the aim of this section to concentrate on the diagnosis and appropriate management, including determination of electrolyte or fluid deficits, pertinent to the ICU setting.

Disorders of Potassium Balance

Potassium abnormalities occur due to two main reasons: (1) potassium intake is greater than excretion or excretion is greater than intake (hyper- and hypokalemia, respectively), and (2) potassium shifts between the extracellular (measured) and intracellular compartments. In the first case, a determination of renal versus extrarenal sources of potassium gain or loss is necessary. This can be accomplished by measurement of the fractional excretion of potassium (Fe_K^+) and the transtubular potassium gradient (TTKG) (see Table 28.4a,b). In hyperkalemia the Fe_K^+ and TTKG are both low or below normal if renal excretion of potassium is causative. Conversely, an extrarenal cause of hyperkalemia exists if the Fe_K^+ and TTKG are high or above normal. These general principals are reversed in hypokalemia. Typically Fe_K^+ and TTKG are low with extrarenal causes of hypokalemia and high with renal causes of hypokalemia (Table 28.4a, b).

Serum potassium levels represent approximately 2–3% of the total body potassium load. The intracellular potassium concentration is approximately 150 mEq/L whereas the extracellular concentration is 4 mEq/L. Thus, small transcellular shifts of potassium may lead to larger fluctuations in the measured extracellular potassium concentration (i.e., if serum [K+] changes due to influx into cells from 4 to 2 mEq/L then the intracellular [K+] would change from 150 mEq/L to 152 mEq/L). The two major driving forces for these transcellular shifts are insulin and epinephrine, both of which tend to cause potassium entry into cells.

Hyperkalemia

Elevation in serum potassium concentration may occur in the ICU setting for several reasons.

- Both acute and chronic kidney disease and adrenal insufficiency are common and lead to decreased potassium excretion in the urine (low Fe_K^+ and TTKG).
- Also, if not monitored closely, potassium added to replacement fluids or in enteral/parenteral preparations may exceed the kidneys' excretory ability with or without normal renal function.
- Rhabdomyolysis causes a transcellular shift into the extracellular compartment as the myocytes breakdown and release potassium directly into the serum.
- Tumor lysis syndrome and neuroleptic malignant syndrome similarly cause hyperkalemia.
- Pseudohyperkalemia (normal serum [K+]) also occurs due to transcellular shift of potassium when the cellular components of the laboratory blood specimen hemolyze before measurement of potassium concentration.
- Medications such as angiotensin converting enzyme inhibitors, angiotensin receptor blockers, heparin, and the azole-class of antifungals inhibit aldosterone production leading to hyperkalemia. NSAIDs indirectly inhibit aldosterone production via blocking normal prostaglandin-stimulated renin production. Beta-blockers inhibit cellular uptake of potassium in the presence of epinephrine (seen with nonselective beta-blockers).

The treatment of hyperkalemia utilizes methods to enhance transcellular shifts, as well as renal and nonrenal excretion of potassium.

- Calcium is administered to stabilize the myocardial membrane if there is electrocardiographic evidence of hyperkalemia (peaked T-waves, prolonged P-R interval, dropped P-waves, or ventricular fibrillation).

■ Insulin, frequently administered with dextrose, infused intravenously can rapidly decrease serum potassium concentration (onset 10–20 minutes) via transcellular shifts into myocytes and hepatocytes primarily. Similarly β_2-agonists can be used (nebulized albuterol). The above mechanisms decrease the serum [K^+] but do not decrease total body potassium levels.

■ Both loop and thiazide diuretics are very effective in increasing excretion of potassium in the urine (as long as there is normal or near normal kidney function).

■ Sodium polystyrene sulfonate (Kayexalate 30–60 grams orally or rectally with lactulose) works by enhancing gastrointestinal potassium loss.

■ Hemodialysis is also effective in removing potassium and should be considered when renal function is absent or severely diminished.

Hypokalemia

Hypokalemia most frequently occurs due to inadequate potassium intake. Loss of total body potassium is seen with vomiting, diarrhea, use of diuretics, and hyperglycemia-related osmotic diuresis. In addition, elevated aldosterone levels (i.e., primary aldosteronism) leads to potassium wasting. Certain defects in renal tubular function also result in renal potassium loss (distal and proximal renal tubular acidosis, Bartter's syndrome, and Gitelman's syndrome). Potassium is transported intracellularly with insulin therapy and epinephrine (catecholamine) release during stress causing transcellular shifts. Either accidental or induced hypothermia can cause intracellular shifts of potassium. This becomes especially important while rewarming the patient as potassium moves to the extracellular compartment.

The treatment of hypokalemia requires halting offending agents (diuretics) if possible and supplementing with either oral or parenteral potassium. The total body potassium deficit reflects both the intracellular and extracellular (measured) compartments. Thus when determining the amount of potassium to supplement one must keep in mind that serum levels account for only 2–3% of the total body stores.

■ The safest method of correcting potassium is via scheduled oral doses (20–40 mEq administered one to three times daily).

■ Parenteral administration of potassium is limited by local venous irritation and concern for over correction with rapid administration. Central venous access is preferred and a rate no faster than 10 mEq/h should be used.

Calcium Disorders

HYPERCALCEMIA

Hypercalcemia is defined as an elevation of ionized (noncomplexed) calcium >1.27 mmol/l or a serum calcium >10.4 mg/dL.

■ Hypercalcemia (especially when developed acutely) may cause neurologic complications such as lethargy, drowsiness, confusion, seizures, or even coma in severe cases.

■ In addition, hypercalcemia causes acute and chronic renal failure, hypertension, a shortened Q-T interval, and multiple gastrointestinal symptoms (nausea, vomiting, constipation, anorexia, pancreatitis, and peptic ulcer disease).

Common etiologies of hypercalcemia include primary hyperparathyroidism, malignancy-associated, thiazide diuretic use, immobilization, and vitamin D intoxication. The frequency of milk-alkali syndrome, a previously common cause, has decreased considerably over the past several years as calcium-based antacids have been replaced by inhibitors of gastric acid secretion.

■ Treatment of symptomatic or severe hypercalcemia ([Ca^{2+}] > 13.5 mg/dL) requires adequate fluid replacement with isotonic saline at rates as high as 200–250 mL/h. This treatment needs to be adjusted to the specific patient's cardiac and renal function (decreased if volume overloaded or in acute congestive heart failure).

■ The addition of intravenous Lasix therapy is advocated by some to help produce a calciuresis once euvolemia is achieved through saline infusion.

■ Additional treatment options are tailored to the specific cause of hypercalcemia and include the use of calcitonin and bisphosphonates and removal of offending agents (thiazide diuretics, calcium or vitamin D supplements).

■ In a patient with severely impaired renal function, dialysis can be used to lower serum calcium.

HYPOCALCEMIA

Hypocalcemia is the most commonly seen electrolyte abnormality in the intensive care setting and is associated with increased mortality.

- Symptoms of hypocalcemia include perioral paresthesias and carpal-pedal spasm in mild cases to whole body tetany (seizures) in more severe cases.
- EKG evidence of hypocalcemia includes prolongation of the Q–T$_c$ and S–T segments, peaked T-waves, arrhythmias, and heart block.
- Clinically, one may elicit Chvostek's (tapping facial nerve evokes a grimace) and Trousseau's (prolonged blood pressure cuff insufflation causes spasms of the outstretched arm) signs to aid in diagnosis.

The increased prevalence of hypocalcemia in critically ill patients may be secondary to calcium precipitation into tissues, complex formation with citrated blood products, decreased renal production of active vitamin D, and suppression of parathyroid gland function.

Treatment of acute onset hypocalcemia is accomplished through the intravenous administration of calcium gluconate or calcium chloride. This can be given in bolus form (1–2 grams) or with a continuous calcium drip. In rhabdomyolysis the hypocalcemia tends to be transient and typically treatment of the primary problem, including fluid resuscitation, is sufficient. Importantly, if acidosis is also present calcium supplementation should precede any attempt at correcting the low pH with bicarbonate therapy. As the pH increases (due to bicarbonate infusion) hydrogen ions on albumin molecules are exchanged for calcium, thereby dropping the ionized calcium level farther. In the more chronic setting oral replacement with calcium carbonate (approximately 1 gram daily) and 1,25-vitamin D$_3$ is appropriate. 1,25-Vitamin D$_3$ enhances the intestinal absorption of calcium but must be used in caution when hyperphosphatemia is present as this may promote extraosseous calcium deposition.

Hypermagnesemia/Hypomagnesemia

Disorders of magnesium balance are also frequently seen in critically ill patients. Hypermagnesemia is almost entirely seen with the combination of ingestion and renal failure (the major site of magnesium handling). Treatment includes the cessation of oral or intravenous supplements and, in severe or symptomatic cases, dialysis may be required. Hypomagnesemia is much more common and, when developed within the ICU, has proven to be an independent risk factor for death. The normal serum magnesium concentration is between 1.5 and 1.9 mEq/L. This concentration represents only 0.3% of the total body magnesium stores. The majority of magnesium resides in the musculoskeletal system (80%) and soft tissues (19%). Hypomagnesemia is associated with both hypokalemia and hypocalcemia via its important role in transmembrane transport and effects on parathyroid hormone secretion respectively. Clinically, low magnesium primarily causes abnormal neuromuscular and cardiovascular sequela. Symptoms seen with magnesium deficiency include: tetany, carpal-pedal spasm, seizures, ataxia, vertigo, muscle weakness, psychosis, ventricular tachycardia, atrial fibrillation, hypertension, and various EKG changes.

The treatment of hypomagnesemia requires oral or intravenous replacement.

- Oral replacement is limited by the gastrointestinal side effects of diarrhea and vomiting with elevated doses.
- In the ICU setting intravenous replacement is preferred. Magnesium is infused slowly over the course of several hours (i.e., 2 grams magnesium sulfate infused over 4–6 hours) to limit the reciprocal renal magnesium wasting seen with more rapid infusions. Up to 8–10 grams (48–56 mEq) of magnesium may be required to correct the deficit.

Treatment of hypomagnesemia is also important when there is corresponding hypokalemia as potassium supplementation alone is often not effective. An entity called normomagnesemic magnesium deficiency is seen with refractory hypokalemia and normal serum magnesium levels. The reason for this phenomenon highlights the skewed distribution of total body magnesium towards the intracellular compartment. Magnesium replacement corrects the refractory nature of this type of hypokalemia. Overall, supplementation requires the periodic assessment of serum magnesium levels to ensure appropriate correction of the deficit.

Hyperphosphatemia/Hypophosphatemia

Phosphate homeostasis is tied tightly to oral intake and both gastrointestinal and urinary excretion of phosphorus. Phosphate plays an integral role in the activity of many biologic pathways. In the acute setting hyperphosphatemia is rarely of clinical significance with the exception of cases of rhabdomyolysis and tumor lysis syndrome. These clinical entities highlight the rapid shift of phosphorus from the intracellular to the extracellular fluid compartments.

- The treatment of severe acute hyperphosphatemia requires adequate hydration (with normal saline) if kidney function is normal and may require dialysis if there is impaired kidney function.
- The management of chronically elevated phosphorus (exclusively seen in patients with advanced kidney disease and end-stage renal disease) has become a major component of outpatient nephrology care and is beyond the scope of this chapter.

Hypophosphatemia, on the other hand, has definite implications for the acutely ill patient. Abnormalities in the cardiovascular, hematological, neurological, and skeletal systems predominate. In particular, patients may have decreased cardiac output, generalized muscle weakness, hemolysis, anorexia, confusion, ataxia, seizures, coma and osteomalacia among many other symptoms. With severe hypophosphatemia (serum levels <1 mg/dL) rhabdomyolysis can develop and mask the underlying total body phosphorus depletion due to the shift of intracellular phosphorus out of damaged myocytes. This is almost exclusively seen in chronically phosphate depleted alcoholic patients during refeeding.

Treating hypophosphatemia requires recognition of the etiology of the phosphate deficit. Hypophosphatemia that develops in the hospitalized setting typically represents translocation of phosphorus from the extracellular to the intracellular fluid compartments. This is seen during the treatment of diabetic ketoacidosis, in severe respiratory alkalosis, as a consequence of refeeding, and in cases of severe burns. Other causes include diminished phosphate intake, increased renal losses, and increased extrarenal losses.

- In the hospitalized patient parenteral administration of phosphate is preferred.
- In patients with severe but asymptomatic hypophosphatemia it is recommended to give 0.08 mmol/kg of body weight over a 6-hour period.
- In symptomatic patients a dose of 0.16 mmol/kg of body weight is recommended.
- Serum phosphate should be checked on all susceptible hospitalized patients.
- Recognition and treatment of hypophosphatemia in the acutely ill patient may reduce both the morbidity and mortality associated with this disorder.

ACID–BASE DISORDERS

Acid–base balance is normally very tightly regulated within the body through a combination of respiratory and renal mechanisms at an arterial blood value of pH = 7.40 ± 0.02. Mixed venous blood is typically only slightly more acidic with a pH = 7.36 ± 0.02, due to the presence of greater amounts of carbon dioxide (pCO_2) in venous blood, which is in equilibrium with carbonic acid (H_2CO_3) by the action of the enzyme carbonic anhydrase. Bicarbonate ion (HCO_3^-) is the principal buffer in blood, protecting the body against sudden changes in pH, particularly abrupt generation of acid loads through various, common metabolic pathways.

The body regulates acid–base balance through both a respiratory pathway (varied ventilation of pCO_2 from the lungs) and a renal pathway (varied recovery of HCO_3^- from urine and secretion of H^+ into urine), and any deviation from normal is characterized in terms of respiratory and metabolic (or renal) components by the partial pressure of carbon dioxide (pCO_2) and HCO_3^- concentrations, respectively. The respiratory response to a disturbance in physiologic pH is normally very rapid (seconds to minutes), but limited in capacity, whereas the renal response takes hours to days, but will persist until normal pH is restored. Consequently, acid–base disorders are defined primarily by the deviation of arterial blood pH, where a below normal pH defines acidosis and above normal pH defines alkalosis. Acid–base disorders are defined secondarily by the deviations from normal values of both HCO_3^- and pCO_2. Other parameters may be critical to defining the

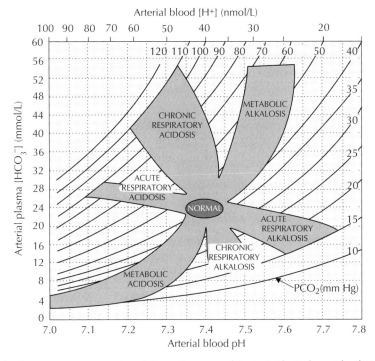

Figure 28.1. Acid–base nomogram (map). From *Brenner and Rector's The Kidney*, 8th ed. (See also figure in color plate section.)

cause and possible physiologic response or compensation to the primary disorders. The most frequently used of these parameters is the anion gap, which is defined as the difference between the sum of major positive ion concentrations (sodium and potassium) and the sum of major negative ion concentrations (chloride and HCO_3^-).

Diagnosis

It is assumed that any compensatory mechanism can never overshoot the normal pH; however, it is important to recognize that patients may exhibit more than one primary disorder. Routinely, the respiratory parameter or pCO_2 is assessed first. Finding an elevation from normal (40 mm Hg) implies that there is a respiratory acidosis component to the disorder due to the increased levels of pCO_2, while finding a below normal value for pCO_2 implies a respiratory alkalosis component. When the change in the respiratory parameter is in the opposite direction as the deviation of pH from normal the respiratory change is typically a primary contributor to the derangement. On the other hand, with respiratory compensation (not the primary

disorder) the respiratory parameter deviates in the same direction as the change in pH. Likewise, the metabolic parameter or HCO_3^- ion concentration is elevated from normal (>30 mEq/L) when a metabolic alkalosis component is present, while finding a below normal value (<23 mEq/L) implies a metabolic acidosis component. The change in HCO_3^- is similarly defined as a primary cause of the disorder when in the same direction as the pH change and a compensatory change when it is in opposition to the pH change. In a simple example, finding a patient with a pH = 7.35, pCO_2 = 25 mmHg, and HCO_3^- = 12 mEq/L would be described as a primary metabolic acidosis (due to the low values for both pH and HCO_3^-) with respiratory compensation (due to the low value of pCO_2).

It should be noted that in diagnosis of acid–base disorders using current blood chemistry parameters as described above does not define the pathway traversed by the patient in reaching that point. In particular, distinguishing an acute respiratory acidosis from a chronic state is determined largely by whether the HCO_3^- level has been adjusted through actions of the kidney or not. This is due to the longer timeframes associated with renal responses. Thus, a patient with chronic respiratory acidosis who is typically fully compensated when stable could develop acute respiratory acidosis from worsening lung function while still displaying blood parameters consistent with chronic respiratory acidosis. More complicated acid–base disorders may require quantitative calculation of the contributions to the measured pH from both pCO_2 and HCO_3^- disturbances, using well-established chemical relationships between these parameters that can be found in many textbooks with more extensive treatments of acid–base disturbances. A simple graphical representation has been published showing the general ranges of the combinations of pH, pCO_2, and HCO_3^- that fall within specifically defined disorders (Fig. 28.1. The major categories of acid–base disturbance are delineated briefly in the following paragraphs.

Metabolic Acidosis

Metabolic acidosis is divided into two large categories: anion gap metabolic acidosis and nonanion gap metabolic acidosis (also known as hyperchloremic metabolic acidosis). Anion gap metabolic acidosis processes are characterized by either the accumulation of nonphysiologic acids or abnormally high levels of normal organic acid components in the blood, where the acid anions account for the excessively large number of unmeasured anions. The most common conditions of this type can be further divided into ketoacidosis (from diabetes mellitus, starvation, ethanol, or inherited errors of metabolism), lactic acidosis from hypoxia (related to either depressed blood delivery, depressed lung function, exercise above anaerobic threshold, seizures, or severe anemia), lactic acidosis without hypoxia (related to depressed liver metabolism, diabetes mellitus, renal failure, various drugs, or inherited errors of metabolism), uremia, toxic anions (methanol, ethylene glycol, paraldehyde, salicylates, or aminocaproic acid), or rhabdomyolysis. Nonanion gap metabolic acidosis is by definition a pure HCO_3^- deficiency from either renal losses or more commonly gastrointestinal losses. Renal mechanisms include the various forms of inherited tubular defects known collectively as renal tubular acidosis, but also include drugs (such as acetazolamide, potassium-sparing diuretics, angiotensin converting enzyme inhibitors, and various toxic agents),

hormones (such as hyperparathyroidism, vitamin D disorders, and mineralocorticoid deficiency or resistance), and toxins (toluene, heavy metals, lithium, and others). Gastrointestinal losses include diarrhea, ureterosigmoidostomy, pancreatic drainage, and cholestyramine.

- Treatment of metabolic acidosis should focus on correction of the underlying condition to the greatest extent possible.
- The most common causes of anion gap metabolic acidosis are consequences of either ingestions or altered physiology, such as diabetes mellitus or conditions causing hypoxia, which must be addressed to correct the acidosis condition.
- Generally, the acidosis will spontaneously improve with correction of the underlying disorder through normal physiologic responses; however, severe acidosis (pH <7.2, or especially <7.0) should be treated with HCO_3^- infusions. Such infusions can be lifesaving by improving cardiac contractility and the response to blood pressure supports.
  - ▷ Large volume infusions of HCO_3^- (usually >200 mEq) may lead to volume overload and/or hypokalemia (due to redistribution of potassium to intracellular spaces with correction of acidosis).
  - ▷ Under less emergent circumstances, HCO_3^- replacements should be given slowly to avoid a paradoxical fall of pH in the cerebrospinal fluid (CSF) related to the relatively slow transport of HCO_3^- across the blood brain barrier, compared to that of pCO_2.
- Dialysis may be required to clear toxins (whether from uremia or ingestions) or to balance blood HCO_3^- levels without volume expansion in severe cases.

On the other hand, most nonanion gap metabolic acidosis conditions are either inherited disorders (such as renal tubular acidosis) or otherwise chronic in nature, and are usually well known features of past medical history in affected individuals. These disorders usually require continuous supplementation of HCO_3^- and other mineral components to limit deviations from normal blood parameters. Absence of these replacements for even a few days can lead to profound acidosis and other mineral derangements.

Metabolic Alkalosis

Metabolic alkalosis conditions are routinely divided into two large categories: conditions associated with volume depletion (chloride responsive) and conditions associated with normal or expanded volume (chloride resistant). Protracted vomiting and prolonged nasogastric suctioning are the two most common causes of volume depletion associated chloride responsive metabolic alkalosis, but prolonged diuretic use, particularly loop and thiazide diuretics, is another frequent cause (known as contraction alkalosis). Alkalosis can also result in the face of chloride depletion in patients on prolonged mechanical ventilation, patients with cystic fibrosis, or in patients with chronic hypercapnia. Classically, urine chloride levels are <10 mEq/L in chloride responsive metabolic alkalosis, but >20 mEq/L in chloride-resistant forms.

Chloride resistant metabolic alkalosis is usually caused by aldosterone excess, such as that found in primary hyperaldosteronism, in the renin–angiotensin system derangements, or in the edema-forming states (liver disease, nephrotic syndrome, or congestive heart failure, where aldosterone is secreted in response to poor renal perfusion despite the overriding relative volume expansion). Chloride-resistant metabolic alkalosis is also found in patients with congenital transport defects in renal tubules (Barter's disease and Gitelman's syndrome), and are usually associated with hypokalemia.

- Treatment for chloride responsive forms of metabolic alkalosis is usually successfully accomplished with volume repletion with saline infusions, though potassium chloride replacement may also be necessary in patients with chronic lung disease.
- Blockade of stomach acid production with either histamine H_2 inhibitors or proton pump inhibitors can correct metabolic alkalosis from prolonged nasogastric suction or vomiting.
- Acetazolamide, a carbonic anhydrase inhibitor, can be used to block HCO_3^- reuptake in the proximal tubules and thereby correct alkalosis in chloride-resistant metabolic alkalosis. Acetazolamide is also useful in the edema-forming states or in chronic hypercapnia, where administration of additional fluids may be undesirable.

- Spironolactone or eplerenone can be used to block excessive aldosterone stimulation in appropriate patients.
- Rarely, acid infusions are given in the form of arginine hydrochloride, ammonium hydrochloride, or even hydrochloric acid to correct alkalosis in patients that are strongly symptomatic with either poor oxygen delivery to tissues (due to increased O_2 affinity for hemoglobin and reduced ventilation) or neuromuscular hyperirritability (manifested as twitching, tetany, or seizures).
- Dialysis can also be useful in corrected severe cases, particularly in the face of renal failure.

Respiratory Acidosis

Chief among causes of respiratory acidosis are conditions that mechanically limit ventilation in the lungs. Chronic obstructive pulmonary disease (COPD) is most common among these conditions, but extensive infiltrative processes (pneumonia or pulmonary edema) or large pleural effusions can also limit alveoli, leading to pCO_2 retention. There can be a mismatch of ventilation and perfusion in the face of a large pulmonary embolism, or there can be ineffective ventilation with a paralyzed diaphragm or flail chest condition, as may occur with multiple rib fractures. Obesity represents an alternative mechanical limit to ventilation. Hypoventilation is a common manifestation of many neuromuscular disorders, is a consequence of the action of drugs (narcotics), or brain stem injury.

- Treatment is more urgent in acute respiratory acidosis while chronic changes are generally well tolerated by patients.
- Therapy is focused on restoring adequate ventilation, which may require intubation and mechanical ventilation.
- In COPD, airway resistance must be reduced if possible, and excessive oxygen replacement should be avoided, since the respiratory drive is more dependent on hypoxia than hypercapnia in many COPD patients. A reasonable target for oxygen supplementation is a blood oxygen pressure of 60 mm Hg in severe COPD, to avoid suppression of respiratory drive.
- Reversal of narcotic suppression with naloxone is appropriate, and the use of respiratory

stimulants (e.g., aminophylline or doxapram) may aid in both centrally medicated and obstructive causes.

■ Typically, bicarbonate replacement to correct respiratory acidosis is reserved for patients that are intentionally hypoventilated to minimize lung injury.

Respiratory Alkalosis

Although it is a common disorder, respiratory alkalosis seldom has a serious impact on patient care and requires little in the way of therapy to reverse hyperventilation. In fact, neurosurgery patients may be purposefully hyperventilated in the postoperative period to exploit the physiologic reduction in cerebral blood flow and consequent decrease in CSF pressure.

The three main causes of respiratory alkalosis are hypoxia, pulmonary diseases, and central nervous system disorders. Hypoxia increases respiratory drive through both central (direct stimulation of the carotid body oxygen receptors) and peripheral (indirect stimulation through formation of lactic acid in peripheral tissues, which then stimulates carotid chemoreceptors) mechanisms. Many pulmonary disorders ultimately trigger hyperventilation through hypoxic mechanisms, but some appear to be caused by other triggers of hyperventilation which persist even in the absence of hypoxia. Central nervous system disorders are among the most common causes, however. Anxiety attacks are commonly associated with hyperventilation, but many intracerebral injuries can also trigger over breathing. Salicylates, theophylline, and progestational hormones are drugs well known for causing hyperventilation. Hyperventilation can be an early sign of gram negative bacterial sepsis, and it also occurs in hepatic coma, possibly due to accumulation of ammonia and amines. Panic, weakness, and a sense of impending doom are common manifestations of respiratory alkalosis, along with neuromuscular irritability (as described above for metabolic alkalosis) and paresthesias.

■ Treatment should address any underlying causes of hypoxia (including anemia) when present, along with discontinuation of offending drugs in appropriate cases.

■ For anxious patients, reassurance and rebreathing respired air from a small paper bag will usually suffice to restore normal respiratory status; correcting the paresthesias and sense of impending doom associated with hyperventilation. Increasing pCO_2 in respired air is not helpful in hepatic causes.

■ Beta adrenergic inhibitors can be helpful in severe cases, as well as specific treatments for anxiety.

■ Acetazolamide could be used in severe, refractory cases to induce a compensating metabolic acidosis.

REFERENCES

Brenner BM, Levine SA. *Brenner & Rector's The Kidney.* Philadelphia: Elsevier Saunders, 2007.

DuBose TD, Hamm LL. *Acid-Base and Electrolyte Disorders A Companion to Brenner & Rector's* The Kidney. Philadelphia: Elsevier Saunders, 2002.

Kraft MD, Btaiche IF, Sacks GS, Kudsk KA. Treatment of electrolyte disorders in adult patients in the intensive care unit. *Am J Health Syst Pharm.* 2005;**62**:1663–82.

Mehta RL, McDonald B, Gabbai F, et al. Nephrology consultation in acute renal failure: does timing matter? *Am J Med.* 2002;**113**:456–61.

Sedlacek M, Schoolwerth AC, Remillard BD. Electrolyte disturbances in the intensive care unit. *Semin Dial.* 2006;**19**:496–501.

Tong GM, Rude RK. Magnesium deficiency in critical illness. *J Intens Care Med.* 2005;**20**:3–17.

Wesson JA, Effros RM. Acid base disease. In Mason RJ, Murray JF, Broaddus VC, et al. *Mason: Murray & Nadel's Textbook of Respiratory Medicine*, 4th ed. Philadelphia: Elsevier Saunders, 2005, pp 172–97.

Zivin JR, Gooley T, Zager RA, Ryan MJ. Hypocalcemia: a pervasive metabolic abnormality in the critically ill. *Am J Kidney Dis.* 2001;**37**:689–98.

29   An Endocrinology Consult

James A. Kruse, MD, FCCM

HYPOGLYCEMIA

A critically low blood glucose concentration is an emergency because severe and prolonged hypoglycemia can potentially cause permanent neurologic deficits. Most cases of hypoglycemia in the ICU represent isolated or short-term events. Common causes in this setting are excessive insulin administration, sepsis, hepatic or renal dysfunction, adrenal insufficiency, and abrupt cessation of parenteral nutrition formulas. A number of drugs may cause hypoglycemia, including ethanol, sulfonylurea agents, and β-adrenergic blockers. Pancreatic islet cell tumors and other unusual causes may require diagnostic evaluation of insulin levels, C-peptide levels, or insulin antibodies; however, these etiologies are comparatively rare and do not need to be pursued unless the hypoglycemia recurs over a more prolonged period.

Whipple's triad encompasses the classic diagnostic criteria for hypoglycemia:

■ Hypoglycemia, i.e., blood glucose concentration <50 mg/dL
■ Clinical signs and symptoms ascribable to hypoglycemia
■ Abatement of symptoms following dextrose administration

Clinical manifestations are due either to the resulting hyperadrenergic reaction or to neuroglycopenia. The former can result in tremulousness, diaphoresis, anxiety, tachycardia, palpitations, nausea, and vomiting; whereas the latter can cause headache, confusion, behavioral changes, stupor, coma, and seizures.

Treatment of acute hypoglycemia in the ICU patient consists of three measures:

■ Intravenous (IV) injection of concentrated dextrose, e.g., 50 mL of 50% dextrose solution. Hypoglycemia may recur once this dextrose load is metabolized.
■ Initiation of a continuous IV infusion of dextrose. If the patient is already receiving IV dextrose, the administration rate should be increased.
■ Serial blood glucose testing at frequent intervals, e.g., every 1 hour initially, to detect recurrences and allow titration of IV dextrose administration. This monitoring is particularly important in ICU patients who are sedated or have underlying alterations in their sensorium.

Glucagon (1 mg) may be given intramuscularly as emergency treatment for patients who initially lack intravenous access and are unconscious or otherwise unable to take oral glucose.

HYPERGLYCEMIA AND DIABETIC KETOACIDOSIS

Elevated blood glucose concentration can occur in patients with underlying diabetes, or in some critically ill nondiabetic patients. Evidence is accumulating to suggest that even mild to moderate hyperglycemia may have deleterious short-term effects on immune function, length of ICU stay, and survival. Randomized controlled trials have shown that maintaining blood glucose in the range of 80–110 mg/dL is associated with improved survival in surgical ICU patients, and less morbidity in medical ICU patients.

Inadequate insulin production results in hyperglycemia. However, ketoacidosis does not commonly occur unless there is near total lack of circulating insulin. Diabetic ketoacidosis (DKA) most often occurs in insulin-dependent juveniles and young adults but is uncommon in older adults. Manifestations include:

- Symptoms: Malaise, fatigue, thirst, polydipsia, polyuria, nausea, vomiting, and abdominal pain
- Physical signs: Kussmaul respirations, tachycardia, orthostatic or supine hypotension, acetone odor on the breath, abdominal tenderness, and sensorial alterations

A precipitating factor is common and should be sought in all cases. In newly admitted patients the most common precipitants are noncompliance with insulin therapy, and infection or other intercurrent illness. For patients that develop DKA while in the hospital, the cause is most often inadequate insulin therapy, nosocomial infection, or worsening severity of illness. Important laboratory findings include:

- Hyperglycemia, typically in the range of 400–800 mg/dL
- Metabolic acidosis with an elevated anion gap
- Ketonemia and ketonuria
- Hyperkalemia, initially, followed by hypokalemia after administration of insulin

An osmotic diuresis results from glycosuria and leads to hypovolemia and kaluresis. In spite of the latter, most patients are hyperkalemic at presentation as a result of hypoinsulinemia. Once insulin is administered, serum potassium levels fall rapidly resulting in hypokalemia, which can be severe.

Treatment consists primarily of IV insulin and vigorous IV fluid administration.

- Normal saline: As rapidly as possible for 1–2 L, typically followed by 1 L/h for 1 h, then 500 mL/h for 1 to 2 hours, then 200–300 mL/h until hypovolemia and interstitial volume depletion is corrected. To minimize hyperchloremic acidosis, hypotonic saline can be substituted once intravascular volume is repleted, typically after the first several liters of IV fluid.
- Regular insulin: An initial IV bolus of 0.15 units/kg, followed by a continuous IV infusion of 0.1 units/kg per hour titrated against hourly blood glucose measurements.

- Potassium supplementation: Typically started as soon as the serum potassium concentration falls to within the normal range.
- Phosphate supplementation: Only if hypophosphatemia is present. Potassium phosphate can be used to correct concomitant hypokalemia and hypophosphatemia.
- Sodium bicarbonate: Usually unnecessary, but may be considered if acidemia is severe, e.g., arterial pH <7.00.

If blood glucose does not fall by at least 50 mg/dL in the first hour, double the insulin infusion rate. When blood glucose concentration reaches 200–250 mg/dL, decrease the insulin infusion rate to 0.05–0.1 units/kg per hour, and substitute normal saline (or half-normal saline) containing 5% dextrose for IV fluid administration to allow continued IV insulin infusion without causing hypoglycemia. The IV insulin administration rate may be decreased, but it should not be discontinued until the ketoacidosis resolves as shown by normalization of the serum anion gap.

In addition to monitoring glucose hourly, close monitoring of serum electrolytes, particularly serum potassium, and acid-base status are necessary. Serum potassium, serum anion gap, and serum CO_2 content or arterial blood gases, should be monitored at no less than 4-hour intervals initially. Specific diagnostic studies are utilized to rule out suspected precipitating factors, such as infection or myocardial infarction. Once the ketoacidosis has resolved and the patient is taking an oral or enteral diet, IV dextrose administration is stopped and subcutaneous regular insulin is given. The IV insulin infusion is discontinued 1 hour after the first subcutaneous insulin dose. Regular insulin is then given subcutaneously at 6-hour intervals as a sliding scale adjusted to the patient's pre-dose blood glucose level. Twice daily doses of intermediate acting insulin or a single daily dose of insulin glargine may also be administered.

The hyperosmolar, nonketotic dehydration syndrome (HONK) is an uncommon form of severe hyperglycemia that occurs in patients that secrete enough insulin to prevent ketoacidosis but have insufficient insulin to prevent hyperglycemia. As with DKA there is usually a precipitating factor, but unlike DKA this disorder occurs more frequently in elderly patients. Therefore, among potential precipitating factors are acute stroke and myocardial infarction, as well as infection. The manifestations are similar to DKA but with several important differences:

- Patients may have a history of non–insulin-dependent diabetes, or no prior history of diabetes.
- Extreme hyperglycemia can occur, often >1000 and sometimes >2000 mg/dL. As with DKA, the resulting glycosuria leads to volume contraction, but the degree of fluid deficit is often more severe in HONK.
- Marked sensorial depression or coma occurs due to the hyperosmolar state caused by severe hyperglycemia.
- Although there is absence of ketoacidosis by strict definition, overlap between DKA and HONK occurs and some patients with HONK have mild ketoacidosis.

Severe hyperosmolality causes osmotically mediated cellular dehydration and results in brain shrinkage, which is responsible for the sensorial depression or coma.

Treatment of HONK is similar to that of DKA, but larger fluid replacement volumes are often required. Initially the choice of IV fluid is always isotonic crystalloid, such as normal saline, to ensure rapid correction of hypovolemia. Once extracellular volume is repleted, hypotonic IV fluids can be substituted and the intracellular dehydration corrected at a slower pace.

HYPOTHYROIDISM AND MYXEDEMA COMA

Etiologies of hypothyroidism include thyroiditis, prior thyroidectomy or radioactive iodine ablation with inadequate thyroid replacement therapy, and drugs such as propylthiouracil (PTU), amiodarone, or lithium. Myxedema coma is a life-threatening state representing the extreme manifestation of hypothyroidism. This syndrome can develop in patients with previously mild, moderate, or compensated hypothyroidism, and it is usually precipitated by an acute illness or injury. Manifestations of hypothyroidism can include:

- Symptoms: Fatigue, difficulty concentrating, cold intolerance, daytime somnolence, constipation, and myalgias.

- Physical findings: Hypothermia, apathetic affect, lethargy, goiter, alopecia, dry skin, bradydysrhythmias, periorbital edema, hoarseness, weakness, and hypoactive or absent deep tendon reflexes. Sensorial depression, ascribable to underlying hypothyroidism, is required for hypothyroidism to qualify as myxedema coma.
- Laboratory findings: Hypercapnia, hypoxemia, hyponatremia, hypoglycemia, elevated creatine phosphokinase, hyperlipidemia, elevated thyrotropin (TSH) levels and decreased free thyroxine (T_4) levels.

Critically ill patients often have abnormal thyroid function test results even in the absence of clinical hypothyroidism, which is known as the euthyroid sick syndrome. Most authorities advise against thyroid hormone supplementation to patients with this syndrome. Differentiating the false positive thyroid function tests found in the euthyroid sick patient from true hypothyroidism can be challenging. Most critically ill patients without hypothyroidism will have low levels of free tri-iodothyronine (T_3), so this test is seldom useful in the ICU setting. Some ICU patients without thyroid disease will have mildly elevated T_4 levels, although depressed T_4 levels are more often seen in the most severely ill ICU patients. TSH is the most reliable test for true hypothyroidism in ICU patients, but even TSH levels can be mildly affected by the euthyroid sick syndrome. Elevations of reverse T_3, an isomer of the physiologic form of T_3, are characteristic of the euthyroid sick syndrome.

Patients with underlying compensated hypothyroidism who are taking thyroid hormone replacement chronically are generally maintained on their usual hormone dose during an acute illness. For those patients who are unable to take pharmaceutical thyroxine orally or by feeding tube, maintenance therapy can be given IV at half their usual oral dose. Patients with myxedema coma, however, require emergency treatment:

- Thyroxine: One dose of 300 μg IV, followed by 50–100 μg/day IV. The maintenance dose may be changed to the oral or enteral route once the patient is stable and the gastrointestinal tract is functioning normally.
- Hydrocortisone: Given in stress doses for the possibility of concomitant adrenal insufficiency.

Alternatively, one dose of dexamethasone may be given while the rapid cosyntropin stimulation test is performed to exclude adrenal insufficiency (see below).

■ Rewarming: Undertaken for hypothermic patients. Passive methods, such as extra blankets, are usually sufficient. Active rewarming methods risk hypotension by causing vasodilation.

■ Endotracheal intubation: For airway protection in patients with coma or hypercapnia. A low threshold for intubation and mechanical ventilation is important because hypoventilation commonly occurs and rapid progression to respiratory failure can ensue.

THYROID STORM

The term *thyrotoxicosis* describes a clinical syndrome caused by excessive amounts of circulating thyroid hormones, usually caused by hyperthyroidism. Thyroid storm describes an uncommon, life-threatening, extreme form of thyrotoxicosis that is a medical emergency. The usual cause is Graves' disease, an autoimmune disorder that represents the most common etiology of hyperthyroidism. Other causes of thyroid storm include toxic nodular goiter, amiodarone exposure, and, rarely, overdose of thyroid hormone. Progression of compensated hyperthyroidism to thyroid storm is usually triggered by an intercurrent illness or injury. Manifestations of thyrotoxicosis include:

■ Symptoms: Nervousness, fatigue, heat intolerance, dyspnea, palpitations, anorexia, diarrhea, and weight loss.

■ Physical findings: Goiter, sinus tachycardia, atrial fibrillation, atrial flutter, systolic hypertension, wide pulse pressure, hyperreflexia, altered mentation, psychosis, tremors, and findings consistent with high-output congestive heart failure. Proptosis and pretibial myxedema can occur if the cause is Graves' disease.

■ Nonspecific laboratory findings: Hyperglycemia, hypercalcemia, hyperbilirubinemia and other abnormal liver function test results may occur.

■ Free T_4 and T_3 levels: Free T_4 levels are elevated in thyrotoxicosis. Free T_3 levels may be elevated. Rarely, there may be elevated T_3 levels but normal T_4 levels, so-called T_3 *thyrotoxicosis*. Hormone levels tend to be more severely abnormal in cases

of thyroid storm, but there are no specific threshold values that distinguish storm from less severe thyrotoxicosis.

■ TSH level: Serum TSH is low in thyrotoxicosis due to primary hyperthyroidism. TSH levels are elevated in secondary hyperthyroidism, which is due to overproduction of TSH.

The diagnosis of thyroid storm requires the presence of either severe cardiac or central nervous system manifestations.

Patients with thyroid storm are managed in an ICU to provide close cardiorespiratory and neurologic monitoring. Specific treatment of thyroid storm consists of:

■ Stopping hormone synthesis: Accomplished using PTU or methimazole. Lithium and potassium perchlorate have also been used, but the former has a narrow therapeutic index and the latter has caused aplastic anemia. Although radioactive iodine ablation and thyroidectomy also stop synthesis, they have no role in the acute treatment of thyroid storm.

■ Administering iodine: Thyroid hormone stored within the thyroid gland continues to be released for days or weeks even after synthesis stops. Iodine in the form of Lugol's solution, sodium ipodate, or potassium iodide solution, administered orally, or sodium iodide given IV, can be used to stop this release. Iodine containing agents should not be given until at least 1 hour after PTU or methimazole to avoid stimulating thyroid hormone synthesis.

■ Giving a β-blocker: To treat the tachydysrhythmias, hypertension, and hyperadrenergic manifestations. Propranolol can be given in incremental doses by slow IV injection. Atrial tachydysrhythmias are often difficult to control and high doses of β-blockers are often required. The cardioselective agents metoprolol or esmolol can be substituted if there are relative contraindications to β-blockers.

■ Inhibiting T_4 to T_3 conversion: T_4 is converted to T_3 in peripheral tissues, and T_3 has greater activity than T_4. Propranolol, corticosteroids, and sodium ipodate inhibit this conversion, and one of these agents is given for this purpose.

■ Avoiding adrenal crisis: Hydrocortisone administration is recommended to cover the possibility of

Table 29.1. Etiologies of adrenal insufficiency

Primary adrenal failure

   Autoimmune adrenalitis (Addison's disease)

   Congenital causes: For example, adrenoleucodystrophy, familial glucocorticoid deficiency, congenital adrenal hyperplasia

   Infiltrative diseases: For example, neoplasm, amyloidosis, sarcoidosis

   Infectious diseases: For example, tuberculosis, meningococcemia, disseminated fungal infection, septic shock of any etiology, acquired immunodeficiency syndrome

   Drug-induced: For example, etomidate, ketoconazole, metyrapone

   Adrenal infarction or hemorrhage

   Bilateral adrenalectomy

Secondary adrenal failure (adrenocorticotropic hormone deficiency)

   Sudden withdrawal of chronic corticosteroid therapy

   Head trauma or radiation therapy

   Brain tumors or non-neoplastic infiltrative brain diseases

   Stroke or anoxic encephalopathy

   Pituitary surgery

coexisting adrenal insufficiency. Alternatively, one dose of dexamethasone may be given while the rapid cosyntropin stimulation test is performed to exclude adrenal insufficiency (see below).

Supportive measures include providing adequate hydration and treating fever with antipyretics or external cooling measures. Acetaminophen is preferable over aspirin because the latter decreases thyroxine binding to circulating plasma proteins resulting in increased free hormone levels. The precipitating factor leading to transition from thyrotoxicosis to thyroid storm should be investigated and treated.

ADRENAL INSUFFICIENCY

Relative or absolute deficiency of corticosteroid production by the adrenal glands can be attributed to primary or secondary causes (Table 29.1). An intercurrent illness or injury, including surgery, can precipitate adrenal crisis in patients with otherwise compensated underlying adrenal insufficiency. Manifestations may include any of the following:

■ Symptoms: Fatigue, anorexia, nausea, vomiting, diarrhea, abdominal pain, arthralgias, myalgias, lightheadedness, and salt craving

■ Physical findings: tachycardia, orthostatic or supine hypotension, weight loss, abdominal tenderness, hyperpigmentation, vitiligo, and confusion

■ Nonspecific laboratory findings: Hyponatremia, hyperkalemia, hypoglycemia, prerenal azotemia, hypercalcemia, normal anion gap metabolic acidosis, anemia, lymphocytosis, neutropenia, and eosinophilia

■ Random plasma cortisol: Levels <15 μg/dL are abnormal in severely ill patients. Higher levels can occur despite relative adrenal insufficiency in critically ill patients.

■ Rapid stimulation test: Plasma cortisol levels are obtained before, 30 minutes after and 60 minutes after a single 250 μg IV dose of cosyntropin. A peak cortisol rise of >9 μg/dL over baseline signifies adequate adrenal reserve and excludes adrenal insufficiency.

If the diagnosis is not already established, stimulation testing should be accomplished quickly. The cosyntropin stimulation test cannot be performed if hydrocortisone has been given because cortisol assays react with the administered hydrocortisone. Dexamethasone does not interfere with cortisol testing; however, it lacks mineralocorticoid activity.

Adrenal crisis implies that there is hypotension or signs of critical hypoperfusion and constitutes a medical emergency. Acute therapy is focused on hormone replacement, intravascular volume expansion, and treatment of the underlying cause.

- Hydrocortisone is administered as a single 200 mg IV dose followed by either 100 mg IV every 8 hours or a continuous IV infusion of 12.5 mg/h.
- Dexamethasone, as a single 10 mg IV dose, should be given in lieu of hydrocortisone if rapid cosyntropin stimulation testing is to be performed. After the 60-minute poststimulation cortisol sample is obtained, hydrocortisone administration can begin while awaiting the assay results.
- Fluid resuscitation is administered using normal saline and 5% dextrose in normal saline to correct hypovolemia and prevent hypoglycemia.
- Fludrocortisone, a synthetic mineralocorticoid, does not need to be given when high doses of hydrocortisone are used. Once the crisis is over and the hydrocortisone dose is tapered to <100 mg/day, fludrocortisone can be added if adrenal insufficiency persists.

Corticosteroid treatment for the relative adrenal insufficiency associated with septic shock has been studied in randomized, controlled clinical trials. Pharmacologic doses, >300 mg/day, are not beneficial. Studies evaluating doses in the range of 50 mg every 6 hours show conflicting results, but appear to offer survival benefit only in patients with septic shock that is refractory to IV fluid and vasopressor therapy.

PHEOCHROMOCYTOMA

Tumors arising from chromaffin cells within the adrenal medulla are known as pheochromocytoma. Approximately 10% of these uncommon neoplasms are malignant, 10% occur bilaterally, and about 10% occur outside the adrenal glands. Extra-adrenal tumors most often are located in the abdomen, especially in the vicinity of the organ of Zuckerkandl near the aortic bifurcation, but they can occur in the pelvis, chest, head, and neck. In more than 10% of cases the disorder is familial, and there are associations with a number of syndromes, including:

- von Hippel–Lindau disease
- von Recklinghausen's neurofibromatosis
- Types IIa (Sipple's syndrome) and IIb multiple endocrine neoplasia syndromes

Clinical manifestations are due to unregulated production of catecholamines by the tumor and most often include brief episodes of hypertension, which may be severe enough to result in a hypertensive emergency with acute left ventricular dysfunction and pulmonary edema or other serious end-organ dysfunction. Sustained hypertension may occur. Other common manifestations include episodic headache, diaphoresis, anxiety, tremulousness, and palpitations. Extrasystoles, tachydysrhythmias, chest pain, nausea, vomiting, abdominal pain, pallor, visual disturbances, and weight loss may also occur. Uncommonly there is orthostatic hypertension or episodic hypotension. The hypotensive variant is rare and is due to predominate epinephrine secretion by the tumor.

The diagnosis is confirmed by biochemical testing:

- Plasma metanephrines assay. The most useful test if pretest probability is high. Normal plasma metanephrines effectively exclude the diagnosis of pheochromocytoma, but mild elevations can represent false positives.
- Initial testing with 24-hour urine collection assays for epinephrine, norepinephrine, and metanephrines may have good diagnostic value when the pretest probability is low.
- The clonidine suppression test may be useful in selected cases if the above tests are equivocal.
- Plasma catecholamines (epinephrine and norepinephrine) and 24-hour urine collection assay for vanillylmandelic acid are of substantially less value than metanephrine assays.
- Provocative tests using phentolamine, glucagon, histamine, or tyramine are no longer advocated.

Diagnostic testing is confounded in the ICU setting because many forms of critical illness and their treatment interfere with the predictive value of biochemical assays. These include respiratory failure, sepsis, myocardial infarction, congestive heart failure, dehydration, peptic ulcer disease, renal failure, hypoglycemia, and use of diuretics, adrenergic blockers, catecholamines, and vasodilators. Biochemical confirmation is therefore deferred until after the patient is stabilized and out of the ICU. Following biochemical confirmation of pheochromocytoma, the tumor is localized using imaging studies such as magnetic resonance imaging, computed tomography, or radiolabeled m-iodobenzylguanidine scintigraphy.

The definitive treatment is surgical excision, which is usually curative but risky because anesthesia and dissection of the tumor can result in catecholamine release and hypertensive crisis. Surgery is therefore deferred until adequate α-adrenergic blockade is achieved, volume status is normal, the patient is stable, and acute medical conditions are optimally treated. Acute hypertensive crisis due to pheochromocytoma is treated pharmacologically:

■ Phentolamine mesylate, a short-acting α-blocker, is the conventional drug of choice. It is given as sequential IV bolus doses of 2–5 mg at intervals of >5 minutes until the desired degree of blood pressure control is achieved.

■ Sodium nitroprusside, given as a titrated continuous IV infusion starting at 0.1 μg/kg per minute, is an alternative to phentolamine.

■ β-Blockers may be used adjunctively to treat tachydysrhythmias, but only after adequate α-blockade is achieved. If there is inadequate α-blockade, β-blockers are contraindicated because they can precipitate or severely worsen pheochromocytoma-induced hypertension due unopposed α-adrenergic stimulation.

Once the acute crisis is over and the blood pressure controlled, phenoxybenzamine is started orally at 10 mg every 12 hours and titrated up to 20–40 mg two or three times daily. This long-acting α-blocker can be used chronically. Other agents that have been used in pheochromocytoma include labetalol, prazosin, terazosin, doxazosin, and metyrosine .

SYNDROME OF INAPPROPRIATE ANTIDIURETIC HORMONE SECRETION

The antidiuretic hormone arginine vasopressin (AVP) is normally secreted from the posterior pituitary in response to hypovolemia or hyperosmolality. The syndrome of inappropriate antidiuretic hormone secretion (SIADH) is present when a pathologic stimulus or ectopic production site results in release of AVP and causes hyponatremia. The major etiologies include:

■ Neoplasm: For example, lung cancer, mesothelioma, prostate and bladder cancer, thymoma, pancreatic and duodenal cancer, lymphoma, sarcoma

■ Pulmonary disorders: For example, pneumonia, chronic obstructive disease, lung abscess, pulmonary embolism, pneumothorax, positive pressure ventilation

■ Neurologic disorders: For example, cranial trauma; brain tumors; meningitis; encephalitis; subdural, intracerebral or subarachnoid hemorrhage

■ Drugs: For example, vasopressin, desmopressin, oxytocin, opioids, barbiturates, carbamazepine, thiazides, antidepressants, antipsychotics, clofibrate, vincristine, vinblastine, non-steroidal anti-inflammatory agents, theophylline, bromocriptine, ifosfamide

Certain physiologic causes of AVP release other than hypovolemia or hyperosmolality are sometimes included as causes of SIADH, such as pain, nausea, and trauma, including surgery.

Manifestations are due to the underlying cause and the resulting hyponatremia. Hypo-osmolar hyponatremia can cause an osmolar gradient between plasma and brain resulting in cerebral edema. The severity of its effect depends on both the degree of hyponatremia and the rate of its development. Hyponatremia is often asymptomatic, particularly if it is not severe or if it develops slowly. Severe or rapidly developing hyponatremia can cause malaise, apathy, headache, hypogeusia, lethargy, behavioral changes, confusion, agitation, ataxia, myoclonus, stupor, coma, hyporeflexia, seizures, and respiratory arrest. Besides hyponatremia, the key laboratory findings in SIADH are:

■ Abnormally low serum osmolality

■ Inappropriately concentrated urine; i.e., urine osmolality that is >100 mOsmol/kg H_2O in young, otherwise healthy adults

■ Urine sodium concentration usually >30 mEq/L. It may be lower if sodium intake is low or after prolonged fluid restriction.

■ Improvement in the hyponatremia after fluid restriction.

The diagnosis of SIADH requires exclusion of other causes of hyponatremia (Fig. 29.1).

Key aspects of acute treatment for SIADH include:

■ Frequently assessing serum sodium concentration and closely monitoring fluid intake and output.

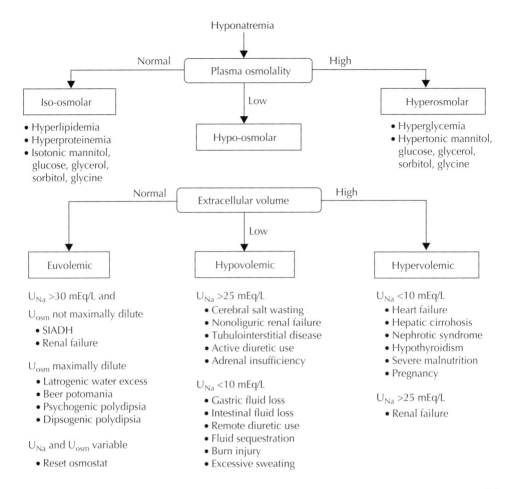

Figure 29.1. Differential diagnosis of hyponatremia. UNa = urine sodium concentration; Uosm = urine osmolality; SIADH = syndrome of inappropriate antidiuretic secretion.
* Some classification schemes omit these generalized forms of tubulointerstitial disease.

- Treating the underlying cause, including stopping drugs that affect ADH secretion.
- Avoiding hypotonic fluid administration and restricting fluid intake to a maximum of 600–1000 mL/day.
- Administering a controlled, time-limited infusion of hypertonic saline if the hyponatremia is severe and associated with neurologic manifestation.

Conivaptan, a V_{1a} and V_2 AVP-receptor blocker indicated for euvolemic hyponatremia, including SIADH, may also be considered. The drug has been shown to raise serum sodium levels by an average of 4 mEq/L in the initial 24 hours of therapy.

The effects of a 1-L infusion of IV fluid on serum sodium concentration can be estimated by:

$$\Delta NA_{serum} = \frac{NA_{infusate} - NA_{serum}}{TBW + 1}$$

where ΔNa_{serum} is the estimated change in serum sodium concentration, $Na_{infusate}$ is the sodium concentration of the IV fluid (e.g., 856 mEq/L for 5% saline, 513 mEq/L for 3% saline, or 154 mEq/L for normal saline), Na_{serum} is the current serum sodium concentration, and TBW is total body water in liters. The latter is estimated by multiplying body weight (in kilograms) by 0.6 for young adult men, 0.5 for women or elderly men, and 0.45 for elderly women. This formula assumes no loss of sodium or water from the body, and no other gain of sodium or water, during the infusion period. Frequent monitoring of serum sodium concentration allows for refinement of the prescription. The IV fluid administration rate must be tailored to avoid overly rapid correction.

The osmotic demyelination syndrome is a potentially devastating neurologic complication of overly rapid correction of hyponatremia. There is controversy regarding the ideal correction rate; however, slowly developing hyponatremia should be corrected slowly whereas acutely developing hyponatremia (over <48 hours) should be corrected more rapidly. For hyponatremia developing over more than 24 hours, which is the vast majority of cases, the risk of myelinolysis can be minimized by striving to limit the rise in sodium concentration to <9 mEq/L per day, and avoiding overshoot hypernatremia. After acutely controlled, chronic treatment may be necessary using demeclocycline, which attenuates the action of AVP on the distal nephron. Lithium, phenytoin, and urea have been used as second line agents.

CEREBRAL SALT WASTING SYNDROME

This syndrome occurs chiefly in patients with subarachnoid hemorrhage, although it has also been described in patients with brain trauma, brain tumors, intracranial hemorrhage, brain infarction, arteriovenous malformation, meningitis, and other central nervous system derangements. It results in hyponatremia, which can range from mild to severe. The mechanism has not been elucidated but may involve alterations in sympathetic tone, elaboration of natriuretic peptides, or release of a ouabain-like compound from the brain, leading to decreased renal sodium reabsorption, natriuresis, and hyponatremia. The resulting volume contraction stimulates AVP secretion, which further worsens the hyponatremia.

Distinguishing CSWS from SIADH can be difficult in practice (Table 29.2). The critical difference is the presence of extracellular volume depletion in CSWS, compared to apparently normal extracellular volume status in SIADH. Key manifestations of the volume contraction occurring in CSWS are dry mucous membranes, negative fluid balance, and signs of hypovolemia, such as flat neck veins, low central venous pressure, oliguria, and orthostatic tachycardia or hypotension. Review of recent fluid intake and output records and weight changes may also help distinguish whether there has been overall mild fluid retention, as is observed during the development of SIADH, or fluid loss, as occurs in CSWS. However, patients with either syndrome may reach a steady state in which fluid balance does not undergo further change.

Once the volume deficit associated with CSWS is corrected, urine osmolality becomes maximally dilute (usually <100 mOsmol/kg H_2O) and the hyponatremia resolves. On the other hand, correction of hyponatremia in SIADH by manipulation of fluid and sodium intake does not normalize renal diluting capacity. The fractional excretion of uric acid (FEUA) has also been proposed as a means of retrospectively distinguishing CSWS from SIADH following normalization of hyponatremia. FEUA is calculated as:

$$FEUA = \frac{urine\ uric\ acid \times serum\ creatinine}{serum\ uric\ acid \times urine\ creatinine} \times 100\%$$

with all concentration units in mg/dL. Normal FEUA is <10%, but higher values are observed in patients with either CSWS or SIADH. After normalization of hyponatremia, FEUA remains high in CSWS but normalizes in SIADH.

Treatment of CSWS consists of:

- Volume expansion using IV isotonic (normal) saline to achieve positive fluid balance.
- Close monitoring of serum sodium concentration, intake and output, and volume status. Central venous pressure monitoring may be helpful. Apply the same caveats to the rate of correction of hyponatremia as in SIADH (see above).
- The mineralocorticoid fludrocortisone has been used to enhance renal tubular sodium reabsorption and thereby minimize further salt loss; however, this hormone can cause hypokalemia, fluid retention, and hypertension.
- Treatment of the underlying neurologic disease.

Restricting fluids in patients with CSWS can exacerbate the hyponatremia. When CSWS is due to subarachnoid hemorrhage, fluid restriction may also precipitate vasospasm.

Table 29.2. Comparison of findings in cerebral salt wasting syndrome (CSWS) and the syndrome of inappropriate antidiuretic hormone secretion (SIADH)

Factor	CSWS	SIADH
Serum sodium concentration	↓	↓
Urine sodium concentration	>40 mEq/L	>40 mEq/L
Extracellular fluid volume	↓	N to ↑
Total body sodium balance	–	= or +
Central venous pressure	↓	N or ↑
Hematocrit	↑	N
Serum albumin and urea nitrogen concentration	↑	N
Serum potassium concentration	N to ↑	N
Serum uric acid concentration	N to ↓	↓
Serum urea nitrogen/creatinine ratio	↑	N
FEUA post-correction of hyponatremia	↑↑	N

↓ = decreased; N = normal; ↑ = slightly elevated; ↑↑ = elevated; + = slightly positive; – = negative; FEUA = fractional excretion of uric acid.

Correction of the hyponatremia requires correction of the extracellular volume deficit and providing sodium to counter continuing urinary losses. This can be accomplished with IV infusion of isotonic saline. In stable patients, enterally administered salt supplementation can be considered. If the hyponatremia is severe or unresponsive to normal saline, a controlled infusion of hypertonic saline may be necessary; however, the same precautions should be observed regarding the rate of correction as with treating SIADH.

DIABETES INSIPIDUS

A major function of the renal collecting ducts is to reabsorb water reaching the distal nephron. However, the ductal membrane is impermeable to water except at sites of aquaporins, channels that allow water reabsorption from the ductal lumen. Aquaporin expression is regulated by the antidiuretic hormone AVP produced by magnocellular neurons of the hypothalamus and secreted by their axons located in the posterior pituitary. Diabetes insipidus (DI) can be due to central causes, in which there is impaired AVP production, or nephrogenic causes, due to refractoriness of the distal nephron to the effects of AVP.

Both forms of the disease have numerous causes (Table 29.3) and result in partial or complete impairment of urinary concentrating ability, which leads to obligatory polyuria (>50 mL/kg per day) and a propensity to develop dehydration. Although the differential diagnosis of polyuria includes DI, there are other causes that must be considered as well. These include excessive IV fluid administration, hyperglycemia, diuretic use (including mannitol), the recovery phase of acute renal failure, primary polydipsia, and after relief of obstructive uropathy. Loss of the normal solute concentration gradient between the renal cortex and medulla can occur after prolonged polyuria of any cause, including excessive IV fluid administration to otherwise normal subjects. This *medullary washout* phenomenon occasionally occurs following overvigorous fluid resuscitation, leading to polyuria, further IV fluid administration, and perpetuation of the polyuria.

DI results in polyuria and polydipsia. Other manifestations reflect either the underlying cause, such as visual field defects from a pituitary tumor, or the effects of dehydration. Excessive loss of water with inadequate replenishment results in elevated plasma solute concentrations, giving rise to hypernatremia and hyperosmolality. Like

Table 29.3. Etiologies of diabetes insipidus

Central diabetes insipidus

Congenital: Wolfram syndrome (diabetes insipidus, diabetes mellitus, optic atrophy and deafness), familial neurohypophyseal diabetes insipidus

Cranial trauma or brain surgery (especially transsphenoidal surgery)

Brain neoplasms: Craniopharyngioma, germinoma, suprasellar tumors, leukemia, lymphoma, brain metastases

Cerebrovascular disease: Brain infarction, intracranial hemorrhage, aneurysm, Sheehan's syndrome

Brain hypoxia: Cardiac arrest, carbon monoxide poisoning

CNS infections: Meningitis, encephalitis, lues, tuberculosis

Granulomatous infiltration: Sarcoidosis, autoimmune lymphocytic infundibulohypophysitis, Langerhans cell histiocytosis, Wegener's granulomatosis

Nephrogenic diabetes insipidus

Congenital causes: V2-receptor or aquaporin-2 mutations

Tubulointerstitial renal disease: Sickle-cell disease, polycystic kidney disease, medullary sponge disease, sarcoidosis, obstructive uropathy, renal amyloidosis, Sjögren's syndrome

Hypercalcemia and hypokalemia

Certain drugs: lithium, demeclocycline, amphotericin B, foscarnet, ofloxacin, vinblastine, cidofovir, ifosfamide, orlistat

polyuria, hypernatremia is not specific for DI, but it has a tendency to occur in ICU patients with DI because critically ill patients frequently have a blunted thirst mechanism, are sedated or have an altered sensorium due to their illness, or do not have self-access to water. Otherwise healthy subjects with DI, on the other hand, act on their polyuria-induced thirst and avoid both dehydration and hypernatremia.

The classic provocative maneuver for diagnosing DI is the water deprivation test. Mild dehydration is induced by withholding water, inducing a rise in plasma sodium and osmolality. This stimulates AVP production, which would normally result in water conservation by the distal nephron. This appropriate response is detectable by monitoring urine output, which should decrease, and urine osmolality, which should increase. Water deprivation testing is dangerous in ICU patients and should not be performed because it can induce hypovolemia and hemodynamic instability. Further, ICU patients with DI often have already developed at least mild hypernatremia spontaneously, which obviates the rationale for water deprivation testing. The finding of an inappropriately low urine osmolality in the face of even very mild hypernatremia signifies the presence of at least partial DI:

- Normal response to hypernatremia: Urine osmolality >800 mOsmol/kg H_2O
- Response in partial DI: Urine osmolality 300–700 mOsmol/kg H_2O
- Response in complete DI: urine osmolality <300 mOsmol/kg H_2O

Once the diagnosis of DI is made, differentiation of central and nephrogenic DI can be made by measuring plasma AVP levels after water deprivation or spontaneous development of mild hypernatremia:

- Normal response to hypernatremia: Plasma AVP concentration >2 pg/mL
- Response in partial DI: Plasma AVP concentration may reach 1.5 pg/mL
- Response in complete DI: Plasma AVP concentration undetectable
- Response in nephrogenic DI: Plasma AVP concentration can exceed 5 pg/mL

Differentiation of central from nephrogenic DI is more commonly achieved by assessing urine osmolality before and after a single dose of aqueous AVP (5 units subcutaneously) or the AVP analog desmopressin (1 or 2 µg subcutaneously or IV):

- Normal response: No more than a 5% increase in urine osmolality
- Response in partial central DI: 10–50% increase in urine osmolality
- Response in complete central DI: At least a 50% increase in urine osmolality
- Response in nephrogenic DI: No change in urine osmolality is expected

The response in central DI may be blunted if there has been down-regulation of aquaporin channels or a significant degree of medullary washout.

DI can cause severe polyuria, in some cases exceeding 20 L/day. If sufficient water intake or hypotonic IV fluid is not provided, profound hypernatremia, hyperosmolality, and dehydration can occur. Hypovolemia is unlikely if the total body water deficit is entirely due to electrolyte free water loss. However, patients with even small degrees of co-existing total body sodium depletion can develop intravascular volume depletion from severe DI. Hypokalemia, hypomagnesemia, and hypophosphatemia can also develop in some patients with polyuria. The following measures can help to avoid these severe derangements:

- Close monitoring of water balance (fluid intake and output)
- Frequent serial measurements of serum sodium, potassium, magnesium, and phosphorus concentration
- Appropriate titration of IV fluids to prevent or correct volume depletion and hypernatremia

Hypotonic IV fluids are administered to correct hypernatremia and hyperosmolality and replenish intracellular volume depletion. For patients with severe fluid depletion and signs of intravascular volume depletion or signs of hypoperfusion, normal saline or other isotonic crystalloid should be given initially even though the patient may be hypernatremic. Once the extracellular volume deficit has been rapidly corrected, the intracellular volume depletion is corrected more gradually to avoid inducing cerebral edema, particularly if significant hypernatremia has been present for more

than 24 hr. Nevertheless, even slow correction of the volume deficit may necessitate a high rate of hypotonic fluid administration if there is ongoing polyuria. Overhydration should be avoided because it will result in a water diuresis that can lead to medullary washout, potentially sustaining the polyuria even if the DI is otherwise controlled or resolves.

Close monitoring of intake and output and titration of IV fluid administration may suffice as treatment for mild DI in the ICU, but patients with central DI and marked polyuria should be given aqueous AVP or desmopressin to control the polyuria and lower the risk of dehydration. Aqueous AVP has a half-life of 2–4 hours and can be given subcutaneously, intramuscularly, by IV bolus, or by continuous IV infusion. It is a potent vasoconstrictor, however, owing to its effect on vascular V_1 receptors, which could pose a risk for critically ill patients by precipitating hypertension or cardiac ischemia.

Desmopressin, a synthetic V_2-receptor agonist, is safer than AVP because it does not affect V_1 receptors and thus avoids vasoconstriction. Its longer half-life, on the order of 8–20 hours, simplifies dosing. These properties make desmopressin the drug of choice for both acute and long-term treatment of central DI. The parenteral form is dosed at 1–2 µg every 8–12 hours, IV or subcutaneously. The drug is also available in oral and intranasal forms that require larger doses and are reserved for noncritically ill patients and chronic use.

AVP and desmopressin are generally not useful in treating nephrogenic DI; however, the same careful attention to fluid balance is necessary in this form of the disease. Treatment for nephrogenic DI consists of stopping any causative drugs, monitoring fluid balance and electrolyte levels, supplying IV fluid, restricting sodium intake, and giving a thiazide diuretic. Sodium restriction and thiazides limit polyuria in nephrogenic DI by causing mild volume contraction, which stimulates sodium and water reabsorption in the proximal tubule and thereby decreases water delivery to the distal nephron. Amiloride has also been used, alone or in combination with a thiazide, particularly when lithium exposure is the cause because amiloride limits lithium entry into tubular cells. Indomethacin and ibuprofen have been employed adjunctively with thiazides to control polyuria. Desmopressin may be tried because a small proportion of patients with nephrogenic DI have receptor mutations that result in a partial effect if high doses are used, e.g., up to 10 µg.

REFERENCES

Annane D, Sebille V, Charpentier C, et al. Effect of treatment with low doses of hydrocortisone and fludrocortisone on mortality in patients with septic shock. *JAMA.* 2002; **288**:862–71.

Bichet DG. Nephrogenic diabetes insipidus. *Am J Med.* 1998;**105**:431–2.

Clayton JA, Le Jeune IR, Hall IP. Severe hyponatraemia in medical in-patients: aetiology, assessment and outcome. *QJM.* 2006;**99**:505–11.

Clement S, Braithwaite SS, Magee MF, et al., and the American Diabetes Association Diabetes in Hospitals Writing Committee. Management of diabetes and hyperglycemia in hospitals. *Diabetes Care.* 2004;**27**:553–91, erratum in 27:1255.

Genuth SM. Diabetic ketoacidosis and hyperglycemic hyperosmolar coma. *Curr Ther Endocrinol Metab.* 1997; **6**:438–47.

Gibson SC, Hartman DA, Schenck JM. The endocrine response to critical illness: update and implications for emergency medicine. *Emerg Med Clin North Am.* 2005;**23**:909–29.

Greenberg A, Verbalis JG. Vasopressin receptor antagonists. *Kidney Int.* 2006;**69**:2124–30.

Kannan CR, Seshadri KG. Thyrotoxicosis. *Dis Mon.* 1997;**43**: 601–77.

Lamberts SWJ, Bruining HA, de Jong FH. Corticosteroid therapy in severe illness. *N Engl J Med.* 1997;**337**:1285–92.

Lenders JW, Pacak K, Walther MM, et al. Biochemical diagnosis of pheochromocytoma: which test is best? *JAMA.* 2002;**287**:1427–34.

Lorber D. Nonketotic hypertonicity in diabetes mellitus. *Med Clin North Am.* 1995;**79**:39–52.

Maesaka JK, Gupta S, Fishbane S. Cerebral salt wasting syndrome: does it exist? *Nephron.* 1999;**82**:100–9.

Maesaka JK, Venkatesan J, Piccione JM, et al. Abnormal urate transport in patients with intracranial disease. *Am J Kidney Dis.* 1992;**19**:10–15.

Pacak K, Linehan WM, Eisenhofer G, Walther MM, Goldstein DS. Recent advances in genetics, diagnosis, localization, and treatment of pheochromocytoma. *Ann Intern Med.* 2001;**34**:315–29.

Palmer BF. Hyponatremia in patients with central nervous system disease: SIADH versus CSW. *Trends Endocrinol Metab.* 2003;**14**:182–7.

Service FJ. Classification of hypoglycemic disorders. *Endocrinol Metab Clin North Am.* 1999;**28**:501–7.

Singer I, Oster JR, Fishman LM. The management of diabetes insipidus in adults. *Arch Intern Med.* 1997; **157**:1293–1301.

Smallridge RC. Metabolic and anatomic thyroid emergencies: a review. *Crit Care Med.* 1992;**20**:276–91.

Tsitouras PD. Myxedema coma. *Clin Geriatr Med.* 1995;**11**:251–8.

van den Berghe G, Wilmer A, Hermans G, et al. Intensive insulin therapy in the medical ICU. *N Engl J Med.* 2006;**354**:449–61.

van den Berghe G, Wouters P, Weekers F, et al. Intensive insulin therapy in the critically ill patients. *N Engl J Med.* 2001;**345**:1359–67.

Verbalis JG. AVP receptor antagonists as aquaretics: review and assessment of clinical data. *Cleve Clin J Med.* 2006;**73**(Suppl 3):S24–S33.

Viallon A, Zeni F, Lafond P, et al. Does bicarbonate therapy improve the management of severe diabetic ketoacidosis? *Crit Care Med.* 1999;**27**:2690–3.

Virally ML, Guillausseau PJ. Hypoglycemia in adults. *Diabetes Metab.* 1999;**25**:477–90.

Yamamoto T, Fukuyama J, Fujiyoshi A. Factors associated with mortality of myxedema coma: report of eight cases and literature survey. *Thyroid.* 1999;**9**:1167–74.

Yoshida D. Thyroid storm precipitated by trauma. *J Emerg Med.* 1996;**14**:697–701.

Index